D1242449

Contemporary Psychotherapies for a Diverse World

Contemporary Psychotherapies for a Diverse World

Editors

Jon Frew
Pacific University

Michael D. Spiegler
Providence College

Chapter Authors

Neil Altman
David J. Cain
Jon Carlson
Matt Englar-Carlson
Kathie Crocket
Teresa McDowell
Pamela Remer
Sandra A. Rigazio-DiGilio
Melba J. T. Vasquez
Clemmont E. Vontress
Robert E. Wubbolding

Lahaska Press
Houghton Mifflin Company
Boston • New York

Dedication

For my children: Gillian, who is a better writer at age 18 than I will ever be, and Ian Michael, my diversity trainer whose presence in my life has transformed my understanding of diversity from my head to my heart   —JF

For my mom, Lillian Spiegler, from whom I learned, among many things to respect and embrace human diversity   —MDS

Publisher, Lahaska Press: Barry Fetterolf
Senior Editor, Lahaska Press: Mary Falcon
Senior Marketing Manager, Lahaska Press: Barbara LeBuhn
Associate Project Editor: Kristen Truncellito
Art and Design Manager: Gary Crespo
Cover Design Manager: Anne S. Katzeff
Senior Photo Editor: Jennifer Meyer Dare
Composition Buyer: Chuck Dutton
New Title Project Manager: Susan Brooks-Peltier
Editorial Assistant: Evangeline Bermas

Cover image: © Lisa Zador

For instructors who want more information about Lahaska Press books and teaching aids, contact the Houghton Mifflin Faculty Services Center at
    Tel: 800-733-1717, x4034
    Fax: 800-733-1810
Or visit us on the Web at **www.lahaskapress.com**.

Library of Congress Control Number: 2006934901

ISBN-10: 0-618-57359-3
ISBN-13: 978-0-618-57359-2

2 3 4 5 6 7 8 9 EB 11 10 09 08 07

Contents

Preface   xvii

About the Authors   xxv

Chapter 1

Introduction to Contemporary Psychotherapies for a Diverse World   1

Jon Frew and Michael D. Spiegler

Counseling and Psychotherapy Approaches in Context   2

     Traditional Contexts   2

     Modern Contexts   3

What Is Psychotherapy or Counseling?   4

Differences in Counseling and Psychotherapy Approaches   5

     Theoretical Foundation   6

     Purpose or Goal   6

     Change Strategy   7

     Internal versus External Factors   9

     Process: What Goes On in Counseling   10

     Evaluation of Effectiveness   11

Present and Future Consumers of Counseling and Psychotherapy   12

Practicing Counseling and Psychotherapy in a Diverse World   13

Choosing the Approach You Will Practice   15

     Choosing Based on Exposure   15

     Choosing Based on Personal Fit   16

     Learning More Before You Choose   16

     Adopting More Than One Approach   17

What You Can Expect in the Remainder of This Book   18

Chapter 2

Ethics for a Diverse World   **20**

Melba J. T. Vasquez

   Brief Overview of the APA and ACA Codes of Ethics   20

   Feminist Multicultural Ethics   24

      Box: The Author's Journey as a Feminist Multicultural Ethicist   25
      Review of Ethical Feminist Multicultural Themes and Principles   27
      Moral Principles   32
      Exceptions to Boundaries   33
      Activism   36

   Summary   37

   Resources for Further Study   39

      Professional Organizations   39
      Professional Journals   39
      Suggested Readings   39
      Other Media Resources   40

Chapter 3

Psychoanalytic Therapy   **41**

Neil Altman

   Origins and Evolution of Psychoanalytic Therapy   42

      Early Development of Freud's Psychoanalytic Theory   42
      Anna Freud and Ego Psychology   45
      Jungian Psychology   46
      Object Relations and Relational Psychoanalysis   47
      *Changes in Response to Feminist and Cultural/Postmodernist
      Theorists   49*
      Context Then—Context Now   50
      Box: The Author's Journey as a Psychoanalytic Therapist   52

   Theory of Psychoanalytic Therapy   55

      Core Theoretical Concepts   55
      Theories of Development   55
      Theory of Change   62

   Practice of Psychoanalytic Therapy   64

      The Client-Counselor Relationship   64
      Classical Psychoanalytic Therapy   64
      Contemporary Psychoanalytic Therapy   66

Transference and Countertransference in the Context of Culture   74
Transference and Countertransference in the Context of Race   78
Some Final Thoughts on Psychoanalytic Practice   80

Evaluation of Psychoanalytic Therapy   82

Evaluation Criteria   82
Process Research   83
Outcome Research   84

Psychoanalytic Therapy: Blind Spots, Limitations, and Challenges   85

Future Development: Psychoanalytic Therapy in a Diverse World   87

Summary   87

Key Terms   90

Resources for Further Study   91

Professional Organizations   91
Professional Journals   91
Suggested Readings   92

Chapter 4

Adlerian Therapy   **93**

Jon D. Carlson and Matt Englar-Carlson

Origins and Evolution of Adlerian Therapy   94

Context Then—Context Now   98
Box: The Authors' Journeys as Adlerian Therapists   100

Theory of Adlerian Therapy   103

Holism   104
Encouragement   104
Subjective or Private Logic   106
Life-Style   107
Basic Mistakes   110
Core Fears   111
Basic Life Tasks   111
Social Interest   112
Compensation for Inferiority   113
Birth Order and the Family Constellation   113
Theory of Change   115

Practice of Adlerian Therapy   117

Therapy Stages   120
Therapeutic Strategies   124
The Client-Counselor Relationship   129

Evaluation of Adlerian Therapy   130

Adlerian Therapy: Blind Spots, Limitations, and Challenges   131

Blind Spots   131

Limitations   132

Challenges   133

Future Development: Adlerian Therapy in a Diverse World   134

Summary   135

Key Terms   137

Resources for Further Study   138

Professional Organizations   138

Professional Journals   138

Suggested Readings   138

Other Media Resources   139

Chapter 5

Existential Therapy   141

Clemmont E. Vontress

Origins and Evolution of Existential Therapy   141

The Evolution of Existential Therapy for a Diverse World   144

Context Then—Context Now   144

Box: The Author's Journey as an Existential Therapist   145

Theory of Existential Therapy   148

The Umwelt (the Natural Environment)   148

The Mitwelt (the Social Environment)   149

The Eigenwelt (the Personal World)   150

Existence and Essence   150

Self-Knowledge   151

Love   151

Responsibility   152

Authenticity   153

Existential Anxiety   154

Courage   155

Unfolding (Becoming)   156

Meaning in Life   158

Practice of Existential Therapy   159

The Client-Counselor Relationship   159

Diagnosis   160

Intervention Procedures 161
Existential Cross-Cultural Counseling 162
Evaluation of Existential Therapy 167
Existential Therapy: Blind Spots, Limitations, and Challenges 169
Blind Spots 169
Limitations 169
Challenges 170
Future Development: Existential Therapy in a Diverse World 170
Summary 172
Key Terms 174
Resources for Further Study 175
Professional Organizations 175
Professional Journals 175
Suggested Readings 176
Other Media Resources 176

Chapter 6

Person-Centered Therapy   **177**

David J. Cain

Origins and Evolution of Person-Centered Therapy 177
Rogers and the Early Development of Person-Centered Therapy 178
After Rogers: Variations in the Evolution of Person-Centered Therapy 182
Existential Influences on Person-Centered Psychotherapy 185
The Evolution of Person-Centered Therapy for a Diverse World 185
Context Then—Context Now 190
Box: The Author's Journey as a Person-Centered Therapist 192
Theory of Person-Centered Therapy 194
Essential Terms of Person-Centered Theory 194
Theory of Change 197
How Change May Come About 198
Practice of Person-Centered Therapy 200
The Client-Counselor Relationship 200
The Therapeutic Endeavor: Relational Attitudes in Action 201
Promoting Client Freedom 201
Empathic Attunement 201
Regard, Acceptance, Affirmation 202

Authenticity 203
Long-Term and Short-Term Applications 213

Evaluation of Person-Centered Therapy 214

Empathy 214
Emotion in Psychotherapy 215
Focusing-Oriented Experiential Psychotherapy 216

Person-Centered Therapy: Blind Spots, Limitations, and Challenges 216

Blind Spots 216
Limitations 217
Challenges 218

Future Development: Person-Centered Therapy in a Diverse World 219

Competency 1: Self-Awareness of One's Own Assumptions, Values, and Biases 220
Competency 2: Understanding the Worldview of the Culturally Different Client 221
Competency 3: Developing Appropriate Intervention Strategies and Techniques 221
Final Comments 222

Summary 223

Key Terms 226

Resources for Further Study 226

Professional Organizations 226
Professional Journals 226
Suggested Readings 226
Other Media Resources 227

Chapter 7

Gestalt Therapy 228

Jon Frew

Origins and Evolution of Gestalt Therapy 229

Early Development of the Approach 230
Evolution of the Approach to the Present 230
The Evolution of Gestalt Therapy for a Diverse World 233
Context Then—Context Now 234
Box: The Author's Journey as a Gestalt Therapist 236

Theory of Gestalt Therapy   239

Philosophical Foundations   240

Theoretical Concepts   242

Practice of Gestalt Therapy   247

Theory of Change   248

Components of Gestalt Therapy Practice   249

The Client-Counselor Relationship   257

Long-Term Versus Short-Term Applications   261

Evaluation of Gestalt Therapy   262

Nomothetic Evaluation   263

Idiographic Evaluation   264

Compatibility of the Approach with Diverse Clients   266

Gestalt Therapy: Blind Spots, Limitations, and Challenges   267

Blind Spots   267

Limitations   267

Challenges   268

Future Development: Gestalt Therapy in a Diverse World   270

Summary   270

Key Terms   272

Resources for Further Study   273

Professional Organizations   273

Professional Journals   273

Suggested Readings   273

Other Media Resources   274

Chapter 8

Behavior Therapy I: Traditional Behavior Therapy

275

Michael D. Spiegler

Origins and Evolution of Behavior Therapy   277

Context Then—Context Now   282

Box: The Author's Journey as a Behavior Therapist   283

Theory of Behavior Therapy   285

Theory of Change   286

Defining Behavior Therapy   288

Practice of Traditional Behavior Therapy   290

Changing Antecedents That Elicit Behaviors: Stimulus Control   291

Changing Consequences to Accelerate Adaptive Behaviors:
Reinforcement 292
Changing Consequences to Decelerate Maladaptive Behaviors 294
Token Economies 297
Exposure Therapy 298
Modeling Therapy 307

To Be Continued 316

Summary 316

Key Terms 319

Resources for Further Study 319

Chapter 9

Behavior Therapy II: Cognitive-Behavioral Therapy   **320**

Michael D. Spiegler

Practice of Cognitive-Behavioral Therapy 320
Cognitive Restructuring Therapies 321
Cognitive-Behavioral Coping Skills Therapies 336

The Client-Counselor Relationship in Behavior Therapy 343

Evaluation of Behavior Therapy 344
Effectiveness of Behavior Therapy 345
Problems and Clients Treated by Behavior Therapy 347
Compatibility of Behavior Therapy for Diverse Clients 348

Behavior Therapy: Blind Spots, Limitations, and Challenges 349
Blind Spots 349
Limitations 350
Challenges 350

Future Development: Behavior Therapy in a Diverse World 351

Summary 353

Key Terms 355

Resources for Further Study 356
Professional Organizations 356
Professional Journals 356
Suggested Readings in Traditional Behavior Therapy 357
Suggested Readings in Cognitive-Behavioral Therapy 358
Other Media Resources 359

Chapter 10

Reality Therapy **360**

Robert E. Wubbolding

Origins and Evolution of Reality Therapy   360

Evolution of Reality Therapy for a Diverse World   363
Context Then—Context Now   363
Box: The Author's Journey as a Reality Therapist   365

Theory of Reality Therapy   366

Philosophical Foundations   367
Theoretical Concepts   367
Theory of Change   372

Practice of Reality Therapy   373

Establishing the Counseling Environment   373
The Client-Counselor Relationship   374
The WDEP System   375
Long-Term Versus Short-Term Applications   388

Evaluation of Reality Therapy   389

Reality Therapy: Blind Spots, Limitations, and Challenges   390

Blind Spots   390
Limitations   391
Challenges   391

Future Development: Reality Therapy in a Diverse World   391

Summary   392

Key Terms   394

Resources for Further Study   394

Professional Organizations   394
Professional Journals   395
Suggested Readings   395
Other Media Resources   396

Chapter 11

Feminist Therapy **397**

Pamela Remer

Origins and Evolution of Feminist Therapy   398

Problems in Specifying the History of Feminist Counseling   398

The Women's Movement Critique of Traditional Therapies 399
First Publications About Feminist Approaches to Counseling 399
Feminist Counseling Milestones 400
Range of Feminist Counseling Approaches 401
Context Then—Context Now 403
Box: The Author's Journey as a Feminist Therapist 405

Theory of Feminist Therapy 407
Foundational Values and Worldviews 408
Theoretical Concepts 409

Practice of Feminist Therapy 420
Feminist Therapy Interventions 420
Theory of Change 425
Long-Term Versus Short-Term Therapy 426
Application of the Four Principles of EFT 426
*General Strengths and Weaknesses of Feminist
Counseling Approaches* 429

Evaluation of Feminist Therapy 432
Feminist Therapy: Blind Spots, Limitations, and Challenges 434
Blind Spots and Limitations 434
Challenges 435

Future Development: Feminist Therapy in a Diverse World 436

Summary 437

Key Terms 439

Resources for Further Study 440
Professional Organizations 440
Professional Journals 440
Suggested Readings 440
Other Media Resources 441

Chapter 12

Family Therapy   **442**

Sandra A. Rigazio-DiGilio and Teresa McDowell

Origins and Evolution of Family Therapy 442
Emergence of Traditional Family Therapy Models 443
*Emergence of Contemporary Family Therapy Models
and Approaches* 444

Context Then—Context Now   446
Box: The Authors' Journeys as Family Therapists   447

Family Therapy: Basic Assumptions   450

Families as Systems   450
Family Development   452
Family Structure   453
Family Culture   454
Family Functioning   455

Traditional Family Therapy: Theory and Practice   455

Psychodynamic/Historical Approaches   456
Cognitive-Behavioral/Interactional Approaches   461
Existential-Humanistic Approaches   465

Contemporary Family Therapy: Theory and Practice   467

Contributions from Postmodern, Ecological, and Integrative Theories   467
Additional Assumptions of Contemporary Family Therapies   468
Theory of Change   470
Systemic Cognitive Developmental Therapy   471

Evaluation of Family Therapy   475

Nomothetic Family Therapy Research: Effectiveness Across Clients   476
*Nomothetic Family Therapy Research: Effectiveness for Specific
Presenting Issues and Populations*   476
Idiographic Family Therapy Research   477
Idiothetic Family Therapy Research   478
Family Therapy and Diverse Populations   479

Family Therapy: Blind Spots, Limitations, and Challenges   481

Psychodynamic/Historical Approaches   481
Cognitive-Behavioral/Interactional Approaches   481
Existential-Humanistic Approaches   482
Contemporary Approaches   482

Future Development: Family Therapy in a Diverse World   483

Summary   484

Key Terms   486

Resources for Further Study   486

Professional Organizations   486
Professional Journals   487
Suggested Readings   487
Other Media Resources   488

Chapter 13

Narrative Therapy   **489**

Kathie Crocket

Origins and Evolution of Narrative Therapy   491
  Context Then—Context Now   493
  Box: The Author's Journey as a Narrative Therapist   495
Theory of Narrative Therapy   499
  Philosophical Foundations   499
  Theoretical Concepts   500
Practice of Narrative Therapy   502
  Externalizing Conversations   502
  Problem Stories and Alternative Stories   503
  The Intentions of Inquiry   504
  Thin and Thick Descriptions   505
  Absent but Implicit   505
  Therapeutic Documents   506
  Audience and Witnessing   507
  A Counseling Conversation: Theory of Change in Action   508
  Role of the Client-Counselor Relationship   521
  Long-Term Versus Short-Term Applications   522
Evaluation of Narrative Therapy   523
  Accountability in Narrative Practice   523
Narrative Therapy: Blind Spots, Limitations, and Challenges   525
  Blind Spots   525
  Limitations   526
  Challenges   528
Future Development: Narrative Therapy in a Diverse World   528
Summary   529
Key Terms   531
Resources for Further Study   532
  Professional Organizations   532
  Professional Journals   532
  Suggested Readings   532
  Other Media Resources   533

Glossary   **G-1**
References   **R-1**
Name Index   **I-1**
Subject Index   **I-14**

Preface

Contemporary Psychotherapies for a Diverse World was inspired by two beliefs and a challenge. Previous generations of graduate students in counseling and clinical psychology chose their theoretical orientation from among the three or four classic approaches, but today graduate students are expected to learn about and choose their preferred therapy approach from among those classics plus many more. Our first belief is that graduate students should be learning about the different theoretical approaches from their champions rather than from one author's interpretation of all the approaches. Our second belief concerns the dramatic shift in demographics of psychotherapy clients in the United States—from a predominantly White, European-American, middle- or upper-class client population to a client base far more diverse. We believe that today's graduate students need to be aware of the difficulties experienced by non-majority (as well as majority) clients and to become skilled in the application of their chosen counseling orientation with these clients.

Based on these two beliefs, the challenge we accepted in writing *Contemporary Psychotherapies for a Diverse World* has been to introduce students to the theory and practice of the major approaches to psychotherapy (both traditional and contemporary in origin) and to illustrate how they are applied to diverse clients. To meet this challenge, we recruited chapter authors who meet two criteria. First, they are at "the top of their game," well-respected, and well-known as leading experts in their chosen approach to psychotherapy. Second, each contributor is interested in the application of his or her approach to diverse clients.[1] The result is a textbook that offers a unique combination of two key features: *authentic contemporary authorship* and *true integration of diversity*.

Although the concept of having experts describe their approaches to psychotherapy is not unique to this book, *Contemporary Psychotherapies for a Diverse World* is the only textbook in which the chapter authors are among *today's* leading spokespersons for their approaches. As a result, both the history of each approach and the latest, cutting-edge theory and practice are presented, affording the reader an insider's perspective, which includes exposure to the style and language used by adherents of the approach. The second unique feature of

---

[1] If you are interested in learning more about the authors of this book, see the About the Authors section following this preface.

Contemporary Psychotherapies for a Diverse World is that it is the first textbook to *fully integrate* discussion and illustration of how the various approaches to psychotherapy are dealing with the ever increasing diversity of the clients of today and the future.

The Organization of This Book

As in other counseling theory texts, the major approaches to counseling are presented in this text in roughly the chronological order in which they were developed. For the older approaches, the chapter authors have presented a continuum of classic to modern versions of the approach. Reading these chapters in order will give students a sense of the evolution of contemporary psychotherapy. However, the chapters are independent of one another, so they can be read in any order.

Chapter 1, Introduction   The introductory chapter was coauthored by the editors. We deliberately made it brief to avoid satiating students on appetizers before they got to the main course. It begins with a thumbnail sketch of the history of psychotherapy and counseling and a broad definition of the field. To prepare students to think critically about each approach, we introduce them to the varieties of psychotherapy that exist and the variables on which they differ, such as purpose, change strategy, process, and approach to evaluating effectiveness. The book's emphasis on treating diverse clients is justified in terms of the changing demographics and the need for counselors to be culturally competent. We also discuss how one goes about choosing an approach to counseling, a process that many students will be beginning as they read this book.

Chapter 2, Ethics for a Diverse World   Ethical principles are essential to the practice of every approach, and so most psychotherapy survey textbooks include a chapter on the subject. The ethics chapter in this book, however, was written by an author with unique expertise especially suited to the goals of the book. Melba Vasquez—an internationally-known expert in the fields of professional ethics, ethnic minority psychology, and the psychology of women—enriches her discussion of the American Counseling Association and American Psychological Association ethical guidelines with multicultural and feminist ethical perspectives.

Chapter 3, Psychoanalytic Therapy   The author of this chapter also is uniquely suited to write about his subject area for this particular book. Neil Altman, a noted relational psychoanalyst, presents the psychoanalytic approach, from classic Freudian theory through object relations to modern relational analysis, with case examples from his own practice that illustrate the application of contemporary relational analysis to ethnically diverse and low-income clients in urban public clinic settings. Dr. Altman presents convincing evidence that psychoanalysis can be relevant today to a widely diverse clientele.

Chapter 4, Adlerian Therapy   Given Adler's abiding interest in the family, who could be better suited to write about his approach than a father–son team of Aderlian therapists? In this chapter, Jon Carlson, one of today's most widely known and respected Adlerians, and Matt Englar-Carlson, whose training as an Adlerian began at birth, introduce us to Adlerian therapy from its earliest formulation to the present day. The practice section of their chapter offers a powerful demonstration of how Adlerian therapy—with its emphasis on prevention and education, multiculturalism, and social justice—continues to be a valuable approach to therapy in a diverse world.

Chapter 5, Existential Therapy   We knew exactly who we wanted to recruit to write this chapter and were delighted when he agreed. The author of this chapter is someone who was there at the beginning, who was inspired as a young student in Paris by Sartre and de Beauvoir, and who participated in the translation of existential philosophy into a psychotherapeutic approach. Clemmont Vontress is an internationally recognized expert both in existential therapy and in cross-cultural counseling. In this chapter, he provides a framework for understanding and applying existential therapy in the 21st century in ways that transcend national, racial, ethnic, and other barriers to effective counseling.

Chapter 6, Person-Centered Therapy   As we built our panel of experts, we asked various colleagues to name the top three people in their field. In our poll of specialists in person-centered therapy, the name they listed first was the same every time: David Cain. In our subsequent discussions with Dr. Cain, we were gratified to learn that he shared our concerns about the need for the integration of diversity into the theoretical training of today's graduate students and was eager to take on the challenge of writing a person-centered therapy chapter with that central purpose in mind.

Chapter 7, Gestalt Therapy   Ask a group of counselors, "When you hear the term *Gestalt therapy*, what is the first thing you think of?" and the two responses you will most likely hear are "Fritz Perls" and "empty chair." In writing this chapter, I (Jon Frew) was determined that the next generation of counselors and psychologists—at least, those I could influence through this book—would instead reply, "Do you mean Gestalt therapy as it was or as it is today?" In this chapter, I present the essential theory of Gestalt therapy and describe the evolution of its practice from the mid-20th century into the 21st century. I have been a participant in that evolution, practicing, teaching, and writing about the approach for 30 years, and I believe this chapter makes a compelling case for the effectiveness of modern-day Gestalt therapy with clients who represent a wide spectrum of diversity.

Chapter 8, Behavior Therapy I: Traditional Behavior Therapy, and *Chapter 9, Behavior Therapy II: Cognitive-Behavioral Therapy*   The field of behavior therapy is just 50 years old, and I (Michael Spiegler) have been a behavior therapy practitioner, researcher, and scholar—as well as a commentator on the field—for 40 of those 50 years. During that time, I have seen behavior therapy change and evolve, most recently in terms of its becoming sensitive to and effective with diverse clients. Behavior therapy is a broad approach that comprises a wide array of treatment strategies and techniques. Thus, I have covered behavior therapy in two sequential chapters. In Chapter 8, I introduce the behavior therapy approach and describe the branch that I have called *traditional behavior therapy,* which includes stimulus control, reinforcement and punishment, exposure therapies, and modeling therapies. In Chapter 9, I continue with *cognitive-behavioral therapy,* which grew out of traditional behavior therapy and employs both traditional techniques that address overt behaviors and newer cognitive techniques that directly modify clients' thoughts and beliefs.

Chapter 10, Reality Therapy   Besides William Glasser, the founder of reality therapy, there is no one more recognized as a proponent of this approach than Robert Wubbolding, today's leading reality therapy practitioner, trainer, and writer. When we learned that for many years Dr. Wubbolding has been working with scholars and teachers around the world to adapt the practice of reality therapy to their cultures, we realized that he would be the ideal person to write about reality therapy for our book. In this chapter, he describes the theoretical foundation of reality therapy, choice theory, which emphasizes personal responsibility for one's behaviors, and the practice of reality therapy.

Chapter 11, Feminist Therapy   We recruited Pamela Remer to write this chapter for two reasons: first, we knew her as the coauthor of one of the most widely read books on feminist therapy, and second, we knew that the focus of her writing is not only women but all subordinate and oppressed groups. In this chapter, Dr. Remer describes the evolution of feminist therapy and shows how feminist therapy educates clients about the cultural contexts that surround and contribute to their counseling issues and enables them to exert influence over the personal, interpersonal, and institutional factors that impact on their well-being.

Chapter 12, Family Therapy   In our search for the right author for this chapter, we turned for a recommendation to Lahaska Press Consulting Editor, Allen Ivey, one of the most widely known and respected figures in the multicultural movement in counseling. He did not hesitate to name Sandra Rigazio-DiGilio, with whom he has collaborated on research and publications aimed at advancing cultural sensitivity in family therapy. She engaged as her chapter coauthor Teresa McDowell, who has published on the important topic of racial equity in family therapy. In this chapter, they survey the gamut of family therapy approaches, from those having their origin in traditional individual therapy orientations to contemporary models that have been informed by feminism, multiculturalism, social constructionism, and evidence-based practice.

Chapter 13, Narrative Therapy   Our survey of approaches to counseling concludes with a chapter on narrative therapy, which not only is the most recently developed approach discussed in this book but also is the only one developed outside Europe or the United States. Narrative therapy originated in Australia and New Zealand, and although it is practiced in other parts of the world, the center of its practice remains in those two countries. It is fitting, then, that the author of this chapter is Kathie Crocket, who practices, teaches, and writes about narrative therapy in New Zealand. Dr. Crocket wrote this chapter with the refreshingly distinctive style and language of narrative therapy, and her case examples are based on work with her own clients, some of whom are members of New Zealand's indigenous population.

Consistent Organization of Each Chapter

Each of the 11 therapy approach chapters has the same basic structure. This consistent chapter organization—combined with our painstaking editing for readability and sound pedagogy—makes this book, written by experts, a cohesive textbook rather than a collection of essays.

Following a brief overview of the therapy, the chapter authors survey how the approach began and how it has evolved, including the broad social context in which it was conceived and in which it exists today. In a special feature called "The Author's Journey," the authors describe what led them to adopt their approach and how their own practice of the approach has evolved over time. Next, the authors present the theoretical foundations of their approach, followed by a discussion of how the theory is manifested in practice. Two sections toward the end of each chapter assess the current status: an evaluation of the evidence validating the approach and a candid appraisal of the approach's blind spots, limitations, and challenges. The two evaluative sections balance the fact that each author is, not surprisingly, an enthusiastic supporter of her or his approach and thus has emphasized its strengths. The final section of each chapter is a commentary on the future development of the approach in a diverse world.

The content of each chapter is followed by a point-by-point summary and an alphabetized list of the key terms that were printed in boldface type when they were defined in the chapter. (A comprehensive glossary of the key terms appears at the end of the book.) Finally, each chapter ends with an annotated "Resources for Further Study" section, including the names and addresses of the main *professional organizations* and *journals* associated with the approach, an extensive list of *suggested readings*, and a list of *other media resources*, such as websites and videos.

A comprehensive list of the references cited in all the chapters appears at the end of the book.

A Personal Note from the Editors on the Process of Writing this Book

Can a Gestalt therapist and a behavior therapist form an unlikely union and invest a substantial portion of their lives for three years collaborating on the conception, writing, and editing of the book you are about to read? The answer is, "Yes they can," and the reason is that we have many more commonalities than differences. We both believe in the value of counseling and psychotherapy and have a passion for teaching students about this noble pursuit. Additionally, we both recognized the need for a truly modern, relevant textbook to help us teach our students about the theory and practice of psychotherapy in a diverse world.

Overriding our very different theoretical orientations to counseling, we share an appreciation of there being diverse approaches to achieving a common goal: alleviating human suffering caused by psychological problems. Just as diversity in people makes the world richer and more challenging and interesting, a comprehensive review of the theory and practice of psychotherapy must be undertaken through the lenses of multiple perspectives. No one perspective provides the best fit and works optimally for all clients, for all therapists, for all problems, and in all contexts.

On a personal level, as editors we recognized that each of us has particular strengths, and we capitalized on them as we collaborated first to conceptualize the book, then to bring together our esteemed team of experts, and finally to orchestrate their writing so that the result is the harmonious symphony that a teaching textbook needs to be.

Instructor's Resources

- *Teaching Ideas*   For each chapter, there are specific suggestions regarding how instructors can draw on and expand what is presented in the textbook in their teaching. Some of these teaching ideas were contributed by the chapter authors and some have been derived from Michael Spiegler's experience class testing the manuscript with his students.

- *Test Bank*   This set of test items includes a chapter-by-chapter compilation of multiple-choice and open-ended questions based on the textbook. The correct answer and the relevant page(s) in the textbook appear after each question. Lahaska Press has made the Test Bank available to instructors as a Microsoft Word file so that they can add, delete, and edit questions to suit their own teaching needs.

- *PowerPoint Program*   The instructor's materials include a set of PowerPoint slides for each chapter of the textbook prepared by the chapter authors.

- *Video Program*   A series of counseling demonstration videos, produced by Lahaska Press, are available free of charge to instructors who have adopted *Contemporary Psychotherapies for a Diverse World*. For instructors seeking information about how to obtain these videos, please see the Lahaska Press contact information on the copyright page of this book.

Acknowledgments

I (Jon Frew) deeply appreciate the able assistance and steady encouragement I received in coediting this book. It is logical that I first thank Allen Ivey; it all began when Allen discovered my interest in the broader issues concerning diversity in psychotherapy, proceeded to introduce me to an editor at Lahaska Press, and deftly planted the seeds of this textbook idea in our heads. Next I want to thank Linda James who provided technical assistance throughout the project to augment my "legendary" computer skills. Thanks as well to Adam Smith, my graduate assistant for the last three years, whose "invisible hand" tracked down countless missing references and bits of information. Conversations with Somphone Khen (Sam) Reynolds were extremely illuminating and enhanced my writing about diversity and Gestalt therapy. I also want to acknowledge the support and encouragement I received from my family of friends: Peg LeVine, David Hutchinson, Michael Matthews, Carl Haefling, Eva Gold, and Steve Zahm. Finally, I received enormous assistance and support from Michael Spiegler who had been down the (textbook) road before and was gracious and patient in lighting my way.

I (Michael Spiegler) want to begin by thanking Jon Frew for engaging my interest in this project and, as we grappled with the myriad details, for gently keeping us focused on the gestalt. I truly appreciate the able assistance of my students and assistants: Jesse Cardozo, Lauren Moses, and Sara Vargas. I am especially grateful for Michael McQuiggin's help; Michael tirelessly and expertly researched numerous issues regarding diverse clients and critically read and made valuable suggestions about early drafts of the chapters in this book (frequently under "I need this yesterday" pressure). Arlene Spiegler was a sounding board for my ideas and read numerous drafts of my writing and editing. As if that were not enough, she listened sympathetically to my frustrations, tolerated my absence during many hours of being ensconced in my study, provided encouragement and social support, and throughout remained my loving wife and friend. Thank you, Arlene. I am grateful for the balance provided by the presence of Amelia and Megan Fink in my life—they will have permanent memories of their zeda at his laptop working on this book. Last and first, I must acknowledge the enduring contribution to all I do from my parents, Lillian and Julie Spiegler, the two people who first picked me up on the hospital stairs (at least that's how they tell the story) and later allowed me the freedom to begin my career as a behavior therapist at the beach (for more on this auspicious beginning, see my Author's Journey in Chapter 8). It is altogether fitting that I have dedicated this book to my mom.

The best way to thank manuscript reviewers is to listen carefully to their advice and counsel. We believe that our reviewers will find plentiful evidence of their hard work in this book. Our thanks go to:

Sylvia Fernandez, University of Miami
Douglas Guiffrida, University of Rochester
Martin Jencius, Kent State University
Natalie Kees, Colorado State University
Jelane Kennedy, College of St. Rose
Beverly Mustaine, Argosy University
Micki Ozbeck, University of Tennessee, Chattanooga
Robert Peterson, Metro State University
Anthony Strange, University of Alaska, Fairbanks
Susan Varhely, Adams State College
Darren Wozny, Mississippi State University, Meridian

Finally, we both want to acknowledge Lahaska Press Senior Editor, Mary Falcon. Simply put, this book would not have been written without her endorsement, her ongoing support, and her perseverance and expertise. Our contributing authors were the orchestra, we were first chairs in the string and brass sections, and Mary was our conductor. She had the extraordinary ability to see the entire piece of music and to hear when the individual instruments were out of tune or not blending with other sections. Like all outstanding conductors, she knew just when to be firm and critical, when to be complimentary and encouraging, and when to step aside to let the authors translate their good ideas and passion into the words you will read in the book. Thank you, Mary, for sharing with us your competence, knowledge, sense of humor, and friendship.

Jon Frew
Michael D. Spiegler

About the Authors

The Editors

Jon Frew, Ph.D., ABPP, is the coauthor of Chapter 1, Introduction, and the author of Chapter 7, Gestalt Therapy. He is Professor of Psychology at the Pacific University School of Professional Psychology where he teaches in both the Clinical Psychology (M.S./Psy.D.) and the Master of Arts in Counseling Psychology programs. He received his doctorate in counseling psychology from Kent State University. Jon has been involved in the training of Gestalt therapists in the United States, Canada, and Australia since 1981, most recently as the codirector of the Gestalt Therapy Training Center Northwest in Portland, Oregon. He is on the editorial board of the *Gestalt Review* and the author of many articles and chapters on a range of topics related to Gestalt therapy. Currently, his primary interest is in the integration of multicultural counseling and Gestalt therapy. He maintains a part-time private practice in which he sees individuals and couples, and he provides consultation and training to groups and organizations.

Michael D. Spiegler, Ph.D., is the coauthor of Chapter 1, Introduction, and the author of Chapter 8, Behavior Therapy I: Traditional Behavior Therapy, and Chapter 9, Behavior Therapy II: Cognitive-Behavioral Therapy. He is Professor of Psychology at Providence College. He received his doctorate in clinical psychology from Vanderbilt University. Michael's contributions to the field of psychotherapy and counseling include conducting pioneering research in filmed modeling therapy and originating the use of skills training as a treatment for chronic psychiatric disorders, an approach now widely used. His books include *The Community Training Center: An Educational-Behavior-Social Systems Model for Rehabilitating Psychiatric Patients; Personality: Strategies and Issues* (8th ed.); and *Contemporary Behavior Therapy* (4th ed.). His research has been in the areas of anxiety and its treatment, assertive behavior, modeling, day treatment of chronic psychiatric disorders, exercise addiction, and active learning. Although primarily an academic clinical psychologist, as a behavior therapist Michael is involved in clinical consultation and has a small private practice, both of which involve working with diverse clients.

The Chapter Authors

Neil Altman, Ph.D., is the author of Chapter 3, Psychoanalytic Therapy. He is Associate Clinical Professor in the Postdoctoral Program in Psychotherapy and Psychoanalysis at New York University. He received his doctorate in psychology from New York University. Neil is coeditor of *Psychoanalytic Dialogues: The International Journal of Relational Perspectives* and on the editorial board of *The Journal of Infant, Child, and Adolescent Psychotherapy*. He is the author of *The Analyst in the Inner City: Race, Class, and Culture through a Psychoanalytic Lens* and coauthor of *Relational Child Psychotherapy*. From 1980 until 1991 Neil worked at Bronx Lebanon Hospital Center in New York City, serving for part of that time as Associate Chief Psychologist and director of the psychology training program. He was a member of the Council of Representatives of the American Psychological Association from 2000 until 2006 and presently serves on the board of directors of The Fostering Connection, a program to provide free psychotherapy to foster children and their families, and of the International Association for Relational Psychoanalysis and Psychotherapy. His primary professional interest is community application of psychoanalytic concepts. He maintains a private practice in New York City.

   David J. Cain, Ph.D., ABPP, CGP, is the author of Chapter 6, Person-Centered Therapy. He has a private psychotherapy practice in San Marcos, California and also teaches at the California School of Professional Psychology, San Diego, of Alliant International University and in the Psychology Department at Chapman University. He received his doctorate in clinical and community psychology from the University of Wyoming. He is the editor of *Humanistic Psychotherapies: Handbook of Research and Practice* and *Classics in the Person-Centered Approach*. David was the founder of the Association for the Development of the Person-Centered Approach and was the founder and editor of the *Person-Centered Review*. He is the psychotherapy editor for the *Journal of Humanistic Psychology* and serves on the editorial boards of *The Humanistic Psychologist, Person-Centered and Experiential Psychotherapies, Person-Centered Journal*, and *Journal of Contemporary Psychotherapy*. He is the current President of the Division of Humanistic Psychology of the American Psychological Association. David's primary professional commitment is the advancement of humanistic psychology and psychotherapy.

   Jon Carlson, Psy.D., Ed.D., ABPP, is the coauthor of Chapter 4, Adlerian Therapy. He is Distinguished Professor of Psychology and Counseling at Governors State University and a psychologist at the Wellness Clinic in Lake Geneva, Wisconsin. He holds doctorates from Wayne State University (in counseling) and from the Adler School of Professional Psychology (in clinical psychology) and holds diplomates in both family psychology and Adlerian psychology. Jon has served as editor of several periodicals, including the *Journal of Individual*

Psychology and *The Family Journal.* He has authored 150 journal articles and 40 books including *Time for a Better Marriage, Adlerian Therapy, The Mummy at the Dining Room Table, Bad Therapy, The Client Who Changed Me,* and *Moved by the Spirit.* He has created over 200 professional training videos and DVDs with leading professional therapists and educators. In 2004, the American Counseling Association named Jon a "Living Legend." Recently, he syndicated an advice cartoon, *On the Edge,* with cartoonist Joe Martin.

Kathie Crocket, Ph.D., is the author of Chapter 13, Narrative Therapy. She is Senior Lecturer and director of counselor education at the University of Waikato, Hamilton, New Zealand. She received her doctorate in counseling supervision from the University of Waikato. The counselor education program that Kathie directs is distinctive in its emphasis on narrative approaches in counseling, family therapy, supervision, and research at the master's and doctoral levels. The focus of her publications is narrative approaches in counseling, supervision, and research. She is coeditor of *Narrative Therapy in Practice: The Archaeology of Hope* and is currently coediting *Ethics in Practice: A Guide for Counsellors,* which is being written for a New Zealand audience. She is a member of the National Ethics Committee of New Zealand Association of Counsellors. Kathie's current teaching focus is counseling practice and supervision. She has a special interest in supervising practitioner research with master's and doctoral students because such research offers opportunities to explore the possibilities the narrative metaphor offers for innovative research practices.

Matt Englar-Carlson, Ph.D., is the coauthor of Chapter 4, Adlerian Therapy. He is Associate Professor of Counseling at the California State University at Fullerton where he teaches courses in theories of counseling, group counseling, family systems, and qualitative research. He holds graduate degrees in health psychology education and counselor education and received his doctorate in counseling psychology from the Pennsylvania State University. A former elementary school counselor, Matt's areas of clinical practice and research focus on men and masculinity, multimodal therapy with children, and social class counseling issues. In reference to men, he is interested in training psychotherapists to understand how masculinity influences well-being, interpersonal relationships, self-identity, and the process of psychotherapy. He is coeditor of *In the Room with Men: A Casebook of Therapeutic Change.*

Teresa McDowell, Ed.D., is the coauthor of Chapter 12, Family Therapy. She is currently Associate Professor and director of the marriage and family therapy master's and doctoral programs at the University of Connecticut. She is also the director of the program's clinic, the Humphrey Center for Individual, Couple, and Family Therapy. She received her master's degree in marriage and family therapy (MFT) from Pacific Lutheran University and her doctorate in adult education with a cognate in MFT from Northern Illinois University. Teresa's contributions to the field of family therapy focus on family therapy education and supervision, systems consultation, diversity and social justice, and global citizenship. She has extensive experience training and consulting with community agencies and family-centered programs.

Pamela Remer, Ph.D., TEP, is the author of Chapter 11, Feminist Therapy. She is Associate Professor in the Department of Educational and Counseling Psychology at the University of Kentucky and serves as director of clinical training for the doctoral program in counseling psychology, which offers a specialization in counseling women and feminist therapy. Pam received her doctorate in counseling psychology from the University of Colorado. She has coauthored two books on empowerment feminist therapy—*Feminist Perspectives in Therapy: Empowering Diverse Women* and *Feminist Perspectives in Therapy: An Empowerment Model for Women*. She is a certified trainer, educator, and practitioner in psychodrama, sociometry, and group psychotherapy and is an editor of the journal *Group Psychotherapy, Psychodrama, & Sociometry*. She has been a member of the executive council of the American Psychological Association's Division 35 (Society for the Psychology of Women) for the past 13 years and is currently the chair of its Committee on Training and Practice. Pam's main areas of focus are women's counseling issues, counseling rape survivors, and researching the effectiveness of social justice-based date rape prevention programs. She is a feminist-diversity therapist who is a licensed psychologist with a small private practice.

Sandra A. Rigazio-DiGilio, Ph.D., is the coauthor of Chapter 12, Family Therapy. She is currently Professor in the marriage and family master's and doctoral programs at the University of Connecticut. She received her master's degree in rehabilitation counseling from the University of Connecticut and her doctorate in counseling psychology from the University of Massachusetts at Amherst. One of her contributions to the fields of psychology, counseling, and marriage and family therapy is the development of the Systemic Cognitive Development Therapy Model and its companion supervision model. She has published on these models and in the areas of multicultural and theoretical foundations and issues of practice in marriage and family therapy training and supervision. Sandra is coauthor of *Community Genograms: Using Individual, Family and Cultural Narratives with Clients* and author of the chapter, "Postmodern Theories of Counseling," in *The Handbook of Counseling*. Her professional practice focuses on end-of-life issues with children and families living through the dying process and on community-network therapy centered around family-community collaborative partnerships.

Melba J. T. Vasquez, Ph.D., ABPP, is the author of Chapter 2, Ethics for a Diverse World. She is a counseling psychologist in full-time independent practice in Austin, Texas. She received her doctorate in counseling psychology from the University of Texas at Austin. She has published extensively in the areas of professional ethics, ethnic minority psychology, psychology of women, and supervision and training. She is the coauthor of *Ethics in Psychotherapy & Counseling: A Practical Guide* and *How to Survive and Thrive as a Therapist: Information, Ideas and Resources for Psychologists in Practice*. Melba is a former president of the Texas Psychological Association (TPA) and of Divisions 35 (Society of Psychology of Women) and 17 (Society of Counseling Psychology) of the American Psychological Association (APA), and she was elected to serve on the APA Board of Directors for 2007–2009. She is a Fellow of the APA and has received numerous awards, including the APA James M. Jones Lifetime Achievement Award in 2004, TPA Psychologist of the Year in 2003, and the APA Senior Career Award for Distinguished Contributions to Psychology in the Public Interest in 2002.

Clemmont E. Vontress, Ph.D., is the author of Chapter 5, Existential Therapy. He is Professor Emeritus of Counseling at George Washington University and has been visiting professor at a number of universities, including Johns Hopkins University, Atlanta University, Kuwait University, and Howard University. "Von" received his doctorate in counseling from Indiana University. A licensed psychologist, he is one of the country's leading authorities on cross-cultural counseling. His 1971 book, *Counseling Negroes*, was the first book to call attention to the impact of culture and race on counseling African Americans in this country. Since that time, he has written more than 100 articles, chapters, and books on existential counseling and psychotherapy, cross-cultural counseling, and traditional healing. A consultant to numerous organizations in this country and abroad, he has traveled widely in the United States, the Middle East, Africa, Europe, and the Caribbean Islands. He has made several field trips to West Africa to study methods used by folk healers to treat patients complaining of physical, psychological, social, and spiritual problems. He also has studied and written about ethno-psychiatry, an approach used in France for counseling immigrants from developing countries.

Robert E. Wubbolding, Ed.D., is the author of Chapter 10, Reality Therapy. He is Professor Emeritus at Xavier University in Cincinnati, director of the Center for Reality Therapy in Cincinnati, and Senior Faculty and director of training for The William Glasser Institute in Los Angeles. Bob received his doctorate in counseling from the University of Cincinnati. He has published extensively on reality therapy, including more than 130 articles, essays, and chapters, 9 videos, and 10 books, including *Reality Therapy for the 21st Century* and *A Set of Directions for Putting and Keeping Yourself Together*. He is an internationally known teacher and practitioner of reality therapy and has taught courses on choice theory and reality therapy in the United States, Europe, Asia, and the Middle East. Bob has consulted with the drug and alcohol abuse programs of the U.S. Army and U.S. Air Force, served as a group counselor at a halfway house for women, an elementary and secondary school counselor, a high school teacher, and a teacher of adult basic education.

Contemporary Psychotherapies for a Diverse World

Chapter 1

Introduction to Contemporary Psychotherapies for a Diverse World

Jon Frew and Michael D. Spiegler

People have been seeking the counsel of others for help with their psychological problems for thousands of years. However, it was not until a little more than a hundred years ago that a formal profession devoted to this endeavor began. In the following pages, you will be introduced to this multifaceted and fascinating field of counseling and psychotherapy.

This is an exciting and challenging time to be entering the profession because there is an important shift taking place in the theory and practice of contemporary psychotherapies. The demographic patterns in the United States are changing rapidly, and those changes are reflected in the clients who are seeking help for their psychological problems. Thus, in addition to learning about theories of counseling and psychotherapy and how they translate into practice, you will need to learn about how they are relevant to and effective with diverse clients. In this book, we incorporate into the concept of *diversity* all factors that differentiate groups of individuals in modern-day society: culture, ethnicity, race, gender, age, sexual orientation, socioeconomic status, educational level, religious and spiritual orientation, and physical ability.

This book pays special attention to the ways in which the major approaches to counseling and psychotherapy are changing to meet the needs of nonmajority clients. The other unique feature of this book is that each counseling approach is presented by a leading contemporary scholar or practitioner of that approach. Thus, you will be learning about the major psychotherapies directly from experts at the forefront of their respective fields.

Counseling and Psychotherapy Approaches in Context

Counseling theories, like theories in all disciplines, originate within a context, a particular set of environmental conditions that exist at a specific time and place. The context in which counseling theories originate inevitably influences the shape and form of those theories. These contexts are often far-reaching and include sociocultural values, political movements, historical events, and economic factors.

The profession of counseling and psychotherapy came of age in the 1950s (Aubrey, 1977). Indeed, if one decade in history had to be singled out as having the most profound impact on counseling professionals, it would be those years. During this period, major breakthroughs in theory, research, and practice occurred; there also were national and worldwide events that shaped the future of the profession.

Traditional Contexts

One of those events occurred in 1944, toward the end of World War II. In response to the large number of returning soldiers who were suffering from combat-related problems, the Veterans Administration offered substantial financial support for public and private institutions to provide counseling to veterans. The counseling profession was further strengthened by the National Defense Education Act (NDEA), which was passed in 1958 in response to the fear that the Russians were getting ahead of the United States in the race to space and other scientific endeavors. The act allotted $7.5 million per year to support counselor education programs and to establish state guidance and counseling testing programs. In the next 5 years, 14,000 counselors were trained with NDEA funding and the number of public school counselors almost tripled (Picchioni & Bonk, 1983).

For the first half of the 20th century, only two major approaches to psychotherapy existed: psychoanalysis and Adlerian therapy. Then, in 1951, Carl Rogers published *Client-Centered Therapy*, a book considered by many to outline the first true theory of counseling. Although Rogers provided a view of abnormal behavior, he emphasized a model of health that captivated the nascent field of counseling and provided an alternative to the darker view of human nature tendered by psychoanalytic theory. Fritz Perls's (with Ralph Hefferline and Paul Goodman) seminal work, *Gestalt Therapy: Excitement and Growth in the Human Personality*, was also published in 1951. Next, with the 1958 publication of *Psychotherapy by Reciprocal Inhibition* by Joseph Wolpe, the counseling profession was introduced to behavior therapy. In the same year, *Existence: A New Dimension in Psychiatry and Psychology*, by Rollo May (with Ernest Angel and Henri Ellenberger) was published; it was the first concise discussion of existential psychotherapy. In the 1960s, Rudolf Dreikurs (1967) resurrected interest in Adlerian psychotherapy in the United States, William Glasser (1965) developed reality therapy, and Albert Ellis (1962) and Aaron Beck (1967) developed their cognitive-behavioral therapies.

With the exception of psychoanalysis and Adlerian theory, all of these theories, along with others described in this book, have common roots primarily in the post–World War II Western European-American experience. The therapists who developed these theories were White males, and the clients for whom they were developing their theories were predominantly White, heterosexual, and middle class. Therefore, the theories embody certain values and assumptions about the goals of therapy (e.g., fostering self-reliance and independence), the methods used to bring about change (e.g., the importance of verbal and emotional expression and disclosure of intimate details of one's life), and the definition of mental health (e.g., a separation of mental health from physical and spiritual health). Given the present diversification of America, the values, beliefs, and assumptions inherent in the fabric of the counseling profession must be reexamined. We have become a nation in which a substantial minority of the population have dual cultural identities and are in various stages of adapting and contributing to the majority U.S. culture. To serve this ever-increasing population, the counseling profession must adapt as well. Our counseling theories and practices must be flexible and broadened so that diverse clients will seek and benefit from our services.

Modern Contexts

Three of the psychotherapy orientations you will read about in this book—feminist therapy, family therapy, and narrative therapy—are newer approaches that were developed as alternatives to the traditional approaches. They differ from the more traditional theories in terms of their basic assumptions, values, or origins. Feminist therapy emerged during the women's movement in the United States in the 1960s and 1970s. From the feminist perspective, women have been socialized by the dominant male culture to be self-sacrificing and passive, and their lives are constrained by the sociopolitical status to which this socialization has relegated them. Feminist therapists have challenged the accuracy and inclusiveness of traditional counseling theories because of their male, gender-biased assumptions and values. More recently, the purview of feminist approaches has been broadened beyond women to other culturally and otherwise diverse groups who have been subject to oppression and discrimination.

Family therapy came into its own in the 1970s and 1980s. In the various forms of the approach, the family is viewed as a system: the complex set of interpersonal dynamics that occur in the family are central, and no individual family member is considered the source of the problem or is identified as the client. Because the more recently developed forms of family therapy also emphasize the crucial role played by the sociopolitical context in which a family lives, they are more closely aligned with the multicultural perspective that focuses on the individual in a much larger, cultural context.

Narrative therapy is the youngest of the approaches discussed in this book. Originating in the late 1980s in New Zealand and Australia, the approach was developed in response to the perception that the traditional psychotherapies reproduced the oppressive and sexist practices of the dominant Western cultures. The central focus of narrative therapy is inquiry into the stories told in families and communities that shape and form individuals' lives and identities—stories of gender, ethnicity, nationality, and class; stories of the life experiences that shape and produce the problems clients encounter. The theory and practice of narrative therapy was, and continues to be, a collaborative enterprise of family and feminist therapists, originally in New Zealand and Australia and more recently in North American and European countries.

What Is Psychotherapy or Counseling?

What is the difference between *psychotherapy* and *counseling?* In the professional literature, distinctions between the terms are narrowing over time but are still being debated in some quarters. Nevertheless, despite any definitional differences, the theories underlying psychotherapy and counseling are the same. Thus, for the purpose of discussing theories in this book, the terms *psychotherapy* (or *therapy*) and *counseling* as well as *psychotherapist* (or *therapist*) and *counselor* will be used interchangeably.

Now for a more difficult question: What is psychotherapy or counseling? More than half a century ago, Raimy (1950) quipped: "Psychotherapy is an undefined technique applied to unspecified problems with unpredictable outcomes. For this technique we recommend rigorous training" (p. 93). This tongue-in-cheek statement intimates that there is no clear-cut, agreed-upon definition of psychotherapy, which was the case in the mid-20th century when Raimy made the observation and still is true today. The lack of one standardized statement of meaning, however, has not deterred therapists from their work. Psychotherapists do what they do, know what they are doing, promote what they do, and believe that what they do works.

All that being said, we would be negligent to begin a book on psychotherapy without providing you with a general definition of the subject matter. So here is a brief, generic definition that fits for most therapies. *Psychotherapy is an endeavor for helping people deal with their psychological problems through a formal, more or less structured interaction between the person(s) seeking help (client[s]) and a trained professional (therapist or counselor).* Although this definition is limited, it does indicate the purpose or aim of psychotherapy, the context in which psychotherapy transpires, and the parties usually involved. In doing so, the definition differentiates psychotherapy from the informal help a person with psychological problems might receive from a caring friend.

Differences in Counseling and Psychotherapy Approaches

The nature of psychotherapy is an enigma for most students taking their first course on psychotherapy, just as it is for clients entering therapy for the first time. This is not surprising because what most people know about psychotherapy is likely to come from three unreliable sources. One source is the depiction of psychotherapy in the media (e.g., movies and TV), which is more dramatic fiction than accurate representation. Then, there are secondhand renditions you may get from friends and relatives who have been in psychotherapy; these provide a hodgepodge of biased and censored glimpses from a very limited sample of clients' experiences. Finally, your knowledge of psychotherapy may come directly from your own experience in therapy, which provides an even narrower view from the perspective of only one client's experience.

The misleading and limited information provided by these sources may shape the picture of psychotherapy with which you start your study of the field. If so, your view of psychotherapy is likely to contain inaccuracies and will certainly be limited. See whether the answers to the following questions surprise you: If there are 32 flavors of Baskin-Robbins ice cream, how many kinds of psychotherapy are there? By one count, there are more than 400 (Gold, 1996). And what do all of them have in common? Actually, just one element: a client. What about a therapist, you may ask? Although most forms of psychotherapy (including the major ones covered in this book) require the presence of a therapist, a few do not. *Bibliotherapy* consists of reading about how to deal with one's problems (e.g., Joshua & DiMenna, 2000). Clients can receive *cybercounseling* that consists of a client's online sessions in which the questions posed to the client and the responses to the client's answers are computer generated (e.g., American Counseling Association, 1999; Bloom & Walz, 2000, 2004). True, these examples of therapist-free counseling are not mainstream interventions. Most psychotherapies involve a therapist and a client. However, in a number of therapies, clients engage in therapeutic tasks outside counseling sessions on their own without direct therapist assistance. In some therapy arrangements, the number of therapists can vary. A single client could have co-therapists or even a team of therapists. And of course, there can be more than one client, as in couple therapy, family therapy, and group therapy. Considering the number of clients and therapists possible, you can already see variety in psychotherapies, and these two variables are just the tip of the iceberg.

Let's look at some of the important variables that all therapies have in common and the ways in which therapies differ with regard to each variable. Although each variable is discussed independently of the others, many of them overlap and are interdependent.

Theoretical Foundation

Every psychotherapeutic *approach* discussed in this book has two components: *theory* and *practice*. Thus far, our discussion has focused on the practice of psychotherapy (i.e., what goes on in psychotherapy to address the problems clients bring to therapy). The practice component of each approach is derived from, or is at least an extension of, an underlying theory. Each theory, or *theoretical orientation*, offers a broad conception of human nature or personality and, more specifically, a perspective on psychological disorders—their nature, their development, the factors that sustain them, and how they can be changed.

The most fundamental difference among psychotherapies is their theoretical orientation; indeed, the wide variety of theoretical approaches is a testament to the radically different ways in which the same human behaviors can be conceptualized. It is as if the theorists came from different worlds, each having its own unique view of human behavior. Of course, there is overlap among theories. But each theory has some, and often many, unique concepts that, in turn, make for unique approaches to psychotherapy.

Purpose or Goal

Although helping clients with the psychological problems for which they seek counseling is the most common purpose, or goal, of counseling, it is not the only one.

Many counselors believe that clients need not have particular psychological problems that are affecting their lives to be in counseling. They consider personal growth and gaining self-knowledge to be legitimate goals for counseling. Advocates of this position think that all people can benefit from psychotherapy because therapy can enhance their strengths and allow them to live more productive and fulfilled lives. Counseling for personal growth would be analogous to consulting a physical trainer in order to remain physically healthy.

A related goal of counseling is specific to counselors in training. Learning more about yourself through counseling, including your strengths and weaknesses, can contribute to personal growth, which will make you better able to deal with your clients' problems. It also may facilitate your ability to separate your own psychological issues from those of your clients. Further, being in counseling yourself gives you firsthand knowledge of the counseling process; not only are you observing the therapist's role and various therapeutic techniques, but you are also learning what it is like to be a client. Some counseling programs require and many recommend that students engage in personal counseling as part of their training to be counselors (cf. Yalom, 2003). And traditional training in psychoanalytic therapy requires that students be in psychoanalysis themselves for an extended period, often several years.

Not all counselors consider personal growth an appropriate goal of counseling. Critics of this goal argue that personal growth and self-knowledge can come about in many other ways, and they consider counseling solely for personal growth to be a luxury. The practice becomes especially egregious when such service deprives people who are in psychological distress from obtaining counseling, an issue that arises when demand for counseling exceeds the availability of counselors. Those who oppose personal growth counseling also believe that personal experience with therapy is not necessary for doing effective counseling (e.g., Macaskill, 1999; Wampler & Strupp, 1976; Wheeler, 1991).

Another aim of counseling is to *prevent*, rather than ameliorate, psychological problems. *Primary prevention* keeps a problem from occurring in the first place (e.g., when a client is taught stress management skills to deal with stress-inducing events that could potentially occur in the future). More often, therapy provides *secondary prevention* that involves early treatment of a problem to keep it from becoming more serious (e.g., interventions that treat a client's substance abuse before the client's drug-related behaviors become substance dependence, which is a more serious disorder). And occasionally, therapy may involve *tertiary prevention*, where the goal is to minimize the long-term effects of a problem (e.g., helping a client who is recovering from dependence on crack cocaine to maintain a job and sustain a family relationship). School counselors often provide individual and group (sometimes schoolwide) prevention interventions and programs for students.

Change Strategy

Approaches to counseling differ in the change strategies they employ, and these strategies are based on the therapy's theory of how change comes about. The five most common strategies are developing insight; increasing awareness; changing cognitions; engaging in adaptive behaviors; and creating systemic change. Each of the approaches to counseling you will be reading about is most closely associated with one of these change strategies, and some approaches employ more than one strategy. However, hypothetically it is possible to construe change that occurs with any counseling approach in terms of any of the six change strategies (and, if you engage in this exercise, you'll increase your understanding of the complexities and nuances of each of the approaches).

Developing Insight

The most frequently employed change strategy is to assist clients in gaining insight (clear understanding) about their problems, such as about the origins of their problems, how their problems developed, and the personal meaning of the problems. Insight in counseling requires both intellectual and emotional understanding. Colloquially, this might mean that a client realizes, "Yes, this explanation of my problems *makes sense*" (intellectual insight), and "This explanation *feels right* to me—it fits for me" (emotional insight). Clients generally gain intellectual insight before emotional insight. But only when emotional insight is also present can clients assimilate and make use of what they have discovered intellectually about their problems and themselves. Insight is critical in such therapies as psychoanalytic therapy (Chapter 3), Adlerian therapy (Chapter 4), existential therapy (Chapter 5), and person-centered therapy (Chapter 6).

Increasing Awareness

Increasing clients' awareness is a major strategy for change in some psychotherapies, most prominently in Gestalt therapy (Chapter 7). This can mean awareness of internal processes (e.g., thoughts, feelings), overt actions and their consequences, the external environment (including people in their lives), and the realities of life (e.g., we are mortal). Increased awareness introduces people to choices and alternatives and, at the same time, may disrupt their level of contentment with a life based on the belief that ignorance (lack of awareness) is bliss.

Changing Cognitions

Many therapies achieve their goals by focusing on clients' cognitions—thoughts, beliefs, attitudes, and broad worldviews—and replacing the maladaptive cognitions that are causing or exacerbating their problems with adaptive cognitions. This change strategy is most closely associated with cognitive-behavioral therapies (Chapter 9). For instance, a client who frequently has self-critical thoughts could be taught to substitute self-praise for self-criticism. On a broader level, narrative therapy (Chapter 13) involves replacing the familial and cultural stories that shape people's lives with alternative stories that better fit the intentions clients have for their own lives.

Engaging in Adaptive Behaviors

The goals of counseling can be achieved by having clients learn and practice new adaptive behaviors to replace their habitual, maladaptive behaviors, a change strategy that is key in traditional behavior therapy (Chapter 8). In cognitive-behavioral coping skills therapies (Chapter 9), clients develop specific coping skills to deal with their problems. Generally, standard coping skills are employed (e.g., muscle relaxation to help deal with stressors in everyday life). Sometimes, however, the coping skills are specially developed for a client with particular needs or characteristics, such as praying daily as a way of alleviating excessive worry for a religiously devout client.

In reality therapy (Chapter 10), clients learn to accept responsibility for their behaviors and for the consequences of their behaviors. This involves taking control of what they *can* control—that is, their own behaviors—and modifying it to more effectively achieve what they want and need in spite of difficult external conditions or events. For example, a married man who complains that his wife is unreceptive to his sexual advances would be asked to consider that perhaps the behaviors he thinks of as "sexual advances" may not be taken as such by his wife.

Creating Systemic Change

On a broader scale than individual change, it also is possible to change the social systems that impact clients. The system changed may involve only two people, as in couple therapy. The system is broader when the interactions of a number of people are dealt with in family therapy (Chapter 12). And in its broadest scale, the system can be sociopolitical, and one of the key goals of therapy may be to engage clients in societal and political change, which is the case in feminist therapy (Chapter 11).

Internal versus External Factors

Psychotherapies differ in their emphasis on *internal* (intrapsychic) and *external* factors, both as contributing to clients' problems and as the focus of therapy. Internal factors may be conscious or unconscious. For example, whereas traditional psychoanalysis focuses on clients' unconscious desires, reality therapy focuses on clients' conscious desires. External factors include clients' environmental (e.g., where they live) and interpersonal (e.g., their social interactions) contexts that influence their lives. For instance, traditional behavior therapy emphasizes environmental factors, and family therapy emphasizes interpersonal factors.

Process: What Goes On in Counseling

What transpires in counseling varies widely with the type of therapy. One way to describe the process is by defining the roles played by the therapist and by the client and how the therapist and client interact. As you will learn, client and therapist roles differ in each counseling approach.

The relationship that develops between the client and therapist is a factor influencing the therapeutic process in all psychotherapies, but the salience of the client-therapist relationship varies among therapies. For example, in person-centered therapy, the client-therapist relationship is the essential element, and specific therapeutic techniques are less critical. In contrast, in behavior therapy, a good therapeutic relationship is seen as necessary but not sufficient; it is specific therapeutic techniques that are considered critical. Most other therapies fit somewhere between these two poles.

Therapies can be placed on a *verbal versus action* continuum. Most methods of counseling require some verbal interchange between the client and therapist, if only to convey information. However, at the verbal end of the continuum, some therapies, such as existential therapy, emphasize client-therapist "conversation" (talking about one's problems) as the modus operandi. At the action end of the continuum, other therapies, such as feminist therapy, stress the client's active engagement in therapeutic tasks (doing something about one's problems).

Therapies also can be placed on an *in-session versus in vivo* continuum that indicates the extent to which therapy occurs in designated sessions in a counselor's office (in-session) versus outside of therapy sessions in the client's everyday environment (in vivo, Latin for *in life*). In verbal therapies, the therapeutic process takes place in sessions, with the exception that clients may think about what was talked about in therapy between sessions. Action therapies involve a combination of in-session work (e.g., learning and practicing coping skills) and in vivo work (e.g., applying coping skills in everyday life).

Locus of Time

Therapies vary in terms of the time frame that is examined. Some consider the past to be of prime importance (e.g., psychoanalysis); some focus on the present (e.g., behavior therapy); and some include the future (e.g., existential therapy). And then there are therapies that emphasize what is being experienced in the moment between the client and therapist, the so-called *here and now* (e.g., Gestalt therapy).

Length of Therapy

Although the specific length of time a client spends in therapy is different for each client, the average length of treatment varies considerably among different psychotherapy approaches. Classical psychoanalysis can extend over several years (generally a minimum of 3 years and sometimes for a dozen or more years) with two to five sessions per week. Most other forms of long-term therapy are not as lengthy, but treatment can take more than a year. Short-term therapies typically require 3 to 9 months of treatment, although some are considerably shorter. Occasionally, clients in short-term therapies can be successfully treated in as few as five sessions, and every once in a while clients are treated in a single session. Although such single-session successes are impressive, they are very much the exception. (Single-session successes should be differentiated from the many single-session dropouts where people come for one session and do not return, although the problem for which they sought therapy remains.)

Short-term therapies may be *time limited* in that they involve a set number of sessions (clients are told the number of sessions at the beginning of therapy). The number of sessions is based on how long it typically takes to treat the specific psychological disorder the client has using the particular psychotherapy. Imposing a time limit may facilitate the counseling process, as both the client and the therapist know that they have just so much time to complete their work and thus cannot waste any of it. Often, the therapist and client will contract for a set number of sessions with the understanding that in the final session they will determine whether or not more sessions are needed.

Short-term therapy has become the norm in recent years because counselors must conform to the requirements of clients' health insurance carriers and managed care companies, which are most interested in cost-effective treatment.

Evaluation of Effectiveness

The bottom line for all therapies is whether they are effective in achieving their goals, whatever those goals are. Effectiveness can be evaluated on two levels. *Idiographic evaluation* concerns how successful treatment has been for a particular client. *Nomothetic evaluation* concerns how effective a particular therapy is for treating many different clients—that is, how effective the therapy is in treating a particular disorder or in general (across disorders). Nomothetic evaluation also is used to assess the relative effectiveness of therapies from different approaches and different specific therapeutic procedures within a particular approach.

There is great disparity in the ways that the effectiveness of therapy is evaluated in different approaches. To begin with, the definition of *effectiveness* differs considerably among therapy approaches. This in turn influences the methods used to evaluate effectiveness, which range from broad, subjective, qualitative assessment to specific, objective, quantitative assessment. Finally, therapists practicing in different counseling approaches vary a great deal in their belief in the importance of evaluation and the extent to which they actually evaluate the effectiveness of their therapy. The result is that a substantial body of evidence in the scientific literature supports the effectiveness of some therapy approaches, whereas very little evidence exists for others.

Present and Future Consumers of Counseling and Psychotherapy

Who are the clients who will be seeking your services as a counselor? The most recent U.S. Census Bureau projections are that the population of the United States will increase from 282.1 million in 2000 to 419.9 million in 2050, which is a 49% increase. However, the European-American population will only increase by 14.6 million, or 7%, which means that by 2050 European Americans will comprise only 50% of the U.S. population. Projections of the U.S. population growth for three ethnic minority groups compared with the growth for European Americans from 2000 to 2050 are shown in Table 1.1.

Table 1.1 Projected Growth of Four Populations (Latinos, Asian Americans, African Americans, and European Americans) in the United States.

Population	Size of the Population in 2000 (millions)	Projected Increase by 2050 (millions)	Projected Percentage Growth	Share of Total U.S. Population in 2000	Projected Share of Total U.S. Population in 2050
Latinos	35.6	67.0	188%	12.6%	24.4%
Asian Americans	10.7	23.0	213%	3.8%	8%
African Americans	35.7	26.0	71%	12.7%	14.6%
European Americans	197.0	14.6	7%	70%	50%

Source: U.S. Census Bureau News, March 18, 2004.

Some other demographic patterns are also worth noting. The elderly population in every state will grow 3.5 times faster than the general population, and by 2030 about 1 in 5 people will be 65 or older. The female population will continue to outnumber the male population and that numerical difference will rise slightly from 5.3 million more women in 2000 to 6.9 million more women in 2050.

Despite the projections about the ethnic demographic shifts in the general population, counseling is and will likely continue for many years to be conducted primarily by White therapists (Negy, 2000) because the proportion of "counselors of Color" is not likely to keep pace with the increasing proportion of diverse clients. To help prepare therapists to bridge this cultural gap, both the American Counseling Association (2002) and the American Psychological Association (2003a) have published a set of multicultural competencies that therapists should have, and these competencies are being taught in graduate counseling and psychology training programs.

Practicing Counseling and Psychotherapy in a Diverse World

Sue and Sue (2003) define *multicultural counseling/therapy* as

> both a helping role and process that uses modalities and defines goals consistent with the life experience and cultural values of clients; recognizes client identities to include individual, group, and universal dimensions; advocates the use of universal and culture-specific strategies and roles in the healing process; and balances the importance of individualism and collectivism in the assessment, diagnosis, and treatment of clients and client systems. (p. 6)

The multicultural movement in the fields of counseling and psychology emerged in the United States in the 1960s and 1970s. Lee and Ramirez (2000) point out that during that era, counselors took one of two stances with culturally diverse populations: either assuming a benevolent role as if helping the less fortunate or recognizing the salience of culture in the counseling process but not abandoning or modifying traditional psychotherapy paradigms to accommodate the role of culture. "The responsibility remained with the culturally different clients to adjust to the psychotherapy process, rather than therapists adjusting models to the needs of clients" (Lee & Ramirez, 2000, p. 280). In the last 30 years, however, the responsibility has shifted to therapists and therapies assuming the burden of adapting to meet the needs of diverse clients, and, as a consequence, multicultural counseling has gained momentum and influence.

As a counseling or psychotherapy student in training, you will be expected to choose a therapy approach and become culturally competent in the practice of that approach. In the context of counseling and psychotherapy—and as it is used in this book—the terms *cultural* and *multicultural* generally have a more inclusive meaning than national identity (e.g., Italian or Cape Verdian).[1] Rather, the terms typically include *diversity* in all its variations, including culture as well as ethnicity, race, age, gender, sexual orientation, socioeconomic status, educational level, religious and spiritual orientation, and physical ability.

Being culturally competent means that you understand and respect the worldviews of culturally diverse clients and develop appropriate intervention strategies and techniques consistent with your clients' cultural identities. To achieve cultural competence, you must become aware of *your own worldview—* that is, your assumptions, values, and biases—*as well as the assumptions, values, and biases of the counseling approach you are using.* Social scientists concerned with multicultural issues point to the fact that traditional psychological notions about human personality, psychological disorders, and change processes were based on the worldviews of the individuals who developed the theories— namely, European-American men who were primarily middle class, middle aged, heterosexual, and physically able. It is no wonder, they say, that the theories of psychotherapy that have been taught in graduate programs since the 1950s are largely irrelevant to minority clients. Sue and Sue (1990) believe that "traditional counseling theory and practice have done great harm to the culturally different" (p. v), and Hall (1997) has referred to traditional counseling practice as "cultural malpractice."

One of the persistent criticisms of traditional theories of counseling is that they assume a *culturally universal perspective* in which good counseling is good counseling, which is to say that sound counseling practice will work for anyone and need not vary in different cultural contexts. This implies that our historical and current counseling practices, conventional definitions of mental health and psychological disorders, and traditional ethical standards are sufficiently applicable to all clients.

Cultural universality is challenged by many in the counseling profession who argue for the use of culture-specific strategies in counseling and psychotherapy (e.g., Herring, 1999; Locke, 1990; Parham, White, & Ajamu, 1999). This *culturally relative perspective* has led to the development of indigenous, or culture-specific, approaches to counseling.

We believe that there are valid aspects of both the culturally universal and culturally relative perspectives, so that "there is a need for models of psychotherapy that balance the benefits of both" (Lee & Ramirez, 2000, p. 286). But it takes time for new theoretical models to be developed and become accepted. In the meantime, future counseling and psychotherapy practitioners need to find that "balance" for themselves within the theories that inform the profession today.

---

[1] See, for example, Ivey, D'Andrea, Ivey, and Simek-Morgan's (2002) *RESPECTFUL* model of counseling and development and Sue and Sue's (2003) Tripartite Development of Human Identity.

The purpose of this book is to present the prominent theories of counseling and to demonstrate how each theory can be applied effectively and sensitively to a wide range of clients, majority and nonmajority. All of our contributors are not only experts in their orientations, but they also share our vision that the traditional theories in counseling and psychotherapy can be adapted to meet the needs of diverse clients. In fact, some of them are actively practicing an adapted version of their primary orientation. For example, Neil Altman, the author of Chapter 3 on psychoanalytic therapy, has for the past 20 years successfully practiced an adapted version of the oldest and most traditional counseling approach in an ethnically diverse and impoverished neighborhood in New York City.

Choosing the Approach You Will Practice

We encourage students preparing for a career in counseling to choose one approach to counseling that they will use. There are 11 major approaches covered in this book. This may raise two questions in your mind. First, how will I know which is the best approach? The answer is that, in general, there is no best approach; many different kinds of psychotherapy are practiced, each with particular strengths as well as limitations. However, there may be a best therapeutic approach *for you*, or at least several optimal approaches for you, and we'll have more to say about that shortly. Second, how will I go about choosing an approach? This choice may seem like a daunting task given that there are many approaches from which to choose, and the approaches appear so different from one another. In fact, the way in which counselors end up adopting a particular approach is probably simpler than you might think. Choosing one's counseling approach is based on two factors: *exposure* and *personal fit*.

Choosing Based on Exposure

In order to make a choice, you first must learn what you have to choose from, which means exposing yourself to a variety of therapy approaches. One of the goals of this book is to begin that exposure process by introducing you to 11 different theoretical approaches used in counseling and psychotherapy. These are not the only approaches, but they are among the most popular or most frequently employed and are a representative sample of the types of therapies that are available to you. Further, five of the approaches presented in the book (psychoanalytic therapy, traditional behavior therapy, cognitive-behavioral therapy, feminist therapy, and family therapy) are broad approaches, with a number of specific subapproaches that are subsumed under each. Accordingly, you will actually be exposed to more than 11 approaches.

Choosing Based on Personal Fit

As you learn about various approaches through reading assignments and associated coursework, you will find yourself particularly drawn to some approaches and turned off by others. For example, you may find yourself thinking, "Of course," "That makes sense," and "That's right" for some approaches and "You've got to be kidding!" "That makes no sense," and "No; that's wrong" for others. This is a good thing because you can use these spontaneous reactions, both positive and negative, as indications of your personal comfort level or fit with each therapy. Your comfort level with a counseling approach is based on your personality characteristics, personal preferences, attitudes, beliefs, values, tastes, and biases. How comfortable you feel with a therapy's basic assumptions and perspective (worldview) and the way the therapy works with clients is a valid measure of the therapy's fit for you. Additionally, your personal belief in the validity or "rightness" of the approach you choose is critical for your ability to practice therapy with confidence as well as to instill confidence in your clients that the therapy will help them.

Given that you are evaluating an approach you will use to help people in distress and not a friend's new shoes or a song you just heard for the first time, it might seem more prudent to rely on a methodical, intellectual evaluation of various approaches. For instance, you could generate a list of pros and cons for each counseling approach that you have been exposed to, in which case the approach you choose to practice would be the one that had the most pluses and the fewest minuses. Such a cerebral exercise is no doubt useful in some ways. However, your most accurate barometer of fit resides in your midsection rather than above your shoulders. And if you think that exposure and personal fit or comfort level are too subjective for choosing something as important as your professional orientation, consider that the same criteria are used to make most of the major decisions in our lives, including selecting a mate and buying a house.

Learning More Before You Choose

Reading the chapters in this book can give you only a taste of each of the major therapies. To really appreciate their nature and practice, you'll need to learn more about the approaches that are appealing or that you are curious about (see the Resources for Further Study at the end of each chapter for good places to start). Next, you should talk to counselors who practice different therapies about their approaches and the factors that influenced their choice. To get you started in this process, in sections called "The Author's Journey as a _____ Therapist," you will read about how the chapter authors came to adopt their therapeutic approaches. Another way to expose yourself to various approaches is to attend workshops on different therapies. Not only will you learn about the approach from the presenters, but you'll also have an opportunity to meet and talk to professionals who use the approach. Once you have sufficient information about and feel for a particular approach that seems to fit well for you, the next step is to get formal training and supervised practice in doing the therapy. Only then will you know that you have found a good therapeutic home.

In your process of choosing an approach to counseling, bear in mind that your initial choice is not set in stone. If, as you use the approach in your counseling, you find that it is not working for you, you certainly can change your approach. In fact, in the stories of their individual journeys, you will see that a number of the chapter authors changed their orientations at some point in their careers.

Adopting More Than One Approach

All we have said about choosing a counseling approach is predicated on your initially selecting a single approach. Indeed, a majority of therapists subscribe to a single theoretical approach and employ therapeutic techniques that are derived from it (Norcross, 2005). However, a substantial minority of counselors adopt more than one approach (Norcross, 2005). This practice is known as *eclecticism*, which involves drawing on theory *(theoretical eclecticism)* or techniques *(technical eclecticism)* from multiple approaches to treat clients. The practice of eclecticism is controversial, but for the purposes of our discussion about beginning counselors choosing a counseling approach, two limitations of eclecticism are especially germane.

First, eclecticism requires being trained and becoming competent in more than one approach. Developing competence in an approach requires considerable time and effort, as well as focused concentration. Accordingly, it is both unrealistic and ill advised for beginning counselors to learn more than one approach at the same time.

Second, to practice eclectically, a therapist must have an overarching or superordinate theory that provides guidelines for making decisions about which approach or unique combination of approaches to use with a particular client. Otherwise, the practice of eclecticism becomes a haphazard, seat-of-the-pants endeavor, which is neither sound nor ethical practice (Lazarus, 1996; Lazarus, Beutler, & Norcross, 1992). Developing a unique overriding theory that encompasses multiple approaches requires extensive experience in practicing psychotherapy, which, of course, new counselors do not have.

Because of both limitations, we believe that you as a new counselor would be better served by adopting a single approach that fits well for you. If, after gaining experience in counseling with a single approach, you decide to seek training in another approach, you will be on firmer ground to do so.

In recent years, a number of therapists have been working on *integrating* divergent counseling approaches (e.g., Gold, 1996; Norcross & Goldfried, 2005; Striker & Gold, 1993). Psychotherapy integration involves identifying the common elements in different approaches to psychotherapy and developing formal theoretical integrations (which is different from individual counselors creating *unique* overarching theories, as may occur in eclecticism).[2] In 1983, the Society for Exploration of Psychotherapy Integration was formed as an international organization. The society's founders prudently chose the words *exploration of* to indicate that psychotherapy integration is a possibility rather than something that exists or that we are certain can occur. What makes psychotherapy integration difficult is the divergent perspectives many approaches have, in terms of both their theories and their techniques of change (Lazarus, 1995). And to be candid, integration also is impeded by political battles among psychotherapists of differing approaches who all believe that their approach is "right."

Another obstacle in the path of formal psychotherapy integration is the lack of a common language among psychotherapists of different orientations. With each theoretical approach having its own terminology, sometimes it is difficult for psychotherapists from different approaches to communicate clearly with one another. Moreover, confusion is created because many terms have multiple meanings. In an effort to overcome these barriers to psychotherapy integration, a dictionary called the *Common Language of Psychotherapy Procedures* is being created by an international task force of therapists representing many approaches (Marks et al., 2005). The entries for each term will (1) focus on what therapists actually do with clients in their practices, (2) include brief illustrations with actual clients, (3) provide cross-references with similar and contrasting procedures, and (4) cite the first known use of the procedure.

What You Can Expect in the Remainder of This Book

The organization of this book is straightforward. In Chapter 2, you will read about general ethical issues in psychotherapy and ethical issues that are specific to therapy provided for diverse clients. Following that are chapters on 11 of the major contemporary approaches to counseling and psychotherapy. Each of these chapters is written by one or two authors, each of whom is a respected expert in and proponent of the approach. Thus, you will be learning about each approach from the horse's mouth, so to speak. These chapters differ in their content, of

---

[2] Despite the differences between the terms *eclecticism* and *integration* (with respect to psychotherapy), therapists use the terms interchangeably. Of the two, *integration* is the more prevalent term (Norcross, Karpiak, & Lister, 2005).

course. There also are differences, some obvious and others subtle, in how the authors write about their approach to psychotherapy. Each author's choice of words and style of expression will give you a sense of how therapists of differing theoretical orientations think and talk about their practice. The approaches are presented in roughly the chronological order in which they were developed, beginning with the earliest, so that reading them in order will give you a sense of the evolution of contemporary psychotherapy. However, the chapters are for the most part independent of one another, so they can be read in any order.

To help you compare and contrast the 11 approaches, Chapters 3–13 are organized in similar ways. Each chapter begins with an overview of the chapter followed by a description of how the approach began and how it has evolved. The author then describes what led him or her to adopt the approach and how her or his practice of the approach has evolved. Next, the author presents the theoretical foundations of the approach, followed by a discussion of how the theory is manifested in practice. The chapter concludes with three sections that assess the current status and future directions of the approach: an evaluation of the evidence validating the approach; a candid appraisal of the approach's blind spots, limitations, and challenges; and the author's commentary on the future development of the approach in a diverse world. These last sections balance the fact that each author is, not surprisingly, an enthusiastic supporter of her or his approach and thus has emphasized its strengths.

Keep in mind, however, that all counseling approaches hone in on aspects of clients and their problems deemed essential by the approach and pay less or even no attention to aspects considered nonessential. They also use particular change strategies and eschew others. Thus, all approaches have their blind spots as well as limitations, which result in challenges. At the end of each theory chapter are a summary, an alphabetized list of the key terms related to the approach (which appeared in boldface type when they were defined in the chapter), and suggested resources and readings for learning more about the approach. At the end of the book, you will find a glossary of all the key terms and a list of the sources cited in the chapters.

When you read any material, it helps to have a purpose to guide your reading and thinking. One purpose of this book is to introduce you to the major contemporary approaches to counseling and psychotherapy as they are used to treat diverse clients. Another purpose is to help you choose your own approach to counseling. Whatever your purpose in reading the book, we hope that your exploration of the fascinating and increasingly diverse world of psychotherapy is worthwhile and stimulating and that it sparks your interest to continue your journey for many years to come.

Chapter 2

Ethics for a Diverse World

Melba J. T. Vasquez

E thics is a very interesting and complex area of professional responsibility. Counseling and psychotherapy are unique and intimate processes. Regardless of theoretical orientation, there exists a power differential, so the risk of exploitation is present. Professional ethics have thus evolved to protect clients, as well as the professional, by informing us of the risks. The American Psychological Association's Ethical Principles of Psychologists and Code of Conduct (APA, 2002) and the American Counseling Association's Code of Ethics (ACA, 2005) both provide various principles and standards to inform us of professional expectations. When individuals make choices regarding the professional counselor or psychologist from whom they will seek services, it is important to know that these professionals are bound by professional ethics that they are obligated to follow.

Brief Overview of the APA and ACA Codes of Ethics

For the first 60 years of its existence, the American Psychological Association had no ethics code. The APA Ethics Committee was formed in 1938, 46 years after APA was founded (APA was founded in 1892, incorporated in 1925). A first, formal ethics code was adopted in 1953 and has been through several evolutions; the current code (2002) is the tenth version. The APA Ethics Committee is charged with reviewing the code every five years to determine the continued appropriateness of the principles and standards; the assumption is that the code is a living document. Attempts to define what it means to engage in "ethical psychological practice" encompass many empirical and theoretical perspectives and ideologies. In particular, the feminist multicultural perspective has had a strong influence on ethical practice, including psychotherapy, research, teaching, consulting, and forensic work, for approximately the last 35 years.

The General Principles of the APA (2002) Ethics Code are designed to be educative, and are aspirational. They are not sanctionable guidelines, but the intent is to guide and inspire psychotherapists toward the very highest ethical ideals of the profession. The General Principles include Principle A: Beneficence and Nonmaleficence, Principle B: Fidelity and Responsibility, Principle C: Integrity, Principle D: Justice, and Principle E: Respect for People's Rights and Dignity. The Ethical Standards, divided into ten sections, evolved from the more general moral principles. Unlike the General Principles, the Ethical Standards do represent obligations and form the basis for imposing sanctions.

The American Counseling Association first formed in 1952 as the National Vocational Guidance Association (NVGA). In 1992, the association changed its name to the American Counseling Association (ACA). The ACA Code of Ethics (2005) has eight sections, each of which begins with an aspirational introduction with regard to ethical behavior and responsibility. It also has an ethical decision-making process.

The ACA Code of Ethics is revised approximately every 10 years for the purpose of examining best practices in light of current issues faced by the profession. The 2005 revision was characterized by increased emphasis on multicultural and diversity issues. For example, the new section A.1.d. Support Network Involvement recognizes the importance of support networks in clients' lives and encourages counselors to consider enlisting family members, friends, and community and spiritual leaders as support resources when appropriate and with client consent. The section on diagnosis of mental disorders recognizes that culture affects the manner in which clients' problems are defined and that clients' socioeconomic and cultural experiences should be considered when diagnosing mental disorders.

Another change reflects a movement in the counseling and mental health professions away from a strict ban on dual or multiple relationships with clients. The 2005 ACA Code states that if a counselor believes that a nonprofessional interaction with a client may be beneficial for the client, the counselor should proceed, while taking care to document in case records (when feasible) the rationale for the interaction, the potential benefits, and anticipated consequences.

Finally, a completely new addition to the 2005 ethics code is Section A.9, which stresses the importance of counselors gaining competence in working with terminally ill clients facing end-of-life issues. While it remains nonspecific about approaches to end-of-life care, ACA is one of the few national mental health–related organizations to address end-of-life care in its code of ethics.

The ethical codes of both the APA and the ACA recognize the importance of diversity and of supporting the worth and dignity of people in the context of their social and cultural environments. Both APA and ACA rely on Kitchener's moral principles (1984, 2000a) to serve as the cornerstone of their respective ethical standards. Those five moral principles are beneficence, nonmaleficence, fidelity, justice, and autonomy.

1. *Beneficence* means that professional counselors and psychotherapists strive to benefit those with whom they work.

2. *Nonmaleficence* means that they take care to do no harm, including inflicting intentional harm and engaging in actions that risk harming others. It is our responsibility to have knowledge about what behaviors have potential for harm. We are urged to safeguard the welfare and rights of those with whom we interact professionally. When conflicts occur among our obligations or concerns, we are encouraged to attempt to resolve these conflicts in a responsible fashion that avoids or minimizes harm. Because our judgments and actions may affect the lives of others, we have to be alert to and guard against personal, financial, social, organizational, or political factors that might lead to misuse of our influence. We are encouraged to strive to be aware of the possible effect of our own physical and mental health on our ability to help those with whom we work.

3. *Fidelity* involves questions of faithfulness, loyalty, and promise keeping. These are issues basic to trust, and fidelity is especially vital to all human relationships, especially the therapist-client relationship. This relationship is dependent on honest communication and the assumption that the contract on which the relationship was initiated obliges both parties to fulfill certain functions.

4. *Justice* in its broadest sense means fairness: dealing with others as one would like to be dealt with oneself, behaving towards others in an impartial manner, and treating others equally. Issues of justice arise because there are conflicts of interest in society over limited goods and services and because human benevolence is limited. So we evolved, in our society, the principle of fairness.

5. *Autonomy* involves the concept that the autonomous person has the responsibility for his or her own behavior, freedom of choice, and making a decision and is at liberty to choose her or his own course of action. It implies a freedom to do what one wants to do, as long as it does not interfere with similar freedoms of others. Professional counselors and psychotherapists respect the dignity and worth of all people, and the rights of individuals to privacy, confidentiality, and self-determination. The concepts of unconditional worth and tolerance for individual differences both imply a respect for clients' rights to make their own decisions. Mutual respect, a basic element of the therapeutic bond for many of us, implies a relationship between autonomous individuals.

Two key imperatives stem from the principle of autonomy. The first is confidentiality. Revered in our profession as a cornerstone to trust in the relationship, *confidentiality* stems from the principle of autonomy and respect for people's rights and dignity. Confidentiality is about the client's right to privacy. It means that the information a client shares with a counselor stays with the counselor unless the client gives permission to release it. Before releasing any client information to others, counselors must first obtain the client's written permission. The ethics codes of both ACA and APA do set certain limits on confidentiality. For example, counselors are ethically and legally obligated to break confidentiality when clients threaten to harm themselves or others.

The second key imperative is *informed consent*, the notion that clients must consent to treatment and be informed of the implications of that consent. This concept also stems from the general principle of autonomy and respect for people's rights and dignity. According to the ACA Code of Ethics (2005), informed consent must occur at the beginning of the counseling relationship. The APA Ethics Code also requires that psychologists obtain informed consent to therapy as early as is feasible in the therapeutic relationship. It includes explaining to the client your treatment approach and any techniques that you may use and your fee and payment requirements. Clients also have the right to receive a clear explanation of their confidentiality rights and to be warned in advance of the limits to confidentiality. Providing sufficient opportunity for the client to ask questions and receive answers is also important.

We are urged to be aware that special safeguards may be necessary to protect the rights and welfare of persons or communities whose vulnerabilities impair autonomous decision making. We must be aware of and respect cultural, individual, and role differences, including those based on age, gender, gender identity, race, ethnicity, culture, national origin, religion, sexual orientation, physical and mental ability, language, and socioeconomic status, and we have to consider these factors when working with members of such groups. We are urged to eliminate the effect on our work of biases based on those factors, and to not knowingly participate in or condone activities of others based upon such prejudices.

Based on these five moral principles, upon which both the APA's General Principles and ACA's aspirational guidelines are derived, clients can expect their counselor or psychotherapist to inform them of the purposes, goals, techniques, procedures, limitations, potential risks, and benefits of all counseling services that they receive. Clients will also be informed about confidentiality and privacy, as well as limits to confidentiality. Financial arrangements related to service are also discussed. All of this information is usually provided in writing and the written statement also includes the therapist's qualifications and specific areas of expertise.

Feminist Multicultural Ethics

Feminist ethics draws from feminist theory to apply lenses to view and analyze dilemmas in various areas of counseling and psychotherapy. Feminist ethics has influenced our profession at least since the early 1970s (Brabeck & Ting, 2000; Brown, 2003). Feminist ethics of professional practice present a mandate for moral action that empowers individuals, creates just social structures, and ensures that all people are attentively cared for to nurture and develop each person's potential within the contexts in which they live.

The multicultural perspective similarly encourages scholars and practitioners to understand racial and ethnic differences and the experiences in society of particular groups of people (Pack-Brown & Williams, 2003; Vasquez, 2005). The APA Guidelines on Multicultural Education, Training, Research, Practice, and Organizational Change for Psychologists (APA, 2003a) that were endorsed as policy of the American Psychological Association by the Council of Representatives were developed over a nearly 40-year period (Constantine & Sue, 2005). The first two of the six multicultural guidelines inform the other four guidelines and encourage psychotherapists to recognize that they may hold attitudes and beliefs that can detrimentally influence their perceptions of and interactions with individuals different from themselves, and to recognize the importance of knowledge and understanding about ethnically and racially different individuals. How have feminist and multicultural ideologies influenced the evolution of the ethics code and ethical practice?

Brown (2003) suggested that the 2002 APA Ethical Principles and Code of Conduct (hereinafter referred to as the APA Ethics Code) principles and standards have become more explicit about some matters of concern to feminists. For instance, *self care,* first articulated as an ethical responsibility by feminists such as Noddings (1984) and Gilligan (1982) is explicitly articulated in the last sentence of General Principle A, Beneficence and Nonmaleficence: "Psychotherapists strive to be aware of the possible effects of their own physical and mental health on their ability to help those with whom they work" (2002, p. 1062). Most of the standards in Section 3, Human Relations, which address discrimination, sexual harassment and other harassment, multiple relationships, and exploitative relationships, have been influenced by feminist multicultural ideologies. Section 7, Education and Training, includes standards that forbid sexual exploitation of students, encourage respect when students disclose personal information, and emphasize the importance of providing informed consent in a program that requires mandatory therapy. Students are also influenced by feminist multicultural tenets that appeal to the importance of respect for clients, including trainees.

The ACA Code of Ethics (2005) also incorporated more emphasis on multicultural and diversity issues facing counseling professionals. In many ways, mainstream ethics has grown closer to feminist and multicultural ethics, and feminist multicultural practitioners should experience less, not more, dissonance when attempting to practice in the context of both. However, in some ways, feminist multicultural ethics diverge from some of the more rigid risk management strategies, according to Brown (2003), Nelson (1993), and others. Risk management strategies are those precautions issued by professional liability insurance companies, based on their views of risky behaviors that can potentially lead to ethical violations, resulting in complaints and lawsuits. For example, a risk management strategy would suggest that a professional never become involved in dual or multiple relationships with clients. Both the APA 2002 Ethics Code and the ACA 2005 Code of Ethics reflect a paradigm shift in recognizing that not all dual or multiple relationships should be avoided or viewed as harmful. However, feminist/multicultural ethicists tend to address the gray areas in professional ethics more directly. Before discussing those diversions, a review of key feminist and multicultural themes and principles that inform ethical practice will help illustrate key points.

The Author's Journey as a Feminist Multicultural Ethicist

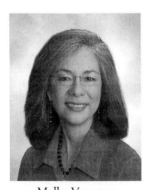

Melba Vasquez

My early experiences as a Latina influenced my interest and affiliation as a multicultural feminist. I grew up in a small central Texas town during the 1950s, and observed and experienced discrimination and sexism before I could articulate the events and describe the consequential feelings and effects. On one hand, I was a firstborn, with the privilege of a considerable amount of attention and regard from parents and a large extended family. The first five or six years of my life were relatively safe; in retrospect, I grew up in a small college community that was socially segregated. I had no substantive contact with the White European community until I entered first grade in the public school system.

However, once I entered public school, the subtle and not so subtle negative attitudes in the schools I attended were clear. We were ignored, spoken to more curtly and harshly than the White children, and some of the children of color (mostly boys, as I recall) were treated harshly (e.g., knocked down on the playground), and insulted with racial epithets. In short, we were treated with significant amounts of disdain and contempt. I remember feeling an immediate identification with and protection from those like me. I remember feeling the

(*continued*)

pain of loss of positive regard at both a personal and group level, but I had no words to describe the loss and sadness and lack of safety and resulting anxiety that emerged. My world—and that of others like me—had become unsafe and harsh. I was frightened and confused about who I was, and about my values, for years.

However, my parents, neither of whom had graduated from high school, were nonetheless self-educated and both activists in our community. They were advocates for civil rights. My mother in particularly was vocal in her challenge of ill treatment of others based on discrimination and was politically active as well. She was a pioneer in that she was the first Latina elected to the school board in the community and has remained active all her life.

These experiences clearly influenced my motivation to understand human behavior, especially in regard to the causes, effects, and cures of bias and discrimination. My parents' role modeling that taking action makes a difference has also shaped my proactive involvement as well. My professional involvement, advocacy, and scholarly interests gravitated toward ethnic minority and feminist issues. My parents' quest for fairness very likely shaped my interest in ethics and moral development.

Thus, my early interest in ethics was actually because of my interest in psychology of women and ethnic minority psychology. In my practice, I began to see women who had been sexually exploited by previous therapists. I became concerned and interested in this ethical violation and began to present relevant papers at conferences and to publish on the topic. In addition, I was interested in the issues relevant to the treatment of ethnic minorities in the psychological literature and research, in education, and in psychotherapy practice. I soon realized that ethical behavior required the development of unique competencies in those applications of psychology. In other words, researchers, educators, and practitioners needed particular knowledge, skills, and attitudes to apply their work competently to ethnic minority populations. It was important to me that our ethics codes reflected these requirements.

In the mid-1980s, I was nominated to run for the American Psychological Association's Ethics Committee. The members of that committee are elected for three-year terms by the APA Council of Representatives. I was elected and served the same three-year term as Ken Pope, 1986–1989. He and I discovered that we were fairly likeminded in our approach to ethics in psychology and decided to write a book, *Ethics in Counseling and Psychotherapy: A Practical Guide* (first edition 1991, second edition 1998, third edition in press, Jossey-Bass/Wiley, publishers). Karen Kitchener was chair of the Ethics Committee during one year of my term, and I came to greatly admire her work, including her application of the bioethical moral principles to psychology, upon which the General Principles of the 2002 Ethical Principles of Psychologists and Code of Conduct are based.

I was appointed to serve on the APA Ethics Committee Task Force to revise both the 1981 Ethics Code (produced as the 1992 Ethical Principles of Psychologists and Code of Conduct) and the 1992 Ethics Code (produced as the 2002 Ethical Principles of Psychologists and Code of Conduct). I frequently provide workshops and training in professional ethics at various meetings and conferences around the country.

Ongoing involvement in ethnic minority and feminist professional activities has continued to inspire my work. In addition, writing with others, serving on relevant journal editorial boards, attending relevant conferences, and involvement in various professional activities have been valuable experiences. I was a co-founder, for example, of the APA Division 45, Society for the Psychological Study of Ethnic Minority Issues, as well as of the original National Multicultural Conference and Summit (with Rosie Bingham, Derald Wing Sue, and Lisa Porche-Burke), which is now held every two years. I have attended various feminist conferences, such as the National Conference on Education and Training in Feminist Practice in Boston in 1993, and have been active in APA Division 35, the Society for the Psychology of Women. I served as president of that division in 1998–1999, and on the APA Committee of Women in Psychology as well.

All of these experiences have inspired the evolution of my thinking and my assumptions as an ethicist in general, especially as a feminist multicultural ethicist.

Review of Ethical Feminist Multicultural Themes and Principles

Themes reflected in the philosophy and assumptions of ethical feminist multicultural therapy include the importance of sociopolitical context, empowerment of clients, social justice, validation of the experience of women and people of color and other diverse groups, the ethic of care, and mutuality and genuineness in the psychotherapeutic relationship. Several basic tenets of feminist theory of psychological practice were developed from the National Conference on Education and Training in Feminist Practice held at Boston College on July 8–11, 1993 (Brabeck & Ting, 2000).

Sociopolitical Context

Brabeck and Ting discuss the fact that women's experiences and subjectivities are constructed within a patriarchy (Brabeck & Ting, 2000). This means that it is ethically imperative to make people aware of how dominance subordinates others. Thus, it is important that the practitioner of feminist ethics engages in analysis of the context and of the power dynamics inherent in that context (Brabeck & Ting). It is critical to assess the way in which the patriarchal society that privileges male insights, experiences, and beliefs has affected the experiences of each client, each consultee, our research participants, and students. For example, one of the most significant differences between ethical feminist psychotherapy and traditional therapies is that feminists not only assess the individual and his or her family history but also examine the overlay of context of the individual's societal experience.

Likewise, the Multicultural Guidelines (APA, 2003a) encourage knowledge of cultural influences on worldview orientations that inform psychotherapists' understanding of how their norms and values may contrast with those of clients who are different from them, and to understand the risks in imposing unconscious biases in their interactions based on societal categorizations. The social construction of gender, ethnicity, social class, and sexual orientation results in insidious internalization of values, role restrictions, and expectations of selves and others. Awareness of these is critical in conducting ethical psychological practice.

In addition to the Guidelines on Multicultural Education, Training, Research, Practice and Organizational Change for Psychologists (APA, 2003a), a variety of aspirational guidelines that recognize the unique sociopolitical experience of marginalized populations have been developed and endorsed by APA as policy. The multicultural guidelines were preceded by the APA Guidelines for Providers of Psychological Services to Ethnic, Linguistic, and Culturally Diverse Populations in 1993. The APA Guidelines for Psychotherapy with Lesbian, Gay, and Bisexual Clients were published in 2000; the Guidelines for Psychological Practice with Older Adults (APA, 2003b) were published in 2003. The Guidelines on Psychotherapy with Women and Girls are in the process of being revised; they were previously produced by a task force of Division 17 but have not yet been endorsed by the entire organization.

Empowerment of Clients

Related to the importance of assessing the effects of patriarchy is the importance of empowering those with whom we work. Most feminist approaches deal with *empowerment* of women and other members of marginalized groups, and some approaches, such as postmodernism, offer feminists' strategies for analyzing power and methods for deconstructing how the role of women has been constructed within the patriarchal society.

Empowerment is considered by many feminists to be an ethical imperative in feminist therapy. Smith and Douglas (1990), for example, propose that empowering women clients involves promoting a feeling of strength and control centered in an individual, as well as promoting skills to engage in societal interactions in a healthy, fulfilling manner. Feminist theory tries to break the silencing of women's voices (Worell & Johnson, 1997).

Kitchener (2000a) discussed how feminist psychology educators are faced with a variety of ethical tensions in their work with students. For example, she points out the tension between not abdicating power and wanting to empower students as well as that between the responsibility to facilitate the development of students and to protect the public from incompetent psychotherapists. Mentoring relationships are one way to facilitate the development of students, yet those relationships often place students and faculty members in overlapping roles. There are opportunities for misunderstanding and exploitation, and feminist faculty must be attentive to those potential risks.

Multicultural Guidelines 3, 4, 5, and 6 encourage psychotherapists to promote multiculturalism in education and training, in research, in practice, and in organizational change as a way of empowering those with whom they work. Support for multiculturalism and diversity in all those psychological activities can help promote affirmation and value of the role of ethnicity and race in developing personal identity.

Social Justice

Feminist ethics is also concerned with achieving *social justice* (Brabeck & Ting, 2000). An ethical person takes action to achieve equity for marginalized persons within existing political, social, and economic structures. Most feminist philosophies propose that feminist awareness must include a stance against the patriarchal status quo, given that "feminine" is a construction within a system in which women are dominated by men. Therefore, one's personal experiences are ultimately a road to political change—thus the often quoted "the personal is political" (Brabeck & Ting, p. 30). McIntyre (2000) described how the underlying tenets of feminism and feminist ethics include the responsibility of becoming and remaining conscious of racism, classism, ageism, anti-Semitism, homophobia, ableism, and other forms of oppression. In addition, feminists have a responsibility to take action on problematic policies and practices that maintain oppression in various institutions and organizations.

The APA (2003a) Multicultural Guideline 6 encourages psychotherapists to use organizational change to support culturally informed organizational policy development and practices. Psychotherapists are encouraged to participate in local, state, and national legislative efforts devoted to promoting equality. Social justice is thus viewed as an important ethical responsibility.

The APA (2002) Ethics Code strengthens the protections of groups that have been historically disenfranchised—for example, 2.01, Boundaries of Competence (b); 9.02, Use of Assessments. Some criticize the code for being less socially responsible than previous codes. Concern about a litigious society has resulted in elimination of vague standards, or those that are not really enforceable, for example, the imperative to provide pro bono services. This is now in the aspirational General Principle B, Fidelity and Responsibility, "Psychotherapists strive to contribute a portion of their professional time for little or no compensation or personal advantage." The ACA 2005 Code of Ethics likewise included increased emphasis on multicultural and diversity issues. For example, E.5.b., Cultural Sensitivity, states that "Counselors recognize that culture affects the manner in which clients' problems are defined. Clients' socioeconomic and cultural experiences are considered when diagnosing mental disorders."

Carolyn Payton criticized the 1992 ethics code for not holding the personal behavior of the psychotherapist responsible to the Ethics Code. She asked, what of the psychotherapist who batters his wife and children? Pipes, Holstein, and Aguirre (2005) pointed out that psychotherapists may, when their professional role is not operative, engage in exploitative relationships and sexual and multiple relationships of their choosing; they may demean individuals of a particular gender or a particular religion with whom they interact only on a personal basis. If it is not illegal, a psychotherapist may own an apartment building and refuse to rent to individuals who are, for example, gay. They may break confidences, be abusive to their romantic partners, lie to their friends, evaluate others unfairly, and generally "act like a louse." Pipes et al. (2005) suggested that the APA ethical standards be applied to professional role behaviors and that the aspirational principles might be applied to personal behavior. This would be a change in the next reiteration of the APA Ethics Code, one that Carolyn Payton and other feminist multiculturalists may likely endorse.

Validation of the Experience of Women and People of Color

Another pervasive theme in ethical feminist multicultural practice has to do with the importance of validation of the experience of women, people of color, and others. Feminist multicultural theory and feminist multicultural practice affirm, attend to, and authorize the experiences of the oppressed in their own voices. A goal of feminist multicultural ethical psychotherapy is thus to believe and trust the reality of the client. It is important to believe and validate the oppression that women and people of color perceive and experience, as a step toward empowerment.

Ethic of Care

Noddings (1984) and Gilligan (1982) proposed that being ethical leads to being caring in relationships with others. Kitchener (2000b) suggested that others have labeled this concept as *compassion* and that acting out of care or compassion means acting out of regard for another's welfare. This stance on the part of a feminist multicultural practitioner means acting out of regard for another rather than simply responding to fixed rules and principles. It requires a mental toughness that allows the caring therapist to feel the other's pain and to see the situation through the eyes of the other but does not mean giving up responsibilities for ethical decision making. One criticism of this ethic of care is that those who take care to its extreme could create dependency and may disempower rather than empower by justifying an inequality in relationships, leading to idealizing relationships in which there is no mutual responsibility. Others (Kitchener, 2000b; Noddings, 1984), however, propose that caring with respect for the other as a full human being would indeed involve setting limits, saying "no," and being strict in judgment, but from a more supportive and compassionate stance.

Pope and Vasquez (1998) suggest that because clients place their trust in professionals, it is critical that caring about the clients' well-being should be a defining characteristic of the professional. We must acknowledge the reality and importance of the individuals whose lives we affect by our professional actions. This means instilling in and reminding ourselves of a care perspective. Caring for the humanity of those whose lives we influence is a cornerstone to our work. Ethical therapy involves the recognition of trust that clients place in us, the power we have over clients, and caring. Often, we forget about the experience of the client and the role we play in clients' lives. When we stay connected to our compassion for each of our clients and the climate for ethical behavior is enhanced.

Mutuality

Most feminist approaches describe *mutuality* as a goal in the professional relationship. Jean Baker Miller (1988) contributes to our understanding of mutuality by defining the importance of being with the client/consumer in an engaging, genuine, present manner rather than maintaining a distant stance. If we are able to successfully engage in mutuality in the therapeutic process, Miller believes that the following five beneficial components are the result (for both professional and consumer): increased zest or well-being that comes with feeling connected to others; the motivation and ability to act in the relationship as well as beyond it; an increased knowledge about oneself and others; an increased sense of self-worth; and a desire for more connection beyond this particular one. A stance of mutuality is important in working with women and other oppressed groups, such as people of color.

The Guidelines for Providers of Psychological Services to Ethnic, Linguistic, and Culturally Diverse Populations (APA, 1993) include a definition of *cultural mutuality*. The definition describes, in part, the importance of relating to women, clients of color, and other oppressed groups in a respectful, connecting manner based on our knowledge of the clients' culture and also on tuning into aspects of the clients' needs that our therapeutic processes may help. Cultural mutuality is an important value for feminist therapists working with persons of color and others who have historically been disenfranchised.

Miller (1988) also describes the importance of connection in promoting mutuality. Most feminist models of therapy are based on the concept that therapeutic healing occurs in the context of loving bonds; when the therapist helps the client learn how to stay in connection through empathy and when the therapist connects with the client (through empathy), something happens inside. An emotional and attitudinal shift can result from this experience and is an essential element of the change process. The client can feel it and is affected. Thus, the therapeutic relationship is a major focus of the therapeutic process; therapy is a special place to work on disconnections and move to reconnections. In fact, therapy outcome research indicates that the success of all techniques depends on the client's sense of connection and alliance with the professional (Frank & Frank, 1991; Wampold, 2000). Special attention on how we distance our clients is an important goal for therapists working from this feminist perspective. It is especially true for women, clients of color, gay, lesbian, and bisexual persons, and the disabled, most of whom have experienced distancing in their lives in the form of discrimination.

Moral Principles

Some feminists criticize a principled approach to ethics (Noddings, 1984) partly because the meaning of moral principles is unclear and shaped by a person's place in the social culture. However, others such as Kitchener (2000a) suggest that principles can provide guidance and that moral principles implicitly underlie many of the ethical decisions feminists make and the beliefs they hold. Kitchener's reframing of bioethical principles to apply to psychology influenced the 2002 revisions of the APA Ethics Code and the 2005 revision of the ACA Code of Ethics. Kitchener's foundational ethical principles, listed earlier, include nonmaleficence, beneficence, autonomy, fidelity, and justice. The APA 2002 Ethics Code's General Principles are now more consistent with the bioethical principles, which are designed to be educative. The General Principles were first made aspirational in the 1992 APA Ethics Code. Their intent is to guide and inspire psychotherapists toward the very highest ethical ideals of the profession. General Principles, in contrast to Ethical Standards, do not represent obligations and should not form the basis for imposing sanctions.

Exceptions to Boundaries

As mentioned earlier in the chapter, Brown and others have been concerned that some of the implications of the tenets and assumptions of feminist multicultural ethics are counter to mainstream practice, despite the inclusion of various feminist and multicultural concerns in the last two codes. Feminist and multicultural theory help us to conceptualize appropriate exceptions to some traditional boundaries. Boundary setting is an important ethical responsibility for psychotherapists. It has evolved as an important strategy in applying the ethical proscription to "do no harm" to our clients. Because the needs of the psychotherapist could potentially obstruct therapy, the mental health professions have established guidelines, often referred to as boundaries, designed to minimize the opportunity for therapists to use their patients for their own needs and gratifications (Pope & Vasquez, 1998). However, I previously (Vasquez, 2005) described how many feminist multicultural ethicists construe boundary maintenance in therapy as a continuous rather than a dichotomous issue. The risk of applying rigid boundaries without careful assessment is the risk of evoking shame and confusion from someone who is often shamed by virtue of ethnicity, gender, or other identity that is marginalized in society.

Verbal Boundaries: Self-Disclosure and Answering Clients' Questions

An ethical responsibility is to ensure that our interactions with clients are in the service of clients and not designed to meet our own needs. We must avoid self-disclosures, for example, that would promote inappropriate multiple relationships or that would potentially exploit the relationship. Therefore, talking about ourselves in psychotherapy, or in other professional contexts, has been discouraged.

However, self-disclosure can be a powerful way to increase mutuality and connection with a client, student, or consultee. Increased professional visibility allows consumers more power in the relationship than they would have with a less forthcoming psychotherapist; it is an expression of genuineness. The consumer may experience validation of her or his own experience as well. Self-disclosure also serves the function of allowing the consumer to reciprocate empathy, which can promote mutuality and empowerment of the client (Nelson, 1993).

From a feminist multicultural perspective in general, the issue is to acknowledge the real and genuine aspects of the human interaction in psychotherapy. Other theoretical perspectives, such as the psychodynamic approach, tend to focus more on the symbolic transaction, in which the therapist puts aside his or her feelings and contributions to the interaction and assumes that all issues that evolve in therapy are those of the client. In the feminist approach, it is also important to not deny various aspects of the symbolic transactions, including the power differential, because doing so is a failure to take responsibility for the roles that clients inevitably attribute to us as therapists. Therefore, in our decision making with self-disclosures, we must be careful that self-disclosures are in the service of the client and not designed to meet our own needs.

The Feminist Therapy Institute Code of Ethics (1990) provides guidelines for therapists' disclosure in the context of the power differential. With the well-being of clients as the overriding principle, the guidelines state: "A feminist therapist discloses information to the client which facilitates the therapeutic process. The therapist is responsible for using self-disclosure with purpose and discretion in the interest of the client" (p. 1). In self-disclosure, analysis of each situation is important. What is therapeutically self-disclosing for one person may not be so for another.

How we respond to the questions of our clients is related to the issue of self-disclosure. In the psychoanalytic model, the goal is to not gratify the client and then process the resulting anxiety from a dynamic perspective. An alternative option is that one may easily answer the question so long as it is within an appropriate, nonprivate realm for the therapist, and then process any significance. One approach fails to gratify the client but risks eliciting anxiety or shame that can then be processed from a dynamic perspective. The other promotes connection, relating on a real, authentic, genuine level, and can also explore the need, anxiety, or symbolic issue behind the question. This latter approach potentially allows for deeper and deeper recycling through issues when the relationship is based on warmth, safety, mutuality, and respect.

Multiple Roles and Life Transitional Events

Circumstances in which feminist multicultural therapists, educators, and others delve into gray areas and perhaps end up feeling like "outlaws" (Nelson, 1993) include multiple roles for those of us from "small communities" or rural areas, including the dilemmas that could attend participation in life transitional events. Small communities include close-knit religious or ethnic minority, gay/lesbian/bisexual/transgender, professional, university communities. Not all multiple relationships are necessarily unethical (APA, 2002; ACA, 2005); the APA Ethics Code and the ACA Code of Ethics suggest that those to be avoided are those that would be expected to cause impairment or risk exploitation or harm. Social roles contain inherent expectations about how a person in a particular role is to behave as well as the rights and obligations that pertain to that role. Role conflicts occur when the expectations attached to one role call for behavior that is incompatible with that of another role (Kitchener, 2000a).

A common situation in which boundary and overlapping relationship issues surface is clients' invitations to special events that, from a multicultural feminist perspective, may be therapeutically meaningful, such as weddings, graduations, performances, and the like. In considering whether to attend such an event, you must recognize that several factors and processes are important, including the fact that the event is somehow related to the work of the therapy. Consulting with colleagues and documenting the decision-making process, conceptualizing the therapeutic benefit of your decision, and recording the outcome in therapy notes are essential.

Bartering, Giving, and Receiving Gifts

The APA's 2002 Ethics Code and the ACA 2005 Code of Ethics allow for bartering unless it is clinically contraindicated or the resulting arrangement is exploitative. The position of the ACA and the APA is an attempt to balance the realities of practices of rural and some ethnic minority communities, in which bartering may be customary, with protection of the consumer from potential exploitation and potential problems created in the therapeutic relationship.

 The context of gift giving and receiving is crucial. Receiving gifts from clients is generally discouraged because clients pay for services; receiving expensive gifts from clients can be exploitation. It can signify that the client does not feel worthy enough unless she or he gives continuously; *or* it can simply be a healthy expression of care on the part of the client. It is important to understand goals, motivations, and expectations when clients provide gifts. The ACA Code of Ethics A.10.e., Receiving Gifts, states:

> Counselors understand the challenges of accepting gifts from clients and recognize that in some cultures, small gifts are a token of respect and showing gratitude. When determining whether or not to accept a gift from clients, counselors take into account the therapeutic relationship, the monetary value of the gift, a client's motivation for giving the gift, and the counselor's motivation for wanting or declining the gift (2005, p. 6).

This is another example of a standard that takes cultural relevance into account.

 In addition, if it is within the cultural norm of the provider of services, the occasional provision of cards or small gifts to clients, usually associated with some major life transitional event about which they worked in therapy, may be meaningful to the client and may promote constructive mutuality. Genuine interactions with clients and other consumers of psychological services reflect several of the feminist multicultural tenets.

Expressions of Care, Including Nonsexual Touch

The ability to assess the need and meaning of hugs for and with the client are important elements in judging hugs and other forms of nonsexual touch with clients. Factors to consider in decision making include the nature of the relationship, the client's personal history, the client's current mental status, the likelihood of adverse impact on the client, and clear theoretical rationale. What does a hug mean to this client in regard to power? Is it a communication of power over her? Or is it a communication of mutuality? It is important to assess whose need it is to hug. Some clients have experienced numerous boundary violations; they may be uncomfortable with touch or must control it to feel safe. What is the client's internal, personal phenomenological experience, and what have physical contacts meant to this client in the social context?

Holroyd and Brodsky (1980) examined whether nonsexual touching of patients is actually associated with therapist-client sexual intimacy. They found no indications that physical contact with patients made sexual contact more likely. They did find evidence that differential touching of male and female clients (touching clients of one gender significantly more than clients of the other gender) was associated with sexual intimacies. It was the differential application of touching, rather than touching per se, that was related to intercourse.

Boundary issues for women therapists are different than those for men therapists. Self-disclosure, especially by men in Western society, can be perceived as weakness and vulnerability and may violate a gender norm. Touch is more dangerous for a male therapist in Western culture. When we discuss these issues, we must acknowledge the realities of the social construction of gender and the differential impact of that construction on women and men therapists as well as on women and men clients. This challenge to the boundaries may be appropriate for women therapists but not necessarily for men therapists.

Activism

One of the Guidelines for Providers of Psychological Services to Ethnic, Linguistic, and Culturally Diverse Populations (APA, 1993), states: "Psychotherapists attend to, as well as work to eliminate, biases, prejudices, and discriminatory practices" (p. 47). Likewise, the APA's (2003a) Multicultural Guideline 6 encourages psychotherapists to use organizational change to support culturally informed organizational policy development and practices. Some of our clients or work situations present problems that require us to shift gears and become activists. The advocacy models provide a conceptualization that allows us to intervene in ways dissimilar to the traditional models. Interventions may involve helping a depressed client get a job, visiting a client in the hospital, or even making house calls. Consultation and supervision from those who have experience and knowledge of the issues in such advocacy, such as our social work colleagues, is an important part of the process. The ACA (2005) Code of Ethics A.6.a., Advocacy, states: "When appropriate, counselors advocate at individual, group, institutional, and societal levels to examine potential barriers and obstacles that inhibit access and/or the growth and development of clients" (p. 5).

At a Harvard Medical School conference entitled "Learning from Women" (2000), Judith Jordan talked about therapeutic failures from the relational cultural perspective. Such failures, she said, occur when the therapist is defensive, when the therapist pathologizes clients, when the therapist uses "outside judges" (old/current supervisors/consultants) against their own voice, and when the therapist tries to control rather than respond, especially in working through dilemmas or conflicts with clients. When we respond with power and control, especially in applying unnecessary boundaries, we risk retraumatizing clients, especially women, people of color, and gay and lesbian individuals whom the dominant culture has oppressed. When we do apply boundaries, we must be sensitive to do so with care and respect. Otherwise, we may elicit shame in our clients. Previously traumatized people are easily shamed, and clients can often feel that "I'm the bad one." Mutuality, genuineness, and respect in our behaviors with clients are core to their empowerment.

These decisions and choices are complex, and occasionally we will face difficult ethical dilemmas. In those cases, engaging in an ethical decision-making model can be helpful. Most models encourage problem identification, from a theoretical perspective; consideration of options; consideration of the client's voice; consultation with colleagues who are ethics experts, attorneys knowledgeable about mental health law, and state board and/or ethics committee members; communication of a decision with the client; and documentation of the process and results throughout.

Feminist multicultural ethics have significantly influenced the current standard of care for our work. There are also gray areas that are sometimes terrifying for those of us who make exceptions because we conceptualize that it is for the greater good, conceptualizing from a feminist multicultural perspective. My hope is that these thoughts have contributed to an attempt to document and publicize these kinds of choices in a context that provides thoughtful legitimacy to the exceptions for boundaries so that ethical feminist and multicultural providers, teachers, researchers, consultants, and any combination thereof can make choices without feeling like outlaws.

Summary

1. Because counseling and psychotherapy are intimate processes and involve a power differential, the risk of exploitation is present. Thus, codes of ethics have evolved to protect both clients and professionals.

2. The APA and ACA codes of ethics recognize the importance of diversity and of supporting the worth and dignity of people in the context of their social and cultural environments. Both codes rely on Kitchener's moral principles, which include beneficence, nonmaleficence, fidelity, justice, and autonomy.

3. Two key cornerstones of the counseling relationship stem from the principle of autonomy and respect for people's rights and dignity: confidentiality (the right to privacy) and informed consent (the notion that clients must consent to treatment and be informed of the implications of their treatment).

4. The codes of ethics urge us to eliminate the effect on our work of biases based on the factors of age, gender, gender identity, race, ethnicity, culture, national origin, religion, sexual orientation, physical and mental ability, language, and socioeconomic status.

5. According to the five moral principles upon which the APA and ACA codes of ethics are based, clients can expect to be informed of the purposes, goals, techniques, procedures, limitations, potential risks, and benefits of all counseling services that they receive and to be informed about confidentiality and the limits thereof.

6. Feminist and multicultural ideologies have influenced the evolution of the ethics code and ethical practice in many ways, including the articulation of therapist self-care as an ethical obligation; cautioning against discrimination, sexual harassment, and exploitative relationships; the emphasis on informed consent; and a strengthening of respect for clients.

7. Themes reflected in the philosophy and assumptions of ethical feminist multicultural therapy include the importance of sociopolitical context, empowerment of clients, social justice, validation of the experience of women and people of color and other diverse groups, the ethic of care, and mutuality and genuineness in the psychotherapeutic relationship.

8. Feminist and multicultural theory proposes exceptions to some of the boundaries of traditional ethics in certain situations. These exceptions include self-disclosure (typically discouraged yet sometimes enhancing mutuality and connection with clients), multiple relationships (traditionally discouraged to maintain strictly professional relationships with clients yet in some cases meaningful to the therapeutic relationship), bartering and gifts (traditionally discouraged to avoid client exploitation yet occasionally acceptable with clients for whom bartering and gift giving/receiving are customary), and physical communications of caring.

9. Feminist multicultural ethics encourages activism and advocacy at the individual, group, institutional, and societal levels when appropriate.

Resources for Further Study

Professional Organizations

American Psychological Association Ethics Office
750 First Street NE
Washington, DC 20002-4242
1-800-374-2721 or 202-336-6009

American Counseling Association Ethics and Professional Standards Office
5999 Stevenson Ave.
Alexandria, VA 22304
1-800-473-2329

Professional Journals

Ethics articles are published in various psychology and counseling journals. The quarterly *Ethics & Behavior*, edited by Dr. Gerald P. Koocher (Simmons College), focused entirely on ethics issues, publishes articles on an array of topics pertaining to various moral issues and conduct. Free sample available at http://www.erlbaum.com. Subscriptions available through

Ethics & Behavior
Journal Subscription Department
Lawrence Erlbaum Associates, Inc.
10 Industrial Avenue
Mahwah, NJ 07430-2262

Suggested Readings

Herlihy, B., & Corey, G. (2006). *ACA ethical standards casebook*, 6th ed. Alexandria, VA: American Counseling Association.

Discusses the latest changes in the 2005 ACA Code of Ethics and how to apply these standards in work with diverse clients.

Nagy, T. F. (2000). *Ethics in plain English: An illustrative casebook for psychologists.* Washington, DC: American Psychological Association.

An interesting and readable ethics casebook for psychotherapists and counselors in training.

Remley, T. P., & Herlihy, B. (2001). *Ethical, legal, and professional issues in counseling.* Upper Saddle River, NJ: Merrill/Prentice-Hall.

A comprehensive text on general ethics for counselors.

Other Media Resources

2005 ACA Code of Ethics
www.counseling.org/Resources/CodeOfEthics/TP/Home/CT2.aspx

2002 APA Ethics Code
www.apa.org/ethics
PBS Frontline, *My Doctor, My Lover* (1991)
www.pbs.org/wgbh/pages/frontline/view/

> Dr. Jason Richter, a psychiatrist, had a sexual affair with his patient Melissa Roberts-Henry, who later sued him for sexual abuse. Frontline examines the history.

The APA Psychotherapy Videotape Series, *Responding Therapeutically to Patient Expression of Sexual Attraction* and *Therapist-Client Boundary Challenges*
www.apa.org

Chapter 3

Psychoanalytic Therapy

NEIL ALTMAN

Classical psychoanalytic therapy was originated by Sigmund Freud (1856–1939) in Vienna, Austria, at the end of the 19th century, and it was developed by him—and by others—over the next 40 years. Trained as a medical doctor, Freud became interested in psychotherapy when he realized that the causes of some of his patients' ailments were more psychological than physical. Intrigued by the work of fellow physician Josef Breuer, who had found that allowing such patients to talk freely about themselves and their thoughts gave them some relief, Freud expanded Breuer's "talking cure" into a therapy that he called *psychoanalysis*. As he worked with these patients, and later as he struggled with his own psychological problems, he developed psychoanalysis as both a system of psychotherapy and as a theory of social and personality development.

Although many of Freud's ideas have been revised or discarded in contemporary psychoanalysis, some of the concepts of classical psychoanalysis are core to the contemporary framework. Freud's psychoanalysis was, in fact, the foundation upon which all modern psychotherapy and counseling was built. Psychoanalytic therapy is presented first in this book (and in most other textbooks on psychotherapy theory and practice) because every other therapy you will read about has either evolved from psychoanalysis or was conceptualized in reaction to psychoanalysis.

In this chapter, I first consider classical psychoanalysis, including the ideas of Sigmund Freud and his daughter, Anna Freud; then I cover post-Freudian perspectives; and finally I examine applications of psychoanalysis in the modern world of cultural diversity.

Origins and Evolution of Psychoanalytic Therapy

By the time I entered the field in the 1980s, the classical psychoanalytic framework was well along in the process of being superseded by a more contemporary framework in which the classical concepts were either abandoned or reframed radically. (One way you will see this contemporary approach illustrated is in the way I address issues of diversity psychoanalytically.) However, some of the classical concepts are core to the contemporary framework, although the meanings of these terms are now very different from the meanings Freud had in mind. Furthermore, some classical psychoanalysts still use these concepts, and even for those who do not, it is still useful to keep the evolution of psychoanalytic theory and technique in mind.

Early Development of Freud's Psychoanalytic Theory

Freud's basic theory can be usefully discussed using three models: the energic, the topographic, and the structural model, each of which I will discuss in turn. As Freud's thinking evolved over the course of his career, he went from one of these models to the next, although concepts from earlier models retained places of importance in later models.

Freud's Energic Model

Freud conceived of his **energic model,** which refers to the functioning of psychic energy, as a consequence of his treating clients with so-called hysterical symptoms (such as paralysis with no identifiable physical origin and various inhibitions) with hypnosis. Freud (Breuer & Freud, 1893–1895) was struck with how frequently hysterical clients under hypnosis—usually young women—recalled sexual advances by older men, often their fathers. Freud's earliest theory, often called his *seduction theory*, was that the hysterical symptoms resulted from the buildup of undischarged sexual energy when a young girl was aroused by the advances of such a man. The energic model reflects the idea that the mind seeks to discharge psychic energy, conceived of as essentially sexual in nature, in order to maintain a preferred state of equilibrium. Freud often used the term **libido** to refer to sexual energy or psychic energy, making all three terms essentially synonymous. When a young girl is subjected to the sexual advances of an older man, her libidinal urges are aroused, but owing to her sexual immaturity and/or the incestuous nature of the relationship, she cannot discharge the energy through orgasm. The buildup of sexual energy is experienced as anxiety. Additionally, Freud thought that the hysterical symptom symbolically represented the conflict the client felt over the sexual impulse that had been aroused. For example, a paralyzed hand might reflect an inhibition about touching the penis of the man in question, or a paralyzed leg might reflect conflict about walking to his house.

Later, acutely aware of the horrors of World War I, Freud (1919) revised his idea that psychic energy was only sexual in nature by adding to his theory the concept of a **death drive,** the fundamental source of aggressive energy. Freud thus postulated a new source of psychic conflict, the conflict between the life-drive, **eros,** which is the source of libido, and the death drive. Freud never elaborated on the course of development, or vicissitudes, of the death drive as he did for the sexual drive. However, one of his followers, Melanie Klein (1975), developed her theory primarily around the idea of the death drive.

It was the symbolic function of his clients' symptoms that Freud considered characteristic of the **unconscious,** the part of the mind that is out of awareness. For Freud, infantile sexual impulses, arising in later childhood and adulthood, arouse intense conflict and anxiety and are subject to **repression,** the process by which impulses and thoughts are moved to the unconscious part of the mind, which means that the person is totally unaware of them. Having been repressed, the sexual impulse exists in the unconscious, where it continues to seek expression in disguised forms. Forbidden impulses cannot be expressed directly because they would arouse too much anxiety, but they can be expressed indirectly. This comes about through a compromise arrived at unconsciously involving various forms of disguise, drawing on the primitive forms of thinking that Freud called *primary process* (as opposed to the *secondary process* of rational, conscious thought). The mechanisms of primary process thought include **condensation** (two ideas expressed with a single image), **displacement** (one idea expressed by a different but related idea), and **reaction formation** (an idea represented by its opposite). Indirect expression also occurs through various universal symbols, such as a house representing the vagina or a snake representing the penis. Dreams are a primary mode of expression of unconscious sexual impulses that exhibit all these forms of disguise. Dream analysis thus assumes a central place in classical psychoanalytic technique, offering a "royal road" to the unconscious. Another hallmark of classical psychoanalytic technique is **free association,** a client's uncensored speech—saying whatever comes to mind, no matter how seemingly unrelated or embarrassing—that presumably allows access to the unconscious mind.

Freud's Topographic Model

In Freud's **topographic model,** he outlined three sections of the mind: the **conscious** mind containing all that we are aware of; the unconscious, which is the repository of repressed impulses; and the **preconscious,** the locus of ideas that are not conscious, but are also not subject to repression, so that they can easily become conscious when pointed out. The process of psychoanalytic therapy described by Freud involved the client's free associating and reporting dreams for analysis so that the analyst could bring to the client's awareness the conflictual material that had been rendered unconscious. Infantile impulses that become unconscious maintain a kind of frozen existence, in Freud's schema, so that the client is unable to mobilize the more mature resolutions of which the adult mind would be capable. Freud believed that if the unconscious could be rendered conscious, mature adult clients would be able to handle their infantile impulses in more satisfactory ways so that symptoms would be unnecessary. For example, the client with an infantile exhibitionistic impulse might productively become an actor, rather than developing a pathological inhibition around public speaking (which is an example of reaction formation).

Early on, Freud, using hypnotic techniques, had regularly uncovered instances of girls having been "seduced" by older men, fathers or father surrogates (nowadays we would call this sexual abuse). At first, he believed that the factor causing illness had been the buildup of undischargable sexual energy, in accord with his energic model. But Freud quickly gave up this seduction theory in favor of the theory that the seductions he was hearing about from his hysterical clients were fantasized rather than real seductions. This led Freud to his theory of the **Oedipus complex,** the idea that boys around the age of 5 universally have sexual impulses directed toward their mother along with murderous impulses toward their father who is their rival for their mother's affection. In the female counterpart, called the **Electra complex,** girls of the same age sexually desire their father and want to eliminate their mother who is their rival for their father's affections. Fantasies of having been seduced by the other-gendered parent, then, reflect wishes rather than facts. In accord with Freud's topographic model, these wishes, along with the associated defenses that keep a person from becoming aware of the wishes, were to be made conscious in *analysis* (the shorthand term for psychoanalytic therapy).

Freud's Structural Model

Following his Oedipal theory, Freud began the development of his **structural model,** which posited a tripartite structure of the mind: the **id,** the repository of the instincts and basic, biological urges; the **superego,** the locus of societal ideals and prohibitions; and the **ego,** the mediating force between id and superego, as well as the mediator between the person and the external world.

Freud coined the term *id* to represent our innate unconscious drives to satisfy the biological needs with which we are born. In infancy and toddlerhood, the drives are oral and anal satisfaction; later, the drives encompass genital sex and aggression.

The superego is formed as part of the solution to the Oedipal or Electra conflict whereby the child internalizes the moral prohibitions about these impulses and, more broadly, the value system of the father. Note that in Judeo-Christian and patriarchal fashion, Freud saw the father as the carrier of moral values and standards. Because girls did not end up identifying with the father, Freud thought that they had weaker superegos and thus weaker moral values. Needless to say, there has been considerable feminist critique of this aspect of Freud's theory.

The ego, the mediating force between id and superego, is also the mediator between the person and the external world. In this latter capacity, the ego looks after the function of adaptation. The ego also is the locus of the **defense mechanisms,** the processes through which people ward off the awareness of threatening (and therefore anxiety-evoking) id impulses. Anna Freud, Sigmund Freud's daughter, was active in defining the functions of the ego and developed the branch of psychoanalysis called **ego psychology.**

Anna Freud and Ego Psychology

In *The Ego and the Mechanisms of Defense* (1966), Anna Freud elaborated on her father's idea of defense mechanisms, but unlike her father, she posited that defense mechanisms can serve healthy, adaptive functions. Chief among the defense mechanisms is repression, the banishment of prohibited impulses from consciousness. Buttressing repression were other defenses such as **denial** (of prohibited wishes), the previously discussed reaction formation (in which one avows the opposite of what one unconsciously wishes for), and **projection** (in which one attributes prohibited impulses that one unconsciously holds to others).

Defense mechanisms vary in their maturity, with repression, for example, being a more mature defense than denial, which is seen as crude and maladaptive because it entails a distortion of reality. Most mature among defense mechanisms is **sublimation,** in which sexual or aggressive energy is transformed into creative and productive activity. An artist, for example, might be seen as having sublimated an exhibitionistic sexual impulse, while a surgeon might be seen as having sublimated aggressive energy. Other important defense mechanisms include **identification** (taking on other people's characteristics), **regression** (repeating behavior that led to satisfaction in an early stage of development), displacement (expressing a threatening idea through a less threatening idea), and **rationalization** (unconsciously making an excuse or rational explanation of unacceptable behavior). In the Oedipal situation, in which considerable anxiety is aroused by the sexual impulses directed toward the mother and aggressive impulses directed toward the father, identification with the father in the process of superego formation serves the defensive purpose of avoiding anxiety. Regression to an earlier psychosexual stage (e.g., from the Oedipal to the anal or oral stage) can also manage the anxiety associated with the later stage. Displacement (e.g., of aggressive impulses from the father to another male figure) defuses some of the anxiety associated with the father. Rationalization of impulse-driven actions, making them seem more reasonable than they are, protects the person from awareness of anxiety-arousing impulses. For example, a boy might rationalize his aggressive impulses toward a male figure, such as a teacher, by thinking and saying, "He's a really bad teacher. No one likes him."

Ego psychologists Heinz Hartmann and David Rapaport furthered Anna Freud's focus on the ego as independent of id energy. They theorized that id energy could be "neutralized" of its sexual quality and transformed into "conflict-free" ego energy so that activities such as sculpting could be engaged in without provoking the conflict around the underlying sexual urges. Inhibition in one's work could be seen as a failure of neutralization. For example, a man with work inhibitions could be seen as having failed to neutralize competitive wishes in relation to his parents (Fenichel, 1945; Robbins, 1939).

Jungian Psychology

Carl Jung, a contemporary of Sigmund Freud, was inspired by Freud's early writings but ultimately went in an alternate direction. Similar to Freud, Jung posited the existence of conscious and personal unconscious realms (the latter was close to Freud's preconscious). However, Jung (1966) added a unique realm, the **collective unconscious.** It was the repository not of one's personal history, which resided in the personal unconscious, but of the history of the entire human species. The collective unconscious contains universal models of human behavior, called **archetypes,** that guide our behaviors. Examples of archetypes include the hero, the wise old man, the earth mother, the shadow (our darker, unacceptable aspects), the animus (masculine characteristics in women), and the anima (feminine characteristics in men). Archetypes appear in ancient myths and fairy tales as well as in modern mythological stories such as the *Star Wars* movie series that pits the hero, Luke Skywalker, against his shadow (and father), Darth Vader. Archetypes provide an explanation for similar cross-cultural behaviors as well as our instinctive understanding of how to play common roles in our lives, such as being a mother. Another way in which Jung's theory is different from Freud's is that Jung did not believe that psychological development culminated at about age 5 with the Oedipal and Electra conflicts. Consistent with his deemphasis of the sex drive, Jung held that at midlife (which in the early 1900s was around age 35 to 40) we strive to reach our full potential and that this period of life is especially significant in our psychological development.

Object Relations and Relational Psychoanalysis

A product of Western European culture, classical psychoanalysis was not very adaptable to other cultures. However, developments in the field over the last 20 to 30 years have begun to change this situation. The first major change in psychoanalytic theory was a movement that replaced Freud's drive-based model with a **relational model** in which mental life is organized by past and present interpersonal relations. Other changes took place in a context of cultural shifts, especially under the influence of feminism and postmodernism.

In 1983 Jay Greenberg and Stephen Mitchell published the book *Object Relations in Psychoanalytic Theory* in which they argued that a fundamental shift from a drive-based model to a relational model had been taking place in psychoanalytic theory. Classical psychoanalytic theory is a drive-based model because it proposes that mental phenomena are derived most fundamentally from drives, specifically sexual and aggressive drives. In classical psychoanalytic theory, psychological development reflects the development of the drives—that is, from a focus on the mouth in the nursing of earliest infancy (the *oral stage*) to a focus on processes of elimination in toddlerhood (the *anal stage*) to a focus on the genitals (the *genital stage*, leading to the Oedipus or Electra complex).

A relational model, by contrast, is one in which mental life is believed to be organized by the interpersonal context in which the person exists. Psychological development in relational models reflects the changing nature of interpersonal relations at various stages of life. Drive-based models see the mind as operating under the influence of forces operating within the individual; the individual person is the basic unit of observation. Relational models see the individual mind in context; the units of observation are the relationships between or among people. Drive models acknowledge that people engage in relationships, but drive models derive the nature of the relationship from the drives that are activated in it. Relational models acknowledge that people have sexual and aggressive drives, but they consider that the nature of the sexual and aggressive drives activated in a relationship depends on the nature of the relationship. In short, drive theories take account of relationships, and relational theories take account of drives, but they prioritize these aspects differently in their explanatory models. For example, in classical psychoanalytic theories other people tend to be called *objects*. This terminology reflects the fact that the place held by other people in a drive theory is as object or aim of a drive. The drive takes priority over the person who is the object of the drive.

Drive models have been called instances of a one-person theory in that the focus is on what occurs within the individual. Interpersonal psychoanalysis, building on the work of Harry Stack Sullivan, puts the emphasis on actual interpersonal relationships and has been called a two-person theory. The theory of Melanie Klein (1975), a Viennese analyst who did most of her work in Great

Britain, occupies an intermediate space between one- and two-person theories, although it tilts strongly toward the one-person side. For Klein, the **inner world** (fantasies containing representations of self and others) consists of **internal objects**—that is, stable representations, schemata, or templates through which other people are perceived. Klein's theory has aspects of both two-person and one-person theory. It is a two-person theory in that the inner world is a representation of the relational world of other people, but it is a one-person theory in that the representation of other people as good or bad, for example, depends crucially on whether libido or aggression is activated in relation to that object. In other words, internal objects take their character from the drive associated with them.

Klein's theory and others that focus on the inner world of object relationships are referred to as **object relations theories.** These theories are more relational than drive theories, but they are incompletely relational to the extent that the inner world is seen as self-contained.

Ronald Fairbairn (1952), a Scottish psychoanalyst, took Klein's theory in a more relational direction by postulating that internal object schemata are formed under the influence of actual experiences with people in the external world. People view others through templates established by their experiences with other people, in particular their early experiences with primary caregivers. Donald Winnicott (1965, 1975), a British psychoanalyst, took an integrative position with respect to the question of how the internal world, emphasized by Klein, and the external world, emphasized by Fairbairn, interact. Winnicott advanced the idea that our perceptions of other people draw on both subjective and objective perspectives simultaneously. Winnicott called this domain in which subjectivity and objectivity coexist *transitional space*. The quintessential transitional object is the child's blankie, which all agree is simultaneously the most precious thing in the world in the child's subjective world and a dirty old piece of cloth in the external world of objectivity.

As an interesting aside, Sigmund Freud had actually begun with a relational model when he started to construct psychoanalytic theory. Recall that the seduction theory posited that hysterical symptoms derived from a damming up of libido because of what we would now call sexual abuse. However, over time, Freud concluded that the memories of "seductions" produced by hysterical young women in hypnosis or through free associations were actually fantasies (perhaps because he could not or would not believe that many seemingly upstanding citizens of Vienna were sexually abusing their daughters). Thus was born the Oedipal theory. While Freud's seduction theory contains elements of a drive model in terms of the emphasis placed on a damming up of libido, it has strong elements of a relational model in terms of the emphasis placed on an actual interpersonal occurrence, sexual abuse. Once Freud's theorizing moved to an Oedipal model, actual interpersonal occurrences were relegated far to the background, while internally generated fantasies that occur relatively independently of context assumed the foreground.

Relational psychoanalysis has also aspired to integrate the one-person and two-person models, finding a place for both an internal world of drives and fantasies and an interaction with an external world of other people. Relational psychoanalysis seeks to demonstrate a circular interaction between the internal and external worlds, such that the internal world of fantasy evolves under the influence of actual interpersonal events, while actual interpersonal events are under the influence of the internal world of fantasy.

Changes in Response to Feminist and Cultural/Postmodernist Theorists

Starting in the late 1960s, additional challenges to psychoanalytic theory came from feminist theory and cultural theory (also referred to as postmodern theory). Feminists pointed out that behind Freud's concept of **penis envy** (women's wish to have a penis and be like a man) lies the assumption of the superiority of the penis and, by extension, masculinity—an assumption that is generalized throughout Freud's theory. One of the impacts of feminism has been to question the supremacy of the stereotypical masculine values of objectivity and detachment, especially when these are valued at the expense of subjectivity and relatedness (e.g., Gilligan, 1982). As the proportion of psychoanalysts who were women increased, it is perhaps not surprising that this cultural shift also occured in psychoanalysis, that is the conception of the analyst began to move from that of a detached and objective observer to a related and emotionally engaged participant.

Cultural theorists framed Freud's assumption of masculine superiority as a manifestation of his embeddedness in a patriarchal society. In a broader criticism launched not only at psychoanalysis but also at all psychologies of Western origin, postmodern philosophers (e.g., Derrida, 1978; Foucault, 1980) questioned claims that knowledge can be absolute and universally valid. According to post-modernists, all knowledge is context specific or *local* (i.e., from people's experiences) and is influenced by the specific cultural surroundings. Notions of rationality and objectivity, too, are seen as culturally based, so that what is seen as objective knowledge in one culture might not be recognized as such in another cultural context. Traditional African healing practices might not seem rationally based to a 21st-century citizen of the United States, but, then again, medical treatments that were regarded as state-of-the-art 50 years ago in the United States might now be regarded as strange, if not harmful (e.g., treating chronic tonsillitis in children with radiation). Postmodernists have also pointed out how claims to knowledge can be deployed in the service of obtaining and maintaining power. For example, the previous classification (until the early 1970s) of homosexuality as a mental disease served to maintain the degraded status of gay people. Such "knowledge" was often the result of theories not being critically scrutinized, as occurred with Freud's idea that genital heterosexuality was the end point of sexual development and thus the very definition of sexual maturity.

The influence of postmodernism on psychoanalysis can be seen in the way in which conceptions of the analyst's knowledge have changed. In classical psychoanalysis, the analyst's authority is based on objectivity and theoretical knowledge, which form the basis of the **interpretations** they make about the meaning of material the client brings forth. In relational psychoanalysis, the analyst's knowledge is a function not only of training and theoretical point of view, but also of subjective experience arising from interaction with a particular client. Thus, the analyst's interpretations are seen as quite personal statements, arising in part out of the analysts' experience with the client. Social constructivism in psychoanalysis (Hoffman, 1991, 1998) makes explicit this notion that psychoanalytic knowledge is constructed in a specific social context, the interaction between a particular client and a particular analyst.

Feminist and postmodern perspectives dovetail with those of postcolonial theorists (Bhabha, 1990; Fanon, 1963) who, building on the idea that knowledge claims serve the interests of entrenched power, noted how the colonial powers based their claims of entitlement to dominate other people on the colonial powers' having a superior culture. In particular, the technological superiority of the European powers was seen as evidence of a general superiority, along with the supposed superiority of the Christian religion. In a sense, the psychoanalytic organization of the mind into the "primitive" and the "mature" corresponded to the colonial division of societies into the same categories. Indeed, defining the id (the primitive part of the mind) as a seething cauldron of unsocialized sexual and aggressive drives, to be dominated by the rational agency of the ego via psychoanalytic treatment, corresponded to colonialism on a psychic level.

With these considerations in mind, we can see how classical psychoanalysis—in the way rationality came to be defined as the very essence of health—enshrined a Western European value system that marginalized people of Third World cultures, which were based more on human connection, emotion, and intuition. From contemporary multicultural, postmodern, and feminist perspectives, we can see how our psychoanalytic forebears unknowingly promoted a theory and practice that was noninclusive cross-culturally.

Context Then—Context Now

At its origins, psychoanalysis was a product of a minority group in Vienna around the turn of the 20th century, the Jews. Sigmund Freud and most of his early followers, with the notable exception of Carl Jung, were Jewish. Until shortly before Freud's time, Jews were not allowed to train as medical doctors in Vienna. When they were finally admitted to medical schools, they were trained with the understanding that they were to treat only Jews. Freud was one of the first Jewish doctors allowed to treat non-Jews. Perhaps because he did not want psychoanalysis to be labeled a "Jewish psychology," Freud was eager to present his theory as having universal applicability. In fact, it was just the opposite; psychoanalytic theory clearly reflected the culture in which it germinated. For example, much of psychoanalytic theory is about the relationships between boys and fathers. Mothers are relatively marginal in his theory, and female development little more than a footnote. This preoccupation with masculinity bespeaks the cultural context of patriarchy in which Freud lived and thought. The centerpiece of his theory, the Oedipus complex, is clearly a product of a patriarchal society in which there is a struggle for possession of women among men. Only recently have some analysts, influenced by our current attention to the cultural location of ideas, noticed the culturally specific nature of Freud's theories.

When psychoanalysis was transplanted to the United States, further developments occurred that resulted in cultural insensitivity on the part of many psychoanalysts. These analysts came to the United States fleeing the Nazis. Having been traumatized by their social world, many of these analysts wanted nothing more than to ensconce themselves in private offices to delve into the workings of individual minds out of social context. Further, as new immigrants, psychoanalysts observed the privileges that would be theirs by "becoming White," a term that I coined (Altman, 2004) following Noel Ignatiev (1995). Jews had actually been called "Blacks" in Vienna (Gilman, 1993), but when they settled in the United States, their clients, with few exceptions, were White. More than that, analysts pursued a privileged place in American society, which for them meant becoming medical entrepreneurs. Analysts set up private practices and adopted the medical model of diagnosis and treatment of psychological disturbance. Freud (1919) had expressed the hope that clinics could be set up in which psychoanalysis would be available to all without regard to financial means; in fact, some of his early followers had set up such low-fee psychoanalytic clinics (Danto, 2005). In the United States, however, psychoanalysis became nearly exclusively a private practice, and a high-fee one at that. Aside from excluding people of limited means, psychoanalysis also came to marginalize people of non-Western European cultural background.

Under the influence of the American medical model, ego psychologists brought into psychoanalysis concepts of relative mental illness and health in terms of the strength of the ego. In the process of defining *ego strength*, the underlying Western European value system already embedded in psychoanalysis was made more explicit. Consider that ego strength was commonly defined in terms of frustration tolerance and the ability to think, rather than act, in response to anxiety and frustration. Ego strength, to this day, is thought of in terms of having achieved a high degree of "separation and individuation" (Mahler, Pine, & Bergman, 1975)—that is, a feeling of psychological separateness and individual identity. A culturally sensitive perspective on this sort of definition of mental health suggests the influence of Calvinist values in terms of the value placed on bearing frustration without acting to seek gratification. The influence of an individualistic culture is seen in the emphasis placed on separation and individuation, as opposed to interconnectedness. To be sure, the differences here are a matter of degree. Ego psychologists might well respond that satisfactory interconnectedness depends on two individuated people coming into relationship. The point of emphasis is telling, however, and results in the value system of psychoanalysis being more appealing to people who have adopted Western European values. People with other value systems—those that prize connection, a "communal self" rather than an "individual self" in the words of Alan Roland (1988)—often did not see the psychoanalytic theory and method as speaking to them. The psychoanalytic method—with its emphasis on verbalization as opposed to action and on the analyst's quiet listening and restraint to the point of anonymity—had always privileged frustration tolerance and the ability to function independently as qualities of a "good client." The good client does not place demands on the analyst to interact, to be friendly and encouraging, to be reciprocally self-revealing. The bottom line was that it took a person with a specific set of values and tolerances to adapt to and derive benefit from the psychoanalytic method.

The Author's Journey as a Psychoanalytic Therapist

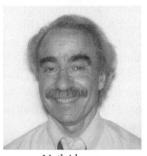

Neil Altman

I grew up without much conscious awareness of culture, even though I was Jewish, in St. Paul, Minnesota, a mostly Irish and Scandinavian city with a small Jewish minority. Minnesotans are notoriously polite, so I was never teased about being Jewish in my mostly non-Jewish elementary school.

I first learned about culture when I went to India in the Peace Corps. I lived in a small remote village in south-central India for two years, learning two Indian languages and becoming quite immersed in the culture by the time I left. Among the culturally significant things I noticed in India was that children and adults slept together. The males in a family slept together (boys and men) and the females slept together (girls and women). I also noted that children were not weaned. They breast fed until they were good and ready to stop. Upon returning to the United States, and especially after having my own children, I became aware of how intent many North American parents are to get their children out of their beds and to wean them. It seemed as if we were afraid that if we did not make our children grow up quick, they would never grow up.

In the big picture, this cultural difference made sense to me, in that Indian village children are not being trained to be able to leave home. North American parents who are middle class or higher usually assume their children will go some distance away from home to college or a job and may not return. They seem to be preparing their children (and themselves) for this separation nearly from birth. The difference in child-parent separation experiences is thus a cultural difference that organizes a whole series of culturally based differences in childrearing practices between North American and Indian people.

In the early 1970s, I entered graduate training in clinical psychology in a program directed by a psychoanalyst who had strong commitments to social justice. Nonetheless, the training we received was almost entirely based on a private practice model. The only required clinical experience was with clients in the program's clinic, and the clinic did not reach out to people in the ethnically and socioeconomically diverse neighborhood nearby. As a result, the clients were mostly White and middle class, even though the program made a strong and successful effort to recruit students of Color. With few exceptions, the clinic supervisors were psychoanalysts in private practice. Of the two supervisors of Color associated with my program, one was a family therapy supervisor and the other was employed in the public sector. Neither had obtained psychoanalytic training, as many White supervisors had. The supervisors I chose were not working in a community-based setting, and my coursework did not address public sector work at all.

Externships in the community were not required and typically were not sought out. But it was important to me to have some community experience, so I worked as a part-time volunteer in a hotel-based outreach program in which most of the tenants were previously homeless, and later in a classroom at a psychiatric hospital for children.

After the completion of our coursework in my program, we were required to do clinical internships. Most of us did our internships in local hospitals, although it was possible to complete this requirement in an outpatient clinic and the ones chosen by students in my program were psychoanalytically based. I did my internship in a Veterans Administration outpatient clinic. My patients were socioeconomically diverse but almost entirely White people, and there were no supervisors of Color. In my internship and in those of my fellow students, the staff attempted to find outpatients whom they considered fit for relatively long-term, psychoanalytically oriented "insight therapy." The model for such a client was the

(*continued*)

young, verbally intelligent person. Although typically it was not explicitly set up this way, most such clients turned out to be White and middle class. Verbal intelligence, of course, was defined in a way that privileged people with certain educational opportunities and cultural backgrounds. The majority of the clients in these inner-city hospital-based clinics were poor people of Color. Most of them were not considered good candidates for insight-oriented therapy because they had pressing "concrete" problems (having to do with poverty) and limited educational opportunities, and so they were passed over as clients for the interns. It seemed clear to me that ultimately we were being trained for private practice work with clients who had money and lots of education and that public-sector work was available primarily for exposure to more severely disturbed patients on the inpatient units. After getting their doctorates, most of my fellow students who were White took jobs in the public sector while building up a private practice. The typical career path was to leave the public-sector jobs as soon as it was possible to have a full-time private practice. The students of Color typically stayed longer, sometimes indefinitely, in their public-sector jobs. As I saw it, psychoanalytically oriented therapists were most likely to gravitate toward full-time private practice with White, middle-class and upper-middle-class clients.

After finishing my doctoral training, I went to work in the South Bronx at the child and adolescent outpatient clinic of a large hospital. At the same time, I was enrolled in postgraduate psychoanalytic training at a program run by the same man who had run my doctoral program. The contrast between the world in which I worked in the Bronx and the world of psychoanalysis could not have been starker. I was always interested in trying to bridge these two worlds, sensing that the psychoanalytic part of me and the part of me that wanted to work in the public sector were linked. The form taken by the intersection of these two parts of me was a determination to provide the highest-quality service I could to people who were usually treated dismissively, to take my work with them as seriously as the work with people who paid top dollar for the service. As far as I was concerned, psychoanalysis was the form of psychotherapy that, in its intensive and painstaking attention to people's experiences was most respectful of their humanity. Thus, I wanted to provide psychoanalytic treatment for my clients in the Bronx and train others to do so. I felt a certain pleasure in defying what I saw as the elitism of psychoanalysis, as well as a psychoanalytic, but also a general societal, dismissal of the poor.

Of course, I was not so deluded as to think that I could provide five weekly sessions of psychoanalysis to people in a public clinic in the Bronx, nor would I have wanted to. What seemed most important to me was to bring to this work a psychoanalytic perspective, especially attentiveness to people's conscious and unconscious experience. At the time, my colleagues in the clinic shared this commitment, so the environment was inspiring. As time went on, however, administrative pressure to see more and more clients (as many as 50) in a 35-hour work week and to bring in more and more revenue to the clinic made working conditions difficult and then intolerable for me. I left after working there for more than 11 years. As I prepared to leave, I began to write about my experience in the Bronx, which led to my formulating a psychoanalytic approach to therapy in public clinics (Altman, 1995).

Theory of Psychoanalytic Therapy

Although most of the foundational concepts of contemporary psychoanalytic therapy were discussed in the section on the origins of psychoanalysis, here I will pause to review the core concepts, then continue with a discussion of one important component of psychoanalytic theory I have not yet discussed: theories of human development.

Core Theoretical Concepts

Up to this point we have discussed, in historical sequence, the development of psychoanalysis, from Freud's original ideas, through the contributions of Anna Freud and the ego psychologists, to the more contemporary ideas of object relations and relational psychoanalytic theorists. Before we continue, you may find it helpful to pause and review Table 3.1 (pp. 56–57), which summarizes the important aspects of these different approaches within the school of psycho-analytic thought.

Theories of Development

Because Freud believed that sexual impulses were at the core of all mental life, his developmental theory was a theory of the development, or evolution, of libido across different ages. In comparison, Erik Erikson (1902–1994), an ego psycholo-gist who studied under Anna Freud, formulated a model of development that included biology as one of three factors that influence psychosocial development throughout the lifespan. The other two factors are the individual's unique life experiences, especially early family experiences, and the cultural and historical forces at work during the individual's lifetime.

Table 3.1 Comparison of Psychoanalytic Approaches

	Classical		Contemporary	
	Freudian	*Ego Psychology*	*Object Relations*	*Relational Psychoanalysis*
Key theorists	Sigmund Freud	Anna Freud, Heinz Hartmann, Erik Erikson	Melanie Klein, Ronald Fairbairn, Margaret Mahler, D.W. Winnicott	Stephen Mitchell, Lewis Aron, Jody Messler Davies, Irwin Hoffman
Focus of theory	Intrapsychic (mental) phenomena derived from basic biological drives (id)	Regulation of drive energy as well as interactions with the outside world (ego)	Intrapsychic representations of people based on early experiences	Integration of the intrapsychic world of object relationships and the external world of interpersonal relationships
Root causes of client problems	Anxiety caused by conflict between infantile impulses and societal dictates and frustration caused by repression (burial in the unconscious) of infantile impulses	Failure to neutralize infantile impulses, which leads to primacy of unhealthy defense mechanisms	Pathological internal object relationships	Disordered interpersonal relationships based on distorted expectations of the interpersonal world
Theory of change	Making conscious what is unconscious allows mature adult clients to handle their infantile impulses in more satisfactory ways so that symptoms are unnecessary	Developing more mature defenses and adaptive ego functions allows adult clients to handle their infantile impulses in more satisfactory ways so that symptoms are unnecessary	Altering the internal world to allow integration of good and bad in human relationships (rather than depicting people as either good or bad) allows clients to deal realistically with people in their lives	Altering expectations and interpretations of human behavior and associated self-fulfilling prophecies in the context of transference and countertransference allows clients to have healthier interpersonal relations

	Classical		Contemporary	
	Freudian	*Ego Psychology*	*Object Relations*	*Relational Psychoanalysis*
Clinical goal	To bring unconscious conflicts and defenses into consciousness	To build ego strength, which is defined in terms of frustration tolerance and the ability to think, rather than act, in response to anxiety and frustration	To develop the capacity to see other people as both good and bad as opposed to either all good or all bad	To be more open and less rigid in human relationships and to be less prone to acting out repetitive self-defeating interpersonal patterns
Client-counselor relationship	Client's job is to relate material to the analyst and gain insight; counselor's job, as a detached expert, is to interpret the material and explain it to the client	Similar to classical psychoanalysis	Counselor's job is to reflect on and interpret the aspects of self that the client projects onto the counselor, which clarifies the client's emotional experiences and makes them more manageable for the client	Client's experience of the relationship with the counselor is the context for altering unproductive interpretations and expectations (including self-fulfilling prophecies) regarding others' behaviors
Clinical techniques	Counselor encourages client to free associate and report dreams; counselor uses that material to bring to the client's awareness conflicts that have been rendered unconscious	Similar to classical psychoanalysis; some pointing out of defense mechanisms	Client free associates and reports dreams, but also induces emotional experiences in the counselor; counselor reflects upon these experiences that are an entrée into the client's emotional experiences	Unpacking of the client's experience of the relationship with the counselor so as to reveal hidden expectations of the behavior of others

57

Freud's Stages of Psychosexual Development

Freud theorized that that libido is expressed through whatever function is the focus of the child's activity at a particular age. In the first year of life, when the child's activities are focused on nursing, libido, or pleasurable sensation, is centered around the mouth, Freud's *oral stage*. In toddlerhood (ages 2–3), when the focus of the child's concerns centers around the anus in toilet training, pleasurable sensations are focused there, Freud's *anal stage*. Next, in Freud's *phallic stage* (ages 4–5), pleasurable sensations are centered on the genital area as the child discovers the pleasure of masturbation. Also at this time, the boy develops fantasies of phallic grandiosity as he discovers that his penis can grow, while girls develop penis envy. The culmination of psychological development occurs in the Oedipus complex, when the male child desires to have sex with his mother and kill his father. These wishes stir up fear of castration in male children because castration is a logical retribution boys might expect from their rival, their father. For boys, the resolution of the Oedipus complex occurs when the boy defensively identifies with his father (following the logic: if you can't beat him, join him) and incorporates his father's value system, the superego (which I discuss in the next section). At this point, he represses his sexual impulses toward his mother, but they live on in the unconscious. Girls have a more complicated job in the Electra complex in that they must overcome their primary attachment to their mothers in order to become symbolically attached to their fathers. For girls, the complex is resolved when they give up their fantasy of having sex with their fathers and accept the fantasy of being impregnated and having a baby as a substitute for the literal possession of their father's penis. Following the phallic stage and the resolution of the Oedipus or Electra complex, Freud theorized that the libido goes dormant (the so-called *latency period*) until puberty, at which point adolescents enter the *genital stage* where their libido refocuses in the genital area, but now libido is directed toward appropriate hetereosexual gratification.

It should be noted that a number of Freud's early followers and colleagues broke their association with Freud and his theory because they strongly disagreed with Freud's giving sexuality an almost exclusive role in determining mental life. Carl Jung was prominent among these dissenters who developed their own theories of personality and counseling, as was Alfred Adler, whose theory is the subject of the next chapter.

Erikson's Theory of Psychosocial Development

Erik Erikson viewed development throughout the lifespan as a series of eight stages. At each stage, we are required to perform new tasks imposed by new interpersonal demands and changing environmental contexts. Each stage is named for the particular *developmental crisis*, or challenge, that the individual must resolve in order to move successfully to the next stage. Successful mastery of the crisis results in personality strength, or *virtue*, that will help the individual meet future developmental challenges (Erikson, 1982; Miller, 1993). Failure to master a crisis leads to feelings of incompetence, psychological distress, and further failure at later stages. Table 3.2 (pp. 60–61) provides a synopsis of Erikson's stages of development.

Erikson did not believe that any one individual could completely master every challenge at every stage in life. Rather, each individual would achieve a more or less favorable balance between trust and mistrust, industry and inferiority, ego integrity and despair, and so forth. Additionally, although each of the eight challenges predominates at a particular time in the lifespan, each of the challenges exist throughout the lifespan. Thus, development is a never-ending process.

Sullivan's Development of Self and Other

The psychiatrist Harry Stack Sullivan (1953) spoke of three categories in self-development: the good-me, the bad-me, and the not-me. The *good-me* consists of those aspects of myself about which I feel good, which I am proud to own as mine. The *bad-me* consists of those aspects of myself about which I feel bad, ashamed, or guilty, but which I nonetheless own as mine. Things get more complicated with the not-me. The *not-me* consists of those aspects of myself that I disown, so that though they are mine, I refuse to accept that they are mine.

The process of disavowing aspects of myself leads into what Melanie Klein and her followers call *projective identification*. Recall that projection refers to the process of attributing disavowed aspects of self to another person. **Projective identification** highlights another aspect of this process: when this aspect of oneself is perceived in another person, there is an unconscious identification with that piece of oneself that one is seeing in the other. One manifestation of this unconscious identification is that one feels one knows what the other is thinking or feeling, or what the other will do. Another manifestation is a preoccupation with that aspect of the other that corresponds to what has been disowned from the self. Finally, one may induce the other to behave in ways that fit with what has been projected so that one's perception of the other will appear to be objectively justified. This sense of objective validity is further enhanced by selective attention to those aspects of the other's behavior that fit with the projection.

The interpersonal aspects of projective identification can be seen most clearly in paranoid people. Paranoid people disavow their own malevolence and attribute it to others. As a result, they only feel victimized while often inducing in others the very antagonistic reactions that allow them to feel that they were right to mistrust the others in the first place. It is an essential part of the paranoid process that paranoid people feel that they know just what other people are

Table 3.2 Erikson's Eight Stages of Development

Stage 1. Infancy (Birth to 1 Year of Age)

Crisis: Trust vs. Mistrust	*Virtue Attained: Hope*

Erikson's theory of psychosocial development begins in infancy with the developmental crisis of trust versus mistrust. Trust is fostered in the infant through the love and attention received from the primary caregiver. The relationship between infant and caregiver is the infant's first experience of connection and intimacy against which all other experiences will be judged. When infants receive consistent loving care, they experience the world as safe and predictable. By contrast, when infants' needs are inconsistently satisfied, they develop feelings of mistrust, and trust becomes harder to achieve in future relationships. Early trust leads to the development of the important virtue of *hope*, the belief that one's wishes are attainable.

Stage 2. Toddlerhood (1–3 Years)

Crisis: Autonomy vs. Shame and Doubt	*Virtue Attained: Will*

During the second stage of psychosocial development, toddlers begin to exercise their autonomy through evolving motor and verbalization skills. Testing limits at every turn, the toddler must find a balance between feelings of confidence resulting from newfound autonomy and feelings of shame and doubt resulting from unsuccessful efforts and disapproval from primary caregivers. The virtue of *will*, or will power, is developed through the experience of both autonomy successes and failures.

Stage 3. The Preschool Years (3–6 Years)

Crisis: Initiative vs. Guilt	*Virtue Attained: Purpose*

Erikson's third stage presents a conflict between initiative and guilt, which occurs as a result of the child's actively engaging in activities outside the family environment. The child initiates exploration of self and others by acting out sexual and aggressive feelings in play and by purposefully pursuing self-initiated tasks and goals. This enterprise enables the development of perspective taking. Guilt results from the child's awareness of disregarding other people's boundaries. If children at this stage are treated respectfully and are helped to formulate and pursue their goals without feeling guilty, they gain the virtue of *purpose* in their lives.

Stage 4. The School Years (6–12 Years)

Crisis: Industry vs. Inferiority	*Virtue Attained: Competence*

As children enter the world of school, they must come to believe in their ability to learn and their ability to be productive if they work hard. When a child's sense of industry is effectively nurtured by significant adults who recognize the positive achievements produced by the child, the child internalizes the virtue of *competence*. Failure to experience mastery and develop competence at this stage leads to one or the other extreme of either social alienation or total conformity.

Stage 5. Adolescence (12–18 Years)

Crisis: Identity vs. Role Confusion	*Virtue Attained: Fidelity*

Identity development is the main task of adolescence. The onset of this stage coincides with the physical changes of puberty and the newly acquired cognitive skill of abstract thinking. This is the time when individuals carve out their uniqueness from the array of values, beliefs, and roles demonstrated around them. The virtue of *fidelity* is achieved when one is able to achieve a coherent self-concept and remain loyal to one's values despite conflicts.

Stage 6. Early Adulthood (18–35 Years)

Crisis: Intimacy vs. Isolation	*Virtue Attained: Love*

At this stage of development, finding another person to develop an intimate relationship with is the goal, and the ability to *love* is the virtue to be attained. The struggle is in the conflict between maintaining one's separate sense of self while simultaneously committing oneself to the intimate relationship.

Stage 7. Adulthood (35–65 Years)

Crisis: Generativity vs. Stagnation	*Virtue Attained: Care*

In Erikson's seventh stage of psychosocial development, the challenge of generativity means that the mature adult achieves personal satisfaction by being useful and effective, contributing to the surrounding world through *care* and concern for others, imparting knowledge to younger generations. The resulting virtue is *care*. Stagnation occurs when life no longer seems purposeful, which precludes further psychosocial development.

Stage 8. Late Adulthood (65–Death)

Crisis: Ego Integrity vs. Despair	*Virtue Attained: Wisdom*

The eighth stage of psychosocial development finds an aging adult entering the twilight of life. The developmental crisis of this stage is to find a balance between integrity and despair. The challenge at this stage is to appreciate and integrate previous life experiences while minimizing feelings of despair or resentment that the end is in sight. Successful resolution brings about the virtue of *wisdom*.

thinking and intend to do to them, thus revealing the extent to which what they perceive is really an aspect of themselves.

A Self Versus Other Explanation of Racism

Given that race does not exist on a biological level, in that intragroup genetic variability is greater than intergroup genetic variability, the concept of racial groups clearly is socially constructed. The question then arises, how and why is the concept constructed as it is? One psychoanalytic explanation is that the construction of racial categories occurs to a great extent under the influence of projective identification. For example, White people who want to construct a self devoid of exploitative sexuality, violent aggression, laziness, criminality, and so on, can project these qualities onto Black people. Once these qualities are projected onto Black people, White people can engage in racist acts free of guilt or anxiety. They can even engage in blatantly aggressive behaviors, such as lynching, while feeling virtuously free of aggression. Racist prejudice and discrimination do, of course, lead to poor ghetto schools, poor employment opportunities, and so on, conditions that foster behaviors that have been projected on to Black people, such as laziness and criminal acts, which allows White racists to believe that they were right about Black people in the first place. And in a racist society, Black people may be induced to identify with derogatory images of themselves that they pick up in contact with White people and in the media, which is consistent with one of the features of projective identification. Such identification further reinforces the images and perpetuates the vicious circle of racism.

I have been speaking so far of relatively blatant manifestations of racism and prejudice, but these can take subtle forms, too, even among well-meaning and consciously anti-racist people. Dismissive and derogatory attributions to people of Color can occur unconsciously among liberal-minded people. In an experiment in which they had college students conduct interviews, Word, Zanna, and Cooper (1974) found that White interviewers, who were consciously liberal and anti-racist, showed more signs of unease when they interviewed Black people than when they interviewed White people. They sat farther away from the Black interviewees, were less verbally fluent, and ended the interview sooner, but they were not conscious of their behavior. When White interviewees were exposed to the same signs of unease on the part of their interviewers, the White interviewees performed less well than when their interviewers were more at ease. Word, Zanna, and Cooper's study demonstrates how the unconscious racist attitudes of a White interviewer can influence a Black job candidate's performance in an interview and result in the faulty conclusion that the Black person is an inferior candidate for the job. This is how racism and prejudice work unconsciously among liberal and well-meaning people who, in an effort to avoid painful feelings of guilt, have a vested interest in keeping these processes unconscious. And the psychoanalytic explanation of racism just described also explains prejudice and discrimination based on ethnicity, gender, sexual orientation, and other forms of cultural diversity.

Theory of Change

Let's consider two different (yet somewhat overlapping) perspectives of the change process from the classical and relational models of psychoanalysis, based on differing conceptions of the nature of the mind and its disturbances. In drive-based classical psychoanalysis, the root of all **neuroses** (the generic term Freud used for psychological problems) is thought to lie in unconscious intrapsychic conflicts regarding sex and aggression that usually begin in early childhood. In order to promote change, clients must first become aware of the intrapsychic conflict underlying their neurosis (singular of *neuroses*). In other words, the unconscious conflict must be brought to the client's conscious awareness. The path to change involves gaining insight about the conflict, both intellectual insight (understanding how the previously unconscious conflict is responsible for present problems) and emotional insight (experiencing the explanation as personally valid). With insight, the client's mature ego can resolve the conflict. For instance, suppose a woman came to feel, early in life, that moves toward independence led to feelings of abandonment by her caretakers. She then developed conflict around her independent impulses, fearing that her impulses would inevitably lead to feeling catastrophically alone. In therapy, she may gain insight into how this conflict came to be and may realize the price she has paid for inhibiting her independence impulses and strivings. Further, in her relationship with her therapist, she may come to learn that feeling independent of the therapist does not necessarily lead to loss of the therapist's support. The various ways in which classical psychoanalysts help clients reveal their unconscious conflicts, gain insight about them, and come to an understanding that promotes change are discussed later.

How people learn from their experiences with the therapist is strongly emphasized by relational analysts. In classical analysis, insight gained from the analyst's interpretations is given the highest priority in promoting change. New experience with the therapist and other people is a secondary factor. Relational analysts see the capacity to have new experiences, outside the box of the patient's limiting expectations of self and others, as the primary factor promoting change. Insight through interpretation is a secondary factor, one that may help the client open up to new experience. Relational analysts consider that insight may follow from new experiences, as well as vice versa. Relational analysts also believe that their behavior toward the client may be a key factor in facilitating new experience. A client may induce behavior in the analyst, such as being overly supportive, that may lead the client to feel that, indeed, the therapist does expect the client to act in a dependent way. The analyst may have to do some soul searching to see if the client has actually picked up on a way in which he or she is indeed supporting dependent behavior. Exploring the analyst's role in reinforcing neurotic assumptions may be important in making the client a full partner in developing change within the analytic relationship, a process that is transferable to other relationships in the client's life. Relational analysts place a premium on the exploration of how clients experience the analyst's behavior and the meanings clients may draw from the analyst's behavior that support their neurotic assumptions. The client's experience of the analyst is not necessarily dismissed as distorted; rather the important thing is that the client's patterns of meaning making become open to exploration. Classical analysts do not see themselves as being so personally involved in an interaction that can promote change. I provide further elaboration of these ideas later in this chapter.

Practice of Psychoanalytic Therapy

In this section, I review how different forms of psychoanalytic theory gave rise to varying forms of psychoanalytic practice and technique. You will see that seemingly arcane differences in theory have important practical implications for how therapy is actually conducted, and particularly for how diversity is handled in the consulting room.

The Client-Counselor Relationship

Classical analysts view the relationship between the client and analyst as principally a source of data for the analyst's interpretations. The analyst's interpretive behavior is viewed as primarily metacommunicative; the analyst remains outside the relationship and gives insight-producing interpretations. For relational analysts, the relationship is much more central; it is the arena in which processes of interpersonal and intrapsychic change can be experimented with and explored by client and analyst together. Analysts attend to their clients' neurotic assumptions about themselves and others as well as clients' interpretations about client-therapist interactions that support these neurotic assumptions. While doing this, the analyst is personally involved in identifying and changing ways in which she or he may be colluding with the patient's neurosis. Recall the example of a therapist's noticing that being overly supportive reinforced the patient's neurotic preconceptions that independent behavior is discouraged by other people.

Classical Psychoanalytic Therapy

Freud saw the process of psychoanalytic therapy as centered around bringing *derivatives* or symbolic representations of repressed impulses into the treatment so that conflict around those impulses could be reopened and resolved using the superior resources of the adult client's mature ego. Unconscious material can enter the treatment in several ways.

First, the client is instructed to free associate, to report all thoughts and feelings that enter his or her mind without censoring any material. Second, the client reports dreams. Freud thought that impulses are as active during sleep as they are during the day, but that defenses are less vigilant during sleep. Unconscious material, related to wishes derived from those impulses, can bypass the individual's normal censoring activities and thus threaten to disturb sleep. The dream arises in order to protect sleep by allowing unconscious wishes to be expressed in disguised form. When dreams are reported in psychoanalysis, the client is asked to free associate to the various elements of the dream. This provides the analyst with access to the client's unconscious thinking behind the dream. Along with the information provided by the client's free associations, analysts use their knowledge of the language of the unconscious to reverse the process of disguise and to discover the unconscious meaning of the dream through interpretation.

The third way in which unconscious material comes out in the analysis is via **transference,** in which clients displace unconscious feelings from the past onto the analyst and the analytic situation. For example, a client may act out toward the analyst unconscious sexual impulses related to her father, as if the analyst were her father. Freud believed that in a properly conducted analysis, the analyst's anonymous, neutral, and abstinent (non-wish-gratifying) stance would elicit the infantile wishes behind the client's neurotic symptoms, but now the wishes are activated in relation to the analyst. In this way, the infantile wishes can be observed in the analytic situation, in what Freud called the *transference neurosis*. The analyst's job was then to interpret that the client's feelings were in fact repetitions of an earlier pathogenic situation and to detail for the client just what the operative impulses and defenses were. Freud believed that the insight clients gained from such information would strengthen their ego and allow them to resolve their impulse-defense conflict in more adaptive ways than through psychopathological symptoms. Corresponding to transference in the client is **countertransference** in the analyst, that is, the reactivation by the client of the analyst's unconscious feelings from the past. Freud believed that countertransference interfered with the analyst's objectivity, and so recommended that all those training to practice psychoanalysis should undergo psychoanalysis themselves to become aware of their own unconscious conflicts.

Freud noted early on, however, that the interpretation of transference does not unfold smoothly. Clients do not accept analysts' interpretations without **resistance,** the process by which a client wards off a therapist's efforts to bring unconscious psychic content to awareness. To some extent, even though transference brings a pathogenic situation to life in such a way that the analyst can comment on it, it also adds to the client's negative attitudes toward the analyst, which in turn, provokes resistance. Unwilling to accept their analysts' interpretations of their feelings as valid, and unwilling as well to remember and reflect on infantile anxiety-producing situations, clients instead press their demands to gratify their sexual wishes toward their analysts (which Freud considered a defensive activity that he called *acting out*). Furthermore, just as clients repress or otherwise defend against awareness of their id impulses in the first place, they resist such awareness when the analyst tries to raise their wishes to the level of consciousness in the analysis. Freud sometimes wrote of intractable resistance as a manifestation of the death drive.

Recognition of the ubiquity of resistance led Freud to introduce the notion that the analyst would often have to call attention to the fact that the patient was resisting the analytic process, such as by not free associating. Interpretation of resistance became a centerpiece of ego psychology because defense mechanisms are a central part of ego functioning, and overly rigid and maladaptive defenses weakened the ego. Too much reliance on denial, for example, could impair the ego's reality-testing function. Ego psychologists also emphasized cultivating a working alliance between client and therapist that would motivate the client to want to accept the therapist's interpretations. Finally, Freud came to recognize that simply calling unconscious impulses to the client's attention once or even a few times was not enough to shake up the client's neurotic systems. The neurotic symptoms would be quite entrenched, and because they functioned to ward off anxiety, clients were reluctant to give them up. Freud then came to recognize that an extended period of working through resistance was required before clients could have a stable reorganization of their neurotic patterns. Accordingly, early analyses, which sometimes took place in a relatively small number of sessions (weeks or a few months rather than years), gave way to extended analyses that often took years.

Contemporary Psychoanalytic Therapy

Greenberg and Mitchell (1983) argued that all schools of psychoanalytic thought had been moving in the direction of a relational model for some time but that often there were intermediate hybrid forms of theory containing both drive and relational elements that were conceptually inconsistent. For example, some analysts who had adopted a relational model in theory continued to adopt a practice stance that was based on a one-person drive theory model. Consider how the psychoanalytic setup and practice model is consistent with, even derives from, the assumptions of such a one-person model. The idea that the analyst should sit behind the client, out of sight, and should say very little with the exception of an occasional interpretation derives from the assumption that the "real action" is located within the client's mind. The analyst strives for a detached, objective perch from which to make observations of the workings of the client's mind. This technical stance is also consistent with the scientific ethos of Freud's day, which demanded that the scientist be as objective as possible.

From a relational point of view, however, the participation of the therapist is a given. It cannot be eliminated. The therapist has an impact on the client and thus influences the object of observation, if only by virtue of the impact of silence. Some therapists give higher priority to the interpersonal world in theory but in practice continue to strive toward an anonymous, or "blank screen," stance with their clients (see Hoffman [1983] for a comprehensive discussion of this phenomenon). For another example, Harry Stack Sullivan argued in theory for the primacy of the interpersonal world in psychological development and in psychopathology. In theory, Sullivan called the therapist a *participant observer*, but in his practice model the therapist was an expert—enlightening the client about aspects of the interpersonal world that the client had failed to take account of—rather than a participant in a more personal way. For Sullivan, therapists were providers of information about the interpersonal world, much like Freudian therapists who provide information about the client's fantasy life in their interpretations.

Later theorists filled out the picture of the therapist as a full participant in the psychoanalytic situation by pointing out (1) that all interventions of therapists, including interpretations, contain elements of therapists' subjective experiences as well as their objective observations and (2) that clients influence therapists' experience as well as vice versa. In this way, an effort was made to integrate the internal and external worlds of both client and therapist in understanding the therapeutic interaction. Through their interaction, the client—and often, incidentally, the therapist—would learn and grow.

Note how the meaning of many of the fundamental concepts in psycho-analysis changes in a relational model. Transference and countertransference refer in a more general way to the nature of the here-and-now interaction, and specifically to the way client and therapist make meaning of, or interpret, each other's behavior. The client's interpretation of the therapist's behavior might be influenced by conflicts deriving from childhood, as Freud thought, but also by the client's general personality style and by plausible constructions of what the therapist is doing. Countertransference likewise can be influenced by the therapist's unresolved childhood conflicts but also by the therapist's theory as well as her or his plausible interpretations of the client's behavior. Inter-pretation, along with everything else the therapist does in the therapy session, is a behavior that can have a therapeutic effect. Thus, interpretation loses its privileged status in relational psychoanalysis.

Relational analysts tend to focus on impasses, or polarized conflicts that develop between client and therapist that amount to enactments of the client's characteristic difficulties in living. When client and therapist can find creative ways to resolve these impasses, this makes it possible for the client to revise internal schemata of self-other relationships in positive ways.

From a relational point of view, the unconscious is not just the repository of drive-defense conflicts. Anxiety-laden interpersonal events can also be rendered unconscious, subject to **dissociation,** in which they are accessible only in certain states of mind. Dissociated interpersonal events might be happenings between client and therapist, or between the client and people in the outside world. Because a client's biases in decoding the behavior of other people reflect the client's internal schemata of interpersonal relationships, the therapist's interpretation of the biases also helps the client to revise her or his internal schemata in positive ways.

From a relational perspective, defenses typically are seen as blind spots around certain kinds of interpersonal events in the service of anxiety avoidance, as opposed to the classical view of defenses as operating to thwart awareness of internal states that would create anxiety. Resistance, in two-person fashion, tends to be seen as requiring "two to tango"—that is, resistance to analytic consciousness raising occurs when both client and therapist collude to avoid anxiety-arousing material.

To summarize this section of the chapter, Table 3.3 encapsulates the differences in psychoanalytic terminology between classical and contemporary relational theories.

Psychoanalytic Practice with Ethnically and Socioeconomically Diverse Clients

Fred Pine (1983, especially chap. 8 and 10) was one of the few psychoanalytically oriented therapists in the 1980s who took therapy with the inner-city poor seriously enough to write about it. He also provided training in the public sector, which included conducting a special seminar for his interns on working with poor, "multi-problem," severely disturbed clients. Considering Pine's work provides an opportunity to note the strengths and weaknesses of ego psychology in addressing clinical practice with ethnically and socioeconomically diverse clients.

Classical psychoanalytic technique relied almost entirely on interpretation. Ego psychology introduced ego-supportive interventions as preparatory to insight-oriented work, which resulted in a dichotomy between "insight-oriented" and "supportive" therapies. Poor clients and clients with limited educational backgrounds were thought to need supportive therapies. Pine (1983), taking supportive therapy far more seriously than most analysts, catalogued a series of ego-building interventions, including naming feelings and helping clients manage their anxiety level by giving them some control over the timing and "dosage" of

Table 3.3 Psychoanalytic Terminology, Then and Now

	Classical	*Relational*
Unconscious	Repository of unconscious impulses	Unformulated expectations of other people
Id	The locus of sex and aggression	Contemporary psychoanalysis does not divide the mind in this way; the focus is more on how human relationships are represented
Ego	The regulating agency in the mind	
Superego	The locus of prohibitions and ideals	
Defense mechanism	Ways of regulating drive energy	Ways of regulating anxiety
Anxiety	Signal of presence of danger from within the mind	Signal of danger from within the mind or the interpersonal world
Transference	Client's distorted interpretation of counselor's behavior, which is based on paradigms carried over from the past	Client's interpretation of the counselor's behavior, not necessarily distorted or carried over from the past
Countertransference	Counselor's distorted interpretation of client behavior based on paradigms carried over from the past	Counselor's interpretation of the client's behavior, not necessarily distorted or carried over from the past

interpretations. He advocated that therapists give clients some warning when they are about to say something that would be difficult to hear and tell clients that they should indicate when they have had enough of an interpretation, at which point the therapist would stop the interpretation (1983, chap. 10).

Pine (1983) made a truly radical move, in a psychoanalytic context, by questioning the dichotomy between insight-oriented and supportive therapy, suggesting that insight could be generated in the context of support from the analyst or in the context of the traditional analytic stance in which the analyst abstains from supporting the client. The kind of work necessary with poor inner-city clients of Color was still considered different from that possible with White, middle-class clients, but at least it was now psychoanalytically valid. Pine further suggested that all clients need support to one degree or another. This was a potentially even more radical step, although Pine never fully developed the implication that, psychoanalytically speaking, one need not consider work with clients of different ethnic and socioeconomic backgrounds as a special case.

In my own writing, I first turned my attention to missed appointments, perhaps the most pervasive fact of life in public clinics. From an ego psychological point of view, missed appointments were viewed as evidence of the client's ego weakness, perhaps to the point of disqualifying the client for psychotherapy at all, and certainly for psychoanalytic therapy. Missed appointments meant poor tolerance for anxiety or a tendency to act out rather than reflect. In the following clinical vignette, which is adapted from my book, *The Analyst in the Inner City* (1995), I show how I came to think psychoanalytically about missed appointments and how I was led to think about the phenomenon of transference in the public sector.

Linda was referred to a public mental health clinic because she had been feeling nervous. She had been brought into a hospital emergency room the previous night by her sister, after Linda had lost her temper and thrown dishes at her boyfriend. She was angry because she suspected that he had another woman. Linda's sister, on her behalf, said that she needed pills for her nerves. Linda had several times in the past received prescriptions for "nerve medicine." She tended to take them irregularly, regardless of how they were prescribed. The emergency room resident, having seen Linda before and knowing that she tended not to follow up on treatment, decided not to give her a prescription that night and to send her to the outpatient clinic the next morning. In the outpatient clinic, a psychology intern talked with her for a long time. The intern heard a story of parental abandonment as a child, of numerous betrayals by parents and boyfriends. Linda expressed a great deal of anger at many people in her life. The intern pointed out that the most recent betrayal, by her boyfriend the previous night, was only the latest in a long series of events and so it struck a very raw nerve. She acknowledged the intern's comment and promised to return the next week to talk with the intern again, without asking for medication. She said that talking to the intern had made her feel much better.

The next week, Linda did not show up, much to the disappointment of the intern, who felt she had established a strong and meaningful connection with Linda in their first meeting. Since Linda had no phone, the intern wrote her a letter. There was no response for 2 weeks from Linda. In the third week, however, the receptionist called the intern to say that Linda was in the waiting room to see her. Linda knew that she had no appointment, but would like to see the intern for just a minute. The intern felt confused, irritated, worried. When Linda came into her office, she apologized for not returning to the clinic and explained that she had been getting the runaround from welfare and that she had decided to apply for SSI (Supplementary Security Income, a Social Security program to provide money to people who cannot work because of a physical or mental disability). Would the intern please send her medical records to the Social Security Administration on her behalf?

The intern felt quite disoriented. Linda's actions seemed to be an indirect yet powerful communication of hostility and despair, provoking similar feelings in the intern. The intern had thought that this woman could benefit from psychotherapy. Linda seemed to be settling for crumbs from life. Why accept the status of a mentally disabled person so easily? Was she trying to exploit the system? Perhaps in her world there were no other options: you either find a secure source of income from the "system" or you do not eat. What should a psychotherapist-in-training say to Linda? The intern felt caught between rejecting her, on one hand, and colluding with her exploitativeness, hostility and despair, on the other. Should she go along with the client's request as a temporary expedient to establish a relationship with her? Would a rejection undermine any chance that Linda would come back? Would acceding to Linda's request be a colluding with Linda's devaluation of herself and with her exploitation of the system? Which course of action would less seriously undermine a therapeutic relationship? Should the intern urge it on her? Linda did not come from a background where people go for therapy when they are in trouble. Perhaps the intern needed to understand and accept Linda's cultural values and gradually work toward becoming a therapist to Linda. But along the way, how does one avoid foreclosing one's ability to take a therapeutic stance in the future?

The intern, trying to deal with all these thoughts, not to mention her feelings and her anxiety, asked Linda about her decision to apply for SSI and whether she saw herself as being able to work. She inquired about how Linda would feel if she got SSI, and she expressed her opinion that the client could benefit from psychotherapy, which might lead to Linda's seeing other options in her life. Linda agreed to give therapy a try and left with another appointment.

The issues raised by working with a client such as Linda can be approached from an object relations perspective by asking, "Who am I in this client's world?" That is, the therapist assumes that the transference comes from the client's previous experiences with other people. For Ronald Fairbairn (1952), for example, a common transference involves the client's seeing the therapist as an *exciting object*[1] (i.e., tempting, promising), as a *rejecting object*, or both. Such transference configurations are elicited in a very powerful way by the situation encountered in public clinics. When a client of lower socioeconomic status such as Linda walks into a public clinic, from her point of view she enters another of the institutions that control crucial aspects of her life. A frame is already established for the therapy that is about to occur. A hospital or a hospital clinic is part of the network of institutions and bureaucracies that include public

---

[1] As noted earlier in the chapter, psychoanalysts originally used the word *object* to refer to the object of a drive, usually another person. Now that many analysts have moved away from drive theory, the term persists but now refers to another person within a transference context—that is, a person is seen through the lens of a set of preconceptions about others that the person tends to apply to interpersonal perceptions. *Internal object relations* refer to templates of self-other interactions. *Bad object* refers to templates of bad experiences with other people; *good object* to corresponding good experiences with others.

assistance, Medicaid, and Social Security. These institutions both provide and frustrate. A person dealing with one of these systems is likely to encounter an overworked, harassed clerk whose mandate is not to provide benefits to anyone who cannot demonstrate impeccable qualifications of need. Could there be an external situation better calculated to evoke an inner world of exciting and rejecting objects? In Fairbairn's picture of the inner world, the self is seen as split in two: a needy, desirous self attached to the exciting object and a need-rejecting self attached to the rejecting object. This depicts the combination of desperate need and hatred of both self and others that is felt by many poor clients as they apply for, or are asked to come for, recertification of their need for public assistance and other benefits.

As Linda requested help from the intern with SSI, the intern found herself identified, despite their conversation about her life, with the entire tantalizing social welfare system. In principle, is this situation different from any other transference situation? Perhaps there are echoes here of what one would presume was Linda's experience with a parent. As one considers the therapeutic possibilities in this situation, Linda herself becomes an exciting and rejecting object. A therapist would like to engage her in an examination of these issues, but she is so elusive. Countertransference is induced, which can be the therapist's entrée into the client's world of inner experience.

Let us examine one likely transference-countertransference configuration that can be created by a client such as Linda when she misses appointments. Such a client can leave the therapist feeling rejected, abandoned, and angry, particularly when there has been a session that stimulates hope for productive work together. The therapist may, after many such experiences, bypass such feelings and say to herself, in effect, "Good. Now I have time to relax or catch up on my reading." She may hesitate to call the client, if calling seems too much like pursuing her. On the other hand, she may feel that she is abandoning the client, perhaps in a retaliatory way, if she does not contact her.

From an object relations perspective—that is, a perspective that focuses on the way people represent their experiences with other people—what we are dealing with here can be seen as the client's way of processing her own experience of unreliability on the part of important people in her life. As the therapist feels rejected, abandoned, or angry in relation to the client, the therapist is sampling something like the client's own experience. The situation provides the opportunity to feel one's way into the client's object world, into her experience. This is a process described by Bollas (1987) as follows: "The client not only talks to the analyst about the self; he also puts the analyst through intense experience, effectively inviting the analyst to know his self and his objects" (p. 250).

Sometimes there is an added twist to this scenario. After missing several appointments, perhaps after the case is closed in the clinic, the client may show up without an appointment, as Linda did. The client may, in addition, be in crisis. With some clients, this pattern can become their modus operandi in the clinic. In extreme cases, clients may come only when they are in crisis and without appointments, while rarely, if ever, keeping the appointments that are offered to them. From an object relations perspective, one can find in such a situation the client's attempt to maintain contact, a connection, with people who are experienced as basically rejecting, unreliable, and ungiving. A crisis coerces a response. A crisis dramatizes the need of the client to such an extent that a caretaking response is virtually guaranteed. Ogden (1986) makes a similar point in stating that self-other boundaries are blurred in a crisis. For Ogden, crises are a way of reestablishing the "unmediated sensory closeness" characteristic of Klein's paranoid-schizoid position. The *paranoid-schizoid position* refers to a situation in which a person keeps "good" and "bad" separate. Thus, other people are experienced as being either all good or all bad. In the *depressive position*, where good and bad coexist, a person can be experienced as both good and bad. This situation gives rise to guilt when bad feelings such as anger are experienced toward a person whom one also loves. Thus, the position is called "depressive." In the paranoid-schizoid position, "objects" are not "whole" in the sense that good and bad are not present together. One's experience of other people is governed by projection rather than by objective perception, in that other people become what one needs them to be in order to keep good and bad separate. Other people are truly separate from oneself only in the depressive position, which is the only position that takes into account the fullness of who others really are.

In the depressive position, whole object relatedness is associated with a sense of isolation, which can be reversed when a crisis brings people together. Ogden (1986) writes: "Crises are not events which take place between separate people. They are events in which client and therapist are 'in it together'" (p. 213). In responding to crises, the therapist experiences the client's way of maintaining, or attempting to maintain, object ties in a depriving environment.

Therapists are in a very uncomfortable position as they begin to empathize with, and sample, the client's experience of abandonment and despair. The burnout that therapists in public clinics struggle with is akin to a generalized burnout that can be observed in poor clients. In other words, one is tempted to give up and withdraw in the face of the anxiety, the sense of futility, and the despair that are engendered both by the client's psychological situation and by the overwhelming social problems that impact him or her. One way of coping with these feelings is to question the suitability of psychoanalytic therapy for inner-city clients. Therapists may thereby justify not engaging the pain of these people's lives while taking the focus off their own sense of helplessness and futility.

From an object relations perspective, missed appointments, crises, and so on are the ways in which the therapist becomes what Greenberg (1986) calls an *old*

object—that is, a modern representative of an object from the past. The therapeutic issue is whether the therapist can also be enough of a *new object* for the
client to allow for change to occur in the client's inner world of representations
as a consequence of the analytic work. In Fairbairn's (1958) terms, can the
therapist avoid being forced to play an assigned role in the client's experience
like everyone else in the client's life?

This is a knotty problem with any client. It is not easy to find the proper
balance between being an "old" and "new" object in the client's world. In the case
of a client from the lower socioeconomic classes, an additional complication is
that deprivation is an ongoing and real factor in the client's life. The therapist's
position as a modern version of the internalized exciting and rejecting object is
reinforced by the socioeconomic differential between client and therapist, by
the therapist's position as part of the social service network, and by the real
power the therapist potentially has as an advocate.

Transference and Countertransference in the Context of Culture

The psychoanalytic concepts of transference and countertransference contain
points of view about the meaning-making activities of client and therapist. As
noted earlier, in classical psychoanalysis *transference* referred to feelings about the
therapist that were "transferred" from the client's primary relationships
(i.e., those with parents) to the therapist. Transference-based perceptions of the
therapist were thus considered to be distorted. Classical analysts believed that
pointing out these distortions to the client, along with their origin in the client's
early life, would have a curative effect by increasing the ego's mastery over the
client's psychic life. In order for transference distortions to be interpretable,
Freud and his early followers believed that the analyst must remain anonymous
so that any perception of the analyst on the part of the client (except a perception
of him as benign and helpful, of course) could be attributed to transference
distortion. Countertransference, which originally meant a reaction to the patient
transferred from the analyst's early life, potentially contaminated the field by
reducing the analyst's objectivity. Countertransference was to be kept in check
through the analyst's own personal analysis and ongoing self-analysis.

Merton Gill (1982) complicated this view of transference and countertransference by claiming that all transference perceptions of the therapist have a
plausible basis in the therapist's actual behavior. Transference is thus not entirely
distortion, but contains at least a grain of truth. The therapist's perceptions of
the client, likewise, came to be seen as drawing on a complex mixture of
objective perception, theory-driven ideas, and the therapist's personal and
subjective reactions, deriving in part from the therapist's own history. The task
of analysis, then, is not to point out the client's distortions from an objective

perch, but rather to sort out with the client the various factors contributing, consciously and unconsciously, to their interaction, including, but not limited to, what was classically referred to as transference. In the process, the client's self-awareness is enhanced (along with the therapist's). If we add the client's and the therapist's cultures to the mix of factors influencing the client-therapist interaction (or, in the jargon, the *transference-countertransference interaction*), you can see how the psychoanalytic method naturally accommodates the analysis of cross-cultural interaction. In the following clinical example, you will see what a difference a relational perspective makes when culture is a clinical issue.

Rosa was a high school senior who came to the clinic where I worked in the Bronx with panic attacks and severe, intermittent depression, triggered by a recent breakup with a boyfriend. She was a bright young woman who went to an elite high school out of her neighborhood. Her mother and father were first-generation immigrants from Puerto Rico who had lived in New York for about 20 years. Rosa's mother was a bright woman, but moody and sometimes quite depressed, and she had never learned English. She stayed home raising her three children, of whom Rosa was the youngest. The father, an intelligent and energetic man, had worked his way up from being a stock clerk in a store to being the store manager. Rosa began therapy talking mostly about her anger toward her boyfriend who had left her for another young woman they both knew. Rosa was enraged, depressed, and had suicidal thoughts. I began seeing her twice a week.

Following the first few sessions, Rosa began missing appointments. My solution was to wait a day or two to see if she would call; if she did not, I would write her a letter noting that she had missed an appointment and saying that unless I heard otherwise, I would expect to see her a few days hence. Rosa would show up at the next appointment with some concrete reason she had been unable to come to the previous appointment and apologize for not calling me.

After an unusually long period in which Rosa did not respond to my calls and letters, when we finally met I asked Rosa what thoughts she had had about our work in therapy in the interval since our last session. She said she had been feeling better and thought perhaps she did not need to come so regularly. I asked if she had considered contacting me to tell me so. She said she felt uncomfortable about that: she anticipated I would think she needed to continue her sessions and that since I was the doctor, it was not her place to disagree. I asked her how she thought I experienced her absence, and she said that she had actually thought about me at one point and wondered how I would fill the time when she did not show up. When I pressed her to speculate about my state of mind, she said she thought I was probably angry to be "stood up." I said this was probably not unlike what she had felt, although more intensely, when her boyfriend had stood her up, and she agreed.

In a later session, Rosa expressed anger at her mother for insisting that she be home at midnight the previous weekend when she had gone to a party. She felt that her mother could not accept that she was pretty much grown up. What if she wanted to go away to college the next year? Would her mother even let her go? Rosa felt that her mother had no life of her own and that she would go into a depression if Rosa did not stay home with her. I suggested to Rosa that she might feel similarly about me, that she had to hide her thoughts that she might be feeling better and might not need me anymore. Rosa agreed and said that she had been angry at me for pursuing her when she thought she was making it clear by her absence that she did not want to come to her sessions, at least on a regular basis. She expressed her feeling that her mother and I were both standing in the way of her developing autonomy.

Over the next few sessions, none of which were missed, we had the opportunity to explore her guilt about wanting to be more independent. She felt that she was leaving behind her mother, as well as her childhood friends, in going "downtown" to school. In subsequent sessions we also talked about how Rosa had initially seen me as representing her mother, but later saw me as potentially facilitating her growth away from her mother because I was White, a professional, and a man and because together we were trying to remove obstacles to her independent development. Now, however, our work was threatening to her because I had come to represent her upwardly mobile father.

That was another problem. Rosa suspected that her father had a covert sexual interest in her. She felt that her father felt more of a kinship with her than with her mother. For example, the two of them would speak English together, excluding her mother. Anxiety about her father's sexual feelings toward her, and presumably hers toward her father, was thus activated in relation to me as a father-transference object. Rosa denied anxiety about sexual feelings between us, but I suspected that this issue was too threatening to pursue at that time.

Rosa continued her treatment on and off until she graduated from high school. She went to college away from home, dropped out, re-enrolled near home, and called me from time to time when she was in distress about ways in which she felt she was sabotaging her success. I have not seen her for many years as of this writing.

This case example illustrates many aspects of clinical work in impoverished neighborhoods. Issues of socioeconomic status, ethnicity, culture, and gender also contributed significantly to the transference/countertransference matrix within which we worked. Missed appointments and my response to them had a crucial catalyzing function in developing a shared understanding of this matrix.

A multicultural perspective can be valuable in any kind of clinical work by providing an essential context of meaning within which to understand psychic phenomena such as conflict, transference, and resistance. For example, consider how my understanding of Rosa's conflict about being in therapy was enhanced by my understanding of the cultural context. Recall that Rosa's mother was from a small town in Puerto Rico. Partly because of my experience in India, I felt

I could understand her failure or refusal to learn English and to assimilate herself into the mainstream of New York life in the light of her sense of disorientation in North America. I imagined that it seemed quite daunting to her even to attempt to find a place for herself in the fast-moving, high-pressure society around her. Her husband, perhaps because men were traditionally more "out in the world," was more ready to learn English and get a job. I believe that Rosa's conflict about going "downtown" to school and about succeeding in North America is understandable only if one takes into account the discordance between the society in which Rosa lived downtown and the rural Puerto Rican society that her mother was trying to maintain at home. The cultural conflict becomes part of the unformulated, unconscious backdrop to Rosa's behavior and her feelings. My understanding of Rosa and my empathy toward her were enhanced by the depth of my understanding of the cultural conflicts in which she was immersed. Without the cross-cultural perspective, I might have seen Rosa's conflicts about success downtown and loyalty to her mother as simply a separation problem, a developmental lag, a conflict around differentiating herself from her mother, around growing up. From an intrapsychic point of view—that is, one that only considers what goes on within the individual— indeed, Rosa did have such conflicts. One runs the risk of overemphasizing developmental failure and, perhaps, conflicts over aggression and dependence, if one understands and interprets without taking account of the cultural context. A psychoanalytic interpretive approach that does not consider context, either interpersonal or societal, can be skewed in its localization of a problem. An interpretative approach that emphasizes the intrapsychic locus of a problem can lead to overpathologizing the individual and result in iatrogenic (treatment-induced) resistance or compliance on the part of the client.

One might reformulate the cross-cultural misunderstanding that I am describing as a case of projection on the therapist's part. Rosa might have become for me the locus of my own disowned dependence and conflict over separation and independence. Cultural biases contribute to individual identity formation via the particular polarities, with privileged and denigrated poles, that structure the personality. When two people from different cultures meet, there is always the potential for the cultural difference to create the opportunity for self-definition in opposition to the other.

From a cultural point of view, what might appear as "resistance" in therapy often can be formulated as a culturally harmonic behavior. For example, to members of some ethnic groups, arriving up to an hour after an appointed time is considered being on time. To most Western Europeans however, if you arrive more than a few minutes after the appointed time you are late. Is lateness to appointments, then, to be considered resistance? Is the therapist who is annoyed about the lateness under the influence of Western European rigidity? Is it a case of induced countertransference? Is it to be considered an indication that there is conflict between the client's and therapist's sense of what is felt to be late? Consideration of the cultural backgrounds of client and therapist, along with transference/countertransference configurations at a particular time, can enrich the potential field for analytic exploration.

Consider as another example Rosa's missed appointments. Here the possible meanings are numerous. Is one to view the missed appointments as resistance, in relation to some warded-off drive or object relation? As a sign of poor ego strength? As an enactment of abandoning an internal object relation? As a culturally harmonic way of expressing difference or defiance with an authority figure? Is my expectation of consistency and continuity in this professional relationship a function of my personal culture, the psychoanalytic culture, or both? Did Rosa have entirely different expectations based on her culture? Do people who grow up in extended family situations, for example, have less expectation of, and need for, consistency within a dyad? Do I dismiss our common humanity in an overzealous cultural relativism when I consider such possibilities? It seems to me that there are no a priori answers to these questions. Rather, understanding evolves as therapists try out various formulations in keeping with their theoretical predispositions, their countertransference, and their understanding of the current transference/countertransference situation, and as they make interventions based on them.

In Rosa's case, analytic exploration led us to an agreement that missed appointments reflected a wish to wind down or terminate the treatment, which she did not feel free to express directly. I believe that her indirectness of expression has a cultural component; from this point of view, it is important to keep in mind that even as I sought to understand Rosa's behavior from her cultural point of view, I was implicitly challenging this framework and offering or imposing my own. By inquiring about the meaning of the missed appointments and in encouraging an exploration of what Rosa felt and wished to do, I was saying, "You can speak directly to me about what you feel, even if it is in opposition to me." In so doing, I may have stimulated conflicts about deserting her tradition or part of her tradition, which may have needed analysis in its own right.

Transference and Countertransference in the Context of Race

We now turn our attention to the practice of psychoanalytic therapy when race is an issue. Consider the case of Laurence, an African-American, upper-middle-class, gay man who was having difficulty in his personal relationships. At the end of our initial consultation, he said that he wanted to continue working with me. I asked him whether race had played a role in his choice of me as a therapist. (I remind you that I am a White, heterosexual, upper-middle-class, Jewish therapist.) He said that he preferred to work with a White therapist. He thought that a Black therapist would focus too much on racial issues, would assume Black solidarity, and would too quickly assume that his problems were the result of White racism.

The client never returned.

What happened? In retrospect, I think I failed to register that his comments about a Black therapist focusing too much on race actually might have been a commentary on my having brought up the racial issue between us. Perhaps he was saying that he thought I was focusing too much on race. Alternatively, he may have concluded that I was uncomfortable with him as a homosexual because I did not even formulate a question about his sexual orientation.

One might well wonder why I asked about race rather than sexual orientation. I believe that I was being too concrete about myself as a White man to hear the (unconsciously) disguised reference to me as being just like a Black therapist. I think the problem in this case was not that I asked about race, but that I was not tuned in to his response to my preoccupation with race. I *was* preoccupied with race. That was an aspect of my subjectivity that was impacting on our interaction, and he reacted to this personal expression of mine with his own personal expression of discomfort. This is par for the course in therapy interactions; the only problem is that we missed the opportunity to more explicitly explore the interaction together.

This clinical vignette, and my way of understanding it, illustrates a number of points about contemporary relational psychoanalysis and its way of working with sociocultural diversity. First is the emphasis on the therapist's inevitable participation in an interaction with the client. To inquire about race is to participate in one way; not to inquire is to participate in another way. Second is the central importance in the therapeutic process of unpacking the meaning of the interaction to both client and therapist. This, in essence, is what the analysis of transference and countertransference means in contemporary relational psychoanalysis. With respect to the psychoanalytic theory of therapeutic action and technique, implicit here is the idea that the client's symptoms, or problems in living, proceed from the nature of his or her meaning-making system. Further, the exploration of this meaning-making system in an interpersonal context creates the potential for making revisions that will improve the quality of the client's life. If Laurence and I had had a chance to unpack our interaction, we would have explored why the client was uncomfortable with my inquiring about race, how he had experienced my inquiry, and how this might have reflected his interpersonal experience with people at other times in his life. My response to his reaction to my inquiry perhaps would have offered an opportunity to revise, or at least open up and make more flexible, his interpersonal schemata. In terms of projective processes, I might have heard his response about the therapist who is preoccupied with race as an interpretation of my projection onto him. That is, I was attributing to him a concern about race, and he may have been saying to me, in effect, "That's your concern, buddy!" From a psychoanalytic point of view, taking account of diversity in psychotherapy is part and parcel of the project of trying to help the client with his or her problems in living.

Some Final Thoughts on Psychoanalytic Practice

My reflections on missed appointments in public clinics demonstrate a great deal about why contemporary relational psychoanalysis appeals to me. Consider the more traditional ego psychological point of view that views missed appointments as evidence of a deficit in the client, even to the point of disqualifying the person as a suitable client for psychoanalytic therapy. This perspective, it seems to me, is quite dismissive of the client's point of view and tends toward an elitism that is not beneficial for clients and for psychoanalysis as a field. On the other hand, viewing missed appointments as a form of communication, as an effort to induce in the therapist a feeling of being abandoned—just as the client may feel abandoned by the therapist in various ways—puts client and therapist in the same boat emotionally. One might easily imagine that judging the client as lacking in some way could be a retaliatory move on the therapist's part and/or a defensive effort to shift attention away from the therapist's own vulnerability. The contemporary relational perspective that I have outlined acknowledges the shared vulnerability of client and therapist; this point of view appeals to my democratic, anti-elitist sensibility.

However, one should not dismiss the ego psychological perspective altogether. It would be going too far to claim that clients (and therapists) do not have deficits of various kinds. From a relational perspective, seeking to integrate one-person and two-person points of view, a deficit is not only a characteristic of a person; it is equally a characteristic of an interaction with another person. A client may have a generally poor tolerance for frustration as a relatively stable characteristic across various interpersonal contexts. Nonetheless, the client may have considerably more tolerance for frustration with a therapist who is sympathetic to her or his feelings of frustration than with a therapist who gets frustrated in return.

Turning to cross-cultural considerations, failure to consider the client's cultural context of meaning may be coupled with the therapist's absolutism, or assumption that his or her own culturally biased views are universally valid. In the case of Rosa, from a cross-cultural perspective, the therapist's valuation of separation and independence might seem to be skewed toward the independent side in relation to the client's values. A therapist who neglects these considerations might take her or his own values as reflecting simply the natural outcome of successful development and thus view the client's behavior as a deviation, a failure to achieve the norm or the mature state. In this connection, one can see a potential limitation of symptom-focused treatments that do not take account of the meaning-making system that forms the context of the symptomatic picture. Even such a seemingly straightforward therapeutic goal as helping Rosa succeed in school needs to consider what it would mean to Rosa to succeed in school. Otherwise, the client's resistance to the therapist's efforts would not be comprehensible in a way that points toward a further intervention. There is an advantage of a psychoanalytic therapeutic approach that looks past a symptom to the meaning of that symptom. Another advantage of psychoanalytic approaches is that they focus on conflict—that is, the full range of feelings and meanings, sometimes contradictory, that might attach to a given psychic or external event. Rosa had both independent and dependent strivings that sometimes put her in conflict around these issues. A therapeutic approach that makes room for her various contradictory feelings will give maximum scope to the therapist's empathic connection to the client.

Finally, let us turn to the question: Why psychoanalysis? Some of the advantages of a psychoanalytic approach to therapy, such as its orientation to the meaning of behavior, its attention to conflict, and its attention to the wide range of people's sometimes contradictory thoughts and feelings, have already been discussed. Let's now elaborate on some of these points, specifically with respect to diversity issues in psychotherapy.

Cultures are above all meaning-making systems. Whether Rosa goes on to college or not, whether she succeeds or not, her culture will make its impact via the meaning that her behavior will have for her and for those around her. In psychoanalysis, people's lives are enriched through increased awareness, via self-reflection, of the meaning-making activities that drive their behavior. As we saw, therapists' efforts to empathize, to enter the experiential world of their clients, depend on their awareness of their own culture and their awareness of their more personal meaning-making activities and the way they interact with the client's meaning-making activities. Cross-cultural communication is thus a special case of interpersonal communication, and both depend on the ability to tune into the world of meaning (cultural and personal) inhabited by self and other.

Perhaps the most distinctive attribute of psychoanalysis that distinguishes it from other approaches to psychotherapy is the attention paid to the process of therapy and the obstacles that arise in the course of an attempt at cure. Psychoanalysis was born, in a sense, when a hysterical client whom Freud called Anna O. claimed, falsely, to be pregnant with the child of her therapist, Josef Breuer. An alarmed Breuer referred the client to Freud and went on vacation. Freud, undaunted by a seemingly dramatic treatment failure, conceived of the idea of transference to explain what had happened. Ever since, psychoanalysis has been primarily interested in obstacles, impasses, and blind spots, along with ways to transcend them.

Evaluation of Psychoanalytic Therapy

Psychoanalytic therapists for the most part are more comfortable with idiographic evaluation of their treatments than they are with nomothetic evaluation. Psychoanalysts, especially those with an interpersonal or relational point of view, tend to view each individual client and each clinical interaction as unique. Further, those contemporary therapists who subscribe to a social constructivist point of view would argue that there is more than one valid way of understanding or describing a person, a person at a particular moment, or the nature of an interaction between two or more people. These therapists would not make a dichotomy between a subjective and an objective point of view—that is, objectivity, in the context of a contemporary psychoanalytic perspective, involves the use of one's subjective experience.

Consider how diagnosis, a potential variable in empirical research on psychotherapy, is reached. A diagnosis is reached in part through the meaning therapists make of their subjective experience of a client, in the context of the particular client-therapist interaction. For example, a client may behave in a histrionic manner with a therapist who the client experiences as unresponsive in an effort to get the therapist's attention. In diagnosing the client's character, the therapist who elicits this sort of reaction from the client may be more likely to make a diagnosis of histrionic personality disorder than a therapist who is experienced as more responsive. Of course, in making a diagnosis one takes into account a client's behavior and experience in a variety of contexts, and one can learn to take into account one's impact on people in general, thus controlling for that impact to some degree. In this way, one seeks a measure of objectivity in what is inevitably a subjective judgment about a client or a clinical interaction.[2]

Evaluation Criteria

In assessing the value of a particular treatment or a particular interaction, psychoanalytic therapists pay attention both to clients' functioning in the therapeutic interaction itself and in the outside world; it is assumed that a certain kind of behavior with the therapist may result in improvements in their clients' lives outside of therapy. In assessing a client's functioning in the world at large,

---

[2] See the recently issued *Psychodynamic Diagnostic Manual* (Alliance of Psychoanalytic Organizations, 2006) for a psychoanalytically informed approach to diagnosis.

psychoanalytic therapists pay close attention to the client's subjective experience, whether the valued experience is conceived of in terms of happiness or a sense of meaningfulness (which can entail an acceptance of unhappiness). Therapists, like everyone else, have value systems, and these values affect what they conceive of as progress in psychotherapy. One psychoanalytic criterion for successful therapy, attributed to Freud, is an improved ability to "love and work." Speaking intrapsychically, ego psychologists from Freud onward looked for the use of more mature defenses (e.g., sublimation as opposed to denial) and a more adaptive way of handling intrapsychic conflict and anxiety. Neo-Kleinian analysts tend to value the ability to tolerate negative experience, including pain and anxiety, which are conceived of as inherent in human life. In other words, from this point of view, suffering is not to be "cured" by therapy, but rather the individual is to be helped to bear suffering. Neo-Kleinians believe that people get into trouble in life mostly because of the things they do to avoid suffering (such as making other people suffer). Contemporary relational therapists, such as Stephen Mitchell (1993), look to help people achieve a sense of meaningfulness in their lives.

In practice, psychoanalytic therapists tend to value an analytic process in which the client is relatively more expressive of feelings, memories, thoughts, and the like. Expressiveness is valued not only because it produces more material for the analysis but also for its own sake. The ability to know and to express one's thoughts and feelings in words and constructive actions (as opposed to destructive acting out) is valued by most therapists. When the therapist's intervention is followed by the client's becoming more expressive, therapists tend to feel that the process is going well.

Process Research

Analytically oriented *process research* tends to focus on the therapist's behaviors that are followed by the client's being more or less expressive. For example, Weiss and Sampson (Weiss, 1993) hypothesized that clients have pathogenic beliefs and that in therapy they unconsciously test whether the therapist's behavior will or will not be in accord with these beliefs. When their pathogenic beliefs are disconfirmed, Weiss and Sampson hypothesized, a sense of safety is created that is conducive to greater openness on the part of the client. For example, a client may believe that other people cannot tolerate assertiveness. The client may assert himself or herself in some form, unconsciously to confirm or disconfirm this belief. Weiss and Sampson's (1993) research identified instances in which clients created such tests and coded the therapist's response in terms of whether it confirmed or disconfirmed the client's implicit belief. In a series of research studies, they found evidence that clients communicate more openly following therapist disconfirmation of a pathogenic belief.

Outcome Research

Outcome research of psychoanalytically oriented therapy is a complicated matter, more so than outcome research of behavior therapy, for example. First, psychoanalytic therapy is lengthier than behavior therapy, so it takes more time and resources to do psychoanalytic outcome research. Some researchers may eschew studies that take a long time because their academic achievement is based on number of publications. And when the time for psychoanalytic treatment is limited for research purposes (e.g., Paul, 1966), psychoanalytic therapists claim that their best results may not be evident in the short term. Second, selecting criteria for success is a relatively complicated matter in psychoanalytic outcome research, given that valued outcomes are difficult to specify—that is, improvement is measured in terms of subjective experiences that are more difficult to measure than the typical well-defined target behaviors in behavior therapy. Third, to the extent that a premium is placed on standardization of method and technique, outcome research tends to take place in a controlled, contrived setting that may bear little resemblance to the actual clinical situation in which psychoanalytic therapy takes place. For all these reasons, psychoanalytic clinicians tend to give relatively greater credence to the case study method, which presents the richness and complexity of the therapeutic process as revealed by qualitative data. Case studies are more valuable in generating than in testing hypotheses, which is an acknowledged limitation of this research method. At the same time, hypothesis generation is consistent with psychoanalytic treatment methodology in which therapists collaborate with clients to generate hypotheses that may be valuable in promoting self-reflectiveness in clients.

Nonetheless, some systematic and controlled outcome research has been done. In summarizing this research, Luborsky (2001) notes a lack of outcome studies comparing psychoanalytic treatments with other forms of treatment. However, he indicates research evidence that all forms of therapy show benefits to clients, that different rates of improvement between different forms of therapy tend to be nonsignificant, that both short-term and long-term therapies seem effective, and that longer-term therapies seem to be associated with more lasting improvement. Fonagy (2001) claims that there is strong evidence that longer-term therapies are more effective than shorter-term therapies and that more frequent sessions are more effective than less frequent sessions, especially for more disturbed clients.

Psychoanalytically oriented clinicians tend to be skeptical about the use of research to guide practice for many reasons. As already stated, most systematic research, for practical reasons, tends to use contrived, standardized methods and techniques, and most outcome measures focus on limited symptom relief rather than the more wide-ranging life changes and changes in subjective experience sought by psychoanalytic practitioners. Psychoanalytic therapists believe that they carefully track each client's outcome and the effectiveness of their work in the intimacy of a sustained, very personal engagement with each client as an individual. They are more cautious about generalizing their experiences from one client to other clients in the abstract.

Psychoanalytic Therapy: Blind Spots, Limitations, and Challenges

Clients' needs may be the most fundamental blind spot of a therapeutic approach that is primarily process oriented. Sigmund Freud was not always as interested in the therapeutic aspect of psychoanalysis as he was in the scientific, knowledge-gathering, and theory-building aspects. Some writers (e.g., Renik, 2002) have argued that psychoanalysts can be more concerned with the purity of their technique than with doing what is needed to help the client. To some extent, the concern with purity of technique has to do with a determination to maintain a certain notion of scientific objectivity—for example, by maintaining a reserved stance so as to avoid "contaminating" the field of observation with one's own subjectivity. Some psychoanalysts acknowledge that the client needs something other than a purist version of psychoanalytic technique and go on to modify the technique with educative, exhortatory, or behavioral techniques. Eissler (1958) spoke of these modifications as temporary measures in response to a pressing need or a deficit in the client that makes the rigors of pure psycho-analytic technique intolerable for the patient. The problem with this way of framing modifications in technique is that it portrays the resulting form of therapy as a degraded version of psychoanalysis, and the client is seen as deficient. Thus, a judgmental attitude is camouflaged by an authentic belief in the value of psychoanalytic technique.

Another blind spot is that psychoanalysts have been slow to recognize that their theory and technique can be culturally biased. For example, the Oedipal theory is based in a patriarchal family structure. The technical emphasis on the analyst's anonymity fits best with a Western European value system that esteems delay of gratification. When these biases are not recognized, a particular set of values is universalized and people who differ tend to be seen as deficient.

With the emphasis on gaining knowledge about the root causes of the client's problem, some psychoanalysts may underestimate the importance of action and initiative in the change process. Analysts and clients may go on too long hoping that unearthing the origin of a dysfunctional pattern will auto-matically result in the client's being able to develop new behaviors when, in fact, the client may need specific help in making a behavioral change. Furthermore, the focus on childhood antecedents tends to exclude the way problematic patterns may be generated and maintained in the present. It may be helpful for clients to see precisely how they keep these patterns going and to experiment with changing them both in the relationship with the analyst and in the outside world with the analyst's guidance. An intrapsychic focus may exclude or underplay the influence of interpersonal and broader social factors, such as the extent to which living in a dysfunctional family or an oppressive society can lead to behavior problems.

There is a potential for a degree of dogmatism that results from the temptation, unique to the psychoanalytic approach, to claim knowledge of the unconscious. Analysts may present their interpretations as if they are God's truths, without inviting correction or amendments from the client, who may too easily be seen as under the influence of unconscious resistance. Ironically, a psychoanalytic perspective that accepts the ubiquity of the unconscious should lead to humility and openness to blind spots at all times both in interaction with clients and in theorizing.

Psychoanalysis has limitations in that it may not be the most effective or suitable treatment for certain conditions. Specific phobias, for example, may need to be treated with exposure techniques. Frank (1999) and Wachtel (1997) have been strong proponents of including behavioral interventions in the context of a psychoanalytic treatment when needed. Panic disorder may benefit from pharmacological intervention. Major depressive and manic episodes, schizophrenic episodes and chronic schizophrenia, violent behavior, and other conditions may absolutely require pharmacological intervention.

An important limitation of psychoanalysis for students is the difficulty of studying an approach that carries with it so much historical baggage. As psychoanalytic theory has evolved, the meaning of many core concepts has changed, creating a potential for confusion for therapists in training. For example, transference once meant primarily the client's view of the analyst that was *distorted* by a transfer of early childhood schemata onto the analytic relationship. Now, to relational practitioners, transference describes the personal way the client makes meaning of the analyst's behavior, which may or may not involve a degree of distortion. The onus is therefore on students to retain the old definition as part of their understanding of the historical development of the concept while learning to shape their practice around the modern definition of the concept.

Making the therapy more affordable and more culturally relevant are the two major challenges faced by the psychoanalytic profession today. Psychoanalysis in any sort of pure or traditional form is labor intensive, thus expensive and not widely available. It is highly ambitious in terms of aspiring to character change as well as symptom relief, and so tends to take time. While some argue that long-term therapy is cost efficient in terms of lasting results, psychoanalysis is challenged to demonstrate its cost efficiency. When a psychoanalytic approach is taken into the public sector, when it is combined with other forms of treatment, or when efforts are made to use psychoanalytic principles on a short-term basis, the technique may be unrecognizable to purists.

As has been discussed, sociocultural diversity has been a psychoanalytic blind spot. To my mind, there is no more essential challenge for psychoanalysis than to attempt to uncover this blind spot and to raise consciousness about that which had been avoided. Psychoanalysts are challenged to adapt psychoanalytic theory and technique to fit new cultural groups, to find ways to develop a systematic short-term approach, and to develop approaches to the community-based work that increasingly characterizes the mental health field.

Future Development: Psychoanalytic Therapy in a Diverse World

In our multicultural modern world, in which we have come to value awareness of cultural bias, psychoanalysis has itself come under scrutiny for its own biases. This scrutiny is, however, consistent with the basic psychoanalytic value system that favors self-awareness, making conscious that which had previously operated unconsciously. If cultural bias had previously operated unconsciously within psychoanalysis, becoming aware of this state of affairs is a quintessentially psycho-analytic endeavor.

Further development of multicultural awareness will be facilitated to the extent that analytically trained therapists work beyond the bounds of private practice with economically privileged clients to engage a more diverse group of people. This will require more technical flexibility, such as being willing to see people less frequently and for shorter periods of time and for lower fees. As long as the focus of the work is on transference and countertransference and the unconscious, such work will warrant the label "psychoanalytic." Psychoanalytic consultation to case workers, case managers, and other nontherapists will also help make psychoanalysis relevant to work in the trenches in our contemporary diverse world.

Summary

1. Psychoanalysis was founded by Sigmund Freud upon his realization that some of his medical patients' problems were more psychological than physical and that patients found relief discussing such problems. Although many of Freud's ideas have been revised or discarded in contemporary

psychoanalysis, some of the concepts of classical psychoanalysis are core to the contemporary framework. In fact, Freud's psychoanalysis is the foundation of all modern psychotherapy.

2. Freud's basic theory can be usefully discussed using three models Freud developed over time. In the energic model, Freud conceived of the life drive (eros), which is the source of libido, and death drive, which is the source of aggression, to explain how the mind seeks to discharge sexual psychic energy in order to maintain a preferred state of equilibrium. In the topographic model, Freud outlined the three sections of the mind as the unconscious, the preconscious, and the conscious. In the structural model, Freud outlined the tripartite structure of the mind: the id, ego, and superego.

3. Anna Freud, Sigmund Freud's daughter, expanded upon her father's ideas about the ego, including articulation of ego defense mechanisms, and developed the branch of psychoanalysis known as ego psychology.

4. Like Freud, Carl Jung posited the existence of the conscious and the unconscious, but he added to these the concept of the collective unconscious, in which resides the history of the human species and universal models of human behavior, or archetypes, that guide our behaviors.

5. Other psychoanalysts differed from Freud in viewing psychological development as a function of the changing nature of interpersonal relations at various stages of life rather than a function of sexual and aggressive drives. Object relations theorists emphasized the way in which interpersonal relations were conceptualized in a person's mind, whereas relational theorists emphasized actual interpersonal relations in the external world.

6. Additional challenges to Freud's theories were developed by feminist and cultural/postmodern theorists, who challenged Freud's focus on patriarchal, heterosexual, and Western superiority.

7. Freud's theories reflected a Western European value system that favored objectivity and rationality. As a result, psychoanalytic theory and technique evolved in a way that made it culturally discordant with non-Western European peoples. Additionally, in North America in particular, psychoanalysis was integrated into a medical framework as a high-priced specialty, making the treatment inaccessible to most people.

8. Because Freud believed that sexual impulses were at the core of all mental life, his developmental theory involved the evolution of libido across different stages—the oral stage, the anal stage, the phallic stage, and the genital stage.

9. Erik Erikson's developmental theory broke psychological development into eight stages, each involving a developmental crisis to be resolved. The stages in Erikson's theory are infancy (trust vs. mistrust crisis), toddlerhood (autonomy vs. shame and doubt crisis), preschool years (initiative vs. guilt crisis), school years (industry vs. inferiority crisis), adolescence (identity vs. role confusion crisis), early adulthood (intimacy vs. isolation crisis), adulthood (generativity vs. stagnation crisis), and late adulthood (ego integrity vs. despair crisis).

10. Harry Stack Sullivan spoke of three categories in self-development: the good-me (those aspects of myself about which I feel good, which I am proud to own as mine), the bad-me (those aspects of myself about which I feel bad, ashamed, or guilty, but which I nonetheless own as mine), and the not-me (those aspects of myself that I disown, so that though they are mine, I refuse to accept that they are mine). The process of disavowing aspects of myself leads into projective identification in which the person projects the disavowed aspects of self to another and then acts to validate the other person's having those aspects.

11. One psychoanalytic explanation of racism is that it occurs under the influence of projective identification.

12. In classical psychoanalysis, change is thought to be brought about by first making the client aware of intrapsychic conflicts, then helping the client gain both intellectual and emotional insight about the conflict, at which point the client's mature ego can resolve the conflict. Relational analysts see the capacity to have new experiences, outside the box of the patient's limiting expectations of self and other, as the primary factor promoting change.

13. In classical psychoanalysis, the relationship between the client and analyst is primarily a source of data for the analyst's interpretations. The analyst stands outside the relationship, commenting on it and providing insight-producing interpretations. In relational psychoanalysis, the relationship is much more central. It is the arena in which processes of interpersonal and intrapsychic change can be experimented with and explored by client and analyst together.

14. Ego therapist Fred Pine pioneered the practice of psychoanalytic therapy with ethnically and socioeconomically diverse clients using ego-supportive interventions. Pine catalogued a series of ego-building interventions that included naming feelings and giving clients control over the timing and "dosage" of interpretations.

15. Psychoanalytic therapists typically prefer idiographic rather than nomothetic evaluation of their treatments, preferring to view each individual client and each clinical interaction as unique. In assessing the value of a particular

treatment or a particular interaction, psychoanalytic therapists pay attention both to the functioning of clients in the outside world and to their functioning in the therapeutic interaction itself.

16. Psychoanalysis carries with it certain blind spots, limitations, and challenges. Regarding blind spots, psychoanalysts can be more concerned with technique than client needs; they have been slow to recognizing the theory's cultural biases; and with their emphasis on uncovering root causes of client problems, they sometimes underestimate the importance of taking immediate action. As for limitations, psychoanalysis may not be the most effective or suitable treatment for certain conditions such as phobias; also, because the theory is complex and ever-changing, there is a potential for confusion for psychoanalysts in training. As for challenges, psychoanalysis needs to respond to the challenge of affordability, and it needs to be adapted to respond better to problems faced by diverse populations.

Key Terms

archetypes (p. 46)
collective unconscious (p. 46)
condensation (p. 43)
conscious (p. 43)
countertransference (p. 65)
death drive (p. 43)
defense mechanisms (p. 45)
denial (p. 45)
displacement (p. 43)
dissociation (p. 68)
ego (p. 44)
ego psychology (p. 45)
Electra complex (p. 44)
energic model (p. 42)
eros (p. 43)
free association (p. 43)
id (p. 44)
identification (p. 45)
inner world (p. 48)
internal object (p. 48)
interpretations (p. 50)

libido (p. 42)
neuroses (p. 63)
object relations theories (p. 48)
Oedipus complex (p. 44)
penis envy (p. 49)
preconscious (p. 43)
projection (p. 45)
projective identification (p. 59)
rationalization (p. 45)
reaction formation (p. 43)
regression (p. 45)
relational model (p. 47)
repression (p. 43)
resistance (p. 65)
structural model (p. 44)
sublimation (p. 45)
superego (p. 44)
topographic model (p. 43)
transference (p. 65)
unconscious (p. 43)

Resources for Further Study

Professional Organizations

The major professional organization in relational psychoanalysis is:

International Association for Relational Psychoanalysis and Psychotherapy (IARPP)
22 Cortlandt St., 20th Floor
New York, NY 10007
212-669-6123
www.iarpp.org

IARPP sponsors a major international conference every other year and a North American conference in the off years.

Classical psychoanalytic organizations include:

American Psychoanalytic Association (APsaA)
309 E. 49th St.
New York, NY 10017-1601
www.apsa.org

At this website you can learn about training programs affiliated with the association.

International Psychoanalytic Association (IPA)
Broomhills, Woodside Lane
London N12 8UD, United Kingdom
+44-20-8446-8324
www.ipa.org.uk

You can learn about the *International Journal of Psychoanalysis* at this website.

The major training institute in Interpersonal Psychoanalysis is:

William Alanson White Institute
20 W. 74th St.
New York, NY 10023
212-873-0725
www.wawhite.org

Professional Journals

The major journal in relational psychoanalysis is:

Psychoanalytic Dialogues: The International Journal of Relational Perspectives
The Analytic Press
10 Industrial Ave.
Mahway, NJ 07430
1-800-926-6579
www.theanalyticpress.com

Journal of the American Psychoanalytic Association
Available from the American Psychoanalytic Association

Contemporary Psychoanalysis
Contemporary Psychoanalysis Publication Office
The Sheridan Press
PO Box 465
Hanover, PA 17331

Suggested Readings

Adams, M. V. (1996). *The multi-cultural imagination: Race, color, and the unconscious.* London: Routledge.

Treats racial issues from a Jungian point of view.

Altman, N. (1995). *The analyst in the inner city: Race, class, and culture through a psychoanalytic lens.* Hillsdale, NJ: The Analytic Press.

The author's clinical experiences, and theoretical reflections, from his experience of 11 years at a public clinic in the South Bronx.

Aron, L. (1996). *A meeting of minds: Mutuality in psychoanalysis.* Hillsdale, NJ: The Analytic Press.

A clearly written history of the relational movement in psychoanalysis, with the theory and its clinical implications well spelled out.

Kovel, J. (1970). *White racism: A psychohistory.*

A classic study of race from a classical psychoanalytic point of view.

Mitchell, S. A., & Black, M. J. (1995). *Freud and beyond: A history of modern psychoanalytic thought.* New York: Basic Books.

A very accessible history of contemporary developments in psychoanalysis written by two of the leaders in the field. Written for both a professional and a general readership.

Perez-Foster, R., Moskowitz, M., & Javier, R. A. (Eds.). (1996). *Reaching across boundaries of culture and class: Widening the scope of psychotherapy.* Northvale, NJ: Aronson.

A collection of articles on issues of diversity in psychoanalytic psychotherapy.

Roland, A. (1996). *Cultural pluralism and psychoanalysis: The Asian and North American experience.* London: Routledge.

An effort to apply psychoanalysis cross-culturally with specific reference to Asian and North American cultures.

Chapter 4

Adlerian Therapy

JON D. CARLSON AND MATT ENGLAR-CARLSON

Alfred Adler (1870–1937) was a contemporary of Sigmund Freud and, during a 10-year period, Adler and Freud were colleagues in the Psychoanalytic Society in Vienna. As you will learn in this chapter, Adler's thinking intersected with, but then diverged from Freud's. We begin the chapter with an overview of Adler's basic ideas and then consider the development of Adler's theoretical perspective in the context of his life and times. In the second part of the chapter, the discussion turns to Adlerian therapy as it is practiced in today's diverse world.

The Individual Psychology of Alfred Adler is based upon a holistic, phenomenological understanding of human behavior. Adler used the word *individual* in the name of his approach in order to emphasize the indivisible (undivided or whole) nature of our personalities. The Adlerian focus on *holism* means that one cannot understand an individual in parts (reductionism), but all aspects of a person must be understood in relationship. Furthermore, individuals can only be fully understood in connection to social systems (Mosak, 2005). The phenomenological perspective of Adlerian psychology suggests that each person views situations from a unique point of view. We live our life and act "as if" our view of the world is correct. When our views are distorted, our thinking becomes faulty and our behavior becomes inappropriate. Adlerians believe that all behavior has a purpose and occurs in a social context, noting that one's cognitive orientation and life-style (literally, one's style of dealing with life) are created in the first few years of life and molded within the initial social setting, the *family constellation*. Adler coined the term *life-style* to mean the characteristic way that we act, think, and perceive, and the way we live. It is from the life-style that we select the methods for coping with life's challenges and tasks.

Adlerians believe that all behavior is goal directed. People continually strive to attain in the future what they believe is important or significant. Adler believed that for all people there are three basic *life tasks:* work, friendship, and love-intimacy. The work task is addressed when work is meaningful and satis-fying. The friendship task is addressed through satisfying relationships with others. The love or intimacy task is addressed by learning to learn to love oneself as well as another. Adlerians have outlined three additional tasks, suggesting a need to master the recreational and spiritual tasks of life (Mosak, 2005) and also the task of parenting and the family (Dinkmeyer, Dinkmeyer, & Sperry, 1987). Mentally healthy people look to master each of these tasks, or challenges of life.

Adlerian theory maintains that humans are all social beings and therefore all behavior is socially embedded and has social meaning (Watts, 2000a). As one of the first models of psychotherapy, Adler's theory emphasized the importance of relationships, of being connected to others. A hallmark of Adlerian theory is the emphasis on *social interest*, which is a feeling of cooperation with people, a sense of belonging to and participating in the common good. Social interest can be equated with empathy for others, and Adlerians view social interest as a measure of mental health, noting that as social interest develops, feelings of inferiority decrease.

Adlerian psychotherapy is a psychoeducational, present/future-oriented, and time-limited (or brief) approach (Carlson, Watts, & Maniacci, 2006; Watts, 2000a). Adlerians espouse a growth model, noting that our fates are never fixed and that individuals are always in the process of "becoming." Adlerians believe that the person experiencing difficulties in living or psychopathology is not sick, but rather *discouraged* (Mosak, 2005). Psychopathology is a result of mistaken notions and faulty assumptions, low social interest, discouragement, and ineffec-tive life-style. The task of psychotherapy then becomes one of encouraging the client to develop more social interests and a more effective life-style to achieve success in the tasks of life.

Origins and Evolution of Adlerian Therapy

Alfred Adler was a physician, educator, best-selling author, and practical philosopher. Adler's life was one of many contrasts. Though trained as a physician, he became a psychologist and educator as well as an early pro-feminist and skilled public speaker. Adler believed in personal freedom, social responsibility, and the rights of children, women, and workers. While alive, he was more popular than Freud, though over time Freud's fame has far surpassed Adler's. For example, Adler's first book of popular psychology, *Understanding Human Nature*, was a huge success, selling over 100,000 copies in the first six months. This is in contrast to Freud's best-selling book of the time, *The Interpretation of Dreams*, which sold around 17,000 copies over a 10-year period. Now Freud is largely viewed as the founder of modern psychotherapy, yet recently there has been a growing appreciation and understanding of the vast influence of Adler's theories and practice on modern psychotherapy and counseling. Adler's psychological and developmental concepts, such as the inferiority complex, power trips, power conflicts, control, life tasks, life-style, goal-oriented behavior, and social interest, have all entered the common lexicon. Adler's theories and insights into the human personality serve as the foundation of today's most prominent theories of psychotherapy, including many that you will read about in this book: person-centered therapy, existential therapy, cognitive therapy, rational emotive behavioral therapy, reality therapy, and family therapy. In many ways, Adler could be considered the grandfather of modern psychotherapy.

Alfred Adler was born on February 7, 1870, near Vienna, Austria. His parents were Jewish and his father worked as a corn trader. Young Alfred, the second of six children, was not a healthy child. He was subject to frequent bouts of a respiratory disorder and vitamin deficiency, and he almost died from pneumonia at the age of 4. If this was not enough, he was run over twice on the Vienna streets. Academically, Adler struggled in school, was required to repeat a grade level, and was encouraged to enter a trade as an apprentice.

These early experiences with feeling helpless must have led Adler to think about a person's internal sense of inferiority or superiority. Coupled with his father's encouragement, these experiences served as catalysts that moved Adler toward studying medicine. At medical school, Adler studied ophthalmology and then neurology. It is not surprising that he chose to study how people view the world before studying neurology. He gained medical experience working at the Poliklinik, a free medical clinic that served the poor, and he was also drafted for two tours of military service. As a medical student, Adler became interested in philosophy and politics and was drawn toward the socialism of Karl Marx. At the end of the 19th century in Europe, the other prevailing political ideology was nationalism, but there was little room for those of Jewish origin within that movement.

As a socialist, Adler was less interested in economics than in the ways society affects individuals. He became active in the labor movement, advocating on behalf of curtailing dangerous labor conditions for the working poor and suggesting improved housing and a limit on the number of work hours allowed during the week. His first book, *Health Book for the Tailoring Trade*, criticized the labor and living conditions of the workers and their families. When Adler opened his first medical practice specializing in nervous diseases, most of his patients were working-class people.

Adler married Raissa Epstein in 1897, and she clearly had a major influence on his life. Hoffman (1994) noted that Raissa was a strong thinker in her own right as a socialist and early feminist and that she maintained her political activities throughout her marriage to Adler. Among her friends were Leon and Nathalia Trotsky, who soon became close family friends. Raissa, the couple's socialist friends, and the socialist intellectual circles in Vienna had considerable influence on Adler's ideas. Yet Adler was actually more of a humanist than a socialist. Whereas he supported socialist ideas to improve the living conditions of the poor, he also believed in the potential within individuals to change their own lives. He believed education and skill training, rather than revolution, would make it possible for people to solve their problems and live life in a more satisfying fashion. He had a passionate concern for the common person and was against all forms of prejudice (Carlson, Watts, & Maniacci, 2006).

Much has been made of the meeting between Adler and Freud in 1902, their time spent in the Psychoanalytic Society, and their subsequence acrimonious parting in 1911 (Handlbauer, 1998). In 1900, Adler wrote a strong defense of Freud's *Interpretation of Dreams*, and later Freud invited Adler to be the fifth member of his Wednesday night psychoanalytic circle (Mosak & Maniacci, 1999). Adler was already established at this time and thus viewed himself as more of a colleague than a student. Adler's relationship with Freud lasted 10 years before their parting. This separation highlighted the stark differences in these two men in terms of their own development and approach to treatment. Whereas Freud was primarily concerned with biological factors and psycho-sexual development that influence a person's behavior, Adler took a holistic perspective. Freud was deterministic in his thinking, but Adler viewed people as essentially goal directed, with the capacity for being creative and responsible for their own choices. Adler's views diverged from Freud's by placing more emphasis on social, familial, and cultural forces as opposed to biological drives. Adler placed less emphasis on the role of unconscious, infantile sexuality and emphasized social drives over sexual ones.

In 1911, when Adler was president of the Psychoanalytic Society, the growing differences became too much, and Adler and Freud parted ways. Though Adler and Freud attempted reconciliation, it failed. Adler, along with one third of the members of the Psychoanalytic Society, went on to form the Society for Individual Psychology. This was a significant moment in the history of psychotherapy. An alternative school of thought had now been established that acknowledged biological influences *and* social and cultural influences on personality. Further, because of Adler's own experiences with working and "common" people, his model emphasized ethical and practical solutions (Bankart, 1997). Interestingly, Adler's ideas about equity and humanity are compatible with the current ethical guidelines of both the American Psychological Association and the American Counseling Association that relate to treatment regarding issues of race, gender, ethnicity, social class, and sexual orientation (Carlson et al., 2006).

Adler went on to serve as a doctor in World War I and then established 30 child guidance clinics in Austria that were staffed by volunteer psychologists. He became active in school reform, childrearing practices, and public family education. Adler escaped his homeland just before the outbreak of Nazi domination and immigrated to the United States in 1935. For years prior to his immigration, Adler's ideas were becoming well known; he was a premier lecturer and author worldwide, but particularly in the United States. During his lectures, he would give live demonstrations of parenting techniques to crowds of thousands.

Adler chose New York as a base for his clinical and lecturing activities, and he spent the latter part of his life promoting his theory, eventually recruiting others (Ansbacher & Ansbacher, 1956; Dreikurs, 1967) to carry on his work. Adler and Raissa had four children, two of whom followed their father into psychotherapy and practiced in New York City for many years. Their eldest daughter, Valentine, lived in Russia and was politically active like Raissa. She was arrested for her position on social justice, and it was reported that she perished in a Russian gulag. Many speculated that Alfred Adler's heart was broken when he heard of her death. He died shortly thereafter of a heart attack while lecturing in Scotland in 1937.

Adler's early writings up to and during World War I focused primarily on abnormal human behavior and seem rather psychoanalytic in tone. However, following World War I, Adler became more interested in normal human behavior and progressively developed his mature theory, which is more holistic, phenomenological, and socially oriented than psychoanalytic theory. Contemporary Adlerian psychology and psychotherapy, as well as subsequent developments by later Adlerians (e.g., Rudolf Dreikurs), are primarily based on Adler's later period.

Adler was ahead of his time. Kottler (2002) noted that many of Adler's important contributions to current practice might seem rather obvious because they have formed the basis of so many other theories. Adler was the first to incorporate into psychotherapy the relationship between thinking processes and feelings; the impact of early family experiences and birth order on present behavior; the value of constructing specific plans of action; the construction of an egalitarian, collaborative counseling relationship (including having the client and counselor face each other); an assessment of life-style and social behavior as they affect personality development; and the importance of skill training and an educational model of treatment. As previously mentioned, Adler was quite involved in the social rights movements of his day. He advocated for school reform and sex education and was a vocal leader in equal rights for women. Adler proclaimed that he wasn't concerned about people remembering his name in association with his theories; he was more concerned that his theories would survive (Mosak, 2000).

Rudolf Dreikurs founded the first Adler Institute in Chicago as a way to introduce Adler's ideas to emerging psychology professionals, who primarily only knew traditional psychoanalytic thinking. Adler's children, Kurt and Alexandra, created a similar center in New York City. Each of these training institutes nurtured the growth of Adlerian psychology at a time when the dominance of Freudian ideas—and the fact that Adler was often branded as a traitor to the master's original teachings—made this difficult. Although Adler did indeed directly contradict the orthodoxy of Freudian theory, he was consistent in crediting Freud with promoting the role of early childhood experiences, bringing attention to the meaning of dreams, and suggesting that symptoms served some useful purpose (Mosak & Maniacci, 1999). Dreikurs, who shared Adler's vision of child guidance centers, went on to make a considerable impact with his books on childrearing, *Children: The Challenge* (Dreikurs & Stoltz, 1964) and *Discipline without Tears* (Dreikurs & Cassell, 1972). Dreikurs was also instrumental in popularizing Adler's principles within the education system. These principles included encouragement, individual responsibility, democratic rules, social awareness, and the use of natural consequences rather than punishment (Pryor & Tollerud, 1999).

After Dreikurs died in 1972, the Adlerian movement lacked a charismatic leader to continue advancing the theory. There were many competent modern Adlerians such as Don Dinkmeyer, Harold Mosak, Bernard Shulman, and Bob Powers, but there was no one person that could unify the Adlerians as Alfred Adler and Rudolf Dreikurs had. This was a time when Adlerians were undecided about whether to adhere to the original words and theories of the leaders for direction or to pick up where Adler and Dreikurs left off by continuing to adapt and advance the approach in accordance with modern therapeutic practice and mental health trends. Eventually, Adlerians did address the evolution of modern Adlerian theory, as we see in the next section.

Context Then—Context Now

Although Adler was ahead of his time, he was nonetheless limited by the historical era in which he lived. He endured many personal and professional hardships, not to mention discrimination because of his Jewish and Hungarian heritage. Adler lived during a time when Europe was experiencing intense debate about political and social ideologies, ethnic and cultural conflicts, and longstanding historical rivalries, all of which contributed to World Wars I and II. The movement from autocracy to democracy in social life was underway, and Adler found himself at the forefront. He realized that people raised in an autocratic system needed skills to learn to live as equals. Although many believed in the concepts and ideals of democracy, Adler felt, they did not know how to treat one another in a democratic or equal fashion. Men talked down to women, adults to children, bosses to employees, and rich to poor. Inequality based on ethnicity, race, and religion abounded. To make a difference, Adler concentrated on helping parents and teachers educate children effectively. He believed that by changing these basic relationships it would be possible eventually to transform the entire society.

The world of counseling and psychotherapy has changed considerably from the time when Adler was developing his theories. One way to understand the developmental path of psychotherapy has been to view the waves of influence, starting with the psychodynamic approaches as the first force, followed by the second-force models that emphasized cognitive and behavioral theories and interventions, and the third force of existential-humanistic models, and the current recognition of multicultural and systemic models as the fourth force (Seligman, 2001). Viewed in this larger context, the Adlerian model does not fit neatly into any one force, but is more like a chameleon, adapting its "colors" depending on the background of the client and the presenting concern. Though Adler clearly influenced other contemporary psychotherapy practices, some scholars still ask the question, "So what? Is Adlerian counseling useful for today?" (Watts, 2000a).

In many ways, Adlerians have struggled with the issue of relevancy over the last 30 years. In 2000, I (J.C.) asked Adlerians what they wanted to be in the world of contemporary psychotherapy, "Astronaut or Dinosaur? Headline or Footnote?"(Carlson, 2000, p. 3). In recent years, it seems that most Adlerians have chosen to be a continued presence in contemporary psychotherapy. Adler's theory of Individual Psychology is enjoying tremendous popularity because many writers (see Carlson et al., 2006; Carlson & Slavik, 1997; Dinkmeyer & Sperry, 2000; Watts, 2003; Watts & Carlson, 1999) have adapted the original theory to a variety of other applications and settings, each of which puts the original ideas in a fresh package. The *Journal of Individual Psychology* has many articles showing how Adler's ideas can be used in treating a wide variety of clients and problems in numerous settings. Further, authors have explored how Adlerian theory can be used to support clients of various racial and ethnic groups (Carlson & Carlson, 2000; Chung & Bemak, 1998; Herring & Runion, 1994; Kawulich & Curlette, 1998; Perkins-Dock, 2005; Reddy & Hanna, 1995; Roberts, Harper, Tuttle Eagle Bull, & Heideman-Provost, 1998; Roberts, Harper, Caldwell, & Decora, 2003), spiritual and religious backgrounds (Baruth & Manning, 1987; Cheston, 2000; Ecrement & Zarski, 1987; Ellis, 2000; Johansen, 2005; Kanz, 2001; Mansager, 2000; Mansager et al., 2002; Noda, 2000; Watts, 2000b), and other marginalized groups (Chandler, 1995; Hanna, 1998; Matteson, 1995). Keep in mind, however, that some Adlerian therapists still practice the classical form of the therapy today.

One of the ways that Adlerians have remained contemporary is by recognizing how aspects of Adler's original model are theoretically consistent with modern psychotherapy, which in many ways has moved away from allegiance to single theories of personality and change and has readily adopted integrative theoretical models. Clearly, Adlerian psychotherapy fits well within the contemporary integrative zeitgeist of psychotherapy. As Dinkmeyer and Sperry (2000) indicated, "there is increasing interest in emphasizing the commonalities and converging themes among psychotherapy systems" (p. 9), and psychotherapy integration is the prevalent focus among many psychotherapy theorists, researchers, and practitioners. Adlerian therapy is both integrative and eclectic, clearly blending cognitive, psychodynamic, and systemic perspectives while having considerable common ground with postmodern approaches such as constructivist, solution-focused, and narrative therapies (Watts, 2000a).

Most important, for any approach to be considered a relevant psychotherapy for contemporary society, it must successfully address multicultural and social equality issues. It is fitting that Adler developed his original theories and model while campaigning for the social equality of women, contributing to the understanding of gender issues, speaking out for the rights of working-class and poor people, and addressing the rights of minority groups. Within that context, many practitioners of Adlerian therapy were addressing social equality and the use of a contextual framework for understanding people long before multiculturalism became a dominant force in counseling and psychotherapy (Watts, 2000a). Arciniega and Newlon (1999) noted that the characteristics and assumptions of Adlerian psychology are congruent with the cultural values of many minority racial and ethnic groups, and they affirmed that the Adlerian therapeutic process is respectful of cultural diversity. In its continuing efforts to train students to be socially focused and responsible practitioners, the Adler School of Professional Psychology in Chicago has recently updated its curriculum to further highlight larger social issues such as poverty, violence, and discrimination. It appears that Adlerian therapy is alive, well, and poised to address the concerns of a contemporary global society. As Mosak (2005, p. 63) noted, "The Adlerian is not interested in curing sick individuals or a sick society, but in reeducating individuals and in reshaping society."

The Authors' Journeys as Adlerian Therapists

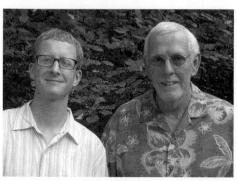

Matt Englar-Carlson and Jon Carlson

Two of Alfred Adler's children (Kurt and Alexandra) became well-known Adlerian psychologists and kept Individual Psychology alive following Adler's death. Rudolf Dreikurs's daughter Eva also became an Adlerian psychologist and continues to build the theory. Adlerian psychologist Don Dinkmeyer's son Don, Jr., followed in his footsteps and promotes the Adlerian model. With a legacy like that, is there any surprise that this chapter would be written by a father and son? Following is a short reflection on our journey and how we embraced Adlerian ideas.

Jon begins:

In graduate school at Southern Illinois University, I learned behaviorism, which was the Zeitgeist current in the mid-1960s. I was not introduced to Adler's works until I was already working as a counselor. My mentor, Don Dinkmeyer, Sr., thought that I should take classes at the Alfred Adler Institute in Chicago. At that time there were Adlerian training centers around the world, but the Chicago Institute, founded by Rudolf Dreikurs, was thought to be the finest. I lasted four classes before I walked out, vowing to never return. For a young behaviorist like me, the Adler Institute seemed like a cult. The students were asking themselves, "What do I believe?" and in many ways seemed more like the patients we were reading about than the practitioners we were hoping to be.

Upon completing my doctorate at Wayne State University, I accepted a position at Governors State University. When I looked for a postgraduate clinical training opportunity, I contacted Gene Gendlin at the University of Chicago and he suggested that I go to the Alfred Adler Institute! Go figure. I began training and within a couple of years had finally grasped Adler's brilliance. During my second go-around with the Adlerians, I was able to see how practical these ideas were with my clients, and I also saw them work with my own family. The philosophy was democratic, positive, and allowed me to use the best of the other approaches that I had studied. I became editor of *The Individual Psychologist*. This publication turned into the *Journal of Individual Psychology*, and my stint as editor turned into 17 years of service.

We moved from Chicago to Ft. Lauderdale and then Honolulu before returning to the Midwest. I returned ten years later to what is now the Adler School of Professional Psychology and completed a Certificate of Psychotherapy (essentially becoming an Adlerian analyst) and a Psy.D. in Clinical Psychology.

I have written from an Adlerian perspective for many years and tackled many topics such as teaching, parenting, couples therapy, consultation, sports psychology, psychopathology, wellness, and health psychology using an Adlerian lens. Yet I also know that many Adlerians are pragmatic and would rather be helping others than writing or doing research. I suppose I am not too different. I have maintained a private practice for over 40 years; I have spent 30 of those years also working as a school counselor/psychologist; and I have conducted hundreds of parent education classes as well as marriage enrichment seminars in my local community and on the national and international stage.

My wife and I found Adlerian ideas useful in the raising of our five children. We enjoyed the numerous challenges the children posed because they forced us to use our creativity. Adlerian ideas were practical and allowed the children to learn how to live in a social world. We practiced logical consequences, provided

(*continued*)

encouragement, and held family meetings. One of my favorite memories of Adlerian parenting in action involved Matt and mowing the lawn:

It was 10:00 p.m. when I finished my last therapy session for the day. I was excited because the next morning at 4:00 a.m. the family was going up north for a weekend of adventure at my brother's northern Wisconsin cabin. As I pulled into the driveway of our home, I noticed that the lawn had not been mowed, which was 10-year-old Matt's main chore. When I came into the house, Matt greeted me with a big smile and pointed to his packed clothes and fishing equipment. I smiled back and said, "I see you've decided not to go up north." Puzzled, Matt said, "No, I plan to go and even have all my stuff ready." I replied, "The lawn needed to be mowed before we go, and you didn't do it." Matt listed all of the reasons (i.e., excuses) why he had not done his job. I replied, "No matter, that was your choice. If the lawn is mowed, you can go."

A few hours later, Matt had duct-taped a flashlight to his baseball hat and was mowing the lawn. Three hours, a few phone calls from the neighbors, and many mosquito bites later, Matt announced he was ready to go. We left in the dark, but the next morning the neighbors gathered around to look at the strange zigzag way the lawn was mowed.

Matt continues:

Yes, I remember the nighttime lawn mowing and the family meetings; in fact, we actually had a family meeting and voted about having another baby in the family! As a child, I knew all about logical consequences, choices, and family meetings on the receiving end, but I didn't know conceptually what my parents were doing. An amazing light bulb experience occurred for me when I was a graduate student at Pennsylvania State University when I had to read *The Parent's Handbook: Systematic Training for Effective Parenting* (Dinkmeyer et al., 1997) for an elementary school counseling course. As I read the book, my childhood flashed before my eyes. I realized that I really didn't need to read the book because my own childhood had taught me the ideas already. In a nutshell, that captures a large portion of my journey: I learned about and knew Adlerian concepts before I ever read an Adlerian textbook or chapter.

When I teach this theory to students, I start the lecture by saying that I was born and raised Adlerian. For me, that meant learning at a young age about social and gender equity. It meant always being encouraged despite the circumstances I was in. It meant understanding that the "whole person" counts, so I trained my mind, body, and spirit. Though I am technically the second born of five children within my family constellation, psychologically and contextually I considered myself the youngest (there is a 10-year gap between my next siblings and myself). The youngest child often struggles to outperform the oldest child, or with encouragement from parents works on charting a new path. I was more of the latter, which maybe is why at the age of 18, I was ready to move to California to start some new adventures. I am the only one of my family of origin not living in Wisconsin.

As a graduate student and psychotherapist, I have not always been specifically drawn to Adlerian ideas. Much of my training occurred in a context that has valued more integrative approaches. I was initially trained in cognitive-behavioral therapies in a master's program in health psychology, followed by two years of training in child multimodal therapy. I then became a voracious learner of narrative and social constructivist therapies while gaining more understanding of culturally appropriate therapies. Over time I have gained a greater appreciation of object relations and existential therapies. Yet at my core, I have always known that Adler made sense to me. A common experience for me, and for other Adlerians, was learning about other therapies and what made them distinct, only to have a reaction and moment of insight along the lines of "Didn't Adler originally say that?" I suppose I have come to realize that as a school of psychotherapy the Adlerian approach may be the most integrative of them all. Further, the Adlerian framework did not require a substantial revision in order to be inclusive for all people—it always has been a theory for everyone.

Now I think that I have come full circle and tend to embrace the Adlerian model. As a scholar and practitioner, I am most interested in gender and social justice issues. What has always resonated with me the most about Adler was his sensitivity to the greater whole of society and his ability to advance social and political issues. I find not only my own mental health, but also that of my clients, to be directly traceable to the personal level of social interest. In today's world of globalization, with vast inequalities in social and economic opportunities and the difficult task of making sense and meaning of the world, it seems that building social interest is a gift Adler has left us.

Now that I am the father of a toddler, once again I realize the utility of Adlerian parenting ideas. Some of the same phrases that come out of my mouth are the identical ones my parents used with me. I am encouraged to see that when my son does not get the outcome he wants, he looks at me and says, "Try again? Try again?"

Theory of Adlerian Therapy

The following concepts provide the foundation for how an Adlerian therapist understands human personality and conceptualizes a client's concerns. Taken together, the concepts form a checklist of those areas that Adlerians consider most critical in their work with clients.

Holism

A central assumption in Adlerian theory is that every person is unique and greater than the sum of his or her parts. Individual Psychology as a concept stresses unity within a person and encourages looking at people as individuals, not as a collection of parts or part functions (e.g., id, ego, drives, emotions, etc.). Adlerian theory proposed **holism,** the notion that understanding a person and her or his behavior necessitates a consideration of all of the components that make up the personality as well as the entire environment in which the person lives.

Rather than looking at polarities (e.g., mind and body, conscious and unconscious, cognition and affect, approach and avoidance, etc.), Adlerians look at the interaction of these components and how clients put them to use. Polarities are only important as subjective experiences of each person (Mosak, 2005). The mind and the body are viewed as interconnected and cannot be understood when considered separately. For example, an Adlerian would look at the "organ jargon" of a client. Organ jargon provides a framework for understanding clients who exhibit physical symptoms, whether or not the symptoms are predominantly organic (Griffith, 2006). It connotes the connection between the physical, emotional, and psychological. Adler (Ansbacher & Ansbacher, 1956) commented that physical symptoms "speak a language which is usually more expressive and discloses the individual's opinion more clearly than words are able to. . . . The emotions and their physical expressions tell us how the mind is acting and reacting" (p. 223). Thus an Adlerian might view a man with a rash as having something emotional "under his skin" that needs to be expressed.

The Adlerian assumption is that a person is unified in action, thoughts, feelings, convictions, attitudes, and so on, and that all of these expressions of uniqueness reflect the person's plan in life to reach self-selected life goals. Adler defined **life goals** as strivings that are not only beneficial to the person, but also beneficial to others. Each person is connected to social systems and interpersonal relationships that interact in a system of reciprocal influence. Regardless of cultural background, each person functions as a member of various groups in daily living (Miranda, Frevert, & Kern, 1998).

The clinical implication is that an Adlerian counselor would look at the "whole person" when doing an assessment. In Adlerian terms, this means exploring the client's world from a holistic perspective that takes into consideration biological, psychological, and social factors.

Encouragement

Encouragement is one of the key words in Adlerian therapy and refers to the process of increasing a person's courage in order to face the difficulties in life.

People can be encouraged or discouraged (Ansbacher & Ansbacher, 1956; Dreikurs, 1967). Encouraged people are willing to take risks and do things that lead toward growth. Because they perceive the world as a benign place, they are willing to risk being wrong because being wrong is not a threat to their **self-concept** (i.e., the sum total of all of the beliefs about "who I am") and **self-ideal** (i.e., ideals about how the world and people should be; Carlson et al., 2006). Discouraged people view the world as a hostile place. Therefore they do not take risks; they become rigid with their convictions and do not look for growth opportunities. For Adler and Dreikurs, psychopathology represented **discouragement,** the feeling of not belonging in a useful or constructive manner. Discouragement can come from within, such as from disturbed cognitions, or from without, from adverse life circumstances and conditions (Ferguson, 2001).

Dreikurs (1967) noted that people's concerns and difficulties in life are based on discouragement and that without "cncouragement, without having faith in himself restored, [the client] cannot see the possibility of doing or functioning better" (p. 62). Thus discouragement from family members, parents, peers, and society can contribute to problems in life by lowering one's self-esteem and self-worth and contributing to feelings of inferiority. Adlerian counselors teach their clients that although they cannot change the past, they can change their attitudes about the past. For many clients, this can be a freeing revelation because the past and their place in it can now be reconfigured in more self-fulfilling ways.

Encouragement serves as a therapeutic stance and technique to initiate change. "In every step of treatment, we must not deviate from the path of encouragement," Adler stated (Ansbacher & Ansbacher, 1956, p. 342). Clients gain courage when they become aware of their strengths, and at the same time they feel less alienated and alone. Encouragement is a process of focusing on a person's resources and giving positive recognition in order to build a person's self-esteem, self-concept, and self-worth (Dinkmeyer, McKay, & Dinkmeyer, 1997). For parents, encouragement means stressing the positive and letting children learn from disappointment. It means recognizing any positive movement, having positive expectations, and valuing children for who they are. Adlerians believe that all children need encouragement and that building children's self-confidence is the best way to promote their development. Children with confidence and courage will meet whatever problem lies ahead as something coming from within that they can alter and control (Carlson et al., 2006). Pampered, overprotected, and physically sick children have their self-esteem undermined by overhelpful adults. This has to be corrected. "Don't do things for children that they can do for themselves" is a helpful rule.

Encouragement begins with acknowledging that life can be difficult and instilling faith in clients that they have the potential to change. As much as possible, the counselor can adopt a positive, optimistic position in order to balance the often greater attention that the client places on distressing life problems. This also includes looking at existing successes and positive resources available to the client.

The emphasis on encouragement can be particularly useful and appropriate for members of populations that have histories and experiences of being marginalized and oppressed in the United States and elsewhere. Many people in the United States experience constant discouragement at the individual, community, and societal level because of prejudice and discrimination associated with gender, race, and ethnicity; sexual orientation; social class; and immigration status. In many ways, entire populations are discouraged and made to feel powerless and invisible in the United States. Within that context, the use of encouragement and acceptance can be an extremely validating and supportive process with sociopolitical ramifications for both the client and the therapist.

Subjective or Private Logic

Freud based his theories on biology and instinctual determinism. Adler thought that Freud's view was too narrow, that people are not merely determined by heredity and environment, but have the capacity to interpret, influence, and create events. Heredity and environment serve as the "frame and influence" within which people work to create their lives. Taking a phenomenological stance, Adlerians look at the individual way that a client perceives the world. Ultimately people have the capacity and choice to grow (Ansbacher & Ansbacher, 1956). Each person creates his or her own reality. This process is uniquely subjective and private rather than objective and universally agreed upon. Foreshadowing the development of cognitive interventions, Adler believed that any experience can have many different possible interpretations, depending on the way a person chooses to look at the situation (Carlson et al., 2006). According to Carlson and Sperry (1998), the realization that individuals co-construct the reality in which they live and that they are also able to question, deconstruct, or reconstruct reality for themselves is a fundamental tenet not only of Adlerian psychotherapy but also of other constructivist psychotherapies.

One's subjective reality includes perceptions, thoughts, beliefs, and conclusions. Adler was significantly influenced by the philosopher Hans Vaihinger's book, *The Philosophy of "As If,"* which emphasized that human cognitive processes serve a purposeful, instrumental, and functional significance for survival and activity in the world. Adler drew upon Vaihinger's work for the notion of *fictions*, or subjective thought constructs that, although not necessarily corresponding with reality, serve as useful tools for coping with the tasks and problems of living. Adler (1931/1992) noted:

> Human beings live in the realm of *meanings*. We do not experience things in the abstract; we always experience them in human terms. Even at its source our experience is qualified by our human perspective. We experience reality only through the meaning we ascribe to it: not as a thing in itself, but as something interpreted. (p. 15)

One's life-style is built upon deeply established personal beliefs or constructs that are referred to as private logic. **Private logic** is composed of ideas developed in early childhood, which may or may not be appropriate to later life. Simply stated, Adlerians believe that you are what you think (Carlson et al., 2006). As people develop, they form ideas about right and wrong based upon subjective personal experience. For example, if early experiences were painful, one may develop mistaken ideas or **faulty logic.** It can begin when a child cannot find a healthy way to feel significant within the family. To achieve some sort of significance, the child learns that the only way to get attention is to act out in useless, negative ways, such as throwing temper tantrums and misbehaving. Even if the attention they receive is painful, for most children, any kind of attention is better than no attention at all. The private logic behind children's attention-seeking behavior is the belief that they do not count or are not important, and that they need to be noticed by others to be somebody. If children develop the faulty logic that the only times they will be noticed by others is when they misbehave, then misbehavior becomes their style of seeking attention even into adulthood.

For Adlerian counselors, subjective and private logic means it is more important to understand a client's perception of past events and how this interpretation of early events has a continuing influence in the client's life. How life is, in reality, is less important to an Adlerian than how an individual client believes life to be.

Life-Style

The Adlerian construct of personality is called the **life-style** or style of life. Unique to each person, life-style is an individual's attitudinal set that includes the basic convictions, choices, and values that influence decisions and behaviors (Ansbacher & Ansbacher, 1956; Shulman & Mosak, 1988; Stein & Edwards, 1998). The life-style describes the individual and that which is created collectively, which are strongly influenced by one's cultural surroundings (Frevert & Miranda, 1998). Life-style is the characteristic way one moves toward life goals and strives for superiority. Created in early childhood within a social context, life-style serves as a blueprint for coping with the tasks and challenges of life. In terms of multicultural counseling considerations, Reddy and Hanna (1995) noted that the Adlerian notion of life-style lends itself to the conceptualization of both the individual and the collective, which is a crucial aspect of effective multicultural counseling. Adlerian theory then emphasizes the influence of subjective individualized psychological processes in the formation of life-style within a homogeneous description of one's culture (Miranda & Fraser, 2002).

Children are also influenced by factors outside the home (Powers & Griffith, 1987). The role of peers, school personnel, neighbors, coaches, friends and their families, and other community and cultural institutions needs to be considered. For many children, the first significant contact with adults other than their parents happens when they go to school and meet teachers. These factors need to be assessed as well, and they often provide clues to understanding the nuances of the life-style.

Adlerians believe that the style of life is fixed at about 5 years of age (Ansbacher & Ansbacher, 1956). Because Adlerian theory is a growth model, Adlerians believe that life-style tends to undergo some refinement throughout life, although for the most part the core life-style remains stable. One way that a person's basic convictions (i.e., the rules governing how to belong) can change is if a therapeutic event occurs. This event does not need to be actual therapy, and often it is not. For example, a man who believes he is unlovable can have a therapeutic-like conversion if he finds someone who loves him.

There are numerous cultural and contextual factors that also influence the development of life-style. Frevert and Miranda (1998) used life-style to conceptualize the effect of migration and immigration on psychological adjustment. For example, they noted that a fifth-generation Mexican American may be exceptionally different from a recent immigrant from Mexico because of acculturation and extended contact with the host culture.

Life-style serves many purposes (Carlson et al., 2006). First, it is a guide to help a person navigate and make sense of life. Life-style is also a limiter of what any one individual will do or not do. For example, imagine a responsible and focused man with a mild-mannered personality. Mild-manneredness limits the range of responses he will master and demonstrate in certain situations. If he were involved in a minor car accident, it would be out of character for him to either leave the scene of the accident or aggressively attack the other driver with a verbal or physical assault. He would not think of it, or even necessarily know how to be irresponsible or violent. Second, life-style provides security and a sort of rhythm to life. As we go through the processes of meaning making and value creating, we need structure and guidance, but we also need predictability and regularity. Our life-style allows us to develop habits—in other words, habitual responses that do not need cortical control. We do not have to think about it, we just respond to events in our habitual way. Thus the life-style can be viewed as the overarching set of rules ("rules of the road") for how humans prepare themselves for life's contingencies (Mosak & Maniacci, 1999). Because Adlerians believe that all behavior is goal directed, once we understand clients' life-styles we can begin to make sense of their experiences, or at the very least, to help them to make sense of their experiences for themselves. One way to understand life-style is to look at how an individual approaches the life tasks of love, friendship, and work.

Life-Style and Emotions

For Adlerians, emotions serve the life-style; they do not interfere with it (Dreikurs, 1967). People do not experience emotions that disrupt their styles; rather, they create emotions in order to facilitate their styles. By knowing the client's life-style, a therapist can see how the client's emotions are being used in service of her or his life-style (Carlson et al., 2006). For instance, anger can be used to push people away or coerce others to submit. Apathy can be used to create power because if people do not care about anything, it is difficult to control them. Love is an emotion generated when people want to move toward something forcefully. Someone whose dominant motive is attachment to others will love people. Another person who has a dominant motive of security will love safety. Adlerians have proposed a number of life-style types. The following are among the most common (Ansbacher & Ansbacher, 1956).

1. *Ruling.* The ruling individual is dominant in relationships. There is a lot of initiative toward others but little social interest in others. This is someone who has to be the boss.

2. *Getting.* These individuals expect things from others and are dependent on them. Little initiative and social interest are shown. They are happy as long as they get what they want.

3. *Avoiding.* These individuals shy away from problems. As with the getting life-style, people with avoiding life-styles show minimal social interest or concern for others. They believe "nothing ventured, nothing lost" and attempt to avoid contact with others and their problems.

4. *Driving.* Individuals with a driving life-style want desperately to achieve. It is a matter of either total success or total failure, with nothing in between. Achievement may result, but at the expense of others' interests.

5. *Controlling.* Such individuals enjoy order, but it must be *their* order. A great deal of activity is expended toward keeping things predictable and avoiding surprises. Social interest is minimal because others in the system are constantly disrupting the controlling individual's plans.

6. *Victimized.* This person feels like a martyr and makes decisions that keep him or her trapped in a victim role, pursuing problems in a self-destructive fashion. The individual lacks social interest and is deeply discouraged.

7. *Being good.* The individual satisfies his or her sense of superiority by being more competent, more useful, more right, and "holier than thou." Heightened activity and interest characterize this club, to which very few can belong.

8. *Being socially useful.* The individual cooperates with others and contributes to their social well-being without self-aggrandizement. Activity and social interest are both significant and constructively directed.

Some Adlerians might use a *life-style inventory* (Kern, 2002) to assess and explore life-style with clients. A life-style inventory will examine a client's connections and roles with siblings and other family members. A life-style assessment will also include the gathering of **early recollections.** Early recollections are the earliest discrete memories (before age 10) an individual can recall. Adlerians believe that people retain these memories as summaries of their current philosophy of life, and thus early recollections can be used to help interpret current behavior.

It is important to reinforce that cultural considerations are crucial in assessment of life-style. If life-style may be determined based on connections with others in and outside the family (Frevert & Miranda, 1998), then life-style assessment needs to be guided by the cultural beliefs and norms of clients to gain an accurate understanding of the clients within their environment. For example, for many African Americans self-identity is related to a wide support network that includes family and friends. Perkins-Dock (2005) suggested that the Adlerian approach is effective for working with African Americans because it explores and accepts "significant others" as part of the family support network.

Basic Mistakes

Basic mistakes are the self-defeating attitudes and beliefs of an individual's life-style. Adlerians believe that people are not so much upset by things and other people as they are upset by the ways they themselves choose to think. Basic mistakes represent examples of cognitions that can be disputed and changed. Basic mistakes often reflect avoidance or withdrawal from others, excessive self-interest, or the desire for power. Mosak (2005) lists five of the more common basic mistakes.

1. *Overgeneralizations.* "There is no fairness in the world," or "Everyone hates me."

2. *False or impossible goals.* "I must please everyone if I am to be loved. Only when I am perfect will people love me."

3. *Misperceptions of life and life's demands.* "Life is so very difficult for me," or "Nobody can enjoy life in Chicago because it is so windy."

4. *Denial of one's basic worth.* "I'm basically stupid, so why would anyone want anything to do with me?"

5. *Faulty values.* "I must get to the top, regardless of who gets hurt in the process."

Core Fears

One additional area in which Adlerian theory has been especially helpful is identifying and addressing core fears. An Adlerian lens can be used to examine the most common fears presented by clients. Those that have been identified most often include the following (Dinkmeyer & Sperry, 2000; Shulman, 1973).

- *Fear of being imperfect.* It is one of our deepest, darkest secrets that each of us is a fraud, hiding our imperfect real selves behind our public facades. Adlerians help their clients to become aware of this phoniness and develop the ability to be truly authentic by embracing who they are.

- *Fear of being vulnerable.* The more we authentically and honestly reveal our thoughts, the more likely it becomes that others will discover what we do not know. We spend our lives pretending to know and understand far more than we really do. With complete genuineness we gain intimacy, but with intimacy we risk rejection. Adlerian therapists create safe settings where clients can honestly share how they think and feel. Clients can learn to be authentic and honest without the fear of being rejected.

- *Fear of disapproval.* Everyone wants to be loved and appreciated almost all the time. Though that might not possible, it appears to be an eternal search. The more people risk connecting with others and showing their true selves, the greater the risk of being hurt. Adlerians help clients realize that it is impossible to please "everyone" and besides, there are many people by whom one may not want to be loved or appreciated.

- *Fear of responsibility.* We all make mistakes in life, some of which we regret. It is easy to think, "If I only could have done things differently. If I only could start over." Adlerians help their clients to choose to move on and stop suffering from past regrets.

Basic Life Tasks

Adlerians believe that the questions and challenges of life can be grouped into major **life tasks**. Adler identified the first three as coping with the problems of social relationships, coping with the problems of work, and coping with the problems of love. Think about it this way. What are the issues that couples generally fight about and bring to therapy for resolution? Most often they are disputes over children, money, and sex, which are variations of the themes that Adler originally identified. Other theorists added two more tasks: coping with self (Dreikurs & Mosak, 1967) and understanding existence (Mosak, 2005). These "existential" dimensions made the Adlerian theory of life tasks more robust because they made space for looking not only at personal issues but also at their meaning within a larger social context. Finally, the tasks of coping with parenting and the family (Dinkmeyer et al., 1987) were added. Even after all the decades since these ideas were developed, there are still precious few frameworks that embrace so many valuable ideas. According to an Adlerian, being healthy means having mastered all of the basic life tasks. Struggles occur with failures in any of the areas. When clients come to therapy, it is often because of difficulties with one or more of the basic life tasks. The goal of therapy often becomes helping clients modify their life-styles to navigate a task more successfully.

Social Interest

Adlerians believe that all individuals have a responsibility to the community, as well as to themselves. **Social interest** is an Adlerian term that is used to measure people's concern for other people. Actually, social interest is an inadequate translation of *Gemeinschaftsgefühl*, the German word used by Adler. The word is more meaningfully translated when broken down into its parts. *Gemein* is "a community of equals," *shafts* means "to create or maintain," and *Gefühl* is "social feeling." Taken together, Gemeinschaftsgefühl means a community of equals creating and maintaining social feelings and interests—that is, people working together as equals to better themselves as individuals and as a community.

Rather than connoting a desire to be "social," the Adlerian term *social interest* is defined as a sense of belonging and participating with others for the common good. It includes the notion of striving to make the world a better place. As social interest develops and increases, feelings of inferiority decrease. Adlerians consider social interest so important that it is often used as a measure of mental health (Carlson et al., 2006). Murderers and others with antisocial personalities would, of course, be seen as having low social interest, as would anyone who is unduly selfish. Adler believed that therapy could play an important role not only to help clients resolve their individual difficulties but also to develop greater concern and compassion for others. Paradoxically, developing greater compassion for others also helps clients resolve their individual problems.

Social interest affects the life-style. When we have social interest, we find our place in life in a way that is good for all (Carlson et al., 2006). Social interest could be viewed as evolving in three stages. The first stage is based on the notion that everyone is born with the potential for cooperation and social living, but one's capacity to feel successful and connected to others is strongly shaped by the parent-child bond and relationships within one's family constellation. At the second stage, the aptitude for social interest has developed into a rudimentary ability to express social interest through social cooperation in various activities. In the third and last stage, one's ability has built to the point where one can integrate social interest into multiple aspects of one's life-style.

Social interest may also be influenced by cultural identity. The Adlerian concepts of an interest in helping others, contributing to the social community, and social belonging support the cultural value system of many African American families (Boyd-Franklin, 1989b; Parham, 2002; Perkins-Dock, 2005). Miranda et al. (1998) studied the mental health of Latinos by looking at the social interest levels of three groups of Latinos: those who were highly acculturated to mainstream U.S. culture, those who were not acculturated, and those who were strongly bicultural and retained connection to beliefs and practices of the native and host cultures. They found that bicultural Latinos had higher levels of social interest than both the Latinos low in acculturation and those high in acculturation. They posited that bicultural Latinos had higher levels of adjustment and were more self-efficacious during the acculturation process because of connections with the host and native communities.

Compensation for Inferiority

Even the most confident of people experience feelings of inferiority some of the time. Inferiority feelings are global, subjective, and evaluative; generalizations that tend to be held onto despite evidence to the contrary. Occasional feelings of inferiority can serve as catalysts, motivating us to strive harder to reach our goals. We see this often in the sports world. For example, the Olympic track star Wilma Rudolph had polio as a child and was never supposed to walk, let alone become the world's fastest woman. The Olympic and major league baseball player Jim Abbott was born with only one arm. He compensated and became a dominant pitcher. However, an **inferiority complex**—an ongoing sense of feeling inferior—can cause an individual to feel discouraged, dispirited, and incapable of proactive development.

Birth Order and the Family Constellation

Today we take it for granted that birth order affects the ways a person develops, but Adler (Ansbacher & Ansbacher, 1956) was among the first to observe that sibling position might be a critical variable to consider. Thus he incorporated the concept of **birth order** into his work. According to Adler, the eldest child does not grow up in the exact same family, nor have the exact same parents, as the younger brothers and sisters. With their firstborn, parents are relatively insecure and unskilled. And for a while at least, the firstborn is the only child in the family. With younger siblings, the parents are more relaxed and knowledgeable, and, of course, younger siblings never experience being the only child. Adlerians have made considerable use of the concept of birth order in their clinical work. Before going any further, however, an important distinction needs to be made. Shulman and Mosak (1988) noted two ways of looking at birth order: (1) ordinal position, the actual order of birth of the siblings, and (2) psychological position, the role the child adopts in her or his interactions with others. Adlerians are interested in the psychological position. Each person interprets his or her place in the family differently. Individuals develop a style of relating to others in childhood and carry this into their adult interactions.

Adlerians discuss five psychological birth order positions: only child, oldest born, second born, middle child, and youngest born.

- *Only child.* Only children never have to share their worlds with other siblings. They grow up using parents (or significantly older siblings) as models. Hence, they tend to be perfectionists who are used to having their way. They set their goals exceedingly high and tend to prefer polite distance from people.

- *Oldest born.* Oldest borns are used to being number one. They are used to doing things independently. They are in charge and like being that way. Oldest borns tend to be analytical, detailed, and methodical; they overvalue control, sometimes expecting unrealistic perfection. It is for this reason that eldest children may have a tendency to try to do what is right. By the time subsequent offspring arrive on the scene, parents have calmed down a bit and have learned they do not have to monitor their children every single moment. This results in the second, middle, or youngest children developing in ways that are different from those of their older siblings.

- *Second born.* Second borns play the teeter-totter game with oldest borns—when one goes up, the other goes down. If the oldest is good in math, the second will typically choose to ignore math and focus upon areas that the oldest ignores, such as sports. Just as this occurs with academic subjects, it also happens with personality traits. Second borns tend to be rebellious, independent, and dislike order. They are responders rather than initiators like their oldest born siblings.

- *Middle child.* Middle children are diplomats; they are people pleasers who dislike conflict but desire fairness and justice for all. They often feel squeezed by their siblings and complain that they receive neither the rights and privileges of oldest borns nor the pampering and attention of youngest borns.

- *Youngest born.* Youngest borns are frequently excitement seekers who crave stimulation and are masters at putting others into their service. They are used to having things done for them, and they know how to play people's emotions quite well. Additionally, youngest borns can often become the most ambitious in the family; feeling so far behind, they desire to catch up to the older ones to prove they are no longer the babies.

The social context of childhood includes both the context of culture and the **family constellation** (Adler's term for the psycho-sociopolitical organization and structure of the primary family group). When considering a client's family constellation, the therapist pays attention to birth order, the individual's perception of self, sibling characteristics, and parental relationships. Children learn about their role within the family and see how their family and others occupy and navigate the world, and thus tend to model their life-style upon these early perceptions and relationships.

Clearly, cultural considerations are important when looking at a person's family constellation. Because the notion of family varies across cultures, Adlerians take steps to define the family constellation based on the client's concept of family and community. Because parenting roles may be shared with grandparents and other adult relatives, adults outside the family, and older siblings, it is important to look at how the client defines her or his family constellation.

Theory of Change

Adler firmly believed that change was both possible and desirable in all people, thus Adlerian therapy optimistically stresses the potential of growth in each client. This suggests that at any given time, each person is at a phase of growth and development. Whereas Adlerians do emphasize the influence of biology and the importance of experience in early childhood, the Adlerian model has more of a "soft" determinism approach, "which is the notion that clients have conscious choices, probabilities, possibilities, and influences, not causes. Whereas Freud was interested in facts, Adler was interested in clients' beliefs about facts" (Sapp, 2006, p. 109). This notion suggests that clients are always in the process of becoming. Adlerians eschew the medical-model orientation to maladjustment and embrace a nonpathological perspective. Clients are not viewed as sick (as in having a disease) or mentally ill, and are not identified or labeled by diagnoses. Because Adlerian theory is grounded in the growth model of personality, clients are viewed as discouraged rather than sick. Therefore, the process of change in

Adlerian therapy is not about curing a client, but rather about encouraging a client's growth and development (Mosak & Maniacci, 1999).

For most clients, the main question is, What needs to be changed? Adlerian therapy is structured to help clients understand how they have a part in creating their problems and they can take responsibility for their behavior. Further, it posits that often one's problems are related to faulty thinking and learning. But ultimately the client can assume responsibility for creating change (Mosak, 2005). When **mistaken goals** are revealed, clients can choose to pursue more appropriate goals with vigor and courage (Carlson et al., 2006). Mistaken goals are goals that are detrimental to others, such as those that run counter to social interest.

The change process in therapy begins with the creation of a positive therapist-client relationship. A good therapeutic relationship is a "friendly one between equals" (Mosak, 2005, p. 69). Adler believed that the client and therapist needed to collaborate in order for change to take place. To emphasize equality, Adler was the first therapist to come out from behind the couch and directly face the client.

In Adlerian therapy, the change process breaks down as follows (Carlson et al., 2006).

1. Through therapy clients can learn about mistaken goals. Once aware of these goals, clients can decide either to change or not to change. Throughout this decision-making process, the relationship between the therapist and client should be one of mutual respect.

2. By knowing their mistaken goals, clients can recognize patterns in motivation and as a result can develop insight. During this process, encouragement helps clients change their behavior.

3. Because the new behaviors may work better in new situations than old behaviors, the client may replace old private logic with a new common sense.

4. As their new common sense grows, clients may show more social interest. More social interest often results in a greater sense of belonging.

5. Feeling a sense of belonging can mean feeling equal to others, which has the effect of being even more encouraged. As this develops, clients feels more confident about their place in the world.

6. Because clients feel better about things, they may take more risks because they are less concerned about making mistakes. The clients have gained the courage to be imperfect.

Thus, in Adlerian therapy change is a process that develops over time. Like a balloon, encouragement fills clients up with hope, expectancy, and the courage to act. Throughout this process, clients are gaining new insights and trying new behavior. Change is bound to follow.

Practice of Adlerian Therapy

Thus far, we have discussed a series of concepts that are central to the Adlerian approach to helping people. The next question we will consider is, How does one apply these ideas to actually doing therapy? A good way to understand Adlerian therapy as a process is to follow a case example. In the remainder of this chapter, we will follow an example of Adlerian counseling in action that looks at both the conceptualization of a client and the many ways in which an Adlerian might intervene. We will initially present the case study details, and later on we will use examples and dialogue from this case to discuss the way an Adlerian constructs the stages of therapy and to highlight different therapeutic interventions.

Antonio Gonzales came to therapy at the request of his wife Rita, to whom he had been married for five years. A third-generation Latino man of Mexican heritage, Antonio had been very unhappy for several months. He willingly completed several assessment inventories that provided background information on his family of origin, life-style, and level of happiness.

By his own report, Antonio came from a "dysfunctional" family. His parents never divorced but did not live together. He was actually raised by his grandfather while his twin brother was raised by his grandmother. The grandparents lived in the same city, but they maintained separate homes so that the brothers grew up attending different schools and seldom saw one another. His grandfather's neighborhood was "not an easy place to grow up." As a teenager, Antonio managed to avoid legal problems but was frequently involved with fights, vandalism, and petty crime. In spite of average grades in high school he was able to enroll in a small private college. He managed to graduate with an accounting degree, although he realized later that he would have really preferred a career in social work. Antonio appreciated all that his grandfather did for him. He worked hard and managed to provide for all Antonio's needs. He and Antonio attended the local parish Catholic Church and were active in the neighborhood social club. When his grandfather died just after his marriage to Rita, Antonio felt as though he no longer had a family. He resented his grandmother and parents for abandoning him and had nothing to do with them or his brother.

Antonio's wife Rita was Latina, also of Mexican heritage, and was very close to her family. They lived on the East Coast so she only saw them once or twice a year, although they talked daily on the phone. Rita had one younger sister, a college student who was also close to the family. Antonio liked Rita's family but had a hard time getting close to them. He found them boring and dull although they were successful and very religious. He felt like they were "better" than he was and couldn't believe that Rita would have ever agreed to marry him.

Both Rita and Antonio worked for the same large accounting firm. Rita was a star and was being promoted at a very rapid rate. Antonio had yet to be promoted and believed that he couldn't advance because of racial discrimination. Rita believed this was just an excuse because she was also Mexican and was not being limited by race. Although it was never determined whether Antonio had actually experienced some racial discrimination, the different views of Antonio and Rita had been causing friction in their marriage and hampered their ability to talk about their work. Further, with Rita's most recent promotion, her salary was now twice that of Antonio. The couple had one child who attended child care at the firm. Jorge was a happy 2-year-old boy and the pride of both his Mom and Dad. They were planning to have more children and discussed the possibility of Antonio's staying home and taking care of the children.

In Antonio's first interview, he expressed being angry and troubled recently. He hated his job and the "poor treatment" he had been receiving. Antonio taught the religion class for adolescents at his church and seemed to really enjoy working with young people. He said he would like to quit his job and go back to school to become a social worker. Rita told him that he should do this, but he didn't seem to be willing to make any changes.

Antonio provided the following early recollections.

> Early recollection 1. "I was 4 years old and I remember there was an ice cream truck going by my house. I really wanted ice cream but just stood and watched it. I remember the bells ringing and the pictures of kids eating ice cream on the side of the truck. The most vivid part was feeling empty as the truck passed me by."
>
> Early recollection 2. "I must have been in first grade, so I was 6 or so. The teacher was picking kids to be the captains for our recess kickball game. I was the best player so I was sure she would select me. She never even looked my way as she picked Paul and Fred. The most vivid part was my sad feeling and thinking that I would not play then, but I am sure I did. It just hurt."
>
> Early recollection 3. "I was 6 or so and we were playing on the playground. Somebody kicked the ball to me and I caught it. When I kicked it back a little kid ran in front of me and the ball hit him so hard he was knocked down and started to cry. I said I was sorry, but no one believed me. The most vivid part was seeing the look on the other kid's face when I was trying to explain that I did not mean it. I felt hurt and all alone."

> T (Therapist): Do you see any pattern or similarity among the three recollections?
>
> C (Client): They seem to be situations where things didn't work out very well for me.

T: Could the pattern be that, "No matter what I do, things never work out the way I want them to"? The goodies in life pass you by, you are the best player but not picked, and no one believes your story.

C: [His eyes become full of tears.] Nothing seems to work for me.

T: I am confused. I thought you had a beautiful and successful wife. A healthy and handsome son. Good health and an okay job. Even your in-laws like you!

C: But not the important things. Why can't I be successful at my job? Why don't I have more friends? Why can't I do what I like doing? I don't even have a family.

T: Although many important things are going well, there still are some big hurts and voids that need to be addressed.

C: Where do you think would be a good place to start?

Although Antonio felt like a total failure, the therapist's encouragement helped him begin to recognize that he might only be a failure in some areas. The therapist also hoped that this reframing would help Antonio to see his problem from a different perspective—that when these feelings occur, he shuts down and lets opportunity pass him by. Antonio acknowledged that this was happening at work. When things didn't go the way he hoped, he would "cop an attitude and piss off everyone in the office." In a subsequent interview with Antonio, the therapist decided to teach him some anger management and relaxation skills.

C (Client): I am just so tense all the time. I get angry at the drop of a hat. Rita says that I need to learn to chill and learn to be calmer . . . especially at work.

T (Therapist): What have you tried to do to help yourself calm down?

C: I try not to react, but that never helps. I thought about taking a yoga class, but I don't have the time.

T: Many people have found that meditation can help to reduce both anxiety and anger. It has something to do with the frontal lobe of the brain. Is that something that might interest you?

C: I would rather do that than take pills like the doctor suggested.

T: Would you be able to free up the first 15 minutes of the day?

C: Sure. Rita usually gets up with Jorge.

> T: Find a quiet place where you can sit in a chair. Begin to focus on your breathing. Breathe in slowly and deeply. As you inhale, say "I am," and when you exhale, say the word "calm." Say it in your mind and not out loud. When you find that your mind has wandered off to other thoughts, just let them go and come back to "I am" . . . "calm."

This was a beginning for Antonio. Other strategies employed by Antonio's therapist follow shortly.

Therapy Stages

The first thing someone new to Adlerian therapy should know about it is that it proceeds in a series of logical, progressive stages. The four stages of Adlerian therapy are as follows.

Stage I: The Relationship

The first step in any therapy encounter is to establish a collaborative relationship. This is an empathic, supportive relationship, one that is based on democratic principles and essential equality. The therapist uses all the standard skills favored by any other professional at this stage, such as well-timed questions and reflections of feeling and content, in order to build a solid alliance. As with most other approaches, it is now considered standard operating procedure to use empathy and support to establish a sense of trust. If that doesn't happen first, subsequent therapeutic efforts are likely to be less than successful.

Stage II: Assessment

In the next stage, the therapist conducts a comprehensive assessment of the client's functioning. This occurs through a combination of inventories, such as a life-style inventory and a clinical interview. In a life-style inventory, the therapist gathers information about how the client is seeking to belong in the social world of family, school, work, friends, and marriage. In this assessment a thorough history is explored, including family background, belief systems, cultural heritage, personal goals, and other facets of being human. The client's basic beliefs are often uncovered through information on the family constellation and the client's early recollections. Client beliefs will also be reflected in the person's current convictions, attitudes, and priorities.

To elicit early recollections, the therapist would ask the client, "I would like to hear about some early memories. Think back to a time when you were very young, as early as you can remember, and tell me something that happened one time. Be sure to recall something you remember, not something you were told about by others." There are three criteria for useful early recollections. First, the early recollection must be a single, one-time event that has a narrative. Second, it must be visualized by the client. Third, two elements must be clearly articulated: the most vivid part of the recollection and how the client felt during the recollection. Generally, eight to ten early recollections are gathered.

Other questions asked during the assessment phase are listed here. As you review each of these basic questions, you might consider asking them of yourself or perhaps discussing them in small groups.

1. *Family constellation.* "What was it like for you growing up?" "What roles did you play in your family?"

2. *Social relationships.* "To whom are you closest?" "What is most satisfying to you about your friendships?"

3. *Work life.* "How do you feel about your job?"

4. *Sexuality.* "What are the most and least satisfying aspects of your sexual relationship with your partner?"

5. *Sense of self.* "How do you feel about who you are and the ways you have developed?"

Of course, in addition to these specific Adlerian-based inquiries, clients would be asked the sorts of questions that any therapist would bring up in a session with a new client regardless of the therapist's theoretical orientation. The goal is to efficiently and quickly gather background information and assess preliminary expectations.

During the assessment stage in Adlerian therapy, the focus is on the person in her or his social and cultural context. Adlerian therapists do not try to fit clients into a preconceived model. Rather, they allow salient cultural identity concepts such age, ethnicity, life-style, and gender differences to emerge in therapy, and then they attend to a client's individual meaning of culture. Adlerian therapists emphasize the value of subjectively understanding the unique cultural world of the individual. With clients from racial or ethnic minorities, subjectively understanding an individual's culture allows the therapist to assess the importance of a macro view of the client's ethnicity within the micro view of the client's individuality. This provides the opportunity to assess acculturation and racial identity within the client's life-style. This can also assist the therapist and the client in identifying culturally specific strengths that may be overlooked in the client's premature judgments (Carlson & Carlson, 2000).

Stage III: Insight and Interpretation

In the third stage, the Adlerian therapist interprets the findings of the assessment in order to promote insight. A therapist might say something like, "It seems like life is unfair and you believe that you can't do anything to change this situation." This, of course, is not just a simple reflection of feeling and content, but rather a confrontation of sorts insofar as the client is asked to examine the validity of the belief in his or her complete powerlessness. Even if the world does sometimes appear to be unfair, is it really true and accurate that you are absolutely powerless?

Adlerian therapists assist clients in developing new orientations to life, orientations that are more fully functioning. For example, although clients might believe that they can't do anything about a particular problem in their lives right now, they can come to realize that they have been successful at dealing with other challenges, many of them far more difficult. A therapist might challenge a client about the client's negativity: "You say that you are powerless with your husband, but I've noticed that you regularly stand up to your parents, your boss, and your children. I wonder what the difference is to you?" Adlerian therapists also try to find out what clients believe they have done wrong in life. For example, a young woman begins counseling believing that if she were more perfect in appearance and behavior, then others would love her even more. She works very hard at doing everything she possibly can to appear fashionable and well groomed; she has a whole library of etiquette books to guide her behavior. Although this may seem like a reasonable self-development plan, it actually makes her rather difficult for others to be around. She doesn't seem to understand that one of the things that makes people attractive to others is not their perfection but their imperfections. Real people make mistakes and have problems. They also have the courage to face their problems. She needs to understand how her quest for perfection and closeness is actually creating distance and contempt from others. A key approach to Adlerian therapy, as it is for the cognitive therapies, is to identify the thought disturbances and core fears that get in the way. In the third stage of therapy, Adlerian therapists are inclined to explore with clients their self-defeating thinking patterns that contribute to distorted perceptions (Mosak & Maniacci, 1999).

Stage IV: Reorientation

Once clients develop sufficient insight into their problems, the therapy shifts to action. Insight can be a wonderful thing, but only if it leads to constructive movement toward desired goals. Sue and Zane (1987) suggested that therapeutic methods of problem resolution must be consistent with a client's culture. In other words, a therapist's goal for a session should be compatible with that of the client. An Adlerian works with the client to create interventions that are culturally and personally congruent.

Because the Adlerian approach is both insight oriented and action oriented, the therapist should not be shy in helping clients to convert their self-declared goals into specific homework assignments or tasks that can be completed between sessions. Adlerian therapists will give specific assignments that involve responding in a different fashion. If a couple is not taking responsibility for their marriage, taking it for granted and not spending quality time together, the therapist might suggest that they plan a "date" together. The therapist might also suggest that the clients do outside reading (i.e., bibliotherapy; see Carlson & Dinkmeyer, 2003) to learn about ways to strengthen their relationship and that they complete weekly structured activities to work on their relationship.

Throughout every step in the process, a collaborative, supportive relationship is used as leverage to keep the client motivated and continuing to making progress. In reorientation, or moving from insight to action, the client is helped to make new choices that are more consistent with desired goals.

One of the things Antonio learned in therapy was that he wanted a career shift. Before therapy, he was aware of these thoughts but was not able or ready to accept them and attempt guided action toward a new career. At the reorientation stage, he was ready for movement.

> T (Therapist): You say you don't really like accounting and would rather be out in the world helping others.
>
> C (Client): I know I say that. I really like helping others but there is no money in that work. I think I can help others through volunteer work.
>
> T: What have you been thinking about?
>
> C: There are lots of things that I can do at church. They are always looking for coaches at the YMCA.
>
> T: So you think that would allow you to feel better by helping others. So what about your job?
>
> C: I don't mind accounting as long as I could be my own boss and make some more money.
>
> T: Can you think of a way to make that happen?
>
> C: I suppose I need to go to school. The people that are getting promoted seem to have master's degrees.
>
> T: Do you need to start an MBA program or something?
>
> C: It is funny you mention that because I have thought that would be a really good idea and they just announced that they are having an MBA cohort group starting right at the company.

The first step in the reorientation stage is to identify clearly what it is that the client wants most. These goals must be realistic and reasonable. A client might say that she wants to have more love in her life. The therapist's next task would be to help her to pinpoint just what it would mean for her to have more love. For one person, it might mean more friends, for another it might mean more dates or perhaps a deeper relationship with a current partner. Through this process the therapist can help the client develop goals that are achievable. Almost any problem-solving method that the client and therapist come up with might be used to create a plan of action.

At this point in the therapy process, the Adlerian practitioner may appear more like a coach or teacher than a therapist. The goal is to help clients to acquire the necessary skills and behaviors to create new patterns in their lives. These behaviors must also be consistent with their life-styles, as defined earlier.

Let's look further at an example of this process in action. A woman comes to counseling with the stated goal of losing weight. "If only I could lose 20 pounds," she explains, "my marriage would be so much better."

"What do you mean by that?" the therapist presses. "How would losing 20 pounds improve your marriage?"

She looks embarrassed, but finally the woman says, "Then my husband would no longer call me lard ass."

Even though it is fairly obvious that the problems she is experiencing in her marriage are hardly connected exclusively to her weight and are far more likely the result of dysfunctional patterns in the couple's communication, the therapist accepts her initial definition of the problem at face value—at least until such time that an alliance can be formed. It is often good policy to avoid challenging clients' inaccurate conceptions of their problems too early.

The therapist and client together devise a structured program in which she works out on a treadmill and adjusts her eating habits. Over time she increases her daily workouts and decreases the calories she consumes. Eventually, of course, her loss of 20 pounds changes very little in the way the couple relates to one another. Instead of calling his wife, "lard ass," the husband just ridicules her in another way. The next step is to get both partners into therapy for some couples work that will allow for direct intervention at a deeper level. This could not have happened earlier in the treatment, not until such time as it could be established that the client's loss of 20 pounds would not really fix the problem (although it has done wonders for the woman's self-image).

Therapeutic Strategies

Throughout the therapeutic stages that have just been described, Adlerians employ a number of unique strategies and techniques. Many of these methods have been borrowed by other approaches, just as contemporary Adlerian therapists use strategies from compatible systems.

Encouragement

Encouragement skills include demonstrating concern for clients through active listening and empathy; communicating genuine respect for and confidence in clients; focusing on client strengths, assets, and resources; helping clients generate alternatives for maladaptive beliefs; helping clients see humor in everyday experiences; and constantly focusing on effort and progress (Ansbacher & Ansbacher, 1956; Carlson & Slavik, 1997; Dinkmeyer & Losconcy, 1980; Watts, 2000a). Put more simply, this strategy means building "courage" in your client. Courage emerges when people become aware of their strengths, feel they belong, and have hope. "I really like that you took time this week to read the meditation book, spent 20 minutes each day in meditation, and drank water in place of alcohol. You have made great progress on your goal of being a more relaxed person." The therapist tells the client exactly what positive things he or she did so that in the future the client can do his or her own self-evaluation.

For Antonio, encouragement was crucial, because he talked as though he had a low opinion of himself.

> T (Therapist): I have listened to you tell me that you are not very successful at work.
>
> C (Client): I don't think that I am.
>
> T: You told me that they have let many people go over the last six years, and yet you have been there for eight years and are not worried about being terminated. You must be doing something right.
>
> C: I guess that I do okay work. At least I get things done on time.
>
> T: It sounds like you are reliable, dependable, and responsible? Those are impressive qualities.
>
> C: I guess I am, but it is hard for me to see.

Reframing

Reframing is a process of helping a client see the same thing from a different perspective. It is a technique commonly used by other kinds of therapists, as you will learn in later chapters. For the Adlerian, the intervention is aimed at helping people to understand that "everything can really be something else."

The therapist might say to a despondent client:

T (Therapist): It seems like your wife doesn't love you because she has been working overtime to get away from you. I wonder if there's another way to look at this?

C (Client): What are you saying? [The client seems confused by the challenge.]

T: I'm just suggesting that there might be other reasons why your wife is not as available as you would prefer—and that this might not necessarily be related to avoiding you, or not loving you.

C: You mean, like, to earn more money?

T: Exactly! You've said before that you have complained to your wife about the financial pressure you are under. Isn't it just possible that one reason she is working all those extra hours is because she does love you and wants to help as much as she can?

Through reframing, clients are helped to look at their situations in more positive ways.

Asking "the Question"

The question is: "What would be different if your problem was gone?" This strategy is used to determine what purpose a problem has in a client's life, for example, the client may be obtaining special treatment or attention from others because of her or his problems. It is also used to determine whether a problem is primarily physiological or psychological. In that case, the question might be phrased more specifically. For example, the therapist might say to a client who has a substance abuse problem: "How would your life be different if you did not do drugs?" The answer will help to determine an area of treatment. The client might say, "Then I would have a good job and somewhere to go." The therapist then realizes that in order to break up the pattern of substance abuse, he or she must help the client to find somewhere meaningful to go each day.

The Push-Button Technique

This technique is used to highlight the control clients can have over their emotions. It is based on the notion that behind each feeling there is an underlying cognition. Simply stated, change the cognition and one can change the emotional reaction. The client is asked to remember a pleasant experience and then an unpleasant one. The therapist helps the client to realize that he or she acts and thinks one way in one situation and a different way in another. It goes like this: "I'd like you to imagine that you have two buttons on your chest. Each button is for a different response. Now picture that however you might respond in any situation, you actually have a choice to push the other button and respond in a very different way. These buttons belong to you. Only you can push them. Only you can choose how you want to respond."

For Antonio, the push-button technique was used to help him learn to respond differently to work situations that made him angry.

> C (Client): I just get so angry at work when I am criticized or not included.
>
> T (Therapist): Yet there are other times, like at church, when you are really calm and focused.
>
> C: Yeah, but what does that have to do with anything?
>
> T: Can you imagine having two imaginary buttons on your chest? One button makes you act like you do at work and the other button makes you act like you do at church.
>
> C: I can picture that.
>
> T: So can you imagine yourself at work, and instead of pushing the work button, you push the church button? Remember, you know how to do both.
>
> C: So you want me to act like I do at church when I'm at work?
>
> T: What do you think would happen if you did that?
>
> C: I would probably get along better with everybody.

Acting As If

This strategy involves suggesting to clients that they act as if they didn't have the problem for a week or two. This pretend exercise allows the client to take actions that previously would have seemed outside the realm of possibility. "For this week," the therapist might say to Antonio, "I want you to act as if you are a good employee. I know that is not the way you have seen yourself until now, nor the way you have been viewed by many others. But just as an experiment, I'd like you to pretend that you really are a good worker. What would that mean?"

Antonio shrugs.

> T (Therapist): Well, how do good employees behave? How do you know one when you see one?
>
> C (Client): I don't know. I guess they show up on time, for one.

T: Good! What else?

C: They seem happy. They do what they're told.

T: What else?

C: I guess most of all they don't have to be told what to do; they just do it on their own.

T: So you know how to *pretend* to be a good worker. Try on this role for a week and see how it fits.

For Antonio, one of his key concerns was class difference. He was aware of his working-class background and his wife's more affluent background. He was also aware of himself as a Latino living in a predominately wealthy town with a European-American majority. He was encouraged to use the "acting as if" strategy to deal with this concern.

T (Therapist): You have mentioned that you feel out of place around Rita's family, as they are better than you. You also mentioned that you live in a wealthy White community and are not sure if people accept you.

C (Client): That is accurate. That is how I feel.

T: I wonder what would happen if the next time you are around Rita's family you would be willing to do something different.

C: I might. Her parents are coming next week for a two-week visit.

T: Would you be willing to act as if they saw you as an equal? Act just like you did when you were around your grandfather.

C: That would be weird, but I would try it if you think it might help.

The Midas Technique

This strategy involves exaggerating the client's neurotic demands. As in the myth of King Midas, who was granted his wish that everything he touched turned to gold, the Midas technique shows clients that their wishes, when taken to their logical extreme, can be absurd. This allows clients to laugh at their own positions. For instance, a client who was busy collecting and investing in material wealth was shocked when the therapist suggested that he buy several more burial plots so that he could take all of his possessions with him into the next life. Then he laughed, "Yeah I see what you mean. I act like I think I'm gonna take it all with me."

Pleasing Someone

Based on the importance of creating social interest in clients, in this strategy the therapist urges the client to do something nice for someone else, an act of grace, a mitzvah, or loving gesture. Sometimes clients, especially those in the throes of depression, spend too much time obsessing about their own situations. They think about themselves constantly, ruminate about the same things, and remain stuck in their "selfness." Such individuals might be encouraged to volunteer their time in service to others, or to make a point of doing something nice for someone everyday, with no expectation of a reciprocal favor.

The Client-Counselor Relationship

How Adlerian therapists behave and what roles they take on can be deduced from the preceding discussion. However, let's review exactly what Adlerian therapy looks like from the perspective of the counselor-client relationship. The many adjectives that describe the Adlerian therapeutic relationship include *cooperative, collaborative, egalitarian, optimistic,* and *respectful* (Watts, 2000a). In addition, an effective Adlerian therapist is one who can convey social interest to the client. Therefore, the Adlerian therapist tries to model caring and empathy.

As noted, Adlerian therapy follows four stages, each of which builds upon the previous stage. The first and most important stage is the relationship stage, wherein therapy occurs in a relational context (Watts, 2000a). The success of subsequent stages rests upon the further development and continuation of a good therapeutic relationship. In this relationship, the therapist creates a safe environment for clients to explore their mistaken beliefs, faulty values, and ineffective behaviors. The subsequent stages (assessment, insight and inter-pretation, and reorientation) all require the counselor to be an active participant in the therapy process. In many ways, because of the level of activity, constant encouragement, and the psychoeducational component, the therapist behaves very much like a coach who is helping someone develop a new life skill.

One aspect that might distinguish Adlerian therapy from other therapies is that at times the psychoeducational component of Adlerian therapy gives the relationship more of a teacher-student feel. Adlerian therapists educate clients about alternative coping styles as a means of dealing with problems. Adlerians might give their clients advice, yet the advice would be offered in the context of a relationship of equals. Adlerian therapists do not decide for clients what their goals should be or what needs to change. This is determined collaboratively. Once goals are identified, Adlerian therapy becomes focused on the goals. Some of the methods of reaching these goals are determined by the therapist, yet the goals themselves rest with the client.

Evaluation of Adlerian Therapy

As was discussed earlier in this chapter, despite the widespread use and adoption of Adlerian ideas, there is a dearth of empirical research on the efficacy of Adlerian therapy. In one of the few studies on the efficacy of Adlerian therapy, Smith, Glass, and Miller (1980) found that Adlerian therapy was parallel to psychoanalytic and person-centered approaches in effectiveness. For a theory of such longevity, the lack of empirical research on Adlerian theory is rather alarming. For the most part, the evaluation of this approach is based more on clinical observations, limited research studies, case studies, and logic. Histori- cally, many Adlerians have preferred more of a case study or idiographic method to support the efficacy of Adlerian therapy (Carlson et al., 2006). In fact, Edwards, Dattilio, and Bromley (2004) suggested that clinical practice and case- based research be included as significant indicators of successful evidence-based practice. For counselors using the Adlerian approach, that means the explicit and conscious use of current best evidence in making decisions about treating clients, with an emphasis on blending individual clinical expertise about Adlerian theory with the best available evidence from external clinical empirical research.

One of the difficulties in conducting empirical research about Adlerian theory is that many of the core concepts are vague and ambiguous, thus hard to define and observe operationally (Slavik, 2006). Slavik and Carlson (2006) brought together Adlerian scholars to address this issue and discuss how to more effectively evaluate Adlerian therapy. There is hope that Adlerians will conduct additional research on the model.

There is a growing body of research that addresses the relationship between certain transtheoretical factors common in many orientations and positive client outcomes (Prochaska & Norcross, 2007). This research involves client factors, therapeutic relationship factors, hope, and technique. One of the rationales suggested by some (Carlson et al., 2006) is that the efficacy of the Adlerian model is indirectly supported by that approach. In terms of client factors, Adlerian therapy emphasizes the importance of attending to what clients bring into therapy, especially their strengths, assets, and resources. In terms of ther- apeutic relationship factors, Adlerian therapy takes a relational approach with specific attention toward creating a solid therapeutic relationship. In terms of hope, Adlerian therapy is an optimistic approach that focuses on encouragement in clients both as an attitude and a way of being. And in terms of model/ technique, Adlerians are generally eclectic in their selection of flexible therapy interventions and techniques and tailor therapy to their client's unique needs and expectations.

Further support for Adlerian therapy comes from the longevity and continued interest in Adlerian concepts and principles. The adoption and integration of Adlerian concepts in other therapies with considerably more empirical support (e.g., cognitive behavioral therapies) does provide some credence for Adlerian therapy.

Adlerian Therapy: Blind Spots, Limitations, and Challenges

As you read subsequent chapters in this book, you will soon realize that Adlerian theory includes a little bit of everything seen in other therapeutic approaches. One reason for this, of course, is that so many other therapists have borrowed and adapted Adler's ideas for their own purposes, often "discovering" many of Adler's fundamental ideas without even knowing it (Kottler, 2001; Watts, 2000a). Without a doubt, Adlerian theory and therapy have been and continue to be significant influences on all forms of therapy. Wilder (Adler & Deutsch, 1956, p. xv, as cited in Mosak, 2005) posed a question more than 50 years ago that appears even more germane today: "Most observations and ideas of Alfred Adler have subtly and quietly permeated modern psychological thinking to such a degree that the proper question is not whether one is an Adlerian but how much of an Adlerian one is." However, despite Adlerian theory's many positive offerings, there are also several blind spots, limitations, and challenges to the application of the model in contemporary society.

Blind Spots

As with most theories that were developed with a Western perspective, the focus of change and responsibility in Adlerian theory rests with the self. This focus on the self may pose a problem for clients from cultures that have a more communal focus. Further, one of the basic tenets of Adlerian theory is that individuals are responsible for their behavior, thoughts, and emotions. Adlerians view not taking responsibility for one's behaviors, thoughts, and emotions as a choice. However, this notion of choice may not be fair when applied to clients who are members of an oppressed minority.

Another blind spot may have to do with the emphasis on assessment that explores detailed personal information about the past (i.e., the life-style inventory). Some clients are put off by questions about the past, including family relationships and early memories. Paniagua (2005) noted that therapists who work with cultural minority populations would be wise to avoid collecting too much personal and family information early in therapy. Because clients' most pressing problems exist in the present, clients may not be interested in— nor will they see the connection with—the past. Instead, the emphasis should be on the presenting problem. As the expression goes, "When you are up to your neck in alligators, you don't want to think about much else." Further, many cultures (particularly Latino culture) have prohibitions about revealing personal and family information (Corey, 2001). Thus the Adlerian who tries to collect too much information may be viewed by such clients as technically and culturally incompetent (Paniagua, 2005). To address this concern, most contemporary Adlerians do not undertake a complete life-style assessment, but they often use brief survey and interviewing techniques to obtain the needed information. Adlerian approaches are thus tailored to the client and rely on verbal interventions, logic, and insights that are dependent on the client's level of understanding in order to focus on client-directed outcomes.

For some cultural minority clients, the fact that the Adlerian approach is a democratic approach, in which an equal relationship is created with the client, may also represent a blind spot of the approach. Adlerians work hard at "not doing for someone what they can do for themselves." Yet some cultures view the therapist as an expert and want to be told what to do. This might be challenging for democratic-minded therapists.

Limitations

One of the criticisms of the Adlerian approach addresses how the theory has evolved over time. Some students, scholars, and practitioners may view the Adlerian approach as an antiquated model that has limited contemporary relevance. Some of the responsibility for that perception must lie with the Adlerian community, which often has such reverence and enthusiasm for Adler's work that the evolution of the model has been overshadowed by allegiance to the past (Carlson, 2000). Manaster and Corsini (1982) observed that very little has been written that contradicts or repudiates the original ideas of Adler. Instead, most Adlerians tend to write additions and supplements to or explanations of Adler's own thoughts without offering a substantial critique or revision. My (J.C.) 1989 editorial in the *Journal of Individual Psychology* titled, "On beyond Adler," was a call to Adlerians to work to evolve the theory into modern practice and recognize how the theory has changed over time. I (J.C.) further suggested that Adlerians look to expand and integrate the model with other systems of therapy in order to avoid exclusivity (Carlson, 2000).

For the most part, Adlerians tend to meet and share writings within a closed community. There is an annual meeting in North America as well as several smaller regional meetings that are not promoted outside the membership. The Adlerian group tends to enjoy its community spirit. Yet as a result of this way of meeting, many Adlerian ideas have not been widely shared with the greater professional community. Further, this inbreeding tends to keep the organization largely White and privileged, and efforts need to be made to create a more diverse membership base that reflects the changing face of therapy. Through a diversity of people and ideas, Adlerian theory and practice can be expanded. Until this occurs, many of the challenges of applying the Adlerian model broadly will not be realized.

Another limitation of Adlerian theory is that Adler himself spent more time training and treating than writing and theorizing. When he did write, he revealed himself to be a mediocre and unsystematic writer. Maniacci (1999) noted that Adler wrote few books for professional audiences. As a result, his language was simple and his style was minimal. An outgrowth of this writing style was that the theory was not especially well defined and was often poorly presented in the existing scholarly literature (Watts, 2000a). Adler's ideas are somewhat vague and general, which makes it hard to research the basic concepts. Further, although Adler had ideas and made observations about how people grow and develop, he did not formulate a theory of development or learning (Mosak & Maniacci, 1999).

Because of the way in which Adlerian theory evolved during Adler's time and subsequently, it is difficult to place Adlerian theory and therapy into a single theoretical category. This, perhaps, may be yet another reason why Adler's theory is often misunderstood and misrepresented. The Adlerian approach can be categorized as cognitive, systemic, existential, and psychodynamic. More recently, some Adlerians have begun describing the approach as a constructivist theory and therapy. This is not so much a result of Adler's trying to make his theory into something for everyone, as it was of his followers' having found ways to do so.

Challenges

The most debilitating limitation for any theory is stagnation of thinking around evolution and theory building (Fall, Holden, & Marquis, 2004). For Adlerians, the challenge exists to continue to develop the model to match the needs of modern society. The history of psychotherapy tends to support the notion that older theories do not necessarily fade away but instead evolve into what appear to be newer theories and approaches (Prochaska & Norcross, 2007). Historically, Adlerian therapy preceded and strongly influenced rational-emotive behavior therapy (Ellis, 1970), which contributed to cognitive-behavioral and cognitive therapies. Whereas Adlerian ideas are alive in other theoretical approaches, there is a question about whether Adlerian theory as a stand-alone approach is viable in the long term. Norcross, Hedges, and Prochaska (2002) asked a panel of experts to forecast changes in theoretical orientations, therapeutic interventions, psychotherapy providers, treatment formats, and future scenarios. They found that cognitive-behavior, culture-sensitive/multicultural, and integrative therapies were expected to expand the most. By contrast, many of the older theories, such as classical psychoanalysis, transactional analysis, and Adlerian therapy, were expected to lose ground in terms of popularity and relevance. Thus, the challenge for Adlerians is quite clear: for the Adlerian model to survive and thrive, it must look at ways to strive for significance. One avenue is to recognize how modern practice is moving toward community involvement and social justice, which are core concepts outlined by both Adler and Dreikurs (Fall et al., 2004).

One of the strengths and continued challenges for Adlerian theory has to do with treating diverse populations and doing social justice work. Perhaps Adler's greatest contribution is that he developed a theory that recognizes and stresses the effects of social class, racism, sex, and gender on the behavior of individuals. His ideas, therefore, are well received by those living in today's global society. Yet acknowledging the utility of Adlerian theory is not enough. The model needs to be continually examined and developed to meet the contemporary needs of all clients.

Another challenge for Adlerians has been adapting the theory for brief and short-term therapy. Because the Adlerian model is a comprehensive approach, it would seem to require a setting and clients conducive to long-term therapy. Nevertheless, the Adlerian approach has been adapted for effective brief therapy (Carlson & Sperry, 1998) with the ability to address the full range of psychopathology (Sperry & Carlson, 1996). Adler believed that he could help most clients in under 20 sessions (Ansbacher & Ansbacher, 1970), and in a survey of Adlerian therapists, Kern, Yeakle, and Sperry (1989) found that 86% of their clients were seen for less than a year and 53% for less than six months. There was a wide variation in the number of sessions, depending on the severity of the problem. A guiding construct is that Adlerians focus on limiting time rather than limiting goals. "Adlerian therapists attempt full and complete therapy in whatever time is available and in the shortest time possible" (Manaster, 1989, p. 245).

Future Development: Adlerian Therapy in a Diverse World

It appears that the basic tenets of Adlerian theory and psychotherapy will continue to be mainstreamed into contemporary thought (Mosak & Maniacci, 1999). This is evident in both the positive psychology movement and in the current emphasis on strength-based therapies for treating diverse populations. Examples include the positive psychology movement's emphases on normal human growth and development; prevention and education rather than merely remediation; lessened reliance on the medical model perspective; focus on mental health and client's strengths, resources, and abilities (rather than on psychopathology and client disabilities); and focus on holism, wellness, multiculturalism, and social justice (Ansbacher & Ansbacher, 1956; Carlson et al., 2006; Mosak & Maniacci, 1999). Because of its emphasis on encouragement and empowerment of clients, Adlerian therapy can have success with populations that are sometimes difficult to reach. Sapp (2006) noted that Adlerian therapy represents a strength-based model that can be effective with at-risk youth.

The Adlerian concept of social interest with an emphasis on helping others, belonging, and focusing on the collective spirit fits well and supports the traditional value system of community-focused minority groups, such as Asian-Americans (Capuzzi & Gross, 1995). Multiculturalism also entails attention to and appreciation of the role of religion or spirituality in the lives of clients. Whereas most schools of psychology have not given much attention to religion or spirituality in clinical work, Adlerian therapy has been quite open to religious and spiritual issues (Mansager, 2000). Adler viewed religion as a manifestation of social interest, specifically calling attention to the tradition of those religions that stress people's responsibility for each other (Mosak, 2005). Contemporary Adlerians also view spirituality as one of the major tasks of life, noting that "each of us must deal with the problems of defining the nature of the universe, the existence and nature of God, and how to relate to these concepts" (p. 55).

Some of the ideas contained in this chapter will come up again in the chapters on other theories that have taken Adlerian concepts and developed them further. Adlerian therapy remains to this day one of the most integrated systems of psychotherapy.

Summary

1. Alfred Adler named his approach Individual Psychology to emphasize the unity of the individual. Adlerian therapists believe that all behavior is goal directed, is socially embedded, and has social meaning. Adlerian psychotherapy posits that people seeking therapy are not sick, but rather discouraged, and therefore need to be encouraged to develop more social interests and a more effective life-style to achieve success in the tasks of life.

2. Adler's early personal experiences with illness and helplessness may have informed his theoretical focus on inferiority and superiority complexes. In addition, his socialism and corresponding beliefs in personal freedom, social responsibility, and the rights of children, women, and workers carried through into his theoretical emphasis on the impact of social, familial, and cultural forces on psychology.

3. Adler was the first to introduce the relationship between thinking processes and feelings, the impact of early family experiences and birth order on

present behavior, the value of constructing specific plans of action, the construction of an egalitarian, collaborative counseling relationship, the assessment of life-style and social behavior as they affect personality development, and the importance of skill training and an educational model of treatment.

4. Adlerian therapy suffered a crisis of relevance after the death of Adler's successor, Rudolf Dreikurs, but modern Adlerians have since adapted the original theory to a variety of other applications and settings. Adlerian therapy has proved to be particularly adaptive to addressing multicultural and social equality issues.

5. Adlerian therapy theory rests on several key concepts: holism (the notion that understanding a person involves consideration of all of the components that make up the personality of the person, as well as the person's environment), encouragement (the process of increasing a person's courage in order to face the difficulties in life), subjective or private logic (the individual way that a client perceives the world), life-style (an individual's attitudinal set that includes the basic convictions, choices, and values that influence decisions and behaviors), basic mistakes (the self-defeating attitudes and beliefs of an individual's life-style), basic life tasks (the questions and challenges of life that influence psychological development), social interest (the notion that all individuals have a responsibility to the community), life goals and belonging (the idea that all behavior is goal directed toward finding a place in the social world), and birth order (the notion that the order in which one was born in relation to one's siblings is a variable in psychological development).

6. The Adlerian theory of change posits that all individuals are always in the process of becoming and that the process of change is not about curing a client, but rather encouraging a client's growth and development. Adlerian therapists pinpoint mistaken goals in order to help their clients reach insight and eventually change their goals.

7. Adlerian therapy proceeds in four stages: the relationship stage (in which a collaborative relationship is established), the assessment stage (in which the therapist conducts a comprehensive assessment of the client's functioning, via such tests as a life-style inventory), the insight and interpretation stage (in which the therapist assists the client in developing new, more fully functioning orientations to life), and the reorientation stage (in which the therapist assists the client in constructive movement toward desired goals, via action-oriented exercises).

8. During the four stages of the therapy process, certain therapeutic strategies may be employed, including encouragement, reframing, asking "the question,"

the push-button technique, acting "as if," the Midas technique, and pleasing someone.

9. The counselor-client relationship in Adlerian therapy could be described as cooperative, collaborative, egalitarian, optimistic, and respectful. In addition, an effective Adlerian therapist is one who can convey social interest to the client.

10. Most Adlerian therapists prefer a case study or idiographic method to support the efficacy of the therapy. Adlerian therapy is difficult to research empirically because many of the core concepts are vague and ambiguous, thus hard to operationally define and observe.

11. Adlerian therapy carries with it a number of blind spots, limitations, and challenges. Blind spots include the Adlerian focus on individual choice (which may pose problems for clients from communal cultures), its emphasis on the client's past history (which may not appeal to some clients), and its egalitarian approach (which may not be effective with clients from cultures that view therapists as experts). Limitations include the tendency of Adlerians to communicate primarily within their closed professional community, the paucity of theoretical literature written by Adler himself, and the difficulty of placing Adlerian therapy into a single category. The challenges for Adlerian therapy are to continue evolving the therapy, to continue creating ways to adapt the therapy for diverse populations, and to further adapt the therapy to brief and short-term therapy.

12. The Adlerian approach is one that shows great respect for all people regardless of gender, ethnicity, race, and sexual orientation. The approach is truly democratic and respects the notion that all people are equal and deserve to be treated in that fashion. Adlerians advocate for social justice and the rights of all people.

Key Terms

basic mistakes (p. 110)
birth order (p. 114)
discouragement (p. 105)
early recollections (p. 110)
encouragement (p. 104)
family constellation (p. 115)
faulty logic (p. 107)
holism (p. 104)
inferiority complex (p. 113)

life goals (p. 104)
life-style (p. 107)
life tasks (p. 111)
mistaken goals (p. 116)
private logic (p. 107)
self-concept (p. 105)
self-ideal (p. 105)
social interest (p. 112)

Resources for Further Study

Professional Organizations

North American Society of Adlerian Psychology (NASAP)
50 Northeast Drive
Hershey, PA 17033
717-579-8795
www.alfredadler.org

   Training Centers: NASAP can provide a list of the 58 Adlerian organizations and institutes.

Adler School of Professional Psychology
65 East Wacker Place, Suite 400
Chicago, IL 60601
312-201-5900
www.adler.edu

   The Adler School of Professional Psychology in Chicago offers fully accredited masters and doctoral programs.

Professional Journals

Journal of Individual Psychology
www.utexas.edu/utpress/journals/jip.html
Also available from NASAP or
University of Texas Press
P.O. Box 7819
Austin, TX 78713-7819
800-252-3206
utpress@uts.cc.utexas.edu

   The *Journal of Individual Psychology* is the journal of the North American Society of Adlerian Psychology. As the premier scholarly forum for Adlerian practices, principles, and theoretical development, it addresses techniques, skills, and strategies associated with the practice and application of Adlerian psychological methods.

Suggested Readings

Ansbacher, H. L., & Ansbacher, R. R. (Eds.). (1956). *The Individual Psychology of Alfred Adler: A systematic presentation in selections from his writings.* New York: Harper Torchbooks.

   This has been the main source of Adler's writings. The editors' comments are very helpful in understanding Adler's theory and practice.

Carlson, J. D., & Slavik, S. (1997) *Techniques in Adlerian psychology*. Philadelphia: Taylor & Francis.

A collection of classic articles from the *Journal of Individual Psychology* that focus on techniques and practice.

Carlson, J. D., Watts, R. E., & Maniacci, M. (2006). *Adlerian psychotherapy: Theory and practice*. Washington, DC: American Psychological Association.

An important book on contemporary Adlerian psychotherapy.

Dinkmeyer, D., Jr., & Sperry, L. (2000). *Counseling and psychotherapy: An integrated, Individual Psychology approach*. Columbus, OH: Merrill.

A good basic text on Adlerian counseling and psychotherapy.

Dreikurs, R., & Stoltz, V. (1964). *Children: The challenge*. New York: Hawthorn.

This has become a classic text on the Adlerian perspective on parenting and raising a child.

Hoffman, E. (1994). *The drive for self: Alfred Adler and the founding of Individual Psychology*. Reading, MA: Addison Wesley.

The best biography on the life of Alfred Adler.

Hooper, A., & Holford, J. (1998). *Adler for beginners*. New York: Writers & Readers.

A fun and easy-to-read primer about the life and contributions of Alfred Adler.

Mosak, H., & Maniacci, M. (1999.) *A primer of Adlerian psychology: The analytic-behavioral-cognitive psychology of Alfred Adler*. New York: Brunner-Routledge.

A good source for the "nuts and bolts" of Adlerian psychology.

Other Media Resources

Carlson, J. D. (1998). *Psychotherapy with the experts: Adlerian psychotherapy* [Video]. Boston: Allyn & Bacon.

Dr. Carlson works with an African-American woman struggling with her divorce and overfunctioning approach to life.

Carlson, J. D. (2002). *Child therapy with the experts: Adlerian parent consultation* [Video]. Boston: Allyn & Bacon.

Dr. Carlson provides an example of both an individual parent consultation with a single mother and a parent group consultation.

Carlson, J. D. (2003). *Brief integrative Adlerian couples therapy* [Video]. Microtraining and Multicultural Development.

Dr. Carlson works with a couple with problems of anger and abuse.

Carlson, J. D. (2004). *Adlerian psychotherapy* [Video]. Washington DC: American Psychological Association.

Dr. Carlson works with a young man with issues of perfectionism. In a brief 45-minute session, significant change occurred.

Kottman, T. (2002). *Child therapy with the experts: Adlerian play therapy* [Video]. Boston: Allyn & Bacon.

Dr. Kottman demonstrates Adlerian play therapy with a 4-year-old boy.

Chapter 5

Existential Therapy

CLEMMONT E. VONTRESS

Since the beginning of human history, people have pondered their existence. They have wondered about the nature of the universe, their place and purpose in the universe, how they should relate to their fellow human beings and nature, who they "really" are, and many other issues that continue to disturb the tranquility of humankind. In 20th-century Europe, ideas pertaining to human existence came to be called *existentialism*. From this construct emerged ideas to understand and help individuals who are troubled by being-in-the-world. These ideas are now referred to as existential counseling and psychotherapy. In this chapter, existential philosophy is discussed briefly, some of the contributors to this philosophy are mentioned, and a few major constructs associated with existential philosophy are defined. Finally, an explanation of how the philosophy can be applied therapeutically is provided.

Origins and Evolution of Existential Therapy

As an unnamed view of life, existentialism dates back to ancient Greece (Kahn, 1982; Mounier, 1947). Socrates (470–399 BCE), the father of Western philosophy, advocated self-knowledge and the courageous confrontation of destiny. Aristotle (384–322 BCE) indicated that the soul and body are inseparable. The Stoics developed a philosophy (300 BCE–200 CE) that taught people to accept unflinchingly suffering and death. The ancient Greeks believed that the wise and happy person is one who lives in harmony with the order of the universe and accepts the commonality of humankind. Although numerous philosophies have emerged in Western culture since the days of Socrates,

Aristotle, and the Stoics, most of them draw upon many of the ideas that ancient Greeks advanced.

Some of the views espoused by ancient Greeks emerged in 20th-century Europe as a philosophical composite called **existentialism** (Christian, 1977). Flew (1979) considers existentialism to be a trend or attitude, not a dogma or system. As such, it eludes precise definition. Most writers resolve the definition problem by listing and explicating a number of themes related to existence. Some of these are being, choice, freedom, death, isolation, and absurdity.

Several philosophers representing different disciplines and attitudes about life contributed to and elaborated on the concepts associated with existentialism. Names most often linked to the philosophical trend are Blaise Pascal (1623–1662), Søren Kierkegaard (1813–1855), Friedrich Nietzsche (1844–1900), Edmund Husserl (1859–1938), Martin Heidegger (1889–1976), Jean-Paul Sartre (1905–1980), Maurice Merleau-Ponty (1908–1961), Martin Buber (1878–1965), and Paul Tillich (1886–1965) (Schneider & May, 1995). Kierkegaard was a major influence on the movement because he was the first to take issue with the highly intellectual and rational philosophy that prevailed during his time (Rychlak, 1981). Contrary to the exclusively rational philosophers, he felt that humans can be understood best when the spontaneous and emotional side of their existence is examined.

Although Martin Heidegger did not regard himself as an existentialist, he contributed significantly to the existential movement. Illustratively, he maintained that an individual's life can only be understood through the description of the individual's **Dasein,** or basic mode of being in the world. According to Heidegger, people illuminate their uniqueness by involvement and participation in their community (Flew, 1979).

In the 20th century, when existentialism came to the forefront as a clearly discernable philosophical stance, Jean-Paul Sartre became one of the most celebrated French existentialists. His novels and essays extolled freedom and individualism. French philosopher Maurice Merleau-Ponty pointed out that there can be no knowledge of things-in-themselves, but only of things as they are perceived by the human being (Olafson, 1967). French writer Albert Camus (1913–1960) fascinated readers with his novel, *L'Etranger* (The Stranger), and many other novels, essays, and short stories that depicted the individual's alienation from the group.

In general, there were two types of existentialist philosophers in the 20th century: the Christians and the atheists. Gabriel Marcel (1889–1973) was a well-known Christian theologian, whereas Sartre and Camus were avowed atheists. Even though these contributors to existential thinking were different, the idea that existence precedes essence permeated most of their views (Droit, 2004). They shared the belief that once in the world, individuals create themselves.

Many European psychiatrists and psychologists applied existential philosophy to helping people with psychological problems. Viktor Frankl (1905–1997) developed **logotherapy,** a systematic psychotherapeutic model based on existential constructs, used to help clients find **meaning** in life. He used **paradoxical intention,** a method that encouraged individuals to do the very thing that caused them anxiety, to relieve anxiety. Another technique he used was **dereflection.** This was a simple approach in which he encouraged clients to focus their attention away from the source of anxiety to assuage it. Ludwig Binswanger (1881–1966), a Swiss psychiatrist, contributed significantly to defining the human condition from an existential and therapeutic perspective (Binswanger, 1991). One of his most important contributions was coining three German words to describe the human situation. The **Umwelt,** or physical world, is the environment that sustains life. The **Mitwelt,** or social environment, protects, nourishes, socializes, and contributes to the individual's psychological well-being. The **Eigenwelt,** or the world of the self, consists of each person's private thoughts, experiences, and uniqueness. Emily Van Deurzen-Smith (1988), a British psychologist, felt that Binswanger had been remiss in not describing another important aspect of human existence. She added the **Uberwelt,** or the spiritual world, to Binswanger's three environments.

Medard Boss (1963) and Martin Buber (1970) both contributed to helping therapists understand anxiety and other mental health problems from an existential perspective. They also highlighted the nature of the psychotherapeutic relationship. Boss declared—among other things—that the therapeutic encounter should be imbued with **psychotherapeutic eros,** the therapist's close feeling for the client. Buber also advocated a friendly and spiritual counselor-client relationship, which he called the **I-Thou.** I-Thou suggests a caring, intimate, and authentic relationship, as opposed to an I-You encounter, which implies a formal respectful involvement, or an I-It relationship, which evokes images of one person relating to the other as if that person were a thing. Like most existential therapists, Boss and Buber considered the therapist and how he or she relates to the client to be especially therapeutic.

In the United States, several therapists have contributed to and advanced the understanding of existential psychotherapy and counseling. Although Carl Rogers (1902–1987) is generally classified as a phenomenologist, many also consider him to be an existentialist. The perception of Rogers as an existentialist probably derives from the fact that most existentialists espouse Kant's view that reality is always subjective, and in like manner, Rogers (Patterson, 1980) emphasized the importance of seeing reality from the client's perspective. His "So you feel" psychotherapeutic inquiries sought to understand the client's inner being. Like Rogers, existentialists also recognize two realities: A perceived object is always different from the object itself. Another American therapist, Rollo May, has done more to promote an understanding of existential therapy than perhaps any other person. He has shown how love, authenticity, and other existential ideas, discussed later in this chapter, promote the well-being of clients. Additionally, Yalom (1980), in discussing life, death, anxiety, responsibility, isolation, and meaning, points out that these and other existential constructs impact psychological states and traits.

The Evolution of Existential Therapy for a Diverse World

American existential therapists tend to stay abreast of the changing needs of society. Bugental (1967) has been for many years a significant contributor to the literature of existential therapy. Ibraham (2003) has developed an existential worldview theory, which aims to allow therapists to transcend national, racial, and ethnic barriers that may impede effective therapy. An advocate of existential cross-cultural counseling, Vontress (1979, 1988) provides a framework for understanding and using existential therapy. He decries the widespread use of psychiatric medicine instead of psychotherapeutic self-examination to help people with problems (Vontress, 2003).

There are similarities between Western existentialism and Eastern philosophies. Rychlak (1981) indicates that exponents of both existentialist and Eastern ideologies recommend that individuals live authentically and stay in tune with life as experienced. People risk becoming alienated when they try to force nature to adjust to them, instead of adjusting themselves to nature. Schneider and May (1995) explain that existentialism draws from and reflects Taoism and Buddhism. For example, Taoists and existentialists maintain that existence should be spontaneous (Watts, 1995a). Additionally, Buddhists and existentialists generally are opposed to reductionism, or the breaking down of the whole into presumed parts to understand it (Rychlak, 1981). Both philosophies hold that individuals can be best understood holistically.

Existentialism is also kin to **animism,** the traditional African view that a single universal spirit or soul unifies all of nature, including human beings. In my 20 years of studying traditional healing in Africa (Vontress, 1991), I have found that the existential therapeutic focus is similar to that of West African village healers. Both advocate holistic procedures that consider clients to be products of their physical, social, psychological, and spiritual environments. The goal of the healer, whether existential or African, is to ensure that the client lives in harmony with the four environments or "worlds," as Binswanger (1991) and Van Deurzen-Smith (1988) call them.

Context Then—Context Now

Because existentialism is a view of human existence, it seems tenable to conclude that it started as an unnamed philosophy at the advent of humankind. We know that it is at least 2,000 years old, because the major scriptures allude to many issues now labeled existential. Birth, life, menacing environmental conditions, and death are common themes of human history. Many scholars associate Socrates with the beginning of existentialism as a therapeutic modality. Others consider 20th-century European philosophers, psychiatrists, and other thinkers as fathers of existentialism and its therapeutic application. The debate is likely to continue because, unlike most psychological counterparts, existential therapy was not started by a single person at a particular place and time.

Today, the basic concepts underlying existentialism remain unchanged. What has changed is the increasing thirst in modern societies for a philosophy that provides meaning for people troubled by a sense of meaninglessness. When applied therapeutically, existentialism offers hope for the hopeless. As philosophical healers seemingly indifferent to methodology, existential therapy theorists often are prodded by general practitioners to develop specialized existential techniques. Existential therapists who submit to such pressuring risk becoming techniques-driven counselors who appear more concerned about adhering to prescribed methods than listening to the problems of their clients.

The Author's Journey as an Existential Therapist

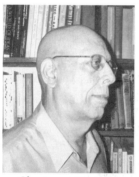
Clemmont Vontress

In retrospect, I realize that all along I have been an existentialist seeking a safe haven, a philosophical sanctuary where I could make myself at home without feeling like an outsider. It took me several years to recognize that I had found the place to be. As a boy growing up in rural Kentucky, I was exposed to the realities of nature—birth, life, maturity, old age, and death. I saw animals in the barnyard doing "the natural," as my father called sexual intercourse. Their offspring grew up, lived out their existence, and eventually died. I saw relatives and friends arrive and others depart life as if my home were a large airport terminal. People were coming and going all the time. I understood that some would stay longer than others, but that eventually we all would leave. Although I reflected on life and death a great deal, I was not always able to get my elders to talk to me about these "twins of human existence."

When I enrolled at Kentucky State University in 1948, I was attracted to English and French literature, especially to poetry about love, suffering, and death. Ralph Waldo Emerson was one of my favorite writers then, as he is today. I was also fascinated by William Shakespeare (1564–1616) and Jean-Baptiste Molière (1622–1673). In their plays, they portray a wide range of emotional issues related to the human journey. It was from reading works by Shakespeare and Molière that I first became interested in philosophy and psychology.

(continued)

After college, I spent two years in the U.S. Army in Germany. Whenever I got leave, I went to Paris, where I met several unforgettable people. One of them was Josephine Baker (1906–1975), the African-American entertainer who left the United States when she was a young woman to search for a life unencumbered by racism. On stage, she drew great applause from French audiences. I had never before seen White people express such appreciation for a Black person. I was affected deeply by the outpouring of love for a person who was rejected in her native country. After one of her performances, I waited an hour backstage to meet her. When I introduced myself, she hugged me and I cried, probably because I realized that she was free of the racial oppression that I still endured.

I accompanied a French friend to a café where I saw and heard Simone de Beauvoir and Jean-Paul Sartre read some of their works to a small audience. Of course, I did not know who they were until years later, when I started reading the writings of the existentialists. People talk a great deal about Sartre today, however, de Beauvoir, his less well known disciple, paramour, and life companion, was also a great thinker and writer. Her book, *Deuxième Sexe* (The Second Sex), was perhaps the first contribution to the feminist movement. In it, she spoke out in support of women's rights, a courageous thing to do in the middle of the 20th century. In Frankfurt, Germany, I met Sidney Bechet (1897–1959), an African-American jazz musician. A clarinetist, saxophonist, composer, and conductor, he was one of the best-known representatives of New Orleans jazz. I remember him because he exuded an unusual radiance, which undoubtedly reflected the freedom he felt in Europe. I saw the same glow of freedom in the faces of other African-American expatriates I met overseas in the early 1950s. I realized that freedom affects people holistically. It is not just the absence of physical hindrance, restraint, confinement, and repression. It is also an attitude or state of mind that overrides externally imposed restrictions.

In 1955, I came back to the United States and enrolled in the master's degree program in counseling at Indiana University. Two counseling theories were the focus of the department. The first was the clinically based and data-driven model developed by E. G. Williamson of the University of Minnesota. The second was the person-centered approach formulated by Carl Rogers, at that time the best-known name in counseling. I was attracted to his theory because it seemed less intrusive on an individual's lifestyle. It permitted each person to elucidate his or her uniqueness.

After completing the program, I took a job with the Indianapolis Public School System as Director of Guidance in a predominantly African-American high school. Because I was trained in Rogerian counseling, I wanted to try it out on my clients. Although polite and eager to benefit from "this thing called counseling," they hardly responded to my repeated "How do you feel?" inquiries. Finally, one of them could no longer restrain his frustration. "What's all this 'how do you feel' stuff?" he blurted out. "I feel like you feel when that happens to you," he said. Even though embarrassed, I understood the client's annoyance. It was then that I thought that there had to be another way to connect with clients who were uncomfortable talking about their feelings. I began to search for a therapeutic supplement to what I had learned in graduate school.

In 1957, I started working on a Ph.D. degree in counseling at Indiana University. One of the highlights of my time in the program was Carl Rogers's visit to the university to deliver a keynote address at a state conference. My professors selected me as one of the three students to sit on the dais with Rogers to ask him questions. In his presentation, he discussed empathy, congruence, and unconditional positive regard as essential ingredients of a therapeutic relationship. When it came time for me to ask my question, I wanted to know how these attitudes could help a counselor establish rapport with hostile and distrustful clients. Dr. Rogers replied that clients' trust is gained when they perceive these qualities in the counselor. Not completely satisfied with the answer, I was motivated to find another way to connect with alienated clients. First, I abandoned therapeutic formulas for establishing rapport, choosing instead to start my counseling sessions as naturally and spontaneously as possible.

When I completed the Ph.D. in 1965, I took a professorship at Howard University, where I organized the university's first master's degree program in counseling. In 1969, I moved to George Washington University to become the institution's first African-American professor. It was during my 28 years there that I conceptualized a complete model of existential counseling. Simultaneously, I made six field trips to West Africa to study traditional healing. Surprisingly, I discovered a close similarity between methods used by traditional healers and those advocated by some existential therapists to help clients. They both consider the individual to be the center of and influenced by the natural, social, personal, and spiritual environments.

In 1985, I proposed to my department a graduate course called "Existential Counseling." I wanted to present a view of existentialism that was not just endemic to Europe, but was common to humanity. Through my presentation of this view, my students came to understand that they could use existential counseling with all clients, no matter where they came from in the world. I offered this course for the first time in 1986. Fifteen doctoral students enrolled in the class. I tried to help them understand that individuals are at the center of and products of four interacting environments: the physical, social, personal, and spiritual. People are "well-adjusted" to the extent that they are in harmony with these forces. The objective of the course was to help students acquire an understanding of how they could take well-known existential constructs and apply them to counseling. They would learn how the concepts could help them to establish a counseling relationship, make a diagnosis, and intervene on behalf on their client.

Theory of Existential Therapy

Over the course of nearly a hundred years, several writers identified with existentialism have posited concepts that define various aspects of human existence. As discussed earlier, Heidegger introduced the German word *Dasein* (being there) to highlight the individual's mode of being in the world (Reese, 1980). Binswanger (Rychlak, 1981) further conceptualized human existence as a holistic unanalyzable entity consisting of the three interactive modes of being-in-the-world: the Umwelt (the natural environment), the Mitwelt (the interpersonal environment), and the Eigenwelt (the self environment).

The Umwelt (the Natural Environment)

Existentially, human beings belong to the universal order (Meek, 1985). It is the physical environment that sustains human life. The *Umwelt* is the world of physical objects. It is also the human being's relationship to the sun, water, moon, mountains, and valleys. Notwithstanding that the natural environment is often taken for granted, all life is connected to and influenced by its rhythms. Night and day dictate sleep patterns. The seasons are associated with planting, sprouting, maturing, and the harvesting of plants. In general, humans, particularly in Western culture, fail to recognize that they are not in charge of nature. They are but a part of and product of it. Nature controls and determines the destiny of all living beings.

Though the concept *Umwelt* was coined by Binswanger (1975), the idea that nature is the support system of the human species is as old as humankind itself. Most of the philosophers of the world have referred to it. Asians thinkers believe that the world is nature (Smart, 1999). For instance, in the Mandarin dialect, *Tao*, one of the major beliefs of Asian philosophy, means "the course of nature" (Watts, 1995a), and the Buddhists teach that everything in the universe depends on everything else (Watts, 1996). Watts (1995b) points out that the behavior of the organism is inseparable from the behavior of its environment. Pachuta (1989) indicates that one of the main differences between Eastern and Western philosophy is that in the East the human being is one with nature. In the West, on the other hand, people tend to isolate and alienate themselves from nature. In the Islamic world, the unity of nature also is recognized (Smart, 1999).

From the existential perspective, the Umwelt and the human spirit are inseparable. Gallagher (1975) declares that the union between the soul and the universe is of the same nature as that between the soul and the body, that there is a human connection with all living organisms, and that this linkage is spiritual. This view of being is evident in the concept of animism, the idea that a single soul unifies all life, a perception of human existence that is especially basic to the African way of life (Vontress, 1991). Similarly, in Islam much of the Koran is devoted to the cosmos and its spiritual nature (Nasr, 2002). What all of these beliefs have in common is that the spirit exists in nature; humankind is a part of nature; therefore, people are gifted with a unifying spirit.

The Mitwelt (the Social Environment)

Human beings enter the world naked and vulnerable to natural forces. The long period of postnatal maturation makes them dependent on people already present when they arrive. Biologically equipped to connect with their fellows, their sexual and speech systems presuppose a mutually beneficial close interpersonal relationship. Binswanger (1975) coined the German word *Mitwelt* to describe human fellowship. Without it, individuals would not even develop a language, a basic requirement for survival. Mitwelt enables two or more people to communicate, in order to pool their strength and resources to cope with and exploit the *Umwelt*.

Although humans need each other, being with others is not without tension. According to the concept of the Mitwelt, individuals are **subject** and **object** at the same time. One person, the subject, sees the other person and initiates action. The other, the object, is seen and acted upon, and is responsive. They each look out from their soul, perceiving the other, the object, as simultaneously similar and dissimilar to themselves. Even though they want to open up to their fellows, they often fear doing so. Servan-Schreiber (1987) explains that anyone who unites emotionally with another loses her or his uniqueness and autonomy. Compatible interpersonal unification necessarily requires a compromise by the members of a dyad. Each relinquishes a little bit of self in the interest of the other.

Even though the Mitwelt may be cause for anxiety, it is simultaneously a source of social pleasure, as Lehman (1993) explains. Love and related emotions are especially contributory to mental health. Sexual relations, satisfying work, a sense of conquest or triumph, and good interpersonal relations all produce a sense of well-being. According to Chessick (1987), the capacity to love and to be loved is the most reliable measure of mental health. Reciprocal love constitutes a pressure valve and buffer to the stresses of life.

Although the Mitwelt is a European existential concept, the idea of human connectedness is universal. In Islam, community implies human collectivity solidified by religious bonds (Nasr, 2002). Believers are taught that God resides in each person. Therefore, the individual and the group are one. Watts (1996) indicates that adherents of the Buddhist belief system recognize that individual separation from the group is an illusion. Smart (1999) agrees with him and adds that the "me" cannot exist apart from the "other." Most Asian belief systems consider individuality to be an illusion. Universally, humans manifest a complex of mental and physical emotions such as love, hate, fear, and anger, which unite and separate them simultaneously. In sub-Saharan Africa, animists believe that a common spirit unifies all humankind (Vontress, 1991). Indeed, the Mitwelt is an interesting and useful existential concept that reflects a significant aspect of the human condition.

The Eigenwelt (the Personal World)

Binswanger referred to human existence as Dasein, or the totality of "being there," as translated from the German (Rychlak, 1981). As discussed, the individual is a product of and related to three interactive worlds—the Umwelt, the Mitwelt, and the Eigenwelt. The last of these three worlds, the Eigenwelt, is the personal world that a person never shares with others. From birth to death, individuals are bound up in an organism, the body, from which there is no escape. It is through the body that people are able to insert themselves into the world of experience, perceptions, and sensations, which together constitute knowledge. People then use their acquired knowledge to manipulate their surroundings in order to ensure and enhance personal existence.

Because each life expires in due course, individuals as a group transmit to the next generation understandings about how to best exist. The content of the transmission is what we commonly call culture. In view of the fact that the individual is a self-contained and closed system, it is difficult for people to communicate to their fellows how they feel about being-in-the-world. Although birth and death are the two most significant events in human existence, neither can be shared consciously with one's fellows (Scheler, 1954). Most people live out their stay on earth trying to get others to understand them as they really are. In existentialist terms, an individual's existence is like being a person locked outside a glass door, through which she or he waves and shouts to the insider, trying to make that person hear the intended message. Unfortunately, the insider, the other person, does not have the key to the outsider's existence.

Existence and Essence

Existence and essence are two ideas basic to the existentialist's understanding of being-in-the-world. **Existence** refers to one's presence on earth. The individual is an organism that lives, matures, and dies like the rest of nature. However, according to most existentialists, individuals must define their own existence. Their definition is called their **essence**. Existence precedes essence (Reese, 1980).

This means that people are responsible for what they make of their lives. In existential philosophy, the notion that individual lives are predetermined is an unacceptable explanation of human behavior. Rather, human beings are free to chart their own destinies (May & Yalom, 1984). Those who refuse to accept this responsibility are usually burdened with a variety of personal problems.

Self-Knowledge

According to Socrates, **self-knowledge** is basic to human existence. In the Socratic view, the essential goal of philosophy is to inculcate self-awareness (Sahakian & Sahakian, 1966). A life without self-inspection is a life not worth living. The same admonition is explicit in the ancient Tao of China and the contemporary teachings of Buddhism (Watts, 1995a). According to these beliefs, ignorance of self is the root of most personal suffering. Likewise, Hindu gurus usually ask their students "Who are you?" Existentialists also emphasize the importance of self-knowledge (Vontress, Johnson, & Epp, 1999). People who do not know their personality traits, abilities, limitations, preferences, and other aspects of themselves are likely to make poor choices in life. Inappropriate personal decisions are apt to contribute to unhappiness and psychological problems.

Love

Love is a strong emotional attachment or devotion to another person or to a religious belief system. Requiring empathy, the existential concept of love presupposes a person's self-awareness. Love starts as early in life as the fetal stage. The most important person to the fetus is the mother, in whose womb it resides. Feeling a oneness with her, the fetus develops a neurological network in which love is basic. After birth, the neonate's organism is affected positively and negatively by the way it is treated during the early stages of life (Janov, 2000).

Binswanger's concept of Mitwelt suggests that interdependence with other human beings is indispensable to life. Love is the glue that ensures human togetherness. The neonate would not survive long without the love, care, and support of the mother. Her hugs release good feeling chemicals in the child's brain. These are the biochemicals of love. As adults, individuals who have experienced love from their parents are apt to transfer it to others. They are inclined to continue to seek love and closeness throughout their existence. For them, intimacy is liberating and healing. Their tie to others gives them a sense of self (Gallagher, 1975). It adds meaning to their lives.

Love is so basic to human existence that being able to exchange it with another person has implications for mental health. According to Ornish (1998), the child's perception of parental love and caring is a powerful predictor of future psychological well-being. Children reared without being hugged and touched early in life have abnormally high stress levels. Those who feel unloved may grow up feeling that indeed they are unlovable. That feeling can lead to depression and a lifelong search for palliatives such as drugs and alcohol to relieve the pain associated with the absence of love.

In his book *Being and Nothingness*, Sartre (1953) discussed love more extensively than other existentialists had before him. To Sartre, love involves the merging of two human beings, each simultaneously a subject and an object. Although individuals usually perceive the other person as an object, mutual lovers, in merging their consciousnesses, overcome the tendency to objectify each other. They become a spiritual unity. Each sees the self, their partner, others, and the world in a more positive light than they did when they were separate and alone.

According to de Beauvoir (1953), genuine love between two people is based on reciprocity and equality. Each person is perceived as equal. Love is spontaneous and mutual. Neither feels superior to the other because of gender, race, nationality, or cultural difference. Love transcends all. What they are as a couple is more important than what they were as individuals. Their togetherness is spiritually uplifting. It transcends their former oneness.

Responsibility

As Binswanger (1991) pointed out, each organism resides in its own habitat, which supports, maintains, and ensures survival. Human beings live in the three interactive and dynamic environments of the Umwelt, the Mitwelt, and the Eigenwelt and therefore have a *responsibility* to protect and care for the environments that care for them.

The Umwelt, or natural environment, is basic to human survival. The natural environment provides soil, water, air, fauna, flora, and many species, ingredients, and conditions that support life on earth. It is humankind's responsibility to respect, love, and cherish its abode. The Umwelt is a veritable Garden of Eden. It is an abundant food chain and storehouse filled with ores, organisms, and countless chemical ingredients that humans use to enhance our existence. We are obliged to protect it. It is our only home in-the-world.

Humans also have a responsibility to the community, or Mitwelt, of which we are participants. We arrive on earth predisposed to respond to the socialization that earlier arrivals (our parents) provided us during our long period of maturation. Our speech and sexual organs suggest that there is an innate will to communicate, cohabit, and propagate with our fellow humans. Our destinies are intertwined. In his novel *La Peste* (The Plague), Camus (1947; 1972), graphically depicts the interdependency of human beings within the Mitwelt. His characters are caught in a community threatened by a deadly virus. Everybody is under quarantine. They are all in the same situation. Nobody can escape. However, their predicament is made easier when they start cooperating with one another.

Authenticity

Authenticity comes from the Greek word *authentes,* which means one who acts with authority or what is done with one's own hand. In existential terms, authenticity is the honesty and courage to be who one really is (Christian, 1977). Being true to oneself is an old idea. In ancient Chinese philosophy, people were admonished to be in harmony with the cosmos (Smart, 1999) and also to be true to themselves. In Korean society, the concept of *cheng,* or sincerity, is an important virtue. So too, the existentialist Rychlak (1981) indicated that people become alienated from self and the group when they refuse to listen to their own dictates.

What is the psychological disadvantage of being inauthentic? Buber (1970) suggested that people who try to be somebody they are not exist in a state of confusion and agony. Individuals who follow the crowd instead of their own dictates live in bad faith. According to Sartre (1983), the inauthentic person is self-deceptive and anxious. The anxiety is usually caused by the individual's failure to recognize and exercise his or her freedom of choice. Kierkegaard (1949) pointed out that individuals become inauthentic when they let the group or their culture define personal choices. People are content only when they are themselves and make their own choices (Rychlak, 1981).

People can be authentic in any society, whether that society is individualistic or collectivistic. In individualistic cultures, individuals generally are socialized to manifest their uniqueness and to individuate themselves from others. Their authenticity is self-centered. Society encourages them to be independent and self-reliant. In collectivistic communities, individuals are less individuated. They derive their personal identities from significant groups, especially their families and the people heading them. In writing their names, they usually place the family name first and the given name last, a practice that reflects their collectivist identities.

According to the existentialists, there are psychological benefits that arise from being authentic. Aristotle (Loomis, 1943) pointed out that the person who knows the self tends to trust that self. Kierkegaard (1949) implied that people who wear one face for self and another for the public threaten their own mental health. The greatest peace of mind comes from listening to one's self. Inauthentic people live precariously. There is always the chance that they will be discovered for who they are. Being true to oneself is psychologically healthy. Living a lie about self is apt to lead to internal conflict.

Existential Anxiety

In the existential view, existence is not fixed. It is dynamic because the interactive environments in which people live are constantly changing. The unpredictability of life causes **existential anxiety** (Watts, 1975). Existentialists use words like *dread, despair,* and *Angst* to describe humankind's uncertainty or "fear and trembling," as Kierkegaard (1949) called it. Hanly (1979) referred to existential anxiety as ontological (being) anxiety, which is intrinsic to human existence. It originates from individuals' need to survive, to preserve their being, and to live out their destiny.

Although existentialists have discussed anxiety from several perspectives, death, freedom, and choice emerge as the main contributing factors to a generalized fear endemic to living. The fear of life is really a submerged apprehension about death, because life and death are inseparable. Death is the human being's most dramatic limit (Koestenbaum, 1971). Once set in motion, life is on a time clock. None of us knows when or where our time will run out. However, one thing is certain: life's movement toward death is unavoidable. From the moment we are born, we are in the process of dying. Yet in spite of the reality of death, it is unreasonable to be afraid of it, because it cannot be experienced. Death is the cessation of experience. Human organisms do not belong to the spirit that inhabits them. Rather, they belong to nature; and nothing in nature has a stable form (Rosenberg, 2000). Existentialists recommend that individuals turn the fear of death into a positive force. That is, we should recognize that our days are numbered. Therefore, we should use wisely and resolutely our time on earth. Events over which we have no control should not detract us from living out our days courageously.

Although existentialists extol humankind's **freedom,** they simultaneously point out that freedom can be a burden and a cause for anxiety (May, 1981; Sartre, 1970). Once in the world, mature individuals are responsible for the courses of their own lives. They create themselves from within. Each person is unique, because there is no master template from which to stamp out identical copies. This uniqueness carries with it an undeniable freedom. Yet many people are inclined to abdicate it willingly in order to relieve themselves of the accompanying anxiety. May (1981) points out that the anxiety that accompanies freedom can be psychologically debilitating. It may paralyze, isolate, and panic people so much that they experience heart problems and other illnesses. Even so, freedom is theirs. Although they are not free from biological, psychological, and sociological conditions that often constrain their existence, they are always free to take a stand toward the circumstances. For example, although Christopher Reeve (1952–2004), one of America's leading actors, was paralyzed in an equestrian competition in 1995, he was free to take a stand toward quadriplegia, his disability. He not only put a human face on spinal cord injury but also motivated neuroscientists around the world to conquer the most complex diseases of the brain and central nervous system. Until his death, he devoted his life to championing the cause of individuals with disabilities.

Freedom inevitably involves making choices, which may be another great source of anxiety for many people (Morano, 1973). We have no choice but to make choices. Once a choice is made, all other possible options may be excluded. The responsibility to choose is often so unnerving that some individuals are inclined to turn the task over to others without realizing that such a course of action can aggravate their problems. Nobody can choose existence for another. For example, personal decisions about college, friends, sexual behavior, marriage, and career are private and often have long-term mental health implications for the person faced with such choices.

Courage

Courage comes from the Latin word *cor*, which means heart. The derivation reveals that courage is an affect or emotion. It is reflected in the way people confront the human condition. Courage is the capacity to keep moving ahead in spite of the misery and despair that may be associated with the movement (May, 1975). Ungersma (1961) defines courage in existentialist terms as the individual's use of all of her or his resources to prevail against the constant threat of nonbeing.

Courage always has been vital to human existence. The Roman emperor and philosopher, Marcus Aurelius (121–180 BCE) advised his soldiers to stand up and fight (Staniforth, 1964) because nobody respects a coward on the battlefield or in life. If success is not achieved on the first try, one should get up and try again. From an existential perspective, each human being is constantly in peril. The three worlds of the Umwelt, Mitwelt, and Eigenwelt constitute both safe havens and threats to human existence. The natural environment, which sustains life, also threatens it. For example, it takes courage for individuals to hunt for food in cold and life-threatening weather. In addition, the societal environment in which individuals protect one another is also a threat, because that environment may at any time be threatened from outside. For instance, individuals may be called upon to exhibit courage to defend their family's or community's sustenance, tools, or arms from outside invaders in a home robbery or war.

Finally, the individual environment can be a threat, insofar as individuals must periodically face frightening aspects of their own lives. For instance, facing one's own death entails courage. Individuals who recognize and accept inevitable death are apt to be fearless in fighting for their existence. In addition, individuals may find that they need to defend their own unique ways of being (Bedford, 1972). For example, gays and lesbians demonstrate courage by demanding the right to be who they are in the face of the malice of people who oppose their fight for equal rights.

According to the existentialists, courage enhances human existence. Courage plays a critical role in every person's life, even if most people are unaware of it. People become fully human only by making choices and committing themselves to their decisions. Paul Tillich (1886–1965), the renowned German-American Protestant theologian, referred to the determination to live as ontological (being) courage (May, 1975).

Unfolding (Becoming)

In general, the laws of nature that govern life are invariable. A seed is planted, it germinates, and after a certain amount of time, life begins to take shape. In due course, it sprouts, grows to maturity, and reproduces itself. Then it ripens, dies, and returns to nature. Human life follows the same pattern. Individually and collectively, people are in a constant state of change. They are obliged to let go of what used to be and to think of what currently is. Every day is a new day because the environments in which people exist are dynamic. According to the teachings of Buddhism, life is a stream of becoming and dying (Durant, 1954). Existence implies impermanence. Likewise, civilization is a product of humankind's unfolding, or **becoming.** Civilization is constantly growing, moving from old discoveries and ways of life to new ones.

Unfortunately, change is often difficult for people to accept. They may be afraid to relinquish the tried and true. Some may resist moving to the next landmark in life—graduation, job, marriage, and the like—because each movement brings them closer to death. They become "stuck," as existentialists describe the trepidation and hesitation associated with unfolding (Vontress et al., 1999). The case of Myson, a 38-year-old African-American man, illustrates a problem related to "stuckness."

In their first session together, Myson defined his problem to the counselor as "not being able to sleep." Over the course of the session, he described his "life so far." The oldest of three children, two boys and a girl, he was slated to fulfill the dream his father set out for him, which was to become a basketball star. As soon as he learned to walk, his father placed a little basketball in his hands. By the time he was 6 years old, he and his father were in the back yard every night after dinner, shooting "hoops." In elementary school, middle school, and high school, he played basketball, winning awards at all levels. To his father's delight, Myson grew to the respectable height of 6 feet 10 inches.

Myson's father was so proud of his son that he never assigned him chores to do at home or encouraged him to get an after-school job. He was expected just to concentrate on the game. When he graduated from high school, he got an athletic scholarship at a major state university. Local, state, and national sports writers praised Myson and his natural ability on the court. His father was pleased that his son was headed for the NBA. Unfortunately, the dream ended during his sophomore year, when Myson had to drop out of college to marry and support his high school sweetheart, whom he had impregnated.

Having never worked before, Myson had problems taking directions and always wound up getting fired. He and his wife had to move in with his parents. They had two children, one after another. When his father died, he became the sole breadwinner of the household. He continued to have trouble finding jobs and, once found, had trouble keeping them. Myson's wife and mother both complained a great deal about his not working.

Desperate, Myson took a job as an exotic dancer in a gay club, where he made good tips. When his wife found out what he was doing for the money he brought home, she divorced him.

> C (Client): Why do you think my wife would pack up the children and walk out, just because I was dancing at a gay club? I was just trying to earn money to take care of her and the kids. Why? [He looked to the counselor for the answer.]
>
> T (Therapist): I have no idea. [Looking the client directly in the eye, the counselor acted as if he were totally bewildered by Myson's inquiry.]
>
> C: It's not as if I'm gay. I know I have a good physique; and I know the gay guys like to look at me and touch me, if I let them. [The counselor kept his gaze on the client. It seemed that two or three minutes passed before Myson continued.] And sometimes I do, when they put money in my sock. But that doesn't make me gay. Does it, Doc?
>
> T: I am confused. You tell me.
>
> C: Damn! That's it! I bet she thinks I have turned gay. That's exactly why I didn't tell her about the club. I knew that she'd think I was on the down low. [Myson was speaking in a low voice as if he were talking to himself. The counselor's body language continued to communicate a lack of understanding.] You know what "on the down low" means, don't you Doc?
>
> T: Perhaps you ought to explain.
>
> C: That's when you mess around with men and women. But I'm no punk.

In later sessions, Myson admitted that he had also prostituted himself in order to earn money to pay child support. By the time he reached 30, he was not able get work as a dancer. At 38, he was not much in demand as a prostitute. His case reflects what can happen to individuals who fail to reflect on their lives as they mature. Although Myson's father contributed to his son's lack of preparation for adulthood, Myson needed to take responsibility for his own "stuckness." He was depressed because he was unable to cope with the demands of adulthood. He ended up selling the only thing he had to sell—his body.

Meaning in Life

The search for *meaning* in life is an essential existential theme. Feeling that one's life has meaning is basic to being human. Frankl (1975) defines meaning as a consuming interest in something or somebody other than oneself that encourages and promotes self-development. Satisfying the need for an object or thing of devotion is humankind's primary motivational force. It requires daily reinforcement. What provides meaning one day may not provide meaning the next; and what has been meaningful to a person throughout life may be meaningless when a person is on his or her deathbed.

Existentialists generally agree that meaning is psychologically beneficial. Watts (1995b) points out that a sense of meaning separates happy and unhappy people. Existence has no purpose unless individuals can attach themselves to a self-transcending entity. Their lives are important to the extent that they are part of a group or significant design. For example, the premise of programs such as Alcoholics Anonymous is that substance abusers can give up their destructive behaviors if they are helped to find real meaning in their lives.

In existential theory, psychological problems are associated with meaninglessness. Yalom (1980) maintains that the absence of meaning contributes to neurosis. Cohen (1994) declares that people devoid of meaning in their lives are apt to be hopeless, depressed, or suicidal. Welwood (2002) indicates that such people may feel an internal disconnection in their being. They feel as if they do not belong to their family, group, or clan. They perceive themselves to be outsiders.

In general, meaning comes from intimate personal relationships, job satisfaction, recreational activities, inner spiritual experiences, and daily pleasures. Because each Dasein is unique, each person must find her or his own meaning. Some may find it through suffering, as Frankl (1967) argues. Individuals learn valuable lessons and acquire a sense of meaning from all experiences, both positive and negative. Even depression can be a blessing in disguise. It often forces the sufferer to take stock of a life previously unexamined (Welwood, 2002).

Practice of Existential Therapy

Grounded in existential philosophy, existential therapy is one of the most radical approaches to healing (Koestenbaum, 1971). It is simply an attempt to teach clients to apply philosophical insights to their existence. It employs a variety of ideas gleaned from observers of human existence down through the ages. Although most existential therapists eschew the use of "techniques," it is appropriate to examine the implications of some existential concepts for the counseling relationship, diagnosis, intervention strategies, and evaluation.

The Client-Counselor Relationship

Several existential ideas suggest the nature and quality of the therapeutic encounter in existential therapy. Two Daseins (beings) come together. Each embodies a unique essence. Both strive to be authentic. Each, although responsible for personal existence, recognizes a responsibility for the other, with whom there is a lifeline. Each is a subject and an object at the same time. They both share the same human condition. This includes a single life support system, the Umwelt, and a similar social system, the Mitwelt. They both also influence the self of the other.

In a counseling relationship, the counselor, the subject, helps the object, the client, to understand the human condition, which impacts the client's existence. The helper is nonpossessive because each person must be free to experience life uniquely. Each must be able to unfold as dictated by an irreplaceable essence. In order to assist without violating the client's existential self, existential counselors should be empathic, identifying with the client while simultaneously recognizing that they are limited in understanding the client's world. Each client resides in a different Eigenwelt and is a different essence. Counselors are at the same time sympathetic toward their clients, because all Daseins share the same human condition, the Umwelt and Mitwelt. They share emotionally their clients' suffering. For example, existential counselors may attend funerals, crying with clients as they mourn the death of loved ones.

In view of the existential constructs just discussed, it is understandable that Boss (1963) used the term *psychotherapeutic eros* to describe an intimate counselor-client relationship and that Buber (1970) described a truly therapeutic encounter as an I-Thou dyad, a caring, intimate, and authentic relationship. In contrast to the I-It of some therapy approaches, in which the counselor relates to a client as if that person were an object, I-Thou reflects the spiritual nature of the existential counselor-client working relationship. It hints of an attitude similar to that of siblings toward each other. Each wants to help the other without hindering the other's growth toward self-sufficiency and independence.

Diagnosis

Diagnosis is the process of defining the client's problem. In traditional psychotherapeutic approaches, diagnosis usually consists of psychological and social norms by which clients are measured. In general, this view of diagnosis is incompatible with existential ideas. In existential therapy, each Dasein (being) is unique and is encouraged to unfold according to the dictates of his or her uniqueness, not according to the dictates of social norms. Existential therapy is philosophical education that aims to facilitate the client's examination of his or her existence. Many of the existential concepts already defined and discussed (e.g., self-knowledge, authenticity, becoming, courage, responsibility, and meaning in life) have significant implications for helping clients to examine their lives. A selection of these existential concepts are employed in a client self-inventory, which provides structure for the existential encounter.

- *Self-knowledge* is a primary item for consideration. Individuals without knowledge of their interests, abilities, values, and ambitions will not be able to make decisions that will enhance their existence.

- *Authenticity* is another idea that can help clients to scrutinize their being. Inauthentic people live in *bad faith*. They deceive themselves as well as others, following the crowd instead of their own dictates and in so doing, risk their psychological well-being.

- *Becoming* is also relevant to existential diagnosis. Life, once set in motion, moves through predictable stages of development, maturation, and demise. Any attempt to interrupt the process is apt to lead to frustration and a sense of failure.

- *Courage* is another significant construct that counselors and clients can use in the philosophical examination of the clients' existence. Individuals who are afraid to make choices are apt to encounter psychological hurdles because they have allowed others to make decisions for them.

- *Meaning in life* invariably comes up in a dialogue in which the focus is self-examination. People devoid of a sense of meaning may feel bored, indifferent to their social surroundings, or depressed (May, 1981).

- *Death*, a much-discussed construct in existentialism, is also an important subject in clients' self-inventories. Clients are asked to consider their fear of nonbeing as the primary cause of their existential anxiety. Some indication exists that there is a relationship between the fear of death and overall mental health (Vontress et al., 1999).

- Finally, *responsibility* is a construct useful in helping clients examine their lives. Everybody needs somebody. Clients are encouraged to think about the construct Mitwelt, of connecting with others in the world by being responsible for themselves and their fellows.

Intervention Procedures

A technique is a procedure, or a way of using basic skills to execute an artistic, scientific, or mechanical operation. At first glance, the word *technique* suggests the opposite of what existentialists hold dear. Wanting most to understand human existence, existentialist therapists believe that the overemphasis on technique blocks the counselor's ability to understand the client's essence (May, 1964). Technique implies that the therapist views the client as an object to be analyzed, manipulated, and adjusted to a norm. Existential therapists prefer to be thought of as philosophical companions, not as people who repair psyches. Like mountain guides, they are familiar with the terrain, human existence (Binswanger, 1991). Although they can teach clients about the lay of the land, they are unable to personally escort each person in her or his own trek up the rocky mountains of life. Because of individual differences such as age, weight, and athletic agility, individuals must negotiate the climb in their own time and in their own way. In existential counseling, therapists should set aside the notion that any one intervention fits all clients. May (1991) recommends that therapeutic techniques be flexible, versatile, and variable from one encounter to the next, even with the same client.

Yet, in spite of reservations about therapeutic techniques, an examination of the existential psychotherapeutic literature reveals that existential therapists do, in fact, use several of the same techniques used by therapists from other schools of thought. The procedure most associated with existential therapy is the **Socratic dialogue** (Ricken, 1991). Socrates believed that each person holds inside himself or herself the solutions to his or her own problems. In a Socratic dialogue, the therapist helps the client explore these solutions without imposing perimeters around the client's thoughts. Self-examination is achieved best when the therapist engages the client while simultaneously resisting the temptation to impose knowledge, advice, and direction on the other.

The Socratic dialogue is also referred to as dialectic, from the Greek *dialektike*, to converse (Christian, 1977). The German philosopher Hegel (Croce, 1910) took the concept further, viewing dialectic as the search for truth, unity, or synthesis through the examination of opposites. To understand anything, one has to consider its opposite: life and death, good and bad, pretty and ugly, happiness and unhappiness, and so on. Thus, counselors employing the Socratic dialogue, or dialectic, coach their clients to examine their own thoughts in light of these opposites and to make personal choices. In a way, the therapist becomes, as Socrates called himself, an "intellectual midwife." This approach to knowledge of self is also known as the **maieutic method,** or hatching method.

Vontress, Johnson, and Epp (1999) advocate the use of the Socratic dialogue in existential cross-cultural counseling because the therapist helps individuals to give birth to the knowledge that they already possess. Myson's counselor was using Socratic dialogue when he responded, "I have no idea," and "I am confused. You tell me." By purposefully feigning ignorance while keeping the conversation on the subject, the counselor steadily led Myson toward his own conclusions regarding the choices he had made in his life.

Frankl's (1967) logotherapy is a therapeutic approach somewhat akin to the Socratic dialogue. Although his approach is based on the assumption that the client has a will for freedom and meaning, it is more structured and authoritarian than straightforward Socratic dialogue. Clients are encouraged to think on (paradoxical intention) or away from (dereflection) the ideas that cause them anxiety. For example, a client who is afraid to speak with others might be asked to go out into the clinic's waiting room and engage the receptionist in a conversation, or an overly self-absorbed client might be asked to volunteer to coach his child's soccer team.

As we have seen, to say that existential therapists are not technique oriented does not mean that they do not use techniques. What differentiates existential therapists from other therapists is their overarching philosophical attitude toward human existence. Their focus is on the Dasein, the human being, and the environments that influence the personal journey. Existential therapists are free to use a variety of psychological techniques, just as long as they do not forget the big picture, the person's whole being in-the-world (Patterson, 1980). Counselors who focus on the client are therapeutic; those who focus only on techniques are apt to be antitherapeutic.

Existential Cross-Cultural Counseling

Because of existentialism's focus on an individual's self-knowledge rather than on any impositions the therapist might bring into the therapeutic relationship, the existential counselor is flexible in relating to, diagnosing, and intervening on behalf of culturally different clients. The following vignettes illustrate two examples of this flexibility.

Olatokundo, an 18-year-old boy, lived in his native Nigeria with an uncle until he was 16. Then he came to the United States to join the rest of his family. Just after Olatokundo was born, his father had moved to the United States to complete a Ph.D. in physics and had become an American citizen. Olatokundo's mother and three older siblings joined his father a few years later. One year after Olatokundo arrived in America, his father died suddenly of a massive stroke. The family was devastated. Nigerian fathers, especially those from the Yoruba tribe, provide strong familial leadership. They are involved in all decisions that each family member makes because the family honor is always at stake. An immigrant family without a father is like a rudderless ship.

When Olatokundo went to see his high school counselor the day after he graduated, the counselor could see from the expression on his face that something was wrong. The counselor soon learned why. The young man was faced with a big decision and his father was not there to help him. His mother had always deferred to his father. Therefore, she could not help him either.

T (Therapist): What's on your mind today?

C (Client): Nothing. [The client replied with his head down, as if he were talking to himself.]

T: Oh, I get the impression that you are troubled.

C: Well, yes, there is a problem. [Olatokundo's voice was hardly above a whisper. He was unaccustomed to elders being so direct. Back home in Nigeria authority figures engage in several minutes of small talk about family, crops, and other such matters before exploring weighty problems. His problem was really heavy on his mind.] You know my father died. [The client continued to speak in a very low voice, still keeping his head down.]

T: Yes, I heard. I am very sorry. I know that it is a terrible loss to you and your family. Your father was a wise man. I extend my condolences. Did you want to talk about that?

C: Sort of. [Out of respect, Olatokundo usually did not make eye contact with elders, but now he looked directly at the counselor.] You know, my father always told us what to do. What next step to take in life. Now he's gone. I have to decide on college and I don't know how to select one or how to pay for my education. And I just know he wants me to go to college. I do not want to displease him.

At first the counselor was perplexed: why did the boy talk about his father as if he were still alive? But he quickly realized that it was cultural, that in some African communities people consider that the dead are still among the living; they are just invisible. He tried to shape his response in a respectful way.

T: Okay! So what do you think your father wants you to do?

C: I don't know.

T: In that case, you need to think about it.

The client appeared confused. He expected the counselor to give him direct advice like his father did.

> T: Olatokundo, why don't you go away and think about your situation and then come back to see me tomorrow. I am sure that we can come up with something.

The next day, the client returned with a smile on his face.

> T: Don't tell me. You found a solution to your problem.

> C: Well, not really. But my father came to me last night and helped me a lot.

> T: Tell me about it.

> C: [In a calm and steady voice.] Well, when I went to bed, I prayed for help and soon fell asleep. During the night my father came to me and told me what I should do, how to go to college.

Then the client went on to tell the counselor that he was going to apply for admission to a nearby community college, that he planned to get a job to pay for his tuition, and that since his mother now was alone, he planned to continue living at home, because it is not in the Nigerian tradition to leave parents alone.

This vignette illustrates therapeutic midwifery or the maieutic method that Socrates used. The counselor aided the client in solving his own problem by encouraging him to think about it. He also revealed knowledge of traditional African culture. He was not shocked when the client told him that his departed father came to him in the night. Instead, he invited the client to relate to him the advice that his father gave him. The way the counselor used the client's reported encounter with the spirit of his father is an excellent example of how the Uberwelt (spirit world) can be used in existential cross-cultural counseling.

Gina was a 16-year-old girl who had recently transferred to the local public high school in a university town in a midwestern state. Almost immediately, this pretty girl with blue eyes and long raven hair became one of the most popular girls in the 1,200-student population. A straight-A student, she became a member of the cheerleaders' squad, sang in the glee club, was elected to the student government, and played clarinet in the school band. By the middle of her first semester at this new school, she was dating the captain of the football team.

However, near the end of the semester, things began to change for her. Her boyfriend broke up with her for "no reason," her girlfriends started shunning her, and she wondered what was happening to her. That was when she went to see Mrs. Holloway, the school counselor, who wanted to know, "What's wrong, honey?"

"I don't really know. That is why I have come to talk with you." At the counselor's urging to talk about herself, Gina explained that she and her family had recently moved to the United States from France. Her father, an American, had played several years of professional basketball in France. Her mother had been a model and part-time actress when she married Gina's father. Gina had two siblings, a younger brother and a young sister, both still in middle school. Her family had come to the United States when her father accepted the position of head basketball coach at the nearby state university.

"What is your father's name?" the counselor asked.

"Sam Johnson," Gina replied.

"You mean Sam Johnson, the head basketball coach at State, is your father?" the counselor inquired excitedly.

"You got it!" Gina confirmed with a slight French accent.

"So your father is African American? Is he your biological father?" Mrs. Holloway rushed the two sentences together. She wanted to be completely sure of the facts.

"Yes, but what has that got to do with anything?" Gina protested.

"I don't know, but we have to find out. May I have your permission to check your files and ask around to see what I can find out about what's going on?" Mrs. Holloway asked.

"Sure, why not?" Gina shrugged.

After Gina left, Mrs. Holloway began her "discovery," as she called her search for answers to her client's problems. First, she went to the Records Office. She wanted to look at Gina's cumulative folder and talk with the intake clerk, the person who enrolled the student the first time she came to the school. She learned from the intake clerk that both parents came to enroll their daughter and that they were excited that she would be attending a school so near the university where her father worked. In examining Gina's folder, she noticed that the girl had been placed in classes that were equivalent to courses she had already taken in her French school. (The counselor, who had taught in French West Africa when she was in the Peace Corps, knew the French school system and the courses equivalent to those in American high schools.)

The counselor also asked some of her other student clients if they knew Gina. She learned that some of the girls who were jealous of Gina's popularity had seen Gina's father drop her off and pick her up. One of the girls who used to date Gina's boyfriend started some vicious rumors about Gina. The counselor understood how all these things might be blown out of proportion to cause her client a great deal of stress, especially in a small insulated community where people are not exposed to many cultural differences.

In their next meeting, the counselor greeted Gina with a smile on her face. "You went to an international school in France, right?" Mrs. Holloway wanted to know again.

"Yes, in Paris," Gina confirmed.

"Did you know that you have already taken some of the courses you are now taking?" Mrs. Holloway informed her. The counselor also told Gina that she had made arrangements through the vice principal for Gina to take some advanced placement tests so that she could go directly to the twelfth grade and graduate in June instead of a year later. Gina was so excited that she embraced her counselor.

"As to your feeling that some students are treating you differently, did your father ever talk to you about the racial situation in the United States?" the counselor inquired.

"Not really. He traveled a lot. My mother talked excitedly about coming to the United States," Gina explained.

Mrs. Holloway then felt that she understood the source of Gina's problem. It was the racism that she knew too well because, she, as an African American, had experienced it throughout her life. "Honey, what do you consider yourself? White or Black?" the counselor asked.

"I am French," Gina shot back.

"But your father is Black, an African American, honey! In this country, you are considered Black if you have only one sixteenth Black blood."

"What are you talking about?" Gina shouted.

"I am talking about racism! You'd better learn about it if you want to survive here." Mrs. Holloway blurted out, as if she was a caring mother who wanted to protect her daughter from hurt. Gina started to sob. The counselor hugged her. She explained to Gina that she had done nothing wrong, that she had to see things the way they really are, the way they have been for too long. Gina wanted to know what she ought to do to be accepted.

"Nothing. Just be yourself, honey," Mrs. Holloway advised her client.

Mrs. Holloway and Gina talked several times thereafter. Gina continued with her extracurricular activities and maintained her A average. Although many of her former "friends" never returned, the few who did were important to her, because they were "real friends," as she put it.

In this case, the counselor was a warm, caring person who related to the client as one human being to another. No psychotherapeutic techniques in the usual sense were evident. Mrs. Holloway did "discovery" work to help her develop a diagnosis that she felt was credible. She took what she discovered and added to it her own experiences as a Black person and as a former Peace Corps member. Then she shared the diagnosis with her client, allowing her to accept or reject it. Throughout her sessions with the client, the counselor was direct but always supportive. The vignette shows that the existential cross-cultural counselor is a companion who is not reluctant to take direct action to help the culturally different client to negotiate an unfamiliar environment.

Evaluation of Existential Therapy

Evaluation is the process of determining the value or efficacy of something. In the scientific community, it usually entails formulating objectives, specifying procedures for measuring their achievement, and establishing indices for their attainment. This understanding of evaluation suggests that existential therapy is not amenable to measurement by the tools of science. The subjectivity of the existential experience precludes its being studied by scientific methods. Concepts such as courage, freedom, authenticity, choice, anxiety, and meaning do not lend themselves easily to statistical manipulation. Change as a result of existential therapy usually takes place outside the counseling relationship (Rychlak, 1981).

In existential therapy, clients report change. With the insights developed in counseling, clients specify before-and-after perceptions and behaviors in terms of how they relate to the Umwelt, Mitwelt, and Eigenwelt. Evaluation is concomitant with therapy. Therapists encourage their clients to assess their personal growth and development during each encounter. Existential therapy is essentially a philosophy for living. As such, it seems illegitimate to compare its outcome with those of psychologically based therapeutic models. The following vignette illustrates how existential therapy is evaluated by the counselor and client on an ongoing basis:

Julio, 30, and Irena, his fiancée, 28, consulted a counselor "about our planned marriage." They had been a couple for six years and had lived together for three. Irena was concerned because Julio was not "very interested in sex." Julio said, "Sex is not everything. Love is not just about sex." They shared the same bed and usually fell asleep in embrace. However, Irena said that she felt ignored, unloved, and at times unwanted. She indicated that she needed confirmation of Julio's love for her before they got married.

A banker, Julio had done well since he graduated from a local Catholic university, where he obtained a degree in accounting. The only child in a Puerto Rican middle-class family, he was an altar boy and had once considered the priesthood. He described himself as "an all-around athlete" who loved to go skiing on weekends with old college friends. Irena usually stayed home. She came from a large Greek-American family of nine children. Also Catholic, she and her siblings had many friends always coming and going to and from their farmhouse in rural Iowa. Julio, on the other hand, grew up in New York City, where he attended an academic high school in the Bronx. His father was a college professor and his mother was a housewife. During several weeks of counseling in which the couple discussed their love for each other, the therapist helped them to examine their ability to merge psychologically and physically. Although Julio did all the right things to convince Irena that he loved her, he was afraid of intimacy. Talking about his attitude toward sex, he said that he could "take it or leave it." He explained that when he approached orgasm, he always held back, fearing that he would lose control.

The therapist helped Julio to recognize that he was experiencing existential anxiety. The real source of it was the fear of death. The anxiety manifested itself in Julio's fear of merging with Irena. Merging completely with her was akin to death. The therapist decided to discontinue couples counseling and to see Julio separately to help him work through his fear.

"I really love my fiancée so much," Julio declared. "But I can't seem to show her how much," he continued.

The counselor looked perplexed. His eyes opened widely, as if he wanted to invite the client to continue; and he did. "I enjoy holding her and falling asleep with her in my arms. And I like waking up and finding her there beside me."

"What are you really saying?" the counselor asked.

"I don't know. It's almost like she's too good to touch sexually. And if I go all the way, it's like I am consumed, like I have lost myself," the client explained.

"And you have lost me," the counselor smiled. "I really don't know where you are going with this."

Now somewhat challenged, the client clarified, "When, you know, when I have sex and have an orgasm, it's like I am losing control, like I am falling into a deep hole or dying. And I am afraid."

"I understand what you are saying, but do you know why this is happening to you?" the counselor wanted to know.

"Well, let me say what I think is happening to me. It seems that I have a deep spiritual bond with Irena, but I am unable to express it physically. Something keeps blocking my ability to be sexual with the one I love," Julio explained.

After engaging him in similar Socratic dialogues for several weeks about death, intimacy, and related issues, Julio emerged from the experience with enough insight and courage to connect with Irena on an authentic and mutually satisfying level. He learned that becoming as one with his lover was similar to unifying with the cosmic order. It was the highest level of completeness. He had to experience the moment and just let it be. The ecstasy of love and sex cannot be controlled; it must simply be experienced. Julio and Irena eventually married and became parents of three children.

Although Julio and Irena were from different backgrounds, they were both second-generation Americans. Cultural differences did not factor into their presenting problem or the resolution of it, however. Their problem transcended culture; it was a part of the human condition. Although existential counselors need to be sensitive to the possible relationship between cultural differences and life challenges, they should always focus on the human condition first and on variations from psychosocial and physical norms second.

Existential Therapy: Blind Spots, Limitations, and Challenges

Proponents of existentialism usually make clear that environmental conditions influence a person's being-in-the-world. Physical, social, individual, and spiritual surroundings are interactive and determine a person's lifelong well-being. As a helping model, existentialism is necessarily multicultural. It recognizes that different geographical conditions produce variations in both the physical and cultural appearance of people, that people are simultaneously similar to and different from each other. Therefore, it is understandable that some blind spots, limitations, and challenges may potentially impede the cross-cultural interventions of existential counselors.

Blind Spots

There is no one single existential philosophy posited by one person. There are only disparate ideas about life from numerous sources that have come to be referred to as existentialism. Therefore, it seems tenable to say that existential therapists experience blind spots in cross-cultural counseling not because they are existentialists but because they are human beings. As such, they, like everybody else, are apt to perceive themselves as the focal point and center of the universe when, in fact, this perception is an illusion. Each human organism is a self-contained entity. People know only what they have learned through their senses, and they can only speculate about things external to themselves. One cannot know directly the experiences of another person. Each person is a subject and object at the same time. We look at others from our place in the world, and they look back at us from their vantage point. Therefore, our vision of others is always blurred by unavoidable blind spots. Even so, existential therapists try to connect with others across cultural, national, racial, and other boundaries on a spiritual level. As therapists, it is a constant struggle because we are all ensnared by the rituals of science, which allow little or no room for the spiritual world. In spite of our protests, many adherents of scientific rigor continue to insist that existentialists fit into their paradigms.

Limitations

There are at least four commonly perceived limitations to existential therapy. First, for some multiculturalists, existentialism is viewed as Eurocentric, just as Buddhism is associated with the Asian continent. Therefore, existential counseling is not considered a useful therapeutic modality outside Europe and other Western societies any more than Buddhism is considered a useful therapeutic modality inside Western societies. Second, existential ideas as expressed by many Western exponents are difficult to understand. Although therapists may be attracted to existentialism, some are turned off by the unnecessarily complicated language with which concepts are expressed. Third, existential therapists usually reject the use of therapeutic techniques because they feel that these may overshadow clients and their problems. Even so, many counselors, especially those fresh out of graduate school, are doubtful of their ability to intervene effectively without techniques. Finally, partly for the reasons just stated, many therapists consider existential therapy to be therapeutic only for highly educated clients.

Challenges

There are two main challenges to existential therapy. The first one is definitional. Because existentialism is an attitude or perspective on human existence, it eludes precise definition. It is also difficult to define the elusive concept of *human existence*. Existentialism as a therapeutic model is more philosophical than psychological. Although it is holistic therapy in that all existential counselors want to understand clients within their natural, social, personal, and spiritual context, existential therapists differ a great deal in how they apply it and clients differ in how they respond to it. Understandably, then, existential therapy is in need of more clarification in the mind of clients and therapists.

The second challenge facing existential therapists is to find ways to integrate their approach with the standard operational procedures for diagnosing and treating client problems that are expected in today's therapeutic environment of HMOs and insurance companies. Even though the theory behind existential therapy departs from the theories behind the standard psychotherapeutic practices, existential counselors are obliged to use the same diagnostic manual that most other therapeutic professionals use (see APA, 2000). This is why existential therapists working within the confines of the expectations imposed on the psychotherapeutic profession often feel constricted. How can they be both existential philosophers and psychotherapists at the same time?

Future Development: Existential Therapy in a Diverse World

A great diversity makes up the comprehensive system that is most often referred to as the universe, world, earth, or the Umwelt, as Binswanger (1975) called it. Diversity always has been a part of the human condition. People are diverse, just as the places in which they live are geographically diverse, differing in terms of nationality, race, and culture; by gender, age, and sexual orientation; and by numerous psychological, physical, and social challenges. During the last 50 years or so, Americans have become increasingly sensitive to human differences. Institutions, organizations, and associations throughout society have instituted measures to ensure equal opportunity for all citizens. During the civil rights movement of the 1960s and 1970s, the counseling profession launched efforts to help counselors to be more effective helping all clients, regardless of differences that set individual clients apart from the general population.

Diversity counseling is an idea now well established in the psychotherapeutic community. Existential therapy is especially suited to helping diverse clients (Vontress, 1985). Existentialism is a philosophy that focuses on the human condition. It encompasses all people, regardless of differences that at first blush might seem to set them apart. Existentialism recognizes and appreciates the human community first and differences second. For example, in counseling a racially different client, the counselor relates to the client as a co-equal. Race is not an issue in the encounter, unless the client presents it as an impediment to her or his situation. Similarly, physically challenged clients should be related to like all other clients, unless they introduce the condition as being problematic for them. A condition or station in life is not as important as the attitude a person takes toward it. Existential counselors are optimistic and supportive of fellow human beings. They encourage clients to discover themselves in order that they may reach their greatest potential.

Interest in existentialism as a foundation for therapy continues to grow. Existential counseling and psychotherapy is a content area included in university courses and in the textbooks written for those courses. Recognizing the widespread malaise and sense of hopelessness at large in the world today, Marinoff (1999) recommends that troubled individuals resort to philosophical counseling instead of psychiatric drugs. Schuster (1991, 1999), Raabe (2001), and Lahav and de Venza Tillmanns (1995) are among the increasing number of psychotherapeutic scholars who promote the use of techniques used by Socrates and other ancient philosophers. The escalating enthusiasm for philosophical counseling reflects a simultaneous interest in existential counseling, because the two approaches are similar. In the future, the public may be able to consult a new category of helpers who encourage clients to focus on the totality of their existence.

Although not always labeled as such, existential ideas are expressed throughout society. Motivational speakers use them to stimulate people to take charge of their lives. Religious leaders draw upon them to prevail upon their followers to respond to others with love and respect. TV talk show personalities strive to get audiences to be authentic. Leaders of self-help groups teach the benefits of responsibility, the profits of living courageously, and the psychological advantages of being in the present. The fact that existential ideas are fast becoming a part of the general culture makes them more understandable and acceptable as a therapeutic model. Therefore, it seems reasonable to predict an increased use of existential counseling in the future.

In view of the current openness to existential counseling, proponents of existentialism need to do more to educate counselors and potential clients to its merits. In the past and continuing in the present, the language used to communicate the essence of existentialism and existential therapy has been unnecessarily complicated. Early works written by Europeans were available primarily in French and German. Their translations in English have not always been easy to understand. For example, Sartre's (1983) *Cahiers pour une morale*, translated as *Notebooks for an Ethics* (Sartre, 1992), is almost as difficult for an Anglophone to read in English as it is in French. Despite this perception of difficulty, existential ideas are simple concepts that most people can understand, appreciate, and relate to their existence. Life, death, love, responsibility, and other such constructs are not new to people. People live them every day.

Summary

1. Humankind always has been concerned with life and death, happiness and unhappiness, meaning and meaninglessness, and other matters related to the human condition.

2. Questions about human existence can be traced to antiquity, when Socrates prodded his interlocutors to examine themselves and their existence. In 20th-century Europe, intellectuals such as Martin Heidegger and Jean-Paul Sartre began to probe the human condition. Their scholarship came to be called *existentialism*.

3. In turn, psychiatrists and psychologists, inspired by existential philosophical concepts, began to apply some of these concepts to their work and facilitated the development of existential psychotherapy. Some of the founding existential therapists included Victor Frankl, the developer of logotherapy; Ludwig Binswanger, who coined the terms *Umwelt*, *Mitwelt*, and *Eigenwelt* to describe the human condition; Medard Boss, who developed the concept of the therapeutic eros, Martin Buber, who further defined the existentialist therapeutic relationship via his concept of I-Thou, and, in America, Carl Rogers.

4. In recent years, existential therapy has responded to the needs of diverse populations. Because existentialism is based on a universal worldview that

has affinities with Eastern Buddhism and African animism, existentialist therapy is in its very nature adaptive to culturally diverse groups.

5. One of the core concepts of existential therapy is that human existence is a holistic un-analyzable entity consisting of the three interactive modes of being-in-the-world, the Umwelt (the natural environment), the Mitwelt (the social environment), and the Eigenwelt (the personal world).

6. Other key concepts in existential therapy include existence and essence (one's presence on earth and one's own definition of one's presence on earth), self-knowledge (which must be attained for psychological well-being), love (which is an essential component of self-knowledge), responsibility (cooperation with the Umwelt and Mitwelt, which leads to psychological well-being), authenticity (the honesty and courage to be who you really are, which also leads to psychological well-being), existential anxiety (an anxiety brought about by the unpredictability of life), courage (which enhances human existence), unfolding or becoming (the constant changes in life that we must all experience), and meaning in life (as opposed to meaninglessness, which leads to psychological problems).

7. In an existential counseling relationship, the counselor (the subject) helps the client (the object) to understand the human condition, which impacts the client's existence. The helper is nonpossessive because each person must be free to experience life uniquely. In order to assist without violating the client's existential self, existential counselors should be empathic while simultaneously recognizing that they are limited in understanding the client's world.

8. Existential therapy in practice is simply an attempt to teach clients to apply philosophical insights to their existence. Existential therapists act as philo-sophical companions, not as people who repair psyches. Diagnosis involves a client's self-inventory of the existential concepts of self-knowledge, courage, authenticity, and others, which provides structure for the existential en-counter. Existential therapy eschews "techniques," but it does employ a variety of ideas gleaned from observers of human existence down through the ages, such as using the Socratic dialogue and encouraging clients to continuously evaluate their interventions.

9. Because of existentialism's focus on the individual's self-knowledge rather than on any impositions the therapist might bring into the therapeutic relationship, the existential counselor is flexible in relating to, diagnosing, and intervening on behalf of culturally different clients.

10. The subjectivity of the existential experience precludes its being studied by scientific methods. Concepts such as courage, freedom, authenticity, choice,

anxiety, and meaning do not lend themselves easily to statistical manipulation. Therapists encourage their clients to assess their own personal growth and development.

11. The blind spot of existential therapy is really a blind spot of being human—one cannot know directly the experiences of another person, so our vision of others is always unavoidably blurred. Existentialist therapy is limited insofar as it is perceived as being a Eurocentric philosophy (though in fact it is not). The philosophy may be at times difficult to understand, it eschews techniques and therefore may be hard for some to practice, and it may only be effective with highly educated clients. The challenges to existentialist therapy include the need to define the therapy more clearly as therapy rather than as philosophy and the need to find ways to integrate the approach with the standard operational procedures for diagnosing and treating client problems expected in today's therapeutic environments.

12. Existential therapy is becoming increasingly acceptable to the general public. Clients who resort to it may be able to avoid or overcome the malaise that is so pervasive in contemporary society. Existential therapy is especially suited to helping diverse clients because existentialism is a philosophy that focuses on the human condition and encompasses all people.

Key Terms

animism (p. 144)
authenticity (p. 153)
becoming (p. 156)
courage (p. 155)
Dasein (p. 142)
dereflection (p. 143)
Eigenwelt (p. 143)
essence (p. 150)
existence (p. 150)
existential anxiety (p. 154)
existentialism (p. 142)
freedom (p. 154)
I-thou (p. 143)

logotherapy (p. 143)
maieutic method (p. 162)
meaning (p. 143)
Mitwelt (p. 143)
object (p. 149)
paradoxical intention (p. 143)
psychotherapeutic eros (p. 143)
self-knowledge (p. 151)
Socratic dialogue (p. 161)
subject (p. 149)
Uberwelt (p. 143)
Umwelt (p. 143)

Resources for Further Study

Professional Organizations

Existential Humanistic Institute
870 Market Street, Suite 463
San Francisco, CA 94102
415-421-3355

> The institute's primary focus is educational. Offering courses in existential-humanistic therapy and theory, it is a forum for mental health professionals, scholars, and students who seek in-depth training in existential-humanistic philosophy, practice, and inquiry.

International Society for Existential Psychology and Psychotherapy
c/o Trinity Western University
Graduate Counseling Psychology Department
7600 Glover Road
Langley, BC V2Y Y1
Canada
604-513-2034

> A multicultural, international, and interdisciplinary organization dedicated to encouraging and advancing research and education in existential psychology and psychotherapy.

Professional Journals

International Journal of Existential Psychology and Psychotherapy
c/o Trinity Western University
Graduate Counseling Psychology Department
7600 Glover Road
Langley, B. C. V2Y 1V1
Canada
604-518-2056

Journal of Existentialism
11 Main Street
Germantown, NY 12526
518-537-4700

Review of Existential Psychology and Psychiatry
11 Main Street
Germantown, NY 12526
518-537-4700

> These three journals are refereed and carry a variety of articles pertaining to existential philosophy, psychology, and psychotherapy.

Suggested Readings

Chessick, R. D. (1982). Socrates: First psychotherapist. *American Journal of Psycho-analysis, 42,* 71–83.

The author argues that Socrates, the ancient Greek philosopher and teacher, was the first person to engage people psychotherapeutically.

Frey, D. H., & Heslet, F. E. (1975). *Existential theory for counselors.* Boston: Houghton Mifflin.

The writers explain how counselors can use existential ideas in their work.

Friedman, M. (1964). Existential psychotherapy and the image of man. *Journal of Humanistic Psychology, 4,* 104–117.

An easy-to-read, thought-provoking article that reveals why existential psychotherapy is a useful helping modality.

Lescoe, F. J. (1974). *Existentialism: With or without God.* New York: Alba House.

A book written by a Catholic priest who excited my interest in existentialism 30 years ago.

Marino, G. (2004). *Basic writings of existentialism.* New York: Modern Library.

A compilation of articles by writers who discuss existentialism from various perspectives.

Singer, I. (1992). *Meaning in life: The creation of value.* New York: Free Press.

The author discusses the psychological implications of meaning in life, a construct basic to existentialism.

Tillich, P. (1944). Existential philosophy. *Journal of the History of Ideas, 5,* 44–70.

This article is one of the first explanations of existentialism written by a renowned European scholar.

Van Kaam, A. (1966). *Existential foundations of psychology.* Pittsburgh: Duquesne University Press.

A book written by one of the first American scholars to explain how existentialism dovetails with therapeutic psychology.

Other Media Resources

Existential Links, Organizations, and Listservs
www.existentialk-therapy.com/Links.htm

Links to several people, organizations, institutes, and services that can help all those interested in increasing their understanding of existential psychotherapy.

Existential Psychotherapy
www.Existential.dsl.pipex.com/Existential/home.htm

Information about lectures, books, research, and consultation provided by existential scholars and therapists.

Chapter 6

Person-Centered Therapy

DAVID J. CAIN

Person-centered therapy, originally developed by Carl Rogers, is based on the assumption that all humans have the innate capacity to solve their own problems and to grow psychologically in an environment that is conducive to such change and growth. Not only is it assumed that all people have this capacity, but also that optimal change and growth occurs when it is self-directed. However, people may only be able to engage in this process when certain conditions prevail, and the fundamental role of person-centered therapists is to establish these conditions for their clients. The conditions involve clients' perceiving that their therapist (1) understands who they are and how they perceive the world (empathetic understanding), (2) accepts them without judgment (unconditional positive regard), and (3) is being genuine in the therapeutic relationship (congruence). Much more will be said about these fundamental conditions of therapy later in the chapter.

Origins and Evolution of Person-Centered Therapy

The name given to the therapy that Rogers developed changed over time. Today *person-centered therapy* is most commonly used and is synonymous with *client-centered therapy*, which was the name Rogers gave to his counseling approach earlier in its development. In this chapter, I primarily use the term *person-centered therapy* unless the earlier term *client-centered therapy* is relevant in an historical context.

Carl Rogers's influence on American psychotherapy is enormous, though often indirect. His fundamental ideas have been absorbed by many diverse approaches to psychotherapy. More than any other theorist, Carl Rogers taught us to listen with sensitivity and caring and to understand that the quality of the client-therapist relationship, in itself, has the potential to foster personal learning and growth in the client.

Rogers and the Early Development of Person-Centered Therapy

Carl Rogers was born in 1902 and raised in a close-knit, religious midwestern family. His parents were exemplars of the Protestant work ethic that was reflected in Rogers's enormous productivity. Rogers originally pursued a career in the ministry. He entered the Union Theological Seminary in New York City in 1924. Kirschenbaum (1979) quotes from Rogers's journal about why he left the seminary and went to Columbia University's Teachers College a few years later.

> My own reason for deciding at that time to leave the field of religious work was that although questions as to the meaning of life and the possibility of the constructive improvement of life for individuals were of deep interest to me, I could not work in a field where I would be required to believe in some specified religious doctrine. I wanted to find a field in which I could be sure my freedom of thought would not be limited. (pp. 51–52)

We can see in this journal entry that Rogers was already moving toward a desire to help individuals improve their lives, but he wanted the freedom to explore more personally compatible ways of doing so. In the fall of 1926, Rogers left Union Theological Seminary and literally walked across the street and entered Teachers College to pursue a degree in clinical and educational psychology. Two years later, he started the next chapter of his life in Rochester, New York.

The Rochester Years (1928–1939)

The roots of person-centered therapy date back to the late 1920s, when Carl Rogers spent his formative years as a child clinical psychologist in Rochester. During this period from 1928–1939, Rogers worked in the Child Study Department of the Society for the Prevention of Cruelty to Children, becoming its director in 1929 at the age of 27. Rogers was a pragmatist. As he found himself faced with the task of choosing a treatment for large numbers of troubled children and parents, his guiding question was, "Does it work?" Rogers's approach to his clinical work was based on careful systematic observation as opposed to trial and error. Not content to rely on his subjective impressions, he carefully evaluated the effect of his work.

In his first book, *Clinical Treatment of the Problem Child* (1939), published toward the end of his Rochester years, Rogers identified some of the basic elements that would form the foundation for client-centered therapy. Rogers's experiences with children and parents led him to begin to realize that "it is the client who knows what hurts, what directions to go, what problems are crucial. . . . It began to occur to me that unless I had a need to demonstrate my own cleverness and learning, I would do better to rely upon the client for the direction of movement in the process" (Kirschenbaum, 1979, p. 89).

Ohio State University (1940–1944)

In 1939, Rogers left Rochester to go to Ohio State University as a full professor in the psychology department. In addition to teaching a full load of courses, he supervised graduate students in counseling, wrote several articles, and counseled several students. Rogers established a practicum in counseling and psychotherapy in 1940 for graduate trainees, apparently the first such supervised training offered in a university setting.

While at Ohio State, Rogers wrote *Counseling and Psychotherapy: Newer Concepts in Practice* (1942), a classic textbook on basic therapeutic issues, methods, the therapy relationship, and the process of change. At the end of the first chapter, Rogers stated the basic hypothesis of his developing approach: "Effective counseling consists of a definitely structured, permissive relationship which allows the client to gain an understanding of himself to a degree which enables him to take positive steps in the light of his new orientation" (p. 18). Rogers originally described his approach to counseling as "non-directive" and referred to the person receiving counseling as a "client" to underscore his belief that the direction and locus of control in therapy were clearly centered in the person seeking help. This was a radical shift away from the interpretive and directive methods that were commonly employed at the time. Rogers was an innovator in the early 1940s, experimenting with and refining the concepts and methods that would emerge as one of the most influential and controversial therapeutic approaches. In his early stages of developing a new approach, a number of his proposals seemed to focus on what Rogers thought the therapist should not do or be. He was adamant in his belief that the therapist should not advise the client, interpret behavior, or attempt to direct or persuade the client to pursue a particular course of action. Rogers objected to these approaches because "they assume that the counselor is the one most competent to decide what are to be the goals of the individual, and what are the values by which the situation is to be judged" (1942, p. 27). Rogers believed that counselor-centered therapy "may serve only to make the counselee more dependent, less able to solve new problems of adjustment" (Kirschenbaum, 1979, p. 116) and more resistant to the counselor.

The therapeutic approach developed by Rogers in the early 1940s had many distinctive characteristics, a number of which continue to be basic to the practice of person/client-centered therapy and other humanistic approaches. Rogers made a major shift in emphasis in therapy by focusing on the person of the client rather than on the problem expressed. Another shift was toward the feelings expressed by the client as opposed to the client's thoughts. The therapist's attitudes of respect for and belief in the client's capacity for self-directed growth resulted in the development of a dramatically different kind of relationship with the client. It was a relationship characterized by disciplined restraint and nonintrusiveness. The therapist attempted to be a careful and understanding listener. To a large extent, the therapist's task was technical in emphasis. While the therapist's acceptance of the client was viewed as critical, the accuracy and effectiveness of the therapist's reflection and clarification of feelings were clearly the primary focus.

Rogers and his students were the first to study the counseling process in depth. In 1940, with the assistance of Bernie Covner, the first audio recordings of a therapy session were made on 78-rpm discs. These live and transcribed recordings provided case studies for training purposes as well as research studies. The case of Herbert Bryan, which constitutes the last 176 pages of *Counseling and Psychotherapy: Newer Concepts in Practice* (1942), was the first verbatim transscript of the phonographic recording of an entire course of psychotherapy ever published. Though today we take for granted the usefulness of reviewing audio and videotapes for training purposes, Rogers was the first to demystify psychotherapy by bringing it out into the open for study.

Rogers was a pioneer in carrying out and publishing research studies in counseling. It is probably fair to say that Rogers was primarily responsible for initiating research in the field of psychotherapy. Early in *Counseling and Psychotherapy: Newer Concepts in Practice*, Rogers stated that the book "endeavors to formulate a definite and understandable series of hypotheses . . . which may be tested and explored" (1942, pp. 16–17). The research tradition established by Rogers and his students during this period has carried forward to the present to ensure the continued development and efficacy of client-centered therapy.

University of Chicago Counseling Center (1945–1957)

In 1945, Carl Rogers left Ohio State to create and direct the Counseling Center at the University of Chicago. There he continued to develop client-centered theory and practice while conducting research on its effectiveness. In his third major book, *Client-Centered Therapy* (1951), Rogers presented applications of the client-centered approach to play therapy, group therapy, leadership and administration, teaching, and counselor training. In this period, Rogers further emphasized the attitudes of the therapist, as opposed to technique, as primary, along with the capacity of the client for constructive change. Rogers and client-centered therapists focused on creating a relationship that would release the client's natural tendency for self-actualization and growth. Increasing emphasis was placed on understanding the client's phenomenal (subjective) world and its meaning.

In 1956, Rogers added *therapist congruence* to *empathic understanding* and *unconditional positive regard* to complete his three fundamental conditions for therapeutic change to occur. Also in 1956, Rogers developed his formulation of what he would call "The Necessary and Sufficient Conditions of Therapeutic Personality Change." This formulation, first published in an article of the same name in 1957, represented the culmination of many years of development in Rogers's thinking and remains foundational to this day.

During the University of Chicago years, client-centered therapy was already addressing issues of culture and diversity. Eugene Gendlin (1986) recalls about that period that the counseling center at the University of Chicago was the only place where a Black person or a gay person could get therapy without encountering extreme prejudice. Rogers trained the counseling center staff to approach each individual in an open-minded way until the client disclosed his or her issues of concern. If race or culture or any form of diversity was an issue for the client, then those aspects of the person's life became an essential part of the therapy. The desire and goal of the client-centered therapist were to hear, comprehend, and respond in a receptive and valuing manner to whatever aspects of that person's life and sociocultural context were relevant.

University of Wisconsin (1957–1963)

In the spring of 1957, Rogers accepted a position at the University of Wisconsin. In 1959, he published the essay "A Theory of Therapy, Personality and Interpersonal Relationships" in Sigmund Koch's *Psychology: A Study of a Science* (1959). This 72-page formal statement of his theory continues to stand as the most complete statement of Rogers's position. His fifth major book, *On Becoming a Person*, was published in 1961. Some of his more provocative and incisive thinking on psychotherapy, education, research, philosophy of science, interpersonal relations, family life, creativity, the process of growth, and the fully functioning person are contained in this book.

La Jolla and Center for the Studies of the Person (1964–1987)

In the summer of 1963, Rogers resigned from the University of Wisconsin and moved to California. For several years starting in 1964, Rogers involved himself in the encounter group movement and became identified with that form of groupwork. He wrote the book *Carl Rogers on Encounter Groups* (1970) in which he outlined how elements of client-centered therapy, such as acceptance of the individual and empathetic understanding, can operate in this type of group.

In the last 15 years of his life, Carl Rogers was increasingly interested in broader social issues, especially peace. Beginning in 1974, Rogers, along with several of his colleagues, initiated a series of large workshops ranging from 75 to 800 participants, sometimes two to three weeks in length, to explore the implications of the person-centered approach for building communities. These workshops would be offered all over the world for the next several years. As they evolved, Rogers and the staff of facilitators provided less and less structure, instead leaving most, if not all, of the decision making to the entire community. Rogers believed that peaceful solutions to difficult problems could be discovered in groups and communities if the leaders established the norms and conditions that facilitate dialogue and the understanding of diverse opinions and worldviews. Rogers believed that groups and communities, like individuals, can solve their own problems when allowed to be self-directed.

In the early 1970s, Rogers introduced the term *person-centered* to describe his work, especially its expansion into areas beyond individual psychotherapy. He also continued to use the term *client-centered* and indicated that he did not see any fundamental distinction between the two terms. Today, I believe it is fair to say that *client-centered* and *person-centered* may be used interchangeably.

In 1986, the *Person-Centered Review*, an academic journal, began publication under my editorship. Up to this point, Rogers had discouraged the creation of client-centered training programs, organizations, or journals, fearing that his approach would become formalized and dogmatic. By 1986, however, Rogers supported and welcomed the journal.

Unfortunately, Carl Rogers was not able to pursue further the strongest commitments of his last years—to contribute whatever he could to the prevention of nuclear war and the accomplishment of world peace. On January 20, 1987, the day Rogers fell and broke his hip, he was nominated for the 1987 Nobel Peace Prize. A few weeks later, on February 4, 1987, at the age of 85, Carl Rogers died as he had hoped he would—with his boots on, and, as always, looking forward. He had been relatively healthy and active until his death.

After Rogers: Variations in the Evolution of Person-Centered Therapy

The founders of any therapeutic system exert an enormous, and often inordinate, influence on the way the therapy is conceived and practiced far beyond its inception. Freud (psychoanalysis), Adler (Individual Psychology), Perls (Gestalt therapy), Ellis (rational-emotive behavior therapy), and Rogers were creative and charismatic founders who attracted many adherents who then extended outward the influence of their adopted system. Adherents tend to practice the therapy in a manner very similar to the founder and defend the originator's views as unshakable truths to be preserved. This happens despite the founder's often-stated desire or belief that, as new discoveries are made, the approach will evolve and be modified conceptually and in practice.

Rogers believed and hoped the person-centered approach would continue to evolve. In fact, he often expressed concern that client-centered therapy would become dogmatic and stifled in its development. Although his thinking did evolve, it is also true that the way Rogers practiced therapy remained fairly constant until he died. Many client-centered therapists, especially the more traditional practitioners, continue to practice as Rogers did or in even more conservative ways. However, Rogers was always receptive to and encouraging of innovative ideas that would advance theory and practice. In 1986, a year before his death, Rogers commented: "I hope . . . we're always on the move, to a new theory . . . to new areas of dealing with situations, new ways of being with persons. I hope that we're always a part of the 'growing edge'" (Cornelius-White & Cornelius-White, 2005, p. 396). Others too believed that client-centered therapy could be modified for the better and proposed newer ideas and varied forms of practice. In a recent publication entitled *The Tribes of the Person-Centered Nation*, the editor (Sanders, 2004) identifies the following versions of the approach.

Classical Client-Centered Psychotherapy

For the classical or traditional client-centered therapist, Rogers's (1959) formal statement remains essentially sacrosanct. In addition, the classical practitioners place a high emphasis on what they characterize as the "nondirective attitude." Rogers (1942) originally described his therapeutic approach as nondirective, emphasizing that the therapist "takes no responsibility for directing the outcome of the process" (p. 115). Rogers believed that the therapies of the 1940s were too focused in the therapist's direction of process and that therapists' suggestions, advice, guidance, persuasion, questioning, and interpretations tended to make the client dependent on the therapist and, consequently, less self-reliant. Rogers wanted clients, not therapists, to be in control of their life goals and means of change. The focus was on the person of the client as opposed to the client's problem or symptoms. In short, Rogers viewed clients as capable, resourceful, and able to develop sufficient insight to understand their current difficulties and to find ways of adapting constructively to them.

As Rogers developed his approach beyond the early 1950s, he rarely used the term *nondirective* and preferred instead to speak of creating conditions that "freed" the client. However, many in the conservative branch of client-centered therapy believe that the truest form of client-centered therapy must be unwaveringly nondirective and have described their view as "nondirective client-centered therapy." In a recent article, Grant (2004), one of nondirective therapy's strongest advocates, argued that the therapist's absolute nondirectiveness forms the ethical basis for the client's inalienable right to self-determination. This conservative group of client-centered therapists essentially views any deviance from this position as some other form of therapy related to but not truly client centered in spirit or practice. That some practitioners should maintain what appears to be a very narrow view of client-centered therapy should not be surprising. There will always be practitioners of a specific approach who truly believe that the original position advanced by the founder will always remain its purest and best form.

Focusing-Oriented Psychotherapy

Focusing-oriented psychotherapy was developed by Eugene Gendlin, a student of Rogers at the University of Chicago Counseling Center during the early 1950s. He later followed Rogers to Wisconsin to research the effectiveness of client-centered psychotherapy with hospitalized schizophrenic persons. Gendlin's original contribution was the concept of *experiencing*, which he later (1996) named *focusing-oriented psychotherapy*. Having observed that successful clients focused on and processed their affective experience, Gendlin gently encouraged his clients to attend to their bodily sense of their problem, believing that the body carries the problem in a physically felt form. By attending to the "felt sense" of the problem in a supportive relationship, along with some guidance from the therapist, the client's experience and its personal meaning would often unfold and become clear. When this sense of clarity was reached, the client's bodily response of relief or release confirmed the "rightness" of the understanding.

Process-Experiential Psychotherapy

Others followed Gendlin's lead and developed a variety of means to assist the client in processing emotional, bodily-felt experiences to illuminate their meanings and implications for growth and change. Laura N. Rice (1974) extended the client-centered response style by developing the method of *evocative reflection*, which she viewed as a more active, vivid, and powerful form of client-centered reflection. The aim of evocative reflection is to "open up the experience and provide the client with a process whereby he can form successively more accurate constructions of his own experience" (p. 290). The goal is to enable the client to reprocess experience in an undistorted manner that results in the reorganization of old and dysfunctional schemes. Rice believes that "if the client can fully explore his reactions to one such situation, and become aware of the elements in a more accurate and balanced form . . . the effect will be to force reorganization of all of the relevant schemes" (p. 294).

Leslie Greenberg, Robert Elliott, and their colleagues have blended the essence of client-centered therapy with elements of Gestalt therapy, existentialism, and Rice's and Gendlin's experiential methods into a therapy they have called *process-experiential therapy*, and more recently *emotionally focused therapy* (EFT). Greenberg and Van Balen (1999) describe process-experiential therapy as both relationally and task oriented. The approach involves the client's working on therapeutic tasks with a process-directive therapist. Greenberg is clear in emphasizing that the client and the quality of the relationship always take precedence over the proposed therapeutic tasks, methods, or goals. The emphasis in process-experiential therapy is on processing emotion and the reconstruction of emotional schemes. "The primary objective in process-experiential therapy is to help clients integrate information from their emotional and cognitive systems to facilitate a more satisfactory adjustment. . . . Process-experiential therapists emphasize the role of emotion in personal development and functioning" (Watson, Greenberg, & Lietaer, 1998, p. 6).

Existential Influences on Person-Centered Psychotherapy

Existential philosophy and psychotherapy, in various forms, have influenced the thinking of client-centered therapists, beginning with Carl Rogers. Rogers had dialogues with existential philosophers Martin Buber in 1957 and Paul Tillich in 1965. Over many years, Rogers corresponded and dialogued in person with Rollo May and had some contact with R. D. Laing. He was also familiar with the ideas of existential philosopher Søren Kierkegaard. Regarding the relationship of existential thought to client-centered therapy, Rogers (1980) wrote, "I felt greatly supported in my new approach, which I found to my surprise was a home-grown brand of existential philosophy" (p. 39).

Mick Cooper (2004, p. 122) summarizes what he sees as the similarities of existential and client-centered views. He suggests that both approaches tend to emphasize the uniqueness and individuality of each client and of each therapeutic encounter. Both approaches understand the client in terms of his or her "subjective," lived experiences rather than from an external, diagnostic perspective. Existential and person-centered approaches see psychological problems as a result of the distortion or denial of experiences and hold that an acknowledgment of one's true being can lead to a greater intensity and fullness of living. Finally, both reject the use of techniques in therapy, emphasizing instead the importance of a genuine, spontaneous human encounter, and both emphasize the importance of accepting and validating clients, however bizarre or maladaptive their behavior might seem.

The Evolution of Person-Centered Therapy for a Diverse World

Diversity is the nature of life. "Each person is, in some respects, like every other person, like some other persons, and like no other person" (Kluckhohn & Murray, 1959, p. 53). The variety of plant life and animal life, including humans, on planet Earth is nothing less than astonishing. As I write, new forms of life are still being discovered. People are infinitely diverse. It is a scientific fact that no two persons, including identical twins, are exactly the same. The diversity of human experience, living conditions, beliefs, customs, cultures, life-shaping events, physical variations, and lifestyles approach incomprehensibility. I suspect that most therapists who have worked with a large number of clients would acknowledge that they still meet clients who present a challenge because of their distinctiveness.

Person-centered therapy is naturally suited to clients in a diverse world. It places a high priority on understanding each unique individual in the broader context of his or her life. Person-centered therapists readily look at all of the variables that are of personal import to clients and focus on those aspects of clients' lives that are most relevant in their daily functioning. A case example illustrates this point.

Roberto is a 60-year-old gay man who was born in Argentina and lived there until he was 17. He currently lives in California with Harry, his partner of 30 years, in what he describes as a relationship devoid of affection. He struggles with severe depression, anxiety, diabetes that has impaired his vision, and chronic back pain. These conditions render him unable to work, though he does assist the visually impaired on a voluntary basis. Roberto sometimes wishes to leave his current life, though he has not been actively suicidal. As I began work with Roberto, I was uncertain whether or how much his cultural heritage or sexual orientation were issues of relevance to therapy, which has now reached one and a half years. I liked Roberto from the outset and easily felt supportive, encouraging, and committed to helping him live as well as possible considering the physical, psychological, and relational challenges he faced. Therapeutically, my first goal was to understand what it was like to be Roberto struggling to get through each day as best he could.

The excerpt that follows is from a recent session in which Roberto grappled with his social isolation and ambivalence about engaging with others or making new friends.

> C (Client): Well, today I had the idea that I would talk about the positive things in my life.

This shift of focus was a slight surprise but seemed to represent something Roberto had been wanting to address, namely, his social relationships over his life span.

> T (Therapist): I'd be happy to hear that. I see a smile on your face. Tell me the positive things in your life.
>
> C: From the beginning or from now?
>
> T: You decide.

C: At 17 I left Argentina, and at 18 I started university. B.Y.U., Utah.

T: Yes. You went to Brigham Young.

C: It was okay. As I look back on those days, I don't know how I survived. I was *so* naïve.

T: Yeah. You were naïve and you're surprised looking back that you did as well as you did.

C: Yeah. People liked me.

I am pleasantly surprised by Roberto's more positive recollections of his life to this point, recollections that focus more on the positive than I had heard in previous sessions, where he focused on being ill and on the difficult aspects of his relationship with his father.

T: People liked you. [Affirmatively.]

C: People have always liked me.

T: People have *always* liked you.

C: With a few exceptions. [Smiling.]

T: With a few exceptions. You have a smile on your face. That's a nice recollection and a nice recognition for you. For the most part, people have always liked you.

These last three interventions may appear to be mindless repetitions of what the client just said, a fundamental misunderstanding about person-centered therapy. In fact, my responses were made with an affirmative inflection that celebrated the client's sense of being liked throughout his life, the first time he had made such comments in the year and a half we had worked together. Furthermore, I personally find this client likable, a factor that lent congruence to my affirmations.

C: It's a type of liking that is light.

T: Light?

C: Yes light . . . . I don't have many deep relationships. But I would like to.

T: Yes, you would, but you feel you are more able to have relationships on a more superficial level? Is that what you mean by "light"?

C: Right. They don't let me come very close.

T: You say *they* don't let you.

C: Or I don't come very close.

T: Or you don't come very close.

C: If it is me, it's because I don't know how.

T: You're not sure you know how to be close? If it's on your end?

C: It is on my end. I think I come through as extremely formal.

T: You imagine your formality is a barrier to someone being close to you.

C: I think people like me and respect me, but from a distance.

T: You can imagine that people would like and respect you, but you think your formality keeps them from being close.

C: Yeah. At least with Americans.

T: With Americans. It might be different with . . . ?

C: South Americans or Europeans. There's a cultural dilemma.

T: A cultural dilemma. How's that?

C: I was brought up in a very formal way. [Describes his formal schooling and lifestyle growing up.]

T: So the culture in which you developed was formal, and so you became formal.

C: Very respectful, very well mannered . . . all that stuff. In this country people are not that formal. I would say even that they're a little scared of that kind of formality.

This is the first hint that Roberto's cultural and family background continue to be factors in the closeness of his social relations.
    A little later:

C: There are some [immigrants] who don't want to change.

T: Aha! So you're thinking, some people come here and don't want to be fully Americanized. And maybe that includes you?

C: Yeah. And there's a price to pay.

T: And there's a price to pay because . . . .

C: You're the outsider.

T: You still feel like the outsider to some degree.

C: Hmm.

T: You were brought up in a different culture that doesn't match American informal culture. So you still remain the outsider. To some degree [C: Yeah.] even though you have been here since you were seventeen.

C: Yeah. That's interesting. Maybe it's a way to be different. Maybe it's a way to have some identity of my own.

Feeling like an outsider is certainly a common experience of many immigrants. Retaining one's cultural identity is also important.

A little later:

C: People used to like . . . that you are a little different from them . . . but it's also a barrier.

T: Well, it's a double-edged sword, you're thinking. [C: Yeah.] There's a certain appeal to your being different, but then on the other side your difference sometimes becomes a barrier because you're unlike some Americans, whose style is less formal.

C: Consciously, I try to do something about it, to become more . . . accepting.

T: You're making a face like that's [accepting] not the right word.

C: No. Because it's not a matter of being accepting . . . because I accept people the way they are . . .

At this point the client mentions that he has made friends with people who are quite different from him but that such relationships are not satisfying because he has little in common with these persons.

C: I have tried to be friends with them . . . and they are friendly with me and with Harry [his partner of 30 years] but more with Harry. And I find that I am not satisfied with the conversation with them. I have nothing in common to talk about with them.

T: Well, you've become aware of the differences: They're not much like me; they come from different experiences. You try to bridge over and converse with them, but it's not satisfying, partly because of the differences.

This case example illustrates how a person-centered therapist would address a client who is struggling with issues related to cultural difference. Roberto believes that the social isolation he feels is, to some degree, a result of the difference between the formality of his upbringing in Argentina and the informality of most Americans. He does not easily form the close friendship he seeks. My goal as the therapist in this excerpt is to understand what it is like to be Roberto and to convey that understanding to him without judgment and with genuine regard. I am not trying to solve the problem. Rather, I endeavor to create an optimal relational atmosphere that will be conducive for Roberto's growth and change. I will talk more about these conditions of therapy later in the chapter.

The culture of the person-centered therapist is also an issue requiring heightened awareness and reflection regarding its possible influence on the therapist's assumptions and therapeutic behavior. This self-scrutiny is especially critical if the therapist is a member of the dominant culture, which is the case for the large majority of person-centered therapists in the United States. For example, with Roberto, I try to be particularly aware of my own formality or informality and how that therapeutic behavior will influence the relationship I have with him.

As I enter each session with a new client, I am aware that there is no one on earth like the client I am about to encounter. Although I know that this client shares at least some aspects of the experiences of other persons who share her or his race, gender, cultural background, age, and other traits, I consciously attempt to lay aside any assumptions I may have about the person before me and any predispositions I may have about how to respond therapeutically. A fundamental question I bring to therapy is, *"What is it like to be you?"* including any and all aspects of the person's life that matter in some meaningful and impactful way. Although I am aware of obvious contextual factors (e.g., race, gender, or disability), I initially make no assumptions about the relative importance of those factors to my client. Client-centered therapy is based in phenomenology, which "looks at immediate experience and attempts to describe it with as little bias or interpretation as possible" (Lindauer, 1998, p. 653). As I embark upon a therapeutic journey with a client, I understand that each client is unique and anticipate that the course of therapy will be as well.

In my view, client-centered therapy offers a potent approach to working with persons with a wide range of cultural backgrounds and diverse experiences. The therapist's core conditions of empathy, unconditional positive regard, and congruence are qualities that are universal or near universal in that they are likely to have a constructive impact on all clients, regardless of their cultural background or other ways they may differ from the hypothetical "mainstream." Compatible with this position, D. W. Sue and D. Sue (1990) agree that "qualities such as respect and acceptance of the individual, unconditional positive regard, understanding the problem from the individual's perspective, allowing the client to explore his or her own values, and arriving at an individual solution are core qualities that may transcend culture" (p. 187).

Context Then—Context Now

From the beginnings of client-centered therapy in the 1940s to the present, the United States has changed enormously, as has the practice of therapy. In the

1950s, the population of the United States was about half as large as it is today and much less diverse. Schools and universities were mostly racially segregated until the early 1970s in most parts of this country. Consequently, the world in which most Americans lived was White, mostly Protestant, and homogeneous in culture. Many White people had relatively little exposure to those of different racial and ethnic groups. Persons who were diverse or different in some substantial way (e.g., handicapped persons, gay and lesbian persons, learning disabled persons) were not part of mainstream culture.

Carl Rogers developed client-centered therapy in the context of a White, midwestern, mostly Protestant, homogeneous culture. He was a product of this culture and his orientation to psychotherapy embraces many of the prevailing values of that era and place, such as the importance of being independent and self-sufficient. The world around Carl Rogers would change considerably from the 1940s and 1950s, when he developed and refined his orientation, to the 1980s, when he turned his attention to promoting peaceful conflict resolution at the global level. His belief and conviction about the essential elements of person-centered therapy—that the client knows best and what is necessary for a client's progress is the therapist's being genuine, empathetically attuned, and demonstrating positive regard—never wavered over the course of his career.

Person-centered therapists today are living and practicing in a world that is increasingly diverse and complex. Person-centered therapy is served by its compatibility with field theory as it responds to the client's immediate and larger context, that is, individuals are seen as being inextricably linked to the larger environment or field that constantly exerts influence on what they think and feel, and how they behave. Person-centered therapists seek to understand how each client is impacted by the field, which, of course, would include the individual's culture, ethnicity, religion, sexual orientation, socioeconomic status, and other aspects of human diversity.

Person-centered therapists utilize their awareness and sensitivity to all of these factors and respond therapeutically to these issues in the therapeutic process. Person-centered therapists are also attuned to how their culture and life experiences may impinge upon and influence their therapeutic responses. "Therapist know thyself" is an important endeavor embraced by person-centered therapists. Self-awareness is one of the three main domains of multicultural competence and is addressed in more detail later in this chapter.

Rogers had the wisdom to foresee that person-centered therapy would need to be continuously examined and refined to stay current as the field and context changed. Many person-centered therapists (including myself) would consider themselves integrative and have explored conceptual modification, a topic discussed further in the sections "Challenges" and "Future Development."

The Author's Journey as a Person-Centered Therapist

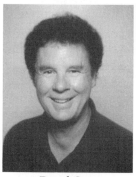

David Cain

I have been a student, practitioner, teacher, and supervisor of person-centered therapy for over 30 years. During my doctoral studies in clinical psychology at the University of Wyoming in the late 1960s and early 1970s, the primary emphasis in that program was behavioral therapy. However, when I saw a film of Rogers engaged with a client, I was struck by the sensitive and perceptive manner in which he listened. He seemed completely immersed in his client and responded with a penetrating understanding. Rogers's gentle but incisive empathic responses seemed to enable his clients to pause and reflect on their experiences and feelings and their meanings. I realized that Rogers represented the kind of therapist that I would like to be and to have if I were a client. Having been exposed to psychoanalytic approaches, to Ellis's rational-emotive therapy, Gestalt therapy, existential therapy, transactional analysis, and a few others, as well as to behavioral approaches, I was most impressed with Rogers's warm and supportive relating to his clients. I went to the counseling program in the education department, took a course in client-centered therapy and felt "at home." Then, as now, client-centered therapy was more accepted in counseling than it was in psychology programs.

In the second year of my doctoral program, I was awarded a stipend to work in the university counseling center under the supervision of Dr. Harry Sharp, a client-centered therapist. Another supervisor, Dr. Leo Sprinkle, was humanistic in style and helped me understand the therapeutic impact of humor. Both supported my developing interest in client-centered therapy. Most of the students I saw for counseling were from Wyoming, a rural state. Consequently, I was exposed to persons who lived in very small towns (mostly with populations of under 5,000 people), many of whom were ranchers and cowboys who had little exposure to city or suburban life.

After completing my doctorate in the early 1970s, I moved to New Haven, Connecticut, and took a position as a child clinical psychologist at Clifford Beers Clinic, a therapeutic environment that was primarily psychoanalytic. While there, I worked primarily with children and their parents and discovered that client-centered play therapy enabled children to thrive in a context where they were able to freely express themselves. Because New Haven was something of a melting pot, I had many clients from various ethnic groups, including Italians,

Hispanics, and African Americans, most of whom lived in inner-city housing projects, and many of whom were on welfare. The value client-centered therapy placed on seeing each person as a unique individual helped me relate to clients with lifestyles considerably different from my own.

In 1980, I took a position in the counseling center at California Polytechnic State University in San Luis Obispo. There I was exposed to a greater range of diversity among students, including many from the Middle East, students with various disabilities, and students from a range of socioeconomic backgrounds. I was the founder, in 1981, of the Association for the Development of the Person-Centered Approach and the founder and editor of the first academic journal based on Rogers's ideas, the *Person-Centered Review*. From 1987 to 1996, I worked primarily in private practice, where I saw clients of all socioeconomic groups, including a large number of graduate students in master's and doctoral programs in psychology. Between 1996 and 2002, I held the position of director of the counseling center at U.S. International University (now Alliant International University), which attracted students from more than 80 different countries. This opportunity enabled me to get a firsthand education working with clients as diverse as a Kenyan woman whose father had more than one wife to a Japanese student who was extremely distraught over the possibility of losing face with his family because he had flunked out of the university. My experience with these diverse clients was that they responded well to person-centered therapy, though there were occasions when I made modifications to fit their needs. For the past four years, I have worked with clients from lower socioeconomic groups, including many chronically and severely mentally ill persons who struggle to get through the day and whose daily functioning is greatly compromised.

Over the years, my thinking has evolved and now includes an integration of person-centered, existential, Gestalt, and experiential concepts and therapeutic responses, as well as the use of my *self* when I am able to bring forth aspects of who I am in ways that allow for a meaningful meeting or encounter with my client. I continue to support person-centered and humanistic organizations around the world and serve on the editorial boards of four person-centered or humanistically oriented journals. I now consider myself an advocate for and supportive critic of person-centered therapy, which I hope will serve to enable this approach to expand and differentiate further while continually increasing its adaptiveness and effectiveness for a wide range of clients and problems.

Theory of Person-Centered Therapy

Carl Rogers published the most complete statement of his approach in 1959 (pp. 184–256), and he never modified it in any significant way. However, the reader should note that Rogers never considered his theory to be a finished product and anticipated that it would be further developed over time.

Essential Terms of Person-Centered Theory

Although the most essential terms of person-centered therapy theory were mentioned earlier as part of the historical narrative, in this section of the chapter I will discuss each term more specifically.

Actualizing Tendency

Rogers (1959) defined the **actualizing tendency** as "the inherent tendency of the organism to develop all its capacities in ways which serve to maintain or enhance the organism" (p. 196). The actualizing tendency, the bedrock on which person-centered psychotherapy is based, suggests that people naturally move toward differentiation, expansion and growth, and effectiveness and autonomy. It includes such notions as a reduction in needs, tensions, and drives as well as an inclination to learn and be creative. A core belief in the actualizing tendency is the basis for the client-centered therapist's trust and optimism in clients' resourcefulness and capacity to move forward and find solutions to their problems. Although life experiences may weaken the actualizing tendency, it is always assumed to exist as a potential that clients can draw on.

Self

The **self** (or self-concept) as defined by Rogers (1959) is the "organized, consistent conceptual gestalt composed of perceptions of characteristics of the 'I' or 'me' . . . together with the values attached to these perceptions" (p. 200). The self is a fluid and changing gestalt that is available to awareness and that is specific and definable in a given moment. The term *self structure* represents an external view of the self. The **ideal self** represents the desired view of self the person would like to be. When the aspects of experience defined as the self are actualized (e.g., I am an athletic person.), the process is one of **self-actualization.** The actualization of the self may be in harmony with the actualizing tendency to maintain and enhance the organism, or it may be at odds with the actualizing tendency, resulting in the development of aspects of the self that may be valued by the person but that may have adverse consequences. For example, the person may develop her or his capacity to be deceptive, thereby increasing his or her ability to gain desired ends from others even though such deception compromises the integrity of the person and her or his trustworthiness.

Congruence and Incongruence

Congruence describes a state in which a person's self-concept and experiences, including thoughts and behavior, are in harmony. That is, the person is integrated, whole, or genuine. Rogers believed that congruence represented an optimal state of functioning or mental health. **Incongruence** represents a state of discord between the self-concept and experience. Rogers (1959) described this state as one of "tension and internal confusion" (p. 203) because people cannot reconcile the discrepancy between their thoughts, feelings, or actions and the way they perceive themselves. For example, a man who views himself as having high integrity will likely experience distress when he realizes that he frequently engages in dishonest behavior.

Openness to Experience

A person who is open to experience readily takes in information arising from within or coming from the external environment without defensiveness. **Openness to experience** is critical to optimal functioning because it enables the person to receive and process any and all experiences and use those experiences to make effective decisions in daily life. Conversely, defensiveness reduces the person's capacity to process, make sense of, and act on experiences that may be threatening to the self. A woman who makes excuses for her boyfriend's failure to make time for her or show much interest in her is failing to assess information critical to her well-being. She may then experience anxiety and depression.

Psychological Adjustment and Maladjustment

Rogers (1959) stated that "optimal **psychological adjustment** exists when the concept of self is such that all experiences are or may be assimilated on a symbolic level into the gestalt of the self structure" (p. 206). Good adjustment occurs when there is congruence of self and experience, which requires openness to experience.

Psychological maladjustment exists when the organism "denies to awareness, or distorts in awareness, significant experiences, which consequently are not accurately symbolized and organized into the gestalt of the self structure, thus creating an incongruence between self and experience" (Rogers, 1959, p. 204). Thus, maladaption is essentially a state of incongruence between one's self and one's experience. The person cannot integrate some experiences (thoughts, feelings, actions) with the self because they don't fit. For example, a young man confidently entering a talent show (seeing the self as talented) may get feedback from credible judges that he has little or no talent. He is thrown into a state of anxiety and disillusionment because he or she cannot reconcile the disheartening feedback with a view of self as talented.

Positive Regard and Unconditional Positive Regard

People experience **positive regard** when they perceive that some aspect of their behavior is genuinely appreciated by another. In this state, the person is likely to feel warmth, liking, respect, or acceptance from others. Rogers (1959) views the need for positive regard as essential to one's well-being. We experience **unconditional positive regard** when we perceive that any self-experience is accepted without conditions by another person. Thus, a person may act in ways of which she or he is not proud but still finds that she or he is accepted by another. According to Rogers, giving someone your unconditional positive regard "means to value the person, irrespective of the differential values which one may place on his specific behaviors" (p. 208). When clients experience unconditional positive regard from their therapists, they are likely to feel accepted and prized, which in turn enables them to develop more tolerant and accepting feelings toward themselves. The desire to be seen accurately and be accepted seems to be a powerful need in people.

Conditions of Worth

Conditions of worth exist in the person "when a self-experience . . . is either avoided or sought solely because the individual discriminates it as being less or more worthy of self-regard" (Rogers, 1959, p. 209). Simply put, an individual may engage in or avoid a behavior based on whether it brings her or him regard from another person. The approval of another may take on such importance that the person disregards whether or not the behavior enhances her or his growth.

Locus of Evaluation

Locus of evaluation refers to the source of a person's values. If the source is internal, the person is "the center of the valuing process, the evidence being supplied by his own senses. When the locus of evaluation resides in others, their judgment as to the value of an . . . experience becomes the criterion of value for the individual" (Rogers, 1959, p. 209).

Organismic Valuing Process

The **organismic valuing process** suggests that persons have a built-in, trust-worthy, evaluative mechanism that enables them to experience "satisfaction in those . . . behaviors which maintain and enhance the organism and the self" (Rogers, 1959, p. 209).

Internal Frame of Reference

The **internal frame of reference** is "all of the realm of experience which is available to the awareness of the individual at a given moment" (Rogers, 1959, p. 209). It is the subjective experience of the person.

Empathy

Empathy exists when one person accurately perceives the internal frame of reference of another, including both the emotional aspects and meaning of the experience. In client-centered therapy, empathy is considered to be both a desirable attitude and a skill that enables clients to clarify and learn from their experiences.

Theory of Change

In his seminal paper "The Necessary and Sufficient Conditions of Therapeutic Personality Change," Rogers described his basic theory of client change in a set of six points.

1. Two persons are in psychological contact.

2. The first, whom we shall term the client, is in a state of incongruence, being vulnerable or anxious.

3. The second person, whom we shall term the therapist, is congruent or integrated in the relationship.

4. The therapist experiences unconditional positive regard for the client.

5. The therapist experiences an empathic understanding of the client's internal frame of reference and endeavors to communicate this experience to the client.

6. The communication to the client of the therapist's empathic understanding and unconditional positive regard is to a minimal degree achieved. (p. 96)

Rogers later amended point 6 of this hypothesis (1967, p. 93) by stating that the "therapist's genuineness (or congruence) must also be perceived by the client as well as his or her unconditional positive regard and empathic understanding." This hypothesis is accepted as the fundamental basis for practice by most client-centered practitioners.

To further explain this process and the mechanisms of change, I begin by describing the ways in which the therapeutic relationship impacts the client. Using Rogers's six "Necessary and Sufficient Conditions" as a starting point, first it is essential for the therapist and client to be in contact and meaningfully engaged in a relationship focused on the client. In this meeting the therapist is fully present with the client. The client is experiencing anxiety about some aspect of his or her life and a sense of incongruence that suggests that the client's experiences (thoughts, feelings, behaviors, beliefs, values) and view of self are not in accord.

In this relationship, the therapist endeavors to listen with fresh ears and see with fresh eyes to understand the client's life and experiences and to grasp what it is like to be the client. The therapist communicates as clearly as possible her or his understanding of the client's world for the client to reflect upon and process further. In a sense, the therapist attempts to paint a vivid, living, multicolored portrait of the client's immediate lived experience. Doing so enables clients to listen to themselves, see themselves more clearly, and make better sense of their experiences and selves, including personal meanings. Person-centered therapists focus their attention intently on their clients' emotions, knowing that emotions signal what is personally important and often what is troubling the person. Identifying emotions also helps clients become aware of their implicit motivations, desires, and needs. By processing emotions, clients elucidate and clarify their experiences in a way that is not possible by focusing solely on the content of their issues.

The therapist's congruence is a critical component of the relationship because it makes the therapist credible and trustworthy to the client. The therapist's unconditional positive regard is likely to have more impact because the client experiences the therapist as authentic and truthful. As the therapist demonstrates through empathic response that he or she sees the client clearly and still prizes the client, the client has the opportunity to look freshly through the therapist's eyes at herself or himself.

How Change May Come About

There are five prominent ways in which client-centered therapy effects change.

1. *The quality of the therapeutic relationship itself promotes client growth.* When clients enter therapy, they often feel stuck in their lives, discouraged about their capacity to change, and have low self-esteem. In short, they are not feeling very good about themselves or how they are living. They need a sense of hope, which is often assisted by the therapist's natural optimism

about their resourcefulness and capacity to change in a constructive direction. Further, when clients feel accepted for who they are, affirmed and valued by their therapists, they become less defensive and fearful and start to feel better about themselves. Being understood without judgment promotes self-acceptance, which diminishes the impact of self criticism. As clients become aware that their therapists see characteristics, strengths, and personal qualities in them, they are able, to varying degrees, to view themselves in a more accurate and positive light. Feeling better about themselves, clients often gain confidence to try out new behaviors.

2. *During the course of therapy, clients engage in self-exploration and self-discovery.* In fact, a major benefit of person-centered therapy is that it facilitates self-definition, or a clearer sense about whom one is, as opposed to whom one thought one was. The self as conceived comes closer to the ideal self, the person the client hopes to be. As the self-concept changes, so does behavior, which now becomes more aligned with a more constructive, capable, and empowered view of self. In other words, clients act in a manner that reflects the way they now perceive themselves.

3. *Clients achieve clarity about their worldviews and their problematic issues.* Through a process of exploration, observation, and reflection on their social worlds, clients' perceptions shift. They become more mindful and see old things in new ways, especially significant relationships. Clients' perceptual range and complexity increases as constricted views are expanded and become more differentiated. New options for alternative behaviors and courses of action become evident. As clients learn to pay closer attention to their experiences, process them more effectively, and achieve a sense of clarity or inner knowing, they become increasingly more confident in their perceptions, judgment, and decision-making ability. Their locus of evaluation gradually moves from an external to an internal one. This shift tends to make clients less dependent on others' views and advice and less vulnerable to conditions of worth imposed by others.

4. *The therapist's empathy facilitates clients' receptivity to and interest in new learning and enables them to move from more superficial and external issues to more personal and internal aspects of the self.* As therapy progresses, clients learn both what they need to learn to move forward in their lives and how to learn it. That is, they identify areas in which their current beliefs and approaches to problems are ineffective, and they realize the need to do something differently. Consequently, they become increasingly inclined to remain open, learn from, and process their experiences more effectively. In this process of learning how to learn, clients come to understand that there are multiple sources of learning, including feelings.

5. *Clients learn to process feelings that reflect the body's interpretation of a situation or experience.* Emotions have an evaluative function. They alert us to

what's wrong and what's needed for our well-being. At the heart of change is the direct experiencing and processing of troublesome emotions. It is not enough to talk *about* feelings. It is essential to take notice that feelings are trying to tell us something of importance and therefore need our careful attention. Improved regulation of emotion often results from processing feelings. Also, once the implicit meanings in feelings are understood, clients often feel a sense of release and relief as the mystery of their problems are transformed into a sense of clarity. Even though what is discovered may be difficult, it is usually helpful to make sense of one's unclear feelings. Processing feelings is also important for effective decision making. When a feeling of rightness occurs, the client is able to act with greater confidence since both a cognitive and a feeling sense of the problem converges. In other words, the body knows; it has its own wisdom that can be tapped. This view contrasts substantially with the view of many current therapies that troublesome feelings should only be regulated or controlled, not processed for their implicit wisdom and guidance.

Practice of Person-Centered Therapy

In the next section, I discuss the practice of person-centered therapy, focusing on the critical role the relationship between client and counselor plays in this orientation to psychotherapy.

The Client-Counselor Relationship

In person-centered therapy, the role of the client-therapist relationship is paramount. The therapist's core qualities of empathy, unconditional positive regard, and congruence, along with the therapist's presence, work synergistically and holistically to create a safe environment for learning and growth. Each quality enhances the impact of the others. For clients to feel accepted and valued, they must perceive that their therapists see them clearly and understand their life experiences. Therapists' accurate empathy is, therefore, critical for clients to feel that they are known. It is also essential that this understanding and prizing be based in the clients' perception that the therapist is congruent, trustworthy, and credible. These attitudes are enhanced to the degree that the therapist is fully present and immersed in the moment-to-moment unfolding of the clients' world. Therapists' implicit and expressed optimism about their clients' resourcefulness and capacity to change also creates a sense of hopefulness while enhancing efforts to move forward.

The Therapeutic Endeavor: Relational Attitudes in Action

How are the most common beliefs, attitudes, and values shared by person-centered therapists put into practice? Person-centered therapists often refer to their therapeutic approach as a "way of being" with clients in which the quality of the relationship itself is considered the primary means of creating optimal conditions for growth and change. An essential desire of the person-centered therapist is to *be present*, fully attentive to and immersed in the person of the client as well as the client's expressed concerns. By being present, the therapist fully brings the person she or he is to the client and concentrates on being receptive to whatever the client addresses. I believe that person-centered therapists also bring their *optimism* about clients' capacity to tap into or develop their internal resources for change. The person-centered therapist brings a strong belief that the client has a natural tendency for actualization that can be manifested in a definable therapeutic environment.

Promoting Client Freedom

Another aspect of the person-centered therapist's endeavor is to support and encourage the client's freedom to choose what will be addressed, how it will be addressed, and when and how the client will make decisions to change. Thus, the person-centered therapist favors a nondirective style of engagement in which the client takes the lead and assumes the responsibility for change. Consequently, person-centered therapists tend to engage very sparingly in behaviors such as advice-giving, suggestion, offering solutions, persuasion, or directing the content of the session. While the client is free to engage in therapy in a manner that best suits her or him, the client is also faced with deciding what to share and how to manage her or his life, albeit in a supportive relationship.

Empathic Attunement

A defining endeavor of the person-centered therapist is to *listen attentively* and to seek to understand the client's world, especially what it is like to be the client. This is an active and involved listening in which the therapist attempts to communicate as clearly and specifically as possible the client's reality in a way that facilitates further reflection and exploration. Sometimes person-centered therapy is misunderstood or caricatured as the therapist's simply saying back or restating what the client has just said. This was never Rogers's intent, nor was it reflected in his behavior. Instead, the person-centered therapist seeks to understand both the stated and intended message of the client, including the implied and tacit meanings that may only be hinted at. Thus, the person-centered therapist strives to bring clarity to what the client articulates as well as illuminate its personal meaning. The purpose of therapists' empathic response is to provide clients with an opportunity to see and hear themselves more clearly and to learn from their own experiences. In a sense, person-centered therapists hold up a magic mirror for their clients that enables them to experience themselves and their perceptions and beliefs more freshly, and in a different way than was previously possible. As clients are able to experience and explore their realities, they often come to see old things in new ways. Frequently, new alternatives for addressing their life concerns become evident during this process of exploration and self-reflection.

Empathic listening and responding are more difficult than they look. Hearing another's experience accurately takes considerable attention and concentration and an ability to "get" the implicit meaning in the client's message. Further, effective empathic responding requires that the therapist use language effectively and precisely. The right words often open up understanding, while less accurate words may not resonate with the client.

Whether they are viewed in videotaped therapy sessions or read in transcriptions of sessions, therapists' empathetic responses may seem to have less impact than they do. Only when one has been listened to attentively while in a troubled state can one fully grasp how therapeutic this experience is. Accuracy of empathic understanding is critical to helping clients hear themselves and process their experiences and learn from them. In teaching empathic listening, I encourage students first to get the content accurately. I call this first step "getting in the ball park." Next, I encourage them to refine their empathy by "getting in the right section," then the "right row," and finally the "specific seat." This process often leads to clients' telling the therapist that he or she feels exactly understood.

Regard, Acceptance, Affirmation

The therapist's unconditional positive regard, acceptance, warmth, lack of judgment, and affirming responses help provide safety and comfort for the client. Clients usually come to therapy when they are distressed and "stuck," when what they are doing isn't working. Most individuals who enter therapy hope that their therapist will be someone with whom they feel comfortable, someone who accepts them as they are. Because so many clients come to therapy with self-doubt, low self-esteem, insecurity about whether they are "okay" or worthwhile, the therapist's genuine acceptance is a vital quality that enables them to open up and disclose problematic and unattractive aspects of themselves. As clients realize, through their therapist's empathic understanding, that they are "seen" and known, they may revise the views they have of themselves in more positive directions. When clients feel better about themselves, they seem to operate more effectively in daily life. As they become more self-accepting, they also tend to be less judgmental of others as well.

Person-centered therapists believe that their nonjudgmental empathy also conveys unconditional positive regard because it is devoid of evaluation. Positive regard for, or prizing, another person may take other forms as well. The therapist may affirm the client in any number of ways, directly or indirectly. For example, in his well-known filmed session with Gloria, Rogers spontaneously commented, "You look to be a pretty nice daughter," a comment that obviously touched her. It is important that such statements are made congruently and without manipulative intent, lest they be experienced as superficial attempts to "help the client feel better."

Authenticity

The therapist's congruence or genuineness lends credibility to everything the therapist does. When the therapist is congruent, she or he is more likely to be perceived as trustworthy and as a person of integrity. Because the therapist is transparent, knowable, credible, and without any desire or intent to act like someone she or he is not, the client is likely to feel safe. Further, the therapist's credibility enhances the impact of her or his positive regard because it is experienced as believable.

Person-centered therapists who are congruent do not play the role of therapist but are naturally themselves in relationship to their clients. Congruent therapists may use themselves in a variety of ways on behalf of their clients. Although person-centered therapists do tend to focus primarily on their clients' experience, there are times when they respond spontaneously as the person they are. For example, the therapist may engage his or her sense of humor with the client, make affirmative or supportive comments to the client, or respond in any other way that fosters the therapeutic process or the client's well-being.

The therapist's congruence may be displayed at times when the therapist is having difficulty with a client. Rogers used as a marker any *persistent* problematic reaction or feeling elicited by the client as a time to share his own feelings with his client. For example, the therapist who feels the client is not disclosing anything of personal relevance may mention this to the client. Or the therapist might initiate a discussion of his or her concern that there is a strain in the relationship that needs attention and/or repair. However, I want to make it clear that being congruent doesn't mean that person-centered therapists have license to say or do whatever they feel simply because it is real or congruent. Expressions of congruence, while authentic, may also be harmful and damaging to the therapeutic relationship. For example, expressing anger at a client for lack of effort during or between sessions may be authentic but runs a high risk of being harmful and should generally be avoided. The bottom line on congruent expression of the therapist's self is whether it is in the best interests of the client.

To further illuminate the concepts I have discussed so far, here are two case examples, one of Rogers's and one of my own. Each illustrates how client-centered therapy is practiced and how issues of diversity are considered when clients present them.

In the first example, a demonstration session in front of a professional audience, Rogers works with a woman in her 40s, Elly, who has been handicapped with polio since childhood. Her body was weakened and deformed by polio and, at times, she is severely incapacitated. Elly came to the interview in a dress that concealed her body and arms. The interview is presented in condensed form by Rogers and Sanford (1989, pp. 1480–1484) along with their commentary in italics.

Rogers: What is it that you would like to talk about?

Elly: It's going to be difficult for me to capsulize it for you, but I'm going to do my best. Very quickly, my background is I think, important. I had polio as a child and was very incapacitated. I was in a hospital for two years before I was 13. I never went to school until college. I had home instruction because of my parents' fear of my exposure to the large world. I was hidden. I had no strength to fight back until something just kind of snapped from somewhere. I was a little less than 17 when 1 finished high school instruction. I had a strong desire to fly—to get out—and I went to college. This was a horrendous experience for me, but I stayed. I married at a very young age, but the marriage was short-lived and I retreated—rejection set in. I went back to my parents' home until I was 24. My second marriage lasted for 12 years—the first 5 were okay but I was beginning to feel numb again. Every once in a while, I'd come out of my shell and fight, but I was feeling near death in my soul.

R: You were kind of withering away inside?

E: Yes. That's right. On and off since I was very young.

Here Elly spoke of her divorce, her second marriage, her fear of being alone, her feelings of despondence, and the urge to run back to a traditional marriage. At the same time, she was feeling happier living with a divorced man in a nontraditional partnership. The words "I seem threatening to people" express her feelings of rejection. Quite openly, she revealed her jealousy of her partner's elder daughter, feeling that he preferred her—"beautiful, young, straight, and talented, the things I would want to be"—to Elly. She was afraid she might lose him and that this jealousy was an obstacle in their relationship.

R: As an obstacle, it's pretty dangerous to you.

E: If I push too much, I could lose him. And that brings me to something else that I work real hard on—that I spent too many years seeing myself through a man, and I don't see myself so much that way anymore.

R: Uh-huh.

E: And I would like to be able not to see myself that way at all. It's good that there's someone important in my life—but I do not see myself as an extension of that person. . . . Still, I get very frightened when I think of being alone.

R: Although you feel stronger than you did, you don't feel strong enough to . . .

E: I prefaced this whole thing with my illness because I'm sure—I never could talk about this, not with all my years of therapy—I could just talk about it here, now. That I can talk about it today is good, but it was awful—2 years alone in a ward—alone—I couldn't move from my neck down, and then hidden for 4 more years. To me, being alone is connected with terrible disaster.

R: Uh-huh.

E: Withering away—withering away.

When the therapist first used the words *withering away*, the client accepted them with "Yes," but seemed not to recognize the impact of the expression. The therapist at that point had not noticed any physical withering: he was responding intuitively to what he had been hearing of her feelings. Without knowing, he had touched on the accurate metaphor. Now the client came back to the phrase, as if hearing it for the first time. Only after the client had experienced the insight, did the therapist move deeper.

E: One of the things you have written about which is important to me is the need to be heard . . .

R: You'd like to be heard?

E: Yes. I think that's what happened in my relationships. No matter how much I tried to talk to them and tell them what I'm feeling, they think I'm off the wall . . . that I'm not reacting to it well is what I want to change.

R: You feel you are not heard, and also you feel that if you *were* heard, they would recognize some of the truth of what you feel?

E: Yes, I want my feelings validated. . . . I feel like I'm shaking.—I feel calm in one way, but on another level, my body is shaking.

R: What is that shaking for you? Can you get in touch with it?

E: Yes. It's the group—it's being observed. *(At this point she looks out at the group, and her gaze was directed toward them several times in the next few moments.)* I haven't had much experience with groups looking at me. My self-image is higher than it was, but it still has a long way to go—a long road ahead.

R: You really dread that they might be observing you?

E: Yes, I'm glad I could tell you this because I don't want to talk about it. I think that's why I shake, because I've been observed—critically and verbally. Even in a group such as this one, where I feel people are sensitive and caring, I'm still shaking.

R: Your shaking is really fear.

E: Uh-huh. I want to get rid of it. This fear is not good for me.

Elly spoke now of the years during which she had turned to meditation, of going back to therapy, and of being unsuccessful in finding the right therapist, and she continued.

E: And when I do meet someone I think I could talk with, I become frightened and don't pursue it.

R: So you say you draw back from people you could share with?

E: Yes. When I get to a certain point of opening up to my pain, I then close up. This is the furthest I've come. In just a few minutes!

R: There's a lot of pain there—pain about the past and pain about the present.

E: Yes, pain about the past because I've never talked about it. . . . Even with my mate, children, and some friends . . . I'll get to a point and I'll close up again.

R: You go so far and then what? You close up, but why?

E: Because I don't want to have to tell them what I'm saying now, here—don't get too close and don't get to know me too much because . . . because . . . because . . . they'll . . . they'll . . . because they'll *see* me. And I'm talking physically. They'll see me more as they get to know me more.

R: So don't get too close because I don't want really to be *seen*. . . . Your eyes grow a little moist at the possibility of people really seeing you.

E: Yes. *(softly.)*

R: Something you want very much and something you dread very much too.

E: Yes . . . *(pause.)*

R: I'm wondering where you want to go next.

E: I'm not sure. I think, if I could have a magic wand, I would want to live alone. Maybe I could fly more. I know I've got it inside me.

R: If you really had the dream you want, you would probably like to be alone, and you would really take off.

E: Yes. I just never was in an independent position. I wonder if I could really take care of myself in that big world.

This interview offers a poignant glimpse into the world of lifelong physical handicap, along with the damage it wreaked on Elly's self/body image, confidence, and ability to live in a world of mostly healthy people. Rogers's sensitive listening and ability to grasp what life has been and is for Elly is remarkable and touching. Rogers's support, acceptance, and understanding enabled her to wrestle with her profound ambivalence about being "seen"—both physically and as a vulnerable person. This appears to be a vital first step toward self-acceptance. Elly (Rogers & Sanford, 1989) commented about the interview:

> What took place in that half hour was a rare experience. . . . I remember saying to Dr. Rogers at the close of the session, "I get the feeling that you're inside of me and that I can talk to you as if I was talking to myself." . . . That one session pulled together for me issues and feelings I had been struggling with for years. (pp. 1484–1485)

Here now is the second case. Juan was a single male in his mid-twenties whom I saw in my private practice in California. He was born in Mexico, where he attended high school and studied for the priesthood in his early twenties. Juan left his priesthood training after a few years because of dissatisfaction with the Catholic Church, especially some of the misconduct he witnessed in other priests. At the time of our work together, he was living in California and was a graduate student in social work. One of his major concerns was his shyness and inexperience with women. He had never had a girlfriend or any sexual experience and found the prospect of dating extremely intimidating.

In the following excerpt, Juan is wrestling with his fears regarding approaching a woman. In the background are Juan's Mexican heritage, his Catholicism, his time in the seminary, and his struggles to define his brand of spirituality. All of these factors are germane now that Juan is living in the United States. His fears about approaching women mix with his sadness and confusion about whether his expectations of having a spiritual connection with a woman are too idealistic.

C (Client): What do you do when you admire a woman and you start to know her?

T (Therapist): What do you do when it gets more personal? Is that what you're asking?

C: Yeah.

T: Because when you're admiring her, you're sort of at a distance?

C: Yeah. But when you're closer. What do you do with those [feelings]?

T: And those feelings are . . . ?

C: Those feelings are . . . like walking on eggshells.

T: You start to get a little tentative, you mean? [C: Yes.] Careful?

C: A lot? Real careful.

A little later:

T: You're trying to figure out, when you have sexual feelings . . . what to make of them and what they mean and how to act on them.

C: Yeah. Well not only sexual feelings but everything . . . anything. Let's don't label that. What do you mean by sexual feelings? Let's start there. I don't want to confuse myself.

Juan reacts to my use of the words *sexual feelings*, which I felt was implied but not yet acknowledged. The person-centered therapist tries to get at both what is evident as well as that which is implicit.

C: It is real scary. And now that I'm finishing my master's it's okay, well, that's one more obstacle I finished, one more step that I advanced. The pool seems real deep and I think I'm gonna drown.

T: The pool of your feelings, you mean?

C: Yeah, the emotions. I'm gonna drown in them.

T: You're afraid you're going to be overwhelmed.

Though Juan is in his mid-twenties, it is clear that he feels more like an inexperienced teenager as he anticipates the possibility of approaching a woman. Here, my nonjudgmental acceptance of his naiveté and fear are important elements in his willingness to share these sensitive feelings.

C: Yes. So where do you go from there. How do you learn . . . what would be the question . . . ?

> T: You're just a beginner is what you're thinking. "So what in the world do I do?"
>
> C: Where do I start?

Notice that I do not attempt to answer such questions directly or offer advice since such responses are not likely to be helpful. I have faith, too, that this client will find his own way.

> T: I guess you already have started, in a sense, by realizing, "My attraction to a woman has changed. It has changed from a sense of admiration from a distance to becoming more personal as I get to know the person." The attraction is partly physical and sexual but also includes a personal attraction to that woman.
>
> C: Yeah.
>
> T: The person she is. So you've started by being aware that "I am attracted." I can be attracted. I'm not in the role of a priest in training anymore.
>
> C: Well, that's it. That's my reality. Even though I left the seminary a few years ago, I still had to finish this goal, get my bachelor's. I had to finish my master's . . . and so I can't think about it.
>
> T: You put it off.
>
> C: Yeah. There was still a barrier there. That was a good excuse. But now I'm out of excuses.

Here Juan realizes that he has found justifications to avoid what he fears, the possibility of an intimate relationship with a woman.

> T: That's right. [We laugh together.]
>
> C: Now it's sink or swim.
>
> T: Yeah. You're feeling intimidated.
>
> C: And now I know I have to swim, I know I want to swim but I don't want to dive in the deep ocean. Where's a safe pool?

A little later:

> T: You mentioned earlier how you were able to avoid this issue by saying, I've got other things to do right now, other things that I want to do. I wonder if this could be sort of the same kind of . . .
>
> C: Yeah, that's the thing I'm asking myself. Am I also avoiding again? If I keep doing it, let's say [until] I'm 80, like, OK . . .

Here I am gently challenging Juan to consider if he is about to fall back into avoidance and good "excuses" (e.g., travel) to deal with his dilemma.

T: Yeah, you could avoid until you're too old!

C: Oh, I don't know, medications might come in.

T: [Laughs.] I guess there's always Viagra. Or something better. [Laughs.]

C: Viagra version 2030. [Mutual laughter.]

T: Right, right!

Here we share a laugh over Juan's fantasy of putting off his anxieties about women until old age. Laughter often brings therapist and client closer as well as providing perspective on an issue.

C: But, I don't know, well at least right now I am feeling a little more relaxed.

T: That's interesting, I wonder what happened?

C: I think . . . it's talking with you . . . disclosing some things, I guess.

T: Just getting it off your chest helps.

C: Yeah, that's it. When somebody helps [by understanding].

T: Yes, yes, I understand. Before it was all churning in you.

This is a nice illustration of the importance to the client of feeling understood and the relief that often follows.

C: Another thing that is scary is, at least for me, is that my [priest] peers, they got married to the first person they knew, or they left the seminary, and knew somebody and immediately married them.

T: You're afraid you would do that?

C: Right now, yeah!

T: Afraid you'd jump before you're ready.

C: Yeah, that's it! So I don't want that without knowing more people.

T: And as you talk about this, there is a mixture of excitement and hesitation and fear. A lot of feelings.

C: Yes, it's not as simple as just physical attraction.

T: It is a whole life change for you, a big life change for you. It's entering a part of your life that you have not entered and not allowed any space for.

C: Yes, but I have to include it. It includes dreams, expectations, aspirations, all that stuff. The thing that is so scary is, are those dreams only dreams? Only illusions?

T: You mean, if I have those dreams, are they beyond my reach?

C: Are my expectations too high or only idealistic?

T: You're wondering, "Am I hoping for something that is beyond me?"

C: Let me calm myself a little bit.

Juan's need to calm himself indicates that he is very close to both his fears and hopes and that the stakes are very high for him.

T: A lot of feelings are coming up.

C: Yes, sadness . . .

T: There is something sad about all this as you think about it.

C: Why should I think that? Let me get my thoughts together. Okay, what was the question again?

This temporary forgetting is not unusual when a client is very close to a sensitive issue and the disconcerting feelings that come with it. At such moments, it is especially important for the therapist be well attuned to the client's feelings and respond with delicacy.

T: You were feeling sad and it wasn't exactly clear what those feelings were about. You were starting to reflect on that sadness.

C: Okay, are my expectations of another person real, in the sense of the relationship. Am I highly influenced by my [seminary] background that I create these expectations [that are] so romantic, [so] idealistic, or, I don't want to label them but [it might be] spiritual [T: Yeah.] in which you encounter another person and you think that you are that other person, but yet you are yourself! I don't know of another way to talk about this except spirituality, where you talk about the divinity and you talk about total freedom and individuality and yet you talk about total communion.

Here it is evident that Juan's Catholicism and spiritual background and beliefs embedded in his Mexican heritage are in play as factors that strongly influence his values and beliefs.

A little later:

T: It's almost as if your whole life comes into play—where you've been, where you were going and where you might go.

C: Yes, well . . . at least I got it off of my chest.

T: It seems to always help you to say these things out loud.

C: Ah. [Groans.] Yes.

T: It seems to release it for you to some degree, even though it's not solved. It helps to release it.

A little later:

C: I don't want to pursue it [a woman] because this is the first time that I feel these crazy emotions. So I don't want to go that fast.

T: Okay. What do you think would feel right for you to do or say in the moment?

C: I don't know . . . be friends. [Hesitantly.]

T: Be a friend first, you mean?

C: Yeah. Be friends. Get to know that person more. See what they're like . . . but the first thing that pops into my mind is infatuation.

T: So you're aware of being infatuated and you're thinking, "Well, I guess I'd like to get to know that woman. I'd like to be friends first."

C: Yes.

Throughout the interview I have resisted giving advice, believing that Juan has a sense of what he'd be willing to do and at what pace. The client is empowered when he sorts this out for himself. These may seem like little steps forward, but for Juan they are risky and intimidating.

A little later:

C: [Long pause.] I don't know. Taking that first step is hard. Do or die.

T: Do or die. It almost feels like death, huh?

C: Yeah. Crash and burn.

T: It is fairly rare that you read in the newspaper that a thirty-something-year-old man crashed and burned from being interested in a woman. [Mutual laughter.] But it sure can feel that way.

C: I'll take it one step at a time.

T: Well, that would be you. One step at a time.

C: Don't rush me, big boy. [Chuckles.]

T: I don't want to rush you and I think you know your own pace quite well. You know your comfort zone [C: Yeah.] and I think you also know that you need to push a little, too, out of your comfort zone or you and I will be having this conversation next year.

Once again it becomes clear that such things cannot be rushed and that the client will need to proceed at his own pace.

C: But that's [Addressing his fears.] a sign of courage.

T: It is a sign of courage. I couldn't have said it better. You are engaging your courage in talking about it, and you are engaging your courage in imagining it and you are engaging your courage in embracing the risky possibility that your dream could be an illusion, could be unattainable.

C: Yeah. [Soberly.]

T: I like your courage.

This last statement is beyond acceptance. It is an affirmation of Juan's courage in beginning to deal with this most difficult challenge in his life.

Rogers's work with Elly and mine with Juan demonstrate person-centered therapy in action with clients who are members of minority groups. Elly's polio set the stage for a lifelong physical disability that had profound implications for her relationships with physically able people. Juan's experience in the seminary in Mexico and his extensive training in Catholicism have similar implications as he examines his fears about dating women in the United States. In both vignettes, the therapist is endeavoring to address the question, *What is it like to be you?* and to be aware of the diversity factors without making assumptions about the relative importance of those factors to the client. In both cases, the therapist's acceptance and affirmation allowed the clients to engage in deeper levels of self-exploration and to achieve more clarity about their worldview and problematic issues.

Long-Term and Short-Term Applications

A common misconception about person-centered psychotherapy is that it is inevitably long-term therapy. It is not. In a recent study, Miller, Duncan, and Hubble (1997) reviewed a range of psychotherapy orientations and concluded that the modal number of sessions clients attend is one and most courses of psychotherapy are six sessions or fewer. The length of person-centered therapy varies from as few as one to more than 100 sessions, depending on the client's goals and severity of problems. I have seen many clients who benefited from a single session, and the majority of clients are satisfied with 10 sessions or less.

There is no fundamental alteration in the way person-centered therapy is practiced to achieve brevity. However, like other brief therapies, brief person-centered therapy may have a more limited focus, which results in the therapist's and client's agreeing to keep their attention and efforts on some circumscribed aspect of the client's problems.

Evaluation of Person-Centered Therapy

Earlier in this chapter, I stated that Rogers was a pioneer in carrying out and publishing research studies in counseling. Rogers and his students were the first to study the process of counseling by subjecting transcripts of counseling sessions to critical examination. His intent was to formulate testable hypotheses about elements of the client-counselor relationship to determine what types of interventions were most effective.

This research tradition has continued and today, 60 years later, person-centered psychotherapists have cause for optimism. In a recent and comprehensive review of research in person-centered therapy, Bozarth, Zimring, and Tausch (2002) concluded:

> In short, psychotherapy outcome research supports the major tenets of CCT. The therapeutic relationship and the client's resources are the crux of successful therapy and the foundation of CCT. It is also clear that Rogers' specific hypothesis of the necessary and sufficient conditions . . . has received much more empirical support than some of the equivocal reviews of the middle 1970s imply. Research has supported the theory that a congruent therapist's experience of empathic understanding of the client's frame of reference and experience of unconditional positive regard are related to positive outcome. (p. 179)

An extensive body of research has been generated and provides support for the effectiveness of person-centered therapy with a wide range of clients and problems of all age groups. The major findings are summarized here in the areas of empathy, emotion in psychotherapy, and focusing-oriented experiential psychotherapy.

Empathy

In recent years, there has been a revival of interest in therapeutic empathy (Bohart & Greenberg, 1997). Watson (2001), reviewing the research on therapist empathy, found that:

1. Research consistently demonstrates that therapist empathy is the most potent predictor of client progress in therapy and an essential component of successful therapy in every therapeutic modality.

2. There are no studies that demonstrate a negative relationship between empathy and outcome.

3. Client ratings of therapist empathy are stronger predictors of successful outcome than the ratings of external judges or therapists.

4. Strong behavioral correlates of empathy include therapist direct eye contact and concerned expression, a forward trunk lean and head nods, a vocal tone that communicates interest and emotional involvement, clarity of communication, and use of emotional language.

5. Therapist interruptions, advisement, and reassurance are negatively correlated with therapist empathy.

Sachse and Elliot's microprocess research (2001) showed that the therapist's empathic responses may deepen, maintain, or flatten client experiential processing and self-exploration. Further, he showed that clients do little experiential processing on their own and do not deepen their processing unless the therapist provides deepening empathic responses.

In more than 30 years of experience as a client-centered therapist, I have yet to hear a client complain about being understood. Both personal and therapeutic experience provide compelling evidence that feeling understood and accepted by important others is conducive to our well-being. Regardless of one's therapeutic approach, the desire to hear our client, enter into her or his experiential world, and communicate that understanding is almost inevitably helpful and never harmful.

Emotion in Psychotherapy

Emotion serves both to provide information to the person about what is important and meaningful, and to energize appropriate action. Research on the therapist's processing of client emotion indicates that the individual's ability to accurately differentiate his or her emotional experience is integral to healthy functioning. Conversely, an inability to access emotional information blocks an individual's attempt to understand the meaning of his or her experiences and make sense of the world.

Research has consistently shown that the depth of experiencing in therapy is related to outcome, especially in person-centered therapy. The literature on clients' processing of emotion reviewed by Greenberg, Korman, and Pavio (2002) concluded that:

1. Processing information in an experiential manner is associated with productive client involvement and predicts successful outcome.

2. Therapies focusing on clients' emotional experience, when successful, are associated with changes, over treatment, in clients' in-session emotional experiences.

3. Emotion is important in reorganizing personal meaning.

Focusing-Oriented Experiential Psychotherapy

Gendlin's focusing-oriented experiential psychotherapy is a close relative of client-centered psychotherapy. Hendricks's review of research on that approach (2002) found that:

1. Higher levels of focusing on their emotional experience by clients correlate positively with successful outcomes in a variety of therapeutic orientations and client problem types.

2. The ability to focus and process emotional experience can be taught to clients.

3. Therapists who themselves focus seem to be more effective in enabling their clients to focus.

Person-Centered Therapy: Blind Spots, Limitations, and Challenges

The paradoxical effect of any psychotherapy theory is that it has the potential to both expand and limit our vision. Thus, it is desirable to examine critically some of the most fundamental premises of the approach. In this section, I discuss person-centered therapy in terms of its blind spots, limitations, and challenges.

Blind Spots

Every system of psychotherapy has blind spots. Generally, those areas where our vision may be impaired are closely tied to the fundamental assumptions that provide the foundation for an approach. For person-centered therapy, the *actualizing tendency* is the bedrock concept upon which the approach is built and is viewed by critics as a controversial concept.

Person-centered therapists take as a given that the individual has a natural tendency toward growth, self-determination, and autonomy. Because that tendency is present in every client, person-centered therapists endeavor to provide the necessary and sufficient conditions of therapy that were outlined earlier in this chapter. If those conditions are present in the therapeutic relationship, the actualization tendency enables clients to tap their resources for constructive growth. However, some have argued that for many clients in our increasingly diverse world, the notion of self-actualization and autonomy is questionable. Many individuals from both the majority individualistic culture and from collectivistic cultures are oriented less toward self-actualization and more toward intimacy and connection with others and toward what is best for the community and the common good.

This concern about the actualizing tendency being biased toward individual fulfillment and autonomy has been addressed in recent years. Friedman (1985) is a humanistic therapist who has suggested that self-actualization has a strong interpersonal component and occurs as a byproduct of a confirming dialogue with another person. Seeman (1988) criticized the concept of self-actualization as being too general and abstract to be tested. Instead, he proposed a human-system model composed of interrelated subsystems that are self-regulating. Seeman's working definition of self-actualization suggests that "persons are maximally actualizing when as total human systems they are functioning at peak efficiency" (p. 309). Both of these reformulations of the actualizing tendency place more emphasis on the role of others in the realization of self-actualization.

Limitations

I have sometimes said to my graduate students, tongue in cheek, that "I never met a client I couldn't help." While this is, of course, untrue, I have always believed that no clients were truly stuck with their troubled past or current life and that all had the capacity to move forward. Despite the optimism person-centered therapists bring to their clients, the approach has its limitations.

Research (e.g., Greenberg et al., 2002) clearly shows that helping clients process their emotional experiences is related to good outcome. However, it is also true that engaging clients' emotion requires considerable sensitivity and relational skill on the part of the therapist since experiencing problematic emotion is often arduous, painful, threatening, and disturbing for many clients. Further, in many cultures emotional expression is minimal, sometimes suppressed, and even unacceptable in some situations. Therefore, person-centered therapists need to be cognizant of these cultural variations and modify the ways they respond to clients' emotion. A possible limitation is that the manner in which the therapist's empathy, congruence, and unconditional positive regard is communicated may need to be modified to fit the needs of persons from different cultures. For example, a therapist's direct expression of empathy might be very uncomfortable for clients who require indirect communication or who find such an expression a violation of the distance they need in the therapy relationship.

As you will recall, Rogers created nondirective psychotherapy in the 1940s because he believed the therapies available at that time tended to be too therapist centered and did not trust the resourcefulness of the client. Some clients, particularly from certain cultural groups, may prefer a more directive therapy because they view the therapist as the "doctor" or expert. The fundamental premise of the therapist's nondirectiveness may also be too constricting for the therapist and client. That is, rigid insistence on nondirectiveness for all clients, regardless of culture, personal preference, learning style, or other forms of diversity, may be experienced as an imposition that does not fit the client's interpersonal and therapeutic learning needs.

The final limitation is related to the need for additional and ongoing research, both quantitative and qualitative, to test the premises and effectiveness of person-centered therapy with diverse clients. As stated earlier, person-centered therapy has reason to be optimistic about research supporting its effectiveness, and I applauded Rogers for being a pioneer in this area. As with other approaches described in this book, however, we need to do to more research to provide evidence that person-centered therapy is effective for majority and nonmajority clients. This research is essential for all therapeutic approaches because the suggested modifications in practice typically suggested by experts in multicultural therapy (e.g., Sue, 1983) are essentially untested in clinical research with diverse populations.

Challenges

Person-centered therapy remains a work in progress. Carl Rogers always took the position that person-centered therapy would and should continue to evolve and change, and he supported such developments. In 1986, a year before he died, he commented on this point. "The approach is paradoxical. It emphasizes shared values, yet encourages uniqueness . . . it encourages those who incorporate these values to develop their own special and unique ways of being, their own ways of implementing this philosophy" (1986, pp. 3–4).

Person-centered therapists do have a shared set of values. Our challenge is to honor those values while advancing the implementation of person-centered therapy with the increasingly diverse and complex range of clients we serve today. One of the primary ways in which person-centered therapists might be more effective is to learn to adapt their therapy to the client rather than attempting to get the client to adapt to the therapist's approach and style. Ideally, therapists constantly monitor whether what they are doing "fits," especially whether their approach is compatible with their clients' manner of framing their problems and their belief about how constructive change will occur. Hubble, Duncan, and Miller (1999) make a compelling case that therapy is more likely to be effective when therapists adopt their clients' view of their problems, their causes, theory of change, and potential solutions. These authors also encourage therapists to develop a positive expectation for change, observe constructive change in the client, validate it when it is evident, and credit the client for her or his part in it. This way of being client centered has been supported in recent years by empirical research demonstrating that approximately 40% of the outcome of psychotherapy can be attributed to clients' qualities, behaviors, and resources (Asay & Lambert, 1999).

Another way in which person-centered therapy could advance is in the expansion of its response repertoire. The predominant response mode of person-centered therapists remains empathic understanding responses. I firmly believe that if a therapist could do only one thing to facilitate growth, the optimal choice would be to respond with empathy. However, if therapy is limited primarily to this response, both the therapist's and client's freedom of movement are constrained. As client-centered therapist and researcher Jules Seeman (1965) noted long ago: "The counselor could lock himself into a verbal response which was anything but spontaneous. And in the end, a situation so much structured for the counselor could not be free for the client" (p. 1216).

Another challenge for person-centered therapists is to bring other therapeutic aspects of themselves to the client. As I said earlier in relating my own journey as a person-centered therapist, over the years my approach as a clinician has evolved to include an increased use of my *self* when I am able to bring forth aspects of who I am in ways that allow for a meaningful meeting or encounter with my client. There are, of course, many ways that therapists could effectively bring aspects of themselves to the therapeutic encounter. In order to do so, client-centered therapists would need to make a slight shift in their view of therapy. They would have to pay more attention to their reactions to their clients and be willing to disclose these responses when it would be fruitful for the client to do so. Maurice Friedman (1986) suggests that therapy might be characterized by "healing through meeting," a description of an I-Thou encounter as described by Buber. Classical client-centered therapy tends to be one-sided in that the therapist primarily strives to communicate his or her understanding of the client's experience and meanings. Friedman believes that person-centered therapy would be strengthened if it recognized more fully that "persons become themselves and reach self-actualization not by directly aiming at these goals but as a byproduct of dialogue" (p. 434).

A final challenge for person-centered therapy is to make the modifications required to be effective in a diverse world. I address that topic in the last section of this chapter.

Future Development: Person-Centered Therapy in a Diverse World

Carl Rogers provided an exemplary style for how person-centered therapy might be practiced. Watching films of Rogers, one readily sees his intent interest, focused listening, and nonjudgmental empathic responding to his client's experienced world. While there is much of value to emulate in Rogers's style, it is also fair to acknowledge that person-centered therapy can be practiced in more diverse ways than is often understood. In this section, I address some of the ways the approach might be modified to accommodate an increasingly diverse world.

I have long argued (Cain, 1989, 1990) that person-centered therapy needs to be adapted when it does not ideally fit the needs of the unique person sitting before the therapist. I believe this can be accomplished while retaining the core values and premises of the approach. Some modifications of assumptions may be desirable to expand the approach's range of effectiveness with clients from other cultures. Sue and Sue (2003) have identified three competencies of the culturally skilled counselor. I believe the Sues' guidelines are also applicable for diversity in clients that extends beyond culture (e.g., sexual orientation, disability, etc.). I address each competency in terms of how well person-centered therapy meets each criterion for diversity and suggest possible modifications as appropriate.

Competency 1: Self-Awareness of One's Own Assumptions, Values, and Biases

Rogers took the position (1977) that clients deserve a "respectful hearing" of all attitudes and feelings, no matter how "extreme" or "unrealistic" (p. 113). To the degree that person-centered therapists embrace these sentiments, they are likely to periodically reassess their own values and assumptions and to make appropriate accommodations in the way they respond to the unique values and needs of clients' individual differences. Nevertheless, the person-centered approach has been criticized for reflecting the values of independence, individualism, and self-determination held by Rogers and many Americans. This position may conflict with that of persons who embrace collectivist views or who are strongly influenced by family values and expectations. To work effectively with such individuals, person-centered therapists would do well to suspend or set aside their own values and be receptive to the powerful influence and merits of the client's family or subculture. For example, in deaf culture enormous pressure is often exerted on deaf children (and later on adults) to embrace sign language as opposed to spoken language. While this stance may run counter to the values of a hearing person-centered therapist, an understanding of this strongly held position and subsequent modifications in the therapist's assumptions about it are appropriate. Regardless of what some person-centered therapists may be tempted to believe are in the deaf person's best interests (e.g., both speech and sign language are valuable and adaptive), the informed decisions of the client deserve acceptance and support.

Competency 2: Understanding the Worldview of the Culturally Different Client

All therapists would serve their clients by learning as much as possible about the worldviews of their clients, whether cultural, those that emerge as a result of the client's experience (e.g., sexual orientation), or those that result from the client's need to cope with a difficult condition (e.g., blindness, physical or mental disability). The sensitive person-centered therapist would seek to understand what it is like to live as a gay, quadriplegic, or mentally challenged person while refraining from adopting stereotyped views and recognizing that persons within a subgroup have diverse experiences and attitudes. Rogers (1951) believed that "the only way to understand another culture is to assume the frame of reference of that culture" (p. 494). MacDougall (2002) commented that Rogers "promoted counselor acquisition of knowledge of clients in their cultural settings, knowledge of cultural anthropology or sociology with actual experiences of living with or dealing with culturally diverse clients" (p. 52).

Competency 3: Developing Appropriate Intervention Strategies and Techniques

In his essay "The Necessary and Sufficient Conditions for Therapeutic Personality Change," Rogers (1957) did not specify how the therapist qualities of empathy, unconditional positive regard, and congruence might be implemented in the therapeutic process. Although Rogers and most client-centered therapists engage primarily in empathic responding, Rogers's theory allowed for variations in how such universal qualities might be provided. Therefore, modifications in therapeutic style are acceptable, desirable, and sometimes necessary to meet the needs of a particular client.

One way in which person-centered therapy might be modified to meet the needs of diverse populations is to modify the extreme view of nondirectiveness advocated by some of its adherents. Although nondirective attitudes and behavior on the part of the client-centered therapist may be seen as freeing the client, they may have the opposite effect. As mentioned earlier, rigid insistence on nondirectiveness for all clients, regardless of culture, personal preference, learning style, or other forms of diverse experience, may be experienced as an imposition that does not fit the client's interpersonal and therapeutic learning needs.

In my view, the optimal form of client-centered therapy would be "client informed" or even "client directed," which suggests that the client plays a strong and collaborative role in how the therapy is implemented. In this approach, the therapist is sensitive to all of the variables that influence the client's life, including cultural and other forms of diversity. MacDougall (2002) has argued that "to be truly person centered, counselors need to allow themselves to be more directive if the culture(s)/circumstances of the client warrant it" (p. 54). I believe that person-centered therapists can make such adaptations to their clients without violating their fundamental values of preserving clients' freedom and autonomy regarding how they live their lives.

Final Comments

In an era characterized by increasing technology, multitasking, overly busy and stressed lives, less personalization, and medication as a first choice for alleviation of a variety of debilitating psychological problems, client-centered therapy becomes increasingly needed and relevant. A therapy that stresses the importance of quality of relationship, that encourages clients to listen to themselves and to live in a more accepting and authentic manner, will always be needed. Good ideas, like good art, endure. Carl Rogers's system of psychotherapy has endured for over 60 years, and the therapist qualities Rogers defined as "necessary and sufficient"— empathy, congruence, and unconditional positive regard—have been acknowledged by almost every major system of psychotherapy as contributors to clients' growth.

Today, the therapeutic trend in the United States is toward cognitive-behavioral therapies. However, this does not diminish the importance of client-centered therapy, which flourishes in the United Kingdom and in parts of Europe, South America, Japan, and increasingly in China. Graduate students in the United States who are exposed to person-centered and other humanistic therapies typically find these approaches quite compelling and lament the fact that they are not taught enough in their master's and doctoral programs.

In a survey of clinical and counseling psychologists published in 1982 in the *American Psychologist* (Smith, 1982), Carl Rogers was identified as the most influential psychotherapist. At present, Rogers's influence on American psychotherapy is still enormous, though often indirect. His fundamental ideas have been absorbed by many diverse approaches to psychotherapy. A substantial number of training programs for graduate students in psychology and counseling typically emphasize the importance of empathic listening and responding skills and attitudes, as well as the critical importance of unconditional positive regard for the client and therapist congruence. Rogers, more than any other therapist, taught us to listen with sensitivity and caring and to understand that the quality of the therapist-client relationship, in itself, has the potential to foster personal learning and growth in the client.

In a 2005 article entitled "The Current Status of Carl Rogers and the Person-Centered Approach," Kirschenbaum (Rogers's biographer) and Jourdan indicate that during the years 1987–2004 there were a total of 777 person-centered publications, including 141 books. This total far exceeds all of the previous publications in this field over the 40-year period from 1946–1986. Further, there are approximately 200 person-centered organizations and training centers worldwide. Kirschenbaum and Jourdan conclude: "By all these indicators, the person-centered approach is . . . alive and well" and "client-centered principles permeate the practice of many, if not most therapists" (p. 48).

Thus, client-centered therapy is as vital and effective as it has ever been and continues to develop in ways that will make it increasingly so in the years to come.

Summary

1. Developed by Carl Rogers, person-centered therapy, originally called *client-centered therapy*, is based on the assumption that all humans have the innate capacity to solve their own problems and to grow psychologically in an environment that is conducive to such change and growth. Not only is it assumed that all people have this capacity but also that optimal change and growth occurs when it is self-directed.

2. The roots of person-centered therapy date back to the late 1920s, when Carl Rogers was a child clinical psychologist. Rogers was adamant in his belief that the therapist should not advise the client, interpret behavior, or attempt to direct or persuade the client to pursue a particular course of action. This was a radical shift away from the interpretive and directive methods that were commonly employed at the time.

3. Rogers made a major shift in emphasis in therapy by focusing on the person of the client rather than on the problem expressed. Another shift was toward the feelings expressed by the client as opposed to the client's thoughts. Rogers emphasized what the therapist should not do, including advise the client and interpret the meaning of behavior.

4. Rogers was already addressing issues of culture and diversity as early as the 1950s. The desire and goal of the client-centered therapist were to hear, comprehend, and respond to whatever aspects of that person's life and sociocultural context were relevant in a receptive and valuing manner.

5. Toward the end of his life, Rogers became increasingly interested in broader social issues, especially peace. He believed that peaceful solutions to difficult problems could be discovered in groups and communities if the leaders established the norms and conditions that facilitate dialogue and the understanding of diverse opinions and worldviews.

6. Like other orientations to psychotherapy, person-centered therapy has evolved and today there are at least three variations in practice: classical client-centered psychotherapy (which adheres closely to Rogers's 1959

formal statement of purpose and places a high emphasis on the nondirective attitude); focusing-oriented psychotherapy (developed by Eugene Gendlin and based on the notion that the client's body carries its problems in a physically felt form); and process-experiential psychotherapy (developed by Leslie Greenberg, Robert Elliott, and colleagues, and involving the client's working on therapeutic tasks with a process-directive therapist).

7. Existential philosophy and psychotherapy have influenced the thinking of client-centered therapists. Both approaches emphasize the uniqueness and individuality of each client; both understand clients in terms of their subjective, lived experiences; both view psychological problems as a result of the distortion or denial of experiences; both reject the use of techniques in therapy; and both emphasize the importance of accepting and validating the client.

8. Person-centered therapists place a high priority on understanding each client as both unique (like no other person) and sharing some aspects of experiences with others. Consequently, this approach is well suited for clients in a diverse world.

9. Carl Rogers developed client-centered therapy in the context of a White, midwestern, mostly Protestant, homogeneous culture. Thus, his approach embraces many of the prevailing values of that era and place, such as the importance of being independent and self-sufficient. However, Rogers had the wisdom to foresee that person-centered therapy would need to be continuously examined and refined to stay current as the field and context changed, and today person-centered therapy responds to a world that is increasingly diverse and complex.

10. Rogers published the most complete statement of his approach in 1959. The key concepts of that statement include the actualizing tendency (the bedrock on which person-centered therapy is based, which suggests that people naturally move toward differentiation, expansion in growth, and effectiveness and autonomy), the self (including self-concept, or the person's view of self; self structure, or the external view of the self; and the ideal self, or the desired view of self), congruence versus incongruence (a state in which the person's self-concept and experiences are in harmony in contrast to a state of discord between the self-concept and experience), psychological maladjustment (a state of incongruence between one's self and one's experience), openness to experience (when one readily takes in internal or external information without defensiveness), psychological adjustment (when there is congruence of self and experience, which requires openness to experience), positive regard (when people perceive that some aspect of their behavior is genuinely accepted by another, which is essential to one's well being), conditions of

worth (which exist when a person engages in or avoids a behavior based on whether it brings him or her regard from another person), locus of evaluation (the source of a person's values), and empathy (when one person accurately perceives the internal frame of reference of another).

11. Rogers believed that clients change when the quality of the client-therapist relationship is healthy, clients engage in self-exploration and self-discovery, clients achieve clarity about their worldviews and their problematic issues, therapists facilitate clients' learning and enable clients to focus on personal/ internal aspects of the self rather than superficial/external issues, and on feelings that reflect the body's interpretation of a situation or experience.

12. In person-centered therapy practice, the role of the client-therapist relationship is paramount. The therapist must be fully attentive to and immersed in the person of the client as well as the client's expressed concerns, must support and encourage the client's freedom, must be empathically attuned to the client via active and involved listening, must express unconditional positive regard as a means of providing safety and comfort for the client, and must be congruent and genuine with the client.

13. An extensive body of research, conducted over a span of more than 60 years, supports the effectiveness of the approach with a wide range of populations and presenting problems.

14. Limitations of person-centered therapy include its acceptance of the foundational concept of the actualizing tendency in all individuals (some individuals may in reality be oriented toward intimacy, connection with others, and what is best for the community and the common good), its focus on emotional exploration (which may not be desirable with clients from some cultures in which emotional expression is not valued), its nondirective approach (some clients may prefer a directive expert type of approach), and the lack of research on the effectiveness of person-centered therapy with diverse clients. Challenges for person-centered therapy include the need to continually evolve the therapy, the need to adapt the therapy to the client rather than attempting to get the client to adapt to the therapist's approach and style, the need to expand person-centered therapy's response repertoire beyond empathy, the need for person-centered therapists to bring other therapeutic aspects of themselves to the client, and the need to make the modifications necessary to be effective in a diverse world.

15. In order to increase the effectiveness of person-centered therapy in a diverse world, person-centered therapists need to focus on three major competencies: gaining self awareness of one's own assumptions, values, and beliefs; acquiring an understanding of the worldviews of culturally different clients; and developing appropriate intervention strategies and techniques for all clients.

Key Terms

actualizing tendency (p. 194)
conditions of worth (p. 196)
congruence (p. 195)
empathy (p. 197)
ideal self (p. 194)
incongruence (p. 195)
internal frame of reference (p. 197)
locus of evaluation (p. 196)

openness to experience (p. 195)
organismic valuing process (p. 197)
positive regard (p. 196)
psychological adjustment (p. 195)
psychological maladjustment (p. 195)
self (p. 194)
self-actualization (p. 194)
unconditional positive regard (p. 196)

Resources for Further Study

Professional Organizations

World Association for Person-Centered and Experiential Psychotherapy and Counseling (WAPCEP)
office@pce-world.org (e-mail)

Association for Humanistic Psychology
1516 Oak St, #320A
Alameda, CA 94501-2947
510-769-6495
www.ahpweb.org
ahpoffice@aol.com (e-mail)

Professional Journals

Person-Centered and Experiential Psychotherapies
www.pce-world.org/idxjournal.htm
Journal of Humanistic Psychology
http://jhp.sagepub.com

Obtain subscription information from the Association of Humanistic Psychology or the publisher's website. For an online search of journal articles, go to the publisher's website.

Suggested Readings

Bozarth, J., Zimring, F., & Tausch, R. (2002). Research in client-centered therapy: The evolution of a revolution. In D. J. Cain & J. Seeman (Eds.), *Humanistic psychotherapies: Handbook of research and practice* (pp. 147–188). Washington, DC: American Psychological Association.

The best review of 60 years of research on person-centered therapy in a text full of person-centered resources.

Cain, D. J. (2002). *Classics in the person-centered approach*. Herefordshire, UK: PCCS Books.

An anthology of some of the best articles available on person-centered theory, research, and practice.

Mearns, D., & Thorne, B. (1999). *Person-centered counseling in action* (2nd ed.). London: Sage.

A well-written introductory text on all major aspects of person-centered theory and therapeutic practice. Full of useful therapist-client dialogue.

Rogers, C. R. (1961). *On becoming a person*. Boston: Houghton Mifflin.

Rogers's best-selling and best-known text.

Rogers, C. R. (1980). *A way of being*. Boston: Houghton Mifflin.

A collection of some of Rogers's most progressive thinking.

Watson, J. C., Goldman, R. N., & Warner, M. S. (2002). *Client-centered and experiential psychotherapy in the 21st century: Advances in theory, research and practice*. Herefordshire, UK: PCCS Books.

A wide-ranging compendium of contemporary experts on person-centered and experiential psychotherapies.

Other Media Resources

Kirschenbaum, Howard. (2003). *Carl Rogers and the person-centered approach* [Video]. (Available at www.howardkirschenbaum.com.)

An excellent VHS video of the highlights of Rogers's life and contributions assembled by his biographer.

Rogers, C. R. (1974). *Carl Rogers on empathy: Parts I & II* [Video]. (Available from the American Counseling Association at www.counseling.org)

A compelling argument for the therapeutic effectiveness of the therapist's empathy.

Rogers, Natalie. (2002). *Carl Rogers: A daughter's tribute* [CD-ROM]. Mindgarden Media. (Available from www.mindgardenmedia.com.)

A wonderful and intimate view of Rogers the man, author, therapist, and family man.

Shostrom, E. (1965). *Three approaches to psychotherapy: A therapeutic interview with Gloria with explanatory comments: Client-centered therapy, Film no. 1* [Video]. (Available from Psychological and Educational Films at www.psychedfilms.com).

Rogers' best-known and most cited therapeutic interview.

Chapter 7

Gestalt Therapy

Jon Frew

Gestalt therapy was founded in the 1940s by Frederick Salomon Perls, M.D., and Lore Perls, Ph.D., who had rejected orthodox psychoanalysis, the dominant therapy of the 1920s and 1930s, because they disagreed with its focus on the client's past and its lack of focus on the client's **environment,** or the context and culture in which the client lives. They based their Gestalt therapy theory on the premise that by focusing on the *present* and expanding their awareness of *self in relation to the environment*, clients would be able to identify their true wants and needs and could then initiate contact with the environment to satisfy those wants and needs.

Today, 60 years after the earliest formulations of the approach were being articulated, Gestalt therapists in the United States and all over the world continue to work with their clients with this premise as their guiding principle. Gestalt therapy is a theory of health, not illness. Individuals have the innate capacity to know what they need and to take the actions necessary to get those needs met in their environment. Of course, disruptions in this natural process are common, and when they occur, individuals are not aware of their needs or able to make effective contact with the environment to get their needs met. Gestalt therapists work with their clients to examine every detail of this relationship between self and environment and to identify the blocks or interruptions in awareness and contact.

The founders of Gestalt therapy immigrated to the United States in 1947 and became known as Fritz and Laura Perls. The story begins prior to that in Germany in the 1930s.

Origins and Evolution of Gestalt Therapy

Gestalt therapy theory began both geographically and conceptually in Germany, simmered for many years in South Africa, and eventually settled in the United States. In Germany during the 1930s, Fritz Perls trained as a Freudian analyst and Laura Perls studied with the existential philosopher Paul Tillich and Max Wertheimer, a research psychologist. Wertheimer and his colleagues were studying human perception in an exciting new way. They had demonstrated that the human brain perceives a cluster of sensory stimuli by organizing it into a **gestalt,** a German word meaning a "form," "whole," or "configuration." As defined by these perceptual psychologists, a gestalt consists of a **figure** that emerges from and is framed by the whole background or **ground.** The figure is the aspect of the environment that stands out to the perceiver. The ground is the backdrop from which figures emerge. This perceptual system enables us to "see" the man in the moon by focusing on those features of the moonscape that contribute to our perception of a face. It also enables us to look at the image in Figure 7.1 and see either a vase or a pair of faces, depending on what you see as figure and ground.

Wertheimer and his colleagues called their study of perception *Gestalt psychology.* Fritz was fascinated by this work, and as his thinking steadily moved away from psychoanalytic theory, he envisioned ways in which the ideas of Gestalt psychology could be adapted to define a new approach to psychotherapy. After moving to South Africa in the late 1930s, Fritz and Laura wrote the manuscript for *Ego, Hunger and Aggression: A Revision of Psychoanalysis,* published in 1947. The term *Gestalt therapy* came a few years later and was chosen by Fritz (over the objections of Laura) to demonstrate his appreciation of the earlier work of the German Gestalt psychologists. Next, Fritz collaborated with Paul Goodman and Ralph Hefferline to produce a second book, published in 1951, titled *Gestalt Therapy: Excitement and Growth in the Human Personality.* This book is regarded as the seminal work on Gestalt therapy theory and practice to this day.

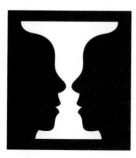

Figure 7.1 A Classic Gestalt Psychology Figure/Ground Image

Early Development of the Approach

As Fritz and Laura Perls developed their new approach, they stepped away from the central concepts of psychoanalysis and its emphasis on structure—the internal mechanisms that influence, or drive, behavior (e.g., ego, id, superego), and the past. In contrast, Gestalt therapy emphasizes **process**—the way in which an individual experiences and interacts with the environment and the present moment. Gestalt therapy is **holistic** in that all aspects of an individual's experience are regarded as equally important and connect to form an organismic whole. The organism/individual is always being impacted by (and is always impacting upon) the environment or, as Fritz called it, the *environmental field*.

In the 1930s and early 1940s, there were only two major psychological schools of thought, psychoanalysis and behaviorism. The former emphasized the individual, the latter emphasized the environment, and both paid little to no attention to the ever-present interaction between the individual and the environmental field. Gestalt therapy was a pioneering approach that required attention to the whole and the parts, the individual and the environment. Borrowing from Gestalt psychology, Fritz and Laura Perls employed the concept of figure and ground to explain how humans strive to maintain their psychological well-being. As with all organisms, humans have the natural capacity for **organismic self-regulation** (OSR), that is, attending to one's most pressing needs and maintaining one's sense of well-being by interacting purposefully with one's environment. Fritz and Laura extended the OSR concept to include the process by which one maintains a sense of *emotional* well-being by attending to the most salient *psychological* need or interest at a particular moment and initiating some interaction with the environment to satisfy that need. The psychological problems that become the focus of therapy were defined by Fritz and Laura as *disturbances* in this process of self-regulation.

Evolution of the Approach to the Present

The 1950s and 1960s were critical years in the evolution of Gestalt therapy. It was during those decades that the approach moved from Laura Perls's living room in New York City (the first Gestalt therapy institute) and emerged as a well-known and popular psychotherapy orientation. Smith (1970) noted that Gestalt therapy was listed as the sixth most common affiliation in the directory of the American Academy of Psychotherapists. This rapid expansion of Gestalt therapy during that era is traced primarily to the efforts of Fritz Perls, efforts that have had far-reaching positive and negative ramifications upon how Gestalt therapy is regarded to this day.

A significant amount of diversity existed among the early framers of Gestalt therapy. The majority of the New York group, including Laura Perls, appreciated the complexity and richness of the theory they were articulating. In early meetings of this group, members discussed and refined the theory while practicing the approach among themselves. Fritz was a man of action, not of words. He grew impatient with the pace and intellectual focus of the New York group. Several members of that original group have reported that Fritz also became jealous of the attention centered on his wife. Fritz was never one to be in the background. He liked to be running the show or directing others. In 1956, Fritz left New York, his wife, and his two children, and set off on a course that ultimately put Gestalt therapy on the map of prominently known and practiced counseling approaches.

After leaving New York, Fritz spent significant amounts of time in Ohio, Florida, California, and Canada. His bombastic, theatrical style attracted a large following, and he became the face of Gestalt therapy, known for his demonstration workshops, and his paperback books (popular literature more easily read than the original works). Because of his proclivities to action and excitement, he was not a disciplined or cohesive writer, and as a result, large portions of these paperback books are simply transcripts of his workshops. However, his brilliance as a therapist and demonstrator of Gestalt therapy eclipsed his shortcomings as a writer and a reflective theoretician. In these demonstrations, he was a master at quickly cutting through the layers of formality and pretense and moving his clients into intense and meaningful pieces of therapy, often in a matter of minutes.

Unfortunately, Fritz popularized Gestalt therapy with a particular spin or skew. Yontef (1993) refers to it as the "boom-boom-boom" style, which was characterized by confrontation, provocative techniques, and pressure for catharsis and quick change. The following excerpt is part of a transcripted session recorded in the late 1960s (Perls, 1969) and is a good example of this provocative style.

C (Client): I want to get . . .

Fritz: "I want"; get out of this seat. You want. I don't want any wanters. There are two great lies: "I want" and "I try."

C: I am fat . . . this is my existence [Whimpering.]. I don't like it and yet I like it. And I constantly bug me with this fact. And this is always with me and I'm tired of crying about it. Do you want me to get off this seat?

Fritz: No.

C: Don't you want me to get off the seat?

Fritz: No. I neither want you to get off nor do I not want you to get off.

> C: Are you going to sit here, Claire, or try to do something about what you are doing? You just want to sit here and stay fat.
>
> Fritz: OK now . . . I think I told you previously my diagnosis.
>
> C: That I'm empty.
>
> Fritz: No. This I find often in fat women, they have no ego boundaries. They don't have a self. They always live through other people and other people become themselves. (pp. 245–246)

In this vignette, Fritz displays a detached, seemingly insensitive style of working with this client. He criticizes her for her language ("I want"), refuses to help her make a decision about staying in the seat to work with him, and diagnoses her as lacking ego boundaries and self because she is a fat woman.

This is the style of Gestalt therapy that has prompted contemporary proponents of culturally sensitive and competent counseling to reject the Gestalt approach. In retrospect, this unconventional and detached style was a product of both the times and the man. The times were the 1960s, and the United States was in the midst of a decade of intense political and social turmoil. It was fashionable to "turn on" and "tune out" anything related to rules, authority, and the establishment.

Fritz Perls spent much of the 1960s in California (1964–1968) at the Esalen Institute and was cast in the role of the aging guru-hippie with his beard and slogans like "Lose your mind and come to your senses" and "You do your thing and I will do mine." Fritz was passionately self-reliant and demanded the same from his patients. He would frustrate or criticize anyone's attempt to gain his (or others') support or favor. He preferred directing others rather than connecting with them, and he directed others by using a set of standard techniques (a **technique** is a standard operating procedure used by a counselor to achieve a particular outcome when certain conditions are present). Two of his favorite techniques were the **top dog–underdog dialogue,** in which unintegrated parts of the individual talk to each other, and the **empty chair,** which allows the client to imagine talking to another who is not present. Laura said that Fritz had always wanted to become a director (he had studied theater in Germany before medical school) and

> that is what he fell back on, in the end. And that is when all the films of him were made. Unfortunately, people think that this is all there is to be done . . . the hot seat and the empty chair. Yet this is just a way in which he could keep himself from getting involved. (Shepard, 1975, p. 73)

Table 7.1 summarizes those aspects of Gestalt therapy theory that were emphasized in Fritz's style of practice and those aspects of the theory that were lost.

Despite the fact that Gestalt therapy continues to be described in many textbooks in terms of the way Fritz demonstrated it in the 1960s, the approach

Table 7.1 Gestalt Therapy as Practiced by Fritz Perls

Emphasized	*Lost*
Individual and intrapersonal conflict	Attention to the interpersonal and environmental field
Independence and self-support	That the fundamental nature of the individual's relationship with the environment is interdependence
Here and now	An interest in and sensitivity to an individual's developmental history, which is part of the background influencing present experience
Techniques	Experiments that are one of a kind because they emerge from unique moments of contact between client and therapist that cannot be repeated
Confrontation	Dialogue or a willingness by the therapist to confirm and validate the client's experience

has emerged from that era and has continued to evolve to reflect the whole of its theory and method. In addition, Gestalt therapy has been able to flex with the changing times and the widening range of clients seen. The Gestalt therapy of today attends to individuals and the environments they inhabit as well as to the contacting processes that occur as individuals interact with their environments. Instead of Fritz's techniques, modern Gestalt therapists engage clients in cooperative dialogue and improvised, one-of-a-kind experiments, which I will expand upon in a later section.

The Evolution of Gestalt Therapy for a Diverse World

Fritz's 1960s style of Gestalt therapy fit a particular demographic of those times. It appealed to a counterculture and individuals ready to cast off the constraints of counseling approaches that were more intellectual, plodding, and academic. After his death in 1970, Fritz's flamboyant style gradually gave way to the more balanced practice of Gestalt therapy that involved attention to awareness, to interpersonal contact, and to the families, communities, and organizations that individuals are an intricate part of and co-create. As Gestalt therapy has evolved and been refined since the late 1970s through writing, practice, and research, two concurrent developments have had a significant influence on the approach.

First, psychotherapy and counseling approaches have become increasingly sophisticated and tied to research and outcome measures. Approaches that were prominent in the 1970s and that occupied space in books like this one (e.g., Jungian analysis and transactional analysis) have been replaced by others (e.g., cognitive-behavioral therapy), which claim to be empirically supported and/or "proven" effective with certain populations and clusters of symptoms.

Second, counseling approaches must accommodate an increasing range of diversity to effectively and sensitively assist clients. As a practicing counselor in the 1970s, I found that most of my clients were a mirror reflecting my own White, straight, physically able image. Times have changed dramatically. Clients and counselors today are less likely to have that mirror between them and more likely to be different from one another in terms of race, ethnicity, sexual orientation, social and economic status, and other factors. These differences call for, actually demand, therapy approaches that can respond to the changing demographics and field conditions.

Context Then—Context Now

It is a legitimate question to ask how the basic tenets of a counseling approach developed by theorists many years ago apply to the contemporary practice of counseling and psychotherapy. Gestalt therapy is a product of an era past. It was created by two theorists who lived in a particular context and were influenced by the worldviews that were commonly held at that time. How can we be sure that the theory and practice of Gestalt therapy has any relevance and value to clients today who are from a wide range of cultural heritages and who have been influenced by very different worldviews? This very critical question is addressed throughout the chapter. At this point, however, some introductory discussion of the context and worldviews of Gestalt therapy, then and now, is fitting.

The theory of Gestalt therapy was crafted as a conscious rejection of the dominant political and psychological worldviews that existed in Germany in the 1930s: fascism and orthodox psychoanalysis. Fritz and Laura Perls were Jewish, and both were active in the anti-fascist movement in Germany in the early 1930s. In 1932, they began to sleep at the homes of friends because their peers and colleagues were being arrested. In 1933, Fritz was listed as a "political opponent" of the fascist regime. In April 1933, Fritz, Laura, and their 2-year-old daughter went into exile, crossing the border (with 100 marks smuggled out in Fritz's cigarette lighter) into Holland.

This experience of being in the minority, being discriminated against, and being oppressed influenced the shape of Gestalt therapy in a very profound way. A fundamental tenet in Gestalt therapy is that individuals and the environments that surround them co-exist in a process of reciprocal influence, each impacting on the other. This principle of reciprocal influence is a rejection of the fascist notion of the individual's adjusting to the majority view of a culture or the view of those in power.

Gestalt therapy was conceptualized as a radical revision of the dominant psychotherapy of the time, psychoanalysis. Emphasis on the therapeutic value of insight was replaced by attention to awareness and the quality of contact with the environment. Focus on the past shifted to attention to the present moment, paralleling such an emphasis in Buddhism and other Eastern traditions. The preeminence of sexuality in psychoanalytic theory was supplanted by an approach that incorporated all aspects of the individual as critical to psychotherapy, including the mind, body, feelings, and spirit. Finally, psychoanalytic drive theory was replaced by a theory that focused on the relationship between the individual and the environment.

The starting point of modern Gestalt therapy theory and practice is the notion that individuals are inextricably part of an environmental field and that to fully understand and assist clients, Gestalt therapists must see each individual as part of a complex matrix of interrelationships, both present and past. Clients experience themselves, more or less, as spiritual, emotional, intellectual, sexual, and physical beings, and their sense of "self" is to some degree fluid and malleable. Gestalt therapy has adopted and expanded upon a biological process that can be observed in infants and children across all cultures. Human beings are born with the innate facility to realize what aspects of self-experience are most salient, and then act and behave in ways to bring these wants, needs, or interests to the attention of their immediate environment. Gestalt therapy also recognizes the thousands of variations that occur within and across cultures that mold and shape the destiny of this natural process of recognizing needs and interests. Gestalt therapy embraces the perspective that there is no objective reality. Rather, it posits that clients have perceptions about the meaning of their experience that must be understood and validated. Finally, Gestalt therapists do not see themselves as the architects of change. Instead, change occurs naturally within clients (not by the hand of the therapist) when sufficient attention is paid to present circumstances, self, environmental support, and readiness.

It is beyond the scope of this chapter to examine the match between these basic tenets and the worldviews of all the different cultural groups you will encounter in your career as a professional counselor. Such an analysis would also require the suspension of a culturally relative (emic) perspective and the adoption of a universal (etic) perspective that there is a commonality of worldviews within particular cultures.

A culturally relative perspective would suggest that individual clients within specific cultural groups seeking counseling will bring a variety of worldviews that may or may not be compatible with the constructs of Gestalt therapy. Gestalt therapy would fit the worldview of clients who view themselves as part of a larger context, including family of origin, community, culture, and current primary relationships. It would fit well with clients who place value on various aspects of their self-experience including thoughts, feelings, and spirituality. Additionally, it would fit well with clients who, over time, come to appreciate that their perceptions of reality and the meanings they ascribe to the events of their lives have validity and value. Finally, with its attention to the relationship between self and environment(s), it would be a good match with clients who are struggling with their sense of self and belonging because they have recently moved to the United States or are alienated by their identification as a minority.

In Gestalt therapy, therapists do not know better than their clients, do not interpret the true meaning of a client's experience, do not dismiss the physical and spiritual as irrelevant to the counseling process, do not conceive of symptoms or mental distress as pathological or abnormal, and do not see themselves as knowing what changes clients must make. Gestalt therapists do not consider clients resistant if they do not talk, are not comfortable with self-disclosure, or do not follow directions.

It is important to note in concluding this section that the worldviews and values of clients are formed not only by culture, but also by a range of factors including religion, gender, social class, and sexual orientation. These worldviews unfold over the course of a counseling relationship and interface with those of the counselor and the fundamental tenets of his or her chosen orientation.

The Author's Journey as a Gestalt Therapist

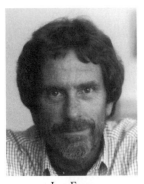
Jon Frew

Every aspiring counselor sets off on a voyage in search of the "right" orientation, the approach that suits her or his values and philosophical beliefs about the nature of the individual (e.g., good, evil, neutral), the most important aspects of the individual (e.g., thoughts, feelings, behavior, dreams, relationships), and how individuals change.

I was on such a journey when I first encountered Gestalt therapy. The year was 1972, and I was beginning a master's degree counseling training program. I quickly identified myself with the existential school of counseling, despite the fact that I vividly remember having absolutely no idea what being an existential therapist actually meant. I had avidly read many existential authors in the late 1960s, including Sartre and Camus, so when I entered counseling training and discovered that existentialism was a counseling approach, it was natural to adopt it as my own. The difficulty I was having at that time was how to translate a very appealing philosophical system into what you do when you sit down to counsel someone.

One of my professors at that time prompted me to look into Gestalt therapy. He described it as a hybrid, part psychoanalytic and part existential-humanistic. So I read a chapter on Gestalt therapy in a theories book and watched a video of Fritz Perls, Carl Rogers, and Albert Ellis demonstrating their respective counseling approaches with a client who identified herself as Gloria. My reaction was something like, "Gestalt therapy is a very powerful and dynamic approach but clearly not for me." I recognized that Fritz (even by Gloria's admission) was the more potent therapist in those tapes, but I was more drawn to Carl Rogers's grandfatherly ways. I couldn't imagine practicing counseling in the "in your face, twinkle in my wise eyes, charismatic" way Fritz did. So my uncharted voyage continued in existential-humanistic waters.

In 1975, having completed my master's degree, a colleague invited me to travel with him to Ohio, to the Gestalt Institute of Cleveland to participate in a weekend-long introductory workshop. The purpose of those workshops was to demonstrate the theory and practice of Gestalt therapy through personal growth groups. I entered my group somewhat skeptically, on the lookout for hot seats and empty chairs, and left three days later as a convert, realizing my journey had finally ended. The Gestalt therapist who led my group bore little resemblance, physically and stylistically, to Fritz. I marveled at his confident presence, his skill level, and his sensitivity to the "other" that I had not previously seen as a part of the Gestalt approach. He did individual therapy work with group members without using standardized Fritz Perls techniques. He facilitated the resolution of interpersonal issues that arose throughout the weekend, and he attended to our group's development.

I left that workshop energized and curious about what I had previously missed about Gestalt therapy. I spent the next seven years reading everything I could find about Gestalt therapy and participating in intensive training to become a Gestalt therapist, training that involved my own therapy with two senior Gestalt therapists. That training and the subsequent years I have spent as a Gestalt therapist and trainer have allowed me to grasp the essence of the theory and practice and to put Fritz into the contemporary context I discussed in the last section.

What appealed to me then and what appeals to me now about Gestalt therapy is the same. Gestalt therapy is a theoretical system that embraces health, not pathology. We do not see our clients as sick, neurotic, or engaging in maladaptive behaviors. Rather, we view every individual as having the capacity to self-regulate and find the best possible solutions to the environmental challenges life offers. We all make accommodations as children (e.g., learning not to cry around a shaming and critical caregiver) that can rigidify, be lost to awareness, and carry into adulthood when they are no longer as necessary in the current context.

(continued)

I have the distinct privilege as a Gestalt therapist to enter into relationships with my clients having no preset agenda in mind other than a genuine desire to support my clients in a process of attending to their awareness (or lack thereof) and how they attempt (or don't attempt) to get needs met in their current environment. As clients regain awarenesses that were lost earlier in their lives and begin to venture into the environment to satisfy their needs, they begin to live more fully in the present field conditions. It is not my job to get them to do anything or to impose upon them my—or the dominant culture's—values and goals. Gestalt therapy is not an adjustment therapy. As a Gestalt therapist with thousands of hours of experience, I have faith that when the logjam of childhood accommodations on the river is cleared, the water will flow again and the water will flow in a direction neither I or my client can predict ahead of time.

I have been trained and train others in a method central to Gestalt therapy called **phenomenological inquiry.** This approach to entering and participating in relationships with my clients has served me very well as I find my clients increasingly to be presenting with life circumstances substantially different than mine. Phenomenological inquiry is a method of both assessment and intervention and is defined as understanding and assisting our clients by encouraging them to describe their experience and the meanings they ascribe to those experiences. The counselor suspends any preconceptions about the meaning or importance of aspects of what clients present and inquires about those meanings without imposing value or diagnosis. Phenomenological inquiry requires an attitude of curiosity, an emphasis on description of experience (not interpretation), and giving up on any notion that I know more about my clients than they do.

In a recent first session with a Laotian woman who had been in the United States for three years, it was clear that we shared almost no life experience. After listening to her description of the feelings, thoughts, and behaviors that were troubling her, I continued my phenomenological inquiry, asking her what meaning she would ascribe to those feelings, thoughts, and behaviors. She hesitated, then told me that my meaning would take precedence over hers because I was older and a male. My phenomenological posture was not what she expected or required at that moment, given her experience of culture, gender, and age. I suggested a compromise. She would tell me what her perspective was on the issues that brought her to counseling first. I would then tell her my perspective and how those issues are usually seen and interpreted in the dominant culture. It was a good beginning.

This vignette illustrates that an approach like phenomenological inquiry, key to Gestalt therapy, may need to be modified to satisfy the most pressing requirements of a counseling relationship at any moment and to flex with the diversity issues inherent in those moments.

Theory of Gestalt Therapy

The theory of Gestalt therapy is built around a fundamental premise that individuals are complex mixes of ingredients that are being continuously impacted by the environments into which those individuals are born, develop, mature, age, and lead their lives. This complex mix includes a genetic history, emotions, spirituality, thoughts, creativity, sexuality, and behaviors. These diverse strands are unique to each person and form a whole that may be called the *self*. In many counseling orientations, particular aspects of the self take precedence over others and are viewed as key to the conceptualization of an individual's distress. In cognitive therapy, for example, irrational beliefs are viewed as leading to anxiety or sadness. In Gestalt therapy, all aspects of an individual's experience are seen as interrelated. No one aspect is viewed as more important than another. The Gestalt therapist attends to a client's feelings or thoughts or dreams or behaviors as they become figural or move into the foreground for the client.

This conceptualization of the interrelationship of all the aspects of self-experience without an externally imposed hierarchy of which aspects are most critical, lends itself well to working with clients in a world of diversity. Clients may lead with their thoughts, feeling, or troublesome behaviors. The Gestalt therapist enters into the client's house through whatever door is provided and is confident that other rooms in the house will eventually become part of the therapy focus.

In the Gestalt view, each individual is in an ongoing relationship with the environment. There is no self that exists and can be defined that is separate from the environment. The interrelationship between the self and environment is vital for survival on a biological and social level. The starting point of the Gestalt approach is the observation and quest for understanding of that ongoing relationship between the individual and the environment. Figure 7.2 illustrates these relationships between parts of the self and between the self and the environment. These concentric circles can be drawn in several ways to include a variety of germane aspects of the self and the environments that influence the self. The lines between sections are fluid and permeable, not fixed boundaries.

The following section outlines and defines the essential theoretical concepts of Gestalt therapy, with brief case examples inserted periodically to illustrate how these concepts come to life in counseling sessions. The section begins with a review of the three philosophical foundations that permeate and underpin the approach (field therapy, phenomenology, and dialogue) and then further theoretical concepts important in Gestalt therapy are discussed.

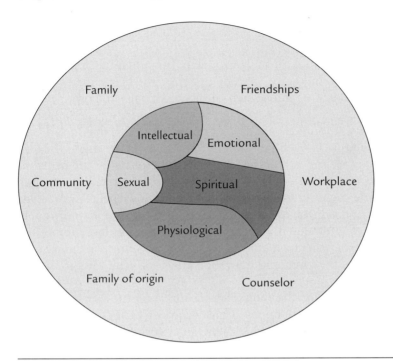

Figure 7.2 Interrelationship Between the Self and the Environment

Philosophical Foundations

Very little is new and original in Gestalt therapy. Rather, Fritz and Laura Perls, along with Paul Goodman and others, borrowed liberally from other disciplines and principles that were part of the environments that influenced them. The three philosophical foundations of Gestalt therapy—field theory, phenomenology, and dialogue—are good examples of this cross-fertilization process.

Field Theory

Field theory originated in the world of physics and was later translated into social psychology and personality theory by Kurt Lewin (1951). Simply put, the **field** is a dynamic interrelated system of relationships, each part of which influences every other part. Current concerns about global warming are a testimony to field theory, as countries around the world are beginning to recognize that regardless of where it originates, the emission of greenhouse gasses into the atmosphere is causing climate change all over the world. No country can exist in isolation from others, and no individual exists in isolation from others. The *field conditions* or contexts, both present and past, are intrinsically woven into the clients whom Gestalt therapists see. Pertinent field conditions that must be considered in a counseling process include (but are not limited to) socioeconomic status, culture, race, and ethnicity—and level of acculturation, if the client has immigrated to the United States. The therapeutic relationship itself is a co-created field, and the counselor is a prominent part of that field. The counselor's goal is to develop a therapeutic environment that will support the client's change process.

Phenomenology

Phenomenology, the second philosophical foundation of Gestalt therapy, was adopted from the writing and work of Martin Heidegger (1962). Phenomenology can be defined as the description of data available to the senses, what is given and evident in any immediate experience. Applied to a counseling approach, it refers to a method of inquiry and a system by which meaning is derived. Gestalt therapists endeavor to suspend any preconceived notions about the client (e.g., my client is elderly and therefore will not be physically active). Rather, they seek to understand the client's experience from the client's perspective. Phenomenological inquiry promotes the description rather than the explanation or interpretation of experience. The counselor says, "I see a tear in your eye," not "You are sad." Only our clients know what their tears mean at any particular moment in a counseling session. Practicing counseling phenomenologically minimizes the error of imposing meaning (a particularly egregious error when seeing non-majority individuals) on the client or conveying that the counselor is the expert. Hearing voices could be a sign of a psychotic process and be subjectively very alarming to a European American seeking counseling. Hearing voices could be a sign of spiritual enlightenment and be perceived as a gift by a Navajo American seeking counseling. Practicing counseling from a phenomenological stance ensures that what is real is determined in the relationship between the observed and the observer, not by an objective standard.

Dialogue

Dialogue, the third philosophical foundation, is the basis of the client-therapist relationship in Gestalt therapy. Dialogue in this context has a particular definition, which was adapted from the work of Martin Buber (1970). Dialogue is a term that describes a relationship between two individuals that alternates between moments of *I-It* relating and *I-Thou* relating. The vast majority of our interactions are in the I-It mode, which involves intentions, task completion, goals, and doing business. For instance, I am in line at the grocery store in a rush to pay for my items and go home. I barely notice the clerk who is assisting me, and she barely notices me. The clerk and I are an I-It moment. I-Thou moments are characterized by presence, no agenda or trying to get somewhere, and a profound sense of connection with the other. In these moments of connection, our sense of self recedes and is replaced by the experience of "we" or I-Thou. Back at the grocery store, the clerk's boss approaches and criticizes her in my presence for taking a long break earlier in the day. When the boss walks away, she and I make eye contact. Time is irrelevant, and there is a palpable connection between us as I smile warmly and she tries to hold back tears. Our I-It relationship was transformed into a few moments of I-Thou. Buber believed that to be "fully human" each individual must have these I-Thou experiences, at least occasionally. Maurice Freidman (1985), who has written about how Buber's work on dialogue has been incorporated by several counseling orientations, has coined the phrase, "healing through meeting."

Laura Perls studied with Buber, and it was Laura, not Fritz, who brought the concept of dialogue to Gestalt therapy through her teaching and demonstrations. Gestalt therapists recognize the therapeutic and healing quality of the relationship, which itself becomes the vehicle for and complements the methods and particular interventions used in a counseling relationship. Following several of Buber's leads, the Gestalt therapist attempts to be fully present (suspending any desire to be seen in any particular way by the client), to experience the relationship as much as possible from the client's perspective, and to confirm the validity of the client's experience. A dialogic approach to counseling tends to eliminate or reduce the traditional vertical hierarchy of counselor above client (e.g., counselor as teacher or expert and client as student or novice) that is present in most counseling orientations, and it blends well with the phenomenological approach.

Theoretical Concepts

Gestalt therapy theory needed to be enriched by concepts that could account for the more sophisticated processes that take place as individuals participate in their inseparable relationships with the environment. The concepts developed by Fritz and Laura included organismic self-regulation, figure formation and destruction, awareness, contact, cycle of awareness and contact, and creative adjustment.

Organismic Self-Regulation

Returning to the term *organismic self-regulation* introduced earlier in the chapter, Gestalt therapy theory is rooted in the proposition that humans, like all organisms, are inherently self-regulating. We seek to maintain ourselves in a state of equilibrium, an overall sense of well-being. When our equilibrium is disrupted, we can identify what we need or want to restore equilibrium and move into the environment to get it. If we are cold, we turn up the heat. If we are frightened, we bolt the door. If we wake up hungry in the middle of the night, we go to the kitchen and rustle up a midnight snack. Think of the infant who cries out to the parent or caregiver. Even at that early age, the infant is aware that something is required to restore equilibrium. Unable to navigate to the kitchen on his own, the infant lets the world know that he is hungry by crying. The only missing component is language, so the caregivers engage in a trial-and-error method (is it hunger, pain, discomfort?) to soothe the child. In short, this capacity to self-regulate comes with the original equipment.

Organismic self-regulation, strictly speaking, is a biological concept and does not comprehensively describe the experience of being human: "I notice I am hungry. I eat. I am no longer hungry" or "I notice I am tired. I sleep. I awake refreshed." The issues and struggles of clients typically transcend the biological and involve social and emotional processes. Their goals and reasons for seeking counseling often go beyond settling for equilibrium and a return to the status quo. They talk to their counselors about a desire to succeed, to grow and to make a difference in their interactions with others (although in some cultures or situations clients may be trying to "fit in" or not stand out).

The principle of organismic self-regulation has profound implications for the practice of Gestalt therapy and drives all the theoretical concepts to be defined next.

Figure Formation and Destruction

According to the Gestalt psychologists of the early 20th century, individuals perceive and organize the environment by focusing on one aspect of the environment at a time. As discussed earlier in this chapter, Gestalt psychologists call the object of focus the *figure*, and everything else becomes the *background* or *ground*. To the midnight snacker with a yen for leftover turkey, the refrigerator is the focus, or the figure, and everything else in the kitchen is ground. If midway through the kitchen the snacker changes her mind and decides to have something sweet, the bowl of apples on the counter becomes the figure and the refrigerator melts away into the background.

Gestalt therapy has extended the **figure formation and destruction** concept beyond visual perception. For the purposes of counseling and psychotherapy, figure formation and destruction is defined as an ongoing process in which individuals become aware of a need or interest and make contact with some aspect of the environment in a way that satisfies or "destroys" that figure, allowing it to recede to the background. This process is typically conceptualized as an inside-out set of phases. First, some aspect of the individual's internal experience becomes figural. This figure represents a need or interest and becomes salient to the individual. As the figure is sharpened or clarified, the individual begins to look out toward the environment, and at that point, certain aspects of the environment related to the need or interest will stand out from the background. An action is taken, and if the need is satisfied, it recedes to the background, making way for a new figure to emerge.

To put this concept into a therapy context, an African-American client sits with a European-American counselor in a first session. The counselor is asking the client a series of questions. The client becomes aware of a pressing need to ask his own question and a growing lack of interest in answering the counselor's. The client interrupts the counselor and says, "I need to know if you have ever worked with an African-American client?" Depending on how the counselor answers the question, the sensitivity expressed in the answer, and what transpires next, that figure of interest may or may not be satisfied. When a figure of interest is pursued and fully satisfied, the client experiences a sense of **closure,** defined as the end point of a figure formation and destruction process. If the figure or need is not completely satisfied, it will linger in the form of rumination, regret, resentment, and unfinished business.

Awareness and the Present Moment

Human beings have the unique capacity to look ahead to the future and look back to past experience. We are also capable of attending to the present moment primarily through our senses. Gestalt therapy recognizes that individuals alternate between these time frames and that certain cultures (see, for example, Kluckhohn & Strodtbeck, 1961) place more or less emphasis on the past, present, or future. The needs, wants, and interests that activate a figure formation process reside in the present. The way present experience is accessed is through awareness.

Awareness is defined as the process of directing your attention to the most salient aspect of the individual/environmental field at the present moment. Healthy functioning requires both awareness of self and awareness of environment. For instance, as I am writing these words I am mostly in my head, not very present. I take a moment and direct my awareness to my physical well-being. I notice that my lower back is stiff. I get up and take a short walk around the courtyard where I am writing. I do a few stretches. My back feels better, and I return to the task at hand. Alternatively, I might notice my stiff back and decide to ignore it, feeling the press of a coming deadline. That short-run gain could lead to long-term pain, when my sore back keeps me up all night and I am too tired to write the next day. Awareness is a powerful concept in Gestalt therapy. It is a necessary but not always sufficient condition for growth and change. It is the primary goal for counseling but not the only one. It is often where Gestalt therapists begin with their clients in each session.

Contact

Another goal of Gestalt therapy is the restoration of **contact** functions that translate the individual's awarenesses into attempts to connect with aspects of the environment in a meaningful way. As noted earlier, infants have no difficulty making contact with their caregivers when they become aware of a need or discomfort. But as we mature, we tend to become less aware of our needs, and even when aware, we may be less able to satisfy our needs. The loss of awareness and contact functions is further discussed in the section on *creative adjustment*. At this point, suffice it to say that in Gestalt therapy theory, contact functions must be restored because they are part of the original equipment.

Contact itself is defined as a "behavior that establishes a relationship with the figure of interest" (Yontef, 1993, p. 207). Technically, we can make contact with an aspect of ourselves (e.g., scratching an itch or recalling a happy memory), but generally speaking, contact refers to the experience of connection with something outside the self, something that is different. Contact is not a steady state. Instead, the process of contacting always involves connecting and separating or contact and withdrawal. The byproduct of contact, if it is informed by awareness and connection with the forming figure of interest, is **assimilation** and growth. Assimilation in the context of Gestalt therapy theory is a subjective experience of being different or changed as a result of contact.

Cycle of Awareness and Contact

Over the years, the concept of figure formation and destruction has been refined by the development of a model and a set of terms that describe the ongoing process of self-regulation or individual-environment interaction with more specificity. The model has been called the cycle of experience or the **cycle of awareness and contact** (Figure 7.3) and was developed by the faculty at the Gestalt Institute of Cleveland.

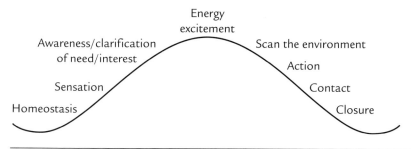

Figure 7.3 The Cycle of Awareness and Contact

The steps outlined in the cycle usually go very smoothly. In fact, we all move through variations of this process many times each day. Imagine that you are sitting on a bench in the park on a beautiful summer afternoon enjoying the sunshine (homeostasis). Your enjoyment is interrupted by a slight flutter in your chest (sensation). You attend to the sensation and identify it as anxiety and realize that you forgot to meet your best friend for lunch two hours ago (awareness and clarification of figure). Wanting to do something to resolve the situation, you get up and begin to pace back and forth (energy and excitement). You decide to call your friend and look around for the nearest pay phone (scan the environment). Spotting a phone by the bus stop, you jog in that direction (action). You call your friend and apologize (contact). She tells you not to worry; you reschedule for tomorrow. Your anxiety dissipates (closure). Other cycles of awareness and contact get derailed and interrupted along the way, and these interruptions become the subject of counseling and psychotherapy.

The concept of the cycle of awareness and contact can be further illuminated via a case study: Martha, a 30-year-old woman, sought counseling after being disowned by her father when she came out to her parents about a lesbian relationship with her partner, whom her parents thought was a friend. At the beginning of a session, her counselor, John, let a few seconds of silence go by, then asked, "At this moment, what are you aware of?" At first Martha replied that she felt fine and nothing was coming into her awareness (homeostasis). Then she noted a clenching of her right fist and a vague sense of tightness in her throat (sensation). Staying with the sensations for several minutes led Martha to realize that she was angry with her father (awareness and clarification of figure). She felt both energized and anxious about doing something with her anger (energy and excitement). She looked out to John (scan the environment), who proposed an experiment: that she express her anger at John, imagining he was her father. Martha liked the idea and began to speak to John about her feelings of anger and resentment (action). After several minutes of expressing her anger, her affect suddenly softened, and she said, "I am angry as hell and I really miss you" (contact). The experiment ended on this note, and Martha no longer experienced the tightness in her fist and throat (closure).

In this vignette, it became evident to John and to Martha that she had feelings about her father that had not been expressed. John assisted Martha in identifying those feelings and encouraged her to talk to her father, thereby creating an opportunity for contact.

Creative Adjustment

If we are all born with the facility to know what we want and need and to call out for it or take our own actions to get it, why would anyone have problems and seek counseling? The answer lies in one of the starting points of Gestalt therapy—field theory. The self is defined, at least partly, as the series of contacts individuals have with the environments into which they are born and raised. Children are embedded in a range of field conditions, and their needs are never completely, or adequately, addressed by their caregivers. Different parents and different customs across cultures have varying philosophies regarding the value of responding to a child's expressed needs. The 2-year-old who cries out to be comforted in the middle of the night may be held by one mother, ignored by another, or yelled at by yet another mother.

There is an innate wisdom in the organism. If a need cannot be met or is met by punishment or disdain, the need will eventually be lost to awareness. Far better to walk through the desert being unaware of your thirst than to be so preoccupied by it you lose all motivation to keep going. This response we all make to the conditions and nuances of our families of origin is called a **creative adjustment.** A creative adjustment is an accommodation made by an individual who is striking a balance between getting a need met and fitting into the dominant field conditions that have power and control over his or her well-being. Creative adjustments are solutions to problems we all face when the current environment cannot or will not respond to our need for contact. They can occur throughout the life span, but Gestalt therapists focus primarily on the ones that occur in childhood. In the United States, for example, the majority population holds certain stereotypes that sometimes fit our clients. Boys who were shamed or criticized when they cried or expressed fears may grow up to be men who have to be tough and who have little access to their tenderness. Conversely, girls who were criticized for being loud, aggressive, or angry may grow up to be women who have difficulty feeling strong and assertive. These prohibitions to feel or behave in certain ways exist in all families to some extent.

Children learn to restrict the awareness of certain feelings and attempts at contact with the environment in order to adjust to a set of field conditions they have no power to change. These creative adjustments are a healthy response to the environment. Unfortunately, these adjustments tend to become reified. Later, when the children become adults, the loss of awareness and contacting ability persists despite the fact that new, more "forgiving" field conditions may exist. Therefore, interruptions in the cycle of awareness and contact occur.

Practice of Gestalt Therapy

The basic tenet of Gestalt therapy is that individuals are in a continuous and complex co-created relationship with their environments. It is a relationship of mutual influence. Gestalt therapy posits that increased awareness of self and environment is generally a good thing and leads to contact with the environment that is satisfying and enhances growth and personal development. In this section, we consider how Gestalt therapy effects client change, then we look at the key components of Gestalt therapy practice.

Theory of Change

Arnold Beisser articulated the theory of change endorsed by Gestalt therapy in 1970. He called it the **paradoxical theory of change,** and it purports that change occurs by more fully experiencing what is, not by trying to get to what is not. Supporting clients to heighten their awareness of what they are experiencing inevitably results in a natural shift in that experience. That shift is an organic one that cannot be predicted and is not imposed by the counselor. A reasonable question might be, "But don't Gestalt therapists want their clients to feel better and have fewer symptoms?" The unequivocal answer is, "Yes, of course we do." We just have a different slant than most other therapeutic orientations have about how that happens. Consider the following example of Consuelo, a 40-year-old Latina, who presents with complaints about anxiety.

> C (Client): I need help getting rid of the anxiety I have been feeling ever since my son was born.

> T (Therapist): Are you experiencing that anxiety right now?

> C: Yes. Can you help make it go away?

> T: I'm not sure I can, but I will try. How are you experiencing your anxiety right now?

> C: I'm not sure what you mean.

> T: Tell me what is happening in your body or your mind that you are calling anxiety.

> C: I have worries that something awful will happen to my son. My stomach is upset and I feel dizzy.

> T: Okay, I'm getting it. I can see why you are so uncomfortable. Let's try something. Put your hands on your stomach and take a few deep breaths very slowly, imagining that the air you are breathing is moving right into your upset stomach.

[Client takes several deep breaths and immediately looks slightly calmer.]

> T: Consuelo, are you still thinking about the bad things that could happen to your son?

> C: Yes, and I don't know how to make the thoughts go away.

T: Would you be willing to tell me about those awful thoughts you want out of your mind?

C: I don't know . . . I have never said them out loud. I am afraid that if I do, they could actually occur.

T: No wonder you keep your fears to yourself, Consuelo.

C: Do you think it would help me to tell you about these thoughts?

T: I don't know for sure, but I have an idea about how to find out. Why don't you tell me one of those awful things and then we'll see how you feel afterwards?

C: Okay, I will try that. [Relates one of the catastrophic events she is worried about.]

T: I appreciate your willingness to tell me about one of the things you worry about. How are you doing?

C: Do you think I am crazy? Is it silly to have such thoughts?

T: I think you love your son so much you can't imagine living without him; that's not crazy. [Client is silent and appears to be much more relaxed and calm.] How is your anxiety now—at this moment?

C: Well, I am not worried about that one thing actually happening to my son, my stomach is calmer, I am not dizzy.

This case example illustrates the paradoxical theory of change and the power of awareness and contact. Consuelo wanted to get rid of her anxiety and her disturbing thoughts. The Gestalt therapist provided both the support and the means to stay with her awareness of both the physiological and cognitive components of her present experience. When the client attended to her upset stomach and took several deep breaths, she appeared to be slightly calmer. When she was able and ready to verbalize one of her awful fears (undoing a self-talk process), contact was made with the therapist, which led to the emergence of another figure of interest for Consuelo. Was she crazy and silly to have these thoughts? The Gestalt therapist's response to this question resulted, by the client's self-report, in a decrease in anxiety. Her disturbing thoughts, at least for that moment, were gone.

Components of Gestalt Therapy Practice

Gestalt therapists effect client change by helping to restore a client's awareness and increasing the quantity and quality of a client's contact with the environment and by illuminating contact boundary disturbances.

Restoring Awareness

To return to our midnight snacker example, awareness is turning on the kitchen light; contact is eating the apple and savoring every morsel of it. Unaware individuals live mostly in the dark. Their interactions with the environment and with other people are superficial and unsatisfying. As awareness is restored, the lights go on and the client sees him or herself more accurately at this moment and sees the contemporary environment with all its potential. The next step is for the client to move into contact in an attempt to derive satisfaction from the environment.

Increasing the Quantity and Quality of Contact

To help a client reach a healthy functioning stage, restoring awareness is a powerful and worthy goal. But, awareness of the environment is not enough—there must also be contact. In Gestalt terminology, increasing contact means being fully aware of the environment and the present moment, being fully engaged in interacting with the environment and the other people in it, and at the same time maintaining a complete awareness of one's own separate self. Contacting the environment requires energy and support, both internal and external. In therapy, internal support comes from within the client and involves simple activities like breathing more deeply or engaging in positive self-talk. External support comes from the counselor and others who are invested in expanding the client's quantity and quality of contact.

Contact is the lifeblood of growth and change (Polster & Polster, 1973). As a general rule, the more diversity or novelty in that which is contacted, the more change and growth will occur. I frequently pose this scenario to my classes: "You have the opportunity to travel by charter bus from Los Angeles to New York. When you arrive at the station, there are two buses to choose from. The first is populated by 40 people just like you in terms of gender, age, ethnicity, and so on. The second bus is bursting with diversity. People in that bus represent a full range of ages, cultures, and languages. Which bus would you take if you wanted to learn and be stretched the most over those three days?" I then remind them that the rapidly shifting demographics in the United States make it more and more likely that, as counselors, they will be working with clients who are on the second bus. The increased diversity lends itself well to enhanced contact possibilities in the counseling relationship.

Contact was defined earlier as a behavior that establishes a relationship with the figure of interest. It is the quality of this relationship that interests Gestalt therapists. Latner (1986) writes, "Good contact is being engaged fully in contacting, so that our absorption in what we are in touch with is thorough and satisfying" (p. 45). Gestalt therapists orient themselves with the belief that individuals are inclined toward growth and change. Good contact results in assimilation, which, as discussed earlier in the chapter, is the subjective experience that one is different or has changed in some way as a result of contact with the environment. When someone assimilates something they have contacted, that something becomes a part of them. I had a powerful moment of contact many years ago with one of my mentors who told me that the Golden Rule, "do unto others as you would have them do unto you," was invalid and possibly discriminatory in the context of working with clients of color. He pointed out the ethnocentric fallacy of the rule, which posits that all others are like us and would want to be treated in the same way. I have never forgotten that moment of contact and have incorporated what I learned from him into all the work I do as a therapist, teacher, and trainer.

Illuminating Contact Boundary Disturbances

In contact, the individual touches some aspect of the environment in a way that facilitates assimilation and growth. When contact occurs between an individual and the environment or another individual, the term used to describe the point of interface is the **contact boundary.** The contact boundary is not a physical location, but it is the meeting point between self and other. The contact boundary is much like the waterline that separates the ocean and the sand, constantly shifting, demarcating the difference between the entities in contact yet permeable, allowing movement across the boundary.

In healthy contact, an individual completes all the steps of the cycle of awareness and contact, which ends with taking action, making contact, and achieving closure. In Gestalt therapy, attention is also paid to disruptions in contact. Referring back to the cycle of awareness and contact, the individual has completed all the steps prior to contact, the last of which is moving into action. On the verge of contact, one of five disturbances can occur.

- **Introjection** is the "swallowing whole" of some aspect of the environment without discrimination. Typically the individual introjects an idea or a behavior. Introjection is a common form of contact in children learning family and cultural values. An example of an idea that might be introjected is that is it wrong to have positive feelings about gays and lesbians. Later the individual's assessment of gays and lesbians will be based on the introjected belief, not actual experience of individuals of those sexual orientations.

- **Projection** is the attribution of a part of the self to the environment such that it is experienced as existing in another, not in the self. If an individual has an introject that she should never be angry, she may project her own feelings of irritation with a colleague's behavior onto the colleague, believing that her co-worker is angry with her.

- **Retroflection** has two definitions. In the first, energy, emotions, and words necessary to make contact with another are cut off and redirected back (retro) toward the self. An example of this type of retroflection would be criticizing yourself when you would rather be criticizing your employer. The second form of retroflection is doing something for yourself rather than allowing someone to do it for you. If I was rubbing out the kinks in my sore neck in the presence of my massage therapist, I would be engaging in this second type of retroflection. Both forms involve doing to or for self rather than making contact with the environment.

- **Confluence** is the denial of any difference between self and environment, a subjective sense that there is no contact boundary. In a fleeting context, confluence is a natural state of intense connection with another (an I-Thou moment), which can occur in lovemaking or intense dialogue. In a chronic context, confluence deprives individuals of meaningful contact because they cannot tolerate the conflict and anxiety of acknowledging how they are different from others. An example would be the person who, when asked by a partner, can never assert the movie or restaurant he or she prefers, out of fear that this desire may be different from the partner's and would lead to conflict and abandonment.

- **Deflection** is the engagement of the environment in an indirect way that diffuses or dilutes the intensity of full-on contact. The many examples of deflection include speaking in the third person, overusing humor, diverting eye contact, and not getting to the point in conversation.

These five processes can be seen as interfering with contact, but it is more accurate to see introjection, projection, retroflection, confluence, and deflection as defining the quality of contact a client is accustomed to experiencing. A Gestalt therapist attempts to illuminate the boundary disturbances as they occur in the therapeutic relationship.

Two final points must be made about introjection, projection, retroflection, confluence, and deflection. First, all these ways of interacting with the environment can also be appropriate and healthy. Learning how to fly an airplane or how to play a musical instrument typically involves swallowing whole (introjecting) the instructions of the teacher. Novelists often project some aspect of themselves onto the characters in their books. Pounding your fist into your hand, not your infant's face, when he won't stop crying is a healthy retroflection. Confluence can be critical to team building or consensus decision making. Finally, humorous deflection may be useful in diffusing a potentially violent confrontation. The key here is that the individual be aware of and intentionally choose introjection, projection, retroflection, confluence, or deflection as the style of contact that best fits the present situation.

The second caveat is that the original conceptualization of these contact styles as disturbances was extremely culture bound. A contemporary Gestalt therapist would not automatically view a client's preferred mode of interacting with the environment as an interruption of contact unless that meaning was derived phenomenologically. For example, a Gestalt therapist would not label averted eye contact (deflection) as a contact boundary disturbance if the client experienced direct eye contact as invasive or a sign of disrespect.

The test of a psychotherapy theory is its versatility and ability to flex with the changing field conditions. Gestalt therapy theory was developed and refined in the United States more than 50 years ago. There have been profound changes in this country since then. One of those changes is the shift in population demographics, which is manifest in the clients counselors are seeing now and will see in the future. With its foundation in field theory and phenomenology, Gestalt therapy allows for a wide range of variations in the awareness and contact process, recognizing the many different experiences that have shaped clients.

The Experiment

Recall that when the client Consuelo asked if speaking her thoughts out loud would help her, the Gestalt therapist made no promises. Rather, the therapist suggested an "experiment" that would answer that question through experience, not through intellect. The **experiment** is defined as a method that shifts the focus of counseling from talking about a topic to an activity that will heighten the client's awareness and understanding through experience. Experiments can happen at any point in a counseling session but commonly are proposed by the Gestalt therapist at the action phase of the cycle of awareness and contact. The counselor and client have identified the figure or primary theme of that particular session, and the counselor might say, "I wonder if you would like to experiment or try something" related to that figure or theme.

The experiment is always one of a kind. Experiments emerge organically and seamlessly in the moment-to-moment contact between a counselor and a client, and they are discovered within that dialogic process. They cannot be replicated because those moments, which are made up of a particular content and set of processes, never occur more than once.

There are many, many types of experiments. In the last case example, Consuelo participated in an experiment when she did something she was afraid to do—say out loud one of the things she worried could happen to her son. What all experiments have in common is that they vitalize a counseling process by moving clients from talking about their ongoing experience of self and environment into performing an action that will heighten awareness or provide a platform to try out certain kinds of contact with the environment (including the counselor). A good experiment remains true to the figure of interest, maintains the energy and interest that has been generated up to that point in the counseling session, and creates an edge of excitement or anxiety in the client. This edge of excitement or anxiety should be a precursor to contact and change without being too much, too soon for the client to undertake. Experiments can be invented and designed either by the counselor or collaboratively by the counselor and the client. The counselor provides the environmental support required by the client to enact the experiment and then debriefs with the client at its completion to maximize the assimilation of the experience. Use of the experiment is demonstrated in the following case of Samuel, who sought out counseling as part of his rehabilitation from a serious automobile accident that left him paralyzed from the waist down. In this session, he was discussing his "confusion" about feedback he had received on several recent job interviews. He was told that he had a subtle "air of bitterness and negativity" that came across in his interpersonal communications. He did not get these jobs and was convinced that he was turned down because of his disability.

> C (Client): I just don't buy this garbage about my negativity. These employers were just looking for an excuse to not hire someone with a disability. [As the client talks about the series of failed interviews, his energy picks up.]
>
> T (Therapist): Samuel, what are you aware of as you are relating these stories to me?
>
> C: I'm not sure, I'm just depressed about my life in general and the bad breaks I've gotten.
>
> T: You don't look depressed. In fact, you look like you have some strong feelings coming up.
>
> C: I guess you're right. There are some feelings.
>
> T: Describe those feelings to me.
>
> C: Actually the feelings are connected to this one image that keeps coming into my head.
>
> T: Okay, imagine you are watching a movie I can't see. Tell me what is happening on the screen.
>
> C: I can't shake this memory. It was the first job I applied for after the accident. I was sure I was going to be hired. But this plant manager, I think his name was Dan, blew me away when he told me I didn't get the job. He seemed sincere when he gave me the feedback about my so-called bitterness—or as he said, the "chip on my shoulder." And then he abruptly ended the meeting and asked if I would mind showing myself out because

he was late for his lunchtime racquetball game. He jumped up, grabbed his gym bag, and literally trotted over to the door. As he left, he propped the door open and said if I needed any help getting to the parking lot to call out for his assistant.

T: Then what happened?

C: You know, I was dumbfounded . . . kind of in shock. I couldn't believe he did that.

T: Did what, exactly?

C: First he denies me a job, then he bounces to his feet and jogs out of the office, and then he assumes I might need help getting his damn door open.

T: Got it. What are you feeling now?

C: I am really pissed off.

T: At Dan?

C: At Dan and everyone else who has legs that work and who assume I am helpless.

T: You know I have legs that work and I just realized that I hold the door open for you every time you leave our sessions. What do you want to say to me about that?

C: It's not fair that you can use your legs and I can't.

T: Anything else?

C: Yes, when I leave today, I will open the door myself.

T: You're right, it isn't fair and from now on you let me know if you want my help with your chair or the door.

C: I appreciate your saying that.

In this case scenario, the bitterness and negativity that potential employers were picking up was out of Samuel's awareness. At first he expressed skepticism about the feedback. The first experiment was anchored in Samuel's description of the image of the end of the first job interview. The elaboration of the story sharpened for Samuel and the therapist the figure of interest, which was Samuel's anger about the insensitivity of others concerning their ablebodiedness and his perceived helplessness. The second experiment created an action Samuel could take, not with Dan, whom he will most likely never see again, but with the therapist. Through this action, Samuel was able to express some of his feelings in the here and now to the therapist. If that proposed experiment had seemed too difficult to Samuel, the therapist could have graded it down to "close your eyes and have a fantasy of telling me what you could say to me." If the therapist enacted the experiment through a fantasy, it would be important to ask Samuel to imagine what he thinks the therapist's reaction would be. In the actual experiment, the therapist gave him the reaction, which provided some closure to that cycle of awareness and contact.

There Is No Concept of Client Resistance in Gestalt Therapy

Another component of the practice of Gestalt therapy that distinguishes it from many other orientations is how Gestalt therapists address what is traditionally called "resistance." In fact, in Gestalt therapy there is no such thing as resistance. Resistance is commonly defined in counseling as an attribute ascribed to clients who are not doing what the therapist wants them to do. The client is labeled as resistant when she or he will not follow the counselor's lead.

Such an attribution is completely foreign to the theory and practice of Gestalt therapy. Rather, to a Gestalt therapist, a client who will not answer a question or participate in an experiment is engaging in a *self-regulating* behavior, a self-protecting behavior that for the moment makes the client feel safe and secure. In Gestalt therapy, saying "no" is often a sign of very healthy functioning. Because a Gestalt therapist is not trying to "get somewhere," a client's reluctance to do something is not viewed as an obstacle. It can be a gateway to increased awareness and understanding. Again, two brief case examples illustrate how a Gestalt therapist might work with what non-Gestalt therapists might call resistance. In the first case example, Devon was referred to the school counselor after an incident in which he punched another boy in the lunchroom.

T (Therapist): So Devon, tell me what happened.

C (Client): I don't think so and you can't make me say anything.

T: You look and sound very determined about keeping your story to yourself.

C: That's right.

T: What's your objection to telling me what happened?

C: Because, whenever I tell anybody my side of a story, nobody believes me.

T: And I will be another "anybody" who won't believe you.

C: That's how I figure it.

T: Makes sense to me. Whenever people don't believe me, I quit talking, too.

The Gestalt therapist stayed out of a power struggle with Devon by exploring why Devon didn't want to answer his question and ultimately supporting Devon's creative adjustment to protect himself from what he saw as another frustrating, invalidating episode.

In the second case example, Sara sought counseling at a college counseling center after several of her professors told her she wasn't speaking up enough in class. She had just moved to the United States from Israel.

> T (Therapist): Hi, Sara. I would like to begin by getting to know you better. Tell me about yourself.
>
> C (Client): My family lives on a kibbutz outside Tel Aviv. The kibbutz began in the 1960s and the community is strong and cohesive.
>
> T: You are introducing yourself by telling me about your family and community.
>
> C: I am not comfortable speaking only about myself or for myself.
>
> T: It must be difficult for you when your professors ask you to express opinions in class.

Sara did not answer the therapist's question in the way it was asked. Her response was consistent with her background and upbringing in a collectivist subculture, and it led quickly to the dilemma she was facing in an individually oriented university system. Interpreting her therapy response or classroom behavior as "resistant" would reflect an insensitive imposition of one set of cultural values over another.

The Client-Counselor Relationship

The client-counselor relationship is the heart and soul of Gestalt therapy. Discussions earlier in this chapter about dialogue, phenomenology, and field theory capture the fundamental and critical role the relationship plays in the theory and practice of Gestalt therapy. The client and counselor are partners in an endeavor that involves increasing awareness, identifying figures of interest, and restoring contacting functions.

All counseling approaches have two dimensions. The first is content. Content is the "what" of counseling: what is talked about, the stories that are told, and the symptoms and circumstances that are described. The second dimension is process. Process is the "how" of counseling: how the client presents the content (e.g., matter-of-factly, rapidly, haltingly), how the client feels as he or she tells the story, how the client perceives the counselor, how the counselor feels and perceives the client, and how the client and counselor relate to one another. The client-counselor relationship is one of the primary processes in counseling and it impacts upon all the others. A Gestalt therapist understands the inextricable relationship between process and content and tracks both very carefully in a counseling session.

Across cultures and individuals there are differences in the extent to which process or content is valued and incorporated into interpersonal relationships. Gestalt therapists have no agenda regarding the relative importance of one or the other. Rather, the task at hand is to develop a relationship with each client and in doing so to seek, using phenomenological inquiry, an understanding of how the client puts content and process together. Generally speaking, majority European-American clients in the United States tend to focus more on content. Process questions like "What's it like to tell me that story" or "Your energy level has picked up" may surprise, confuse and possibly irritate them. However, within the majority U.S. culture, women tend to be more aware of and comfortable with process than men. Clients from other growing minorities in the United States, including Latinos, African Americans, and Asian Americans, may present to counseling with more of a process orientation, but this varies widely within cultures and with different levels of acculturation.

Gestalt therapy embraces the inseparable yin and yang of process and content, but it is primarily a process-oriented counseling approach. The mechanism of change requires attention to awareness and to the quality and nuances of contact with the environment, both of which are processes. However, a counseling relationship cannot proceed without content, the story line that provides points of contact through which the counselor engages the client, exploring and pointing out—if appropriate and timely—the process that attends the content.

Given the rapidly changing demographics in the United States, the wide range of differences our clients embody, including their facility for content and process, how does a Gestalt therapist proceed with building the relationship that is so vital to the successful outcome of the counseling?

1. *Proceed phenomenologically.* Phenomenological inquiry and attitude is almost always key to building and maintaining therapeutic relationships. Suspend, as much as possible, preconceived notions and stereotypes about the clients you see. Enter their world and strive to understand from their perspective how they experience their lives, sorrows, triumphs, and relationships.

2. *Validate the client's experience.* So simple, yet so powerful, validating the client's experience can be healing in and of itself. Most of our clients have been told by people who matter to them things like "You don't really feel that way," or "You shouldn't feel that way," or "You have no right to have that reaction," or "You don't really want that." When a counselor responds to a client by making a statement that conveys that the counselor "gets it" (can feel

it or understand it from the client's side), the client is frequently stunned by this simple act of acceptance and validation. Buber (1967) called this "practicing inclusion," and it is often a necessary and sufficient field condition for therapeutic change.

3. *Foster dialogue with an eye toward diversity.* Buber's concept of dialogue is generally useful in framing a counseling relationship. Counselors try to minimize hierarchy while being cognizant of the inherent power differential that is built into a counseling relationship. Some clients, however, may require a type of hierarchy to feel supported and safe to pursue their counseling goals. They may regard the counselor as an authority or elder, in which case the counselor would not attempt to create a more egalitarian relationship. Also, it must be noted that Buber's notion of the I-Thou moment was embedded in a Western European context that values the individual and interpersonal dimensions of relationship. For some clients, the Thou is a group or community, not another individual.

4. *Find out what the client needs the most.* Gestalt therapy offers a wide range of types of support that a client may receive from the counselor. The art of counseling is to know what need is at the top of the list (most figural) and what type of support to offer from moment to moment. Counselors in training are taught many things *not* to do. For example, "Don't give advice." A Gestalt therapist has a wide range of intervention options born of the moment and related to what type of environmental support the client is seeking. Because Gestalt therapy is experimental, the possibilities are expansive. If a client asks a counselor for advice, the counselor might just give it, but that would only be the beginning of an exchange. The counselor might follow by asking the client what she or he thinks of the advice. Did the client introject the advice? Perhaps the client thought the advice was useless but couldn't express that to the counselor. The therapy work is not about the content of the advice. Rather, it is about the examination of the contact boundary phenomena that are awakened in the exchanges between counselor and client.

5. *Self-disclose when appropriate.* Different therapeutic orientations have different practices about counselor self-disclosure. On one hand, Jourard (1971) coined the phrase "self-disclosure begets self-disclosure," thereby indicating that self-disclosure is a good thing to do. On the other hand, the traditional analytic viewpoint argues that self-disclosure interferes with the critical development of transference. Gestalt therapy's answer to the question, "Is it ever okay for the counselor to self-disclose?" is, "It depends." Zahm (1998) has written the preeminent article about self-disclosure in Gestalt therapy in which he discusses the factors it depends on. It is beyond the scope of this chapter to discuss those factors in detail. A few points, however, are important to keep in mind as you make your own decisions about self-disclosure. A counselor can make two primary kinds of self-disclosure.

The first is the disclosure of past or current personal information (e.g., where you are from, your marital status, or information about your educational background). The second is information about your here-and-now reactions to the counseling process (e.g., sharing a feeling you are having about what the client is discussing). The most important question to ask yourself when making a decision to disclose or not to disclose is this: Will your disclosure add support to what the client is dealing with at this moment? In other words, will it contribute to or detract from the client's process of heightening awareness, clarifying the figure of interest, and making contact? The tricky part is that making the right decision takes years of experience, and even then you won't always know if self-disclosure was the right thing to do until you make the disclosure and attend to its impact. Generally speaking, however, a good rule to keep in mind is that self-disclosures that shift or keep the focus on the counselor are not generally helpful or prudent in any counseling relationship.

Here are examples of two different self-disclosures, one heard as being very supportive and the second as not supportive. In both examples, a client is telling a story about being abused by her uncle.

Example 1

T (Therapist): I feel angry as hell at this moment at your uncle.

C (Client): I approach my anger sometimes, but usually I don't feel like it is okay to be angry at him. Your reaction makes me realize he deserves my anger. [Client views counselor's statement as supportive.]

Example 2

T (Therapist): I feel sad about what happened to you.

C (Client): I did not come to counseling to deal with your sadness. I need you to be steady and strong for me. [Client views counselor's statement as not supportive.]

These two examples illustrate how two self-disclosures by counselors about how they are feeling could go two very different ways, depending on a number of variables or field conditions that exist at the moment the disclosure intervention is made.

The role of the client-counselor relationship is central to the theory and practice of Gestalt therapy. Health and change are a byproduct of the restoration of lost aspects of awareness and opportunities for novel contact with the environment. The therapeutic relationship is the crucible in which awareness and contact occur, and the counselor is the "shepherd" of those processes.

Clients' rigidified and unsuccessful attempts at contact in their out-of-therapy relationships eventually emerge and are replicated and enacted with the counselor. The counseling relationship becomes a kind of laboratory in which these contact processes can be observed and modified as they occur in the moment, and what is learned carries over to the client's other relationships.

Long-Term Versus Short-Term Applications

There has been a trend in the United States in recent years toward short-term counseling. Gestalt therapy has been and can be practiced over a brief or more protracted course of sessions. The key, of course, is to ensure that clients are able to experience the change they seek during their counseling.

Change in Gestalt therapy is conceptualized in two fundamental ways. First, the recovery or heightening of an awareness, which had been lost or blunted to a past creative adjustment, would be a significant change. An example would be a man who enters counseling and presents with concerns about being overly strict and extremely insensitive in his attempt to parent his children. He also reports that he was raised in a physically abusive environment where he learned to shut off his softer feelings. A significant change with this client would be his recovery of feelings of tenderness and love toward his children. Change is also marked by the expansion of the client's range of contacting styles. An example would be a client who tends to introject (swallow whole) the world and the words of the counselor in the first few sessions but tells the counselor in the fourth session, "I don't completely agree with what you just said. It just doesn't make sense to me."

Paradoxically, there are times when clients benefit from a more thorough understanding of why they don't change. Individuals who have recently immigrated to the United States, for example, are often caught between two conflicting sets of field conditions. Their families and culture might require one kind of contact with the environment (cooperative and acquiescent), while their employers and friends are pushing for another (competitive and assertive). The counseling goals in this situation would be increased awareness of the dilemma they experience, not working with clients to choose to comply with one set of field conditions while ignoring the other.

In general, Gestalt therapy is more appropriate for a longer-term counseling framework. There is no quick fix when the goal is increasing awareness and increasing the range and accuracy (appropriate to the immediate situation) of contact styles. Gestalt therapy can, however, also be applied very effectively to a briefer counseling model. One of the ways this occurs is to conceptualize the cycle of awareness and contact as a diagnostic tool and a "self-help" instrument for the client. The American Psychiatric Association's *Diagnostic and Statistical Manual* (*DSM IV-TR*) is useful and widely accepted. However, its user-friendliness is limited. Essentially the manual tells the insurance companies and our clients "what they have" or "what they are." Based on its content diagnosis, we say to our clients, "You are depressed," or "You are anxious," or "You have PTSD." Conversely, in Gestalt therapy the cycle of awareness and contact provides a process diagnosis. In other words, clients in a short-term therapy can begin to understand exactly where on that cycle they tend to get stuck.

- They have sensations that they cannot name or identify accurately.
- They identify what they need but have no energy to take a next step.
- They have energy but don't scan the current environment for what might address the need or interest.
- They scan the environment but fail to take action.
- They take action that never leads to satisfying contact.
- Contact is blocked or diluted by deflection, confluence, retroflection, projection, or introjection.
- Contact is made, but they don't "let go" of the thing that is satisfying and hold on for dear life.

In a short-term therapy, I will frequently give my clients a diagram of the cycle of awareness and contact and work with them collaboratively to identify (using in-session experiments and out-of-session homework) places on the cycle where they characteristically get stuck. After therapy is completed, clients can continue to use this model as a tool on their own.

Evaluation of Gestalt Therapy

One of the most contentious debates in the field of counseling and psycho-therapy over the last 10 years has been about the trend toward identifying, teaching, and practicing empirically supported treatments (ESTs). The debate centers around the fundamental and critical question, "How does a counselor decide what treatment approach is most appropriate and useful for a client?" The Clinical Psychology Division (Division 12) of the American Psychological Association (1995) published a set of guidelines that identified specific treatment approaches, primarily behavioral and cognitive-behavioral, to be utilized with particular "mental disorders." That report and many others that present similar findings and recommendations have been challenged by others (e.g., Beutler, 1998; Garfield, 1998; Norcross, 2001) who caution against the "manualization" of counseling, thereby underestimating or dismissing key variables in the effectiveness of counseling, such as the "therapist-client alliance."

Furthermore, and key to the topic of this book, the vast majority of studies that promote ESTs have been done with only a handful of disorders and with majority population samples. Deegear and Lawson (2003) conclude that "until such a time that research has settled the current EST debate, trainees should be encouraged to develop their own personal style and approach balanced with the unique world view of the client" (p. 275).

There is increasing research support for the effectiveness of Gestalt therapy across a range of clients and presenting concerns (nomothetic evaluation). That research is referenced and summarized in the next section. Gestalt therapists also assess the effectiveness of the orientation and its interventions for individual clients (idiographic evaluation), and those methods are also discussed.

Nomothetic Evaluation

Strümpfel (2004) has published an excellent article that summarizes more than 60 research studies that have been conducted about Gestalt therapy since 1973. These studies, which focus on a range of diagnoses and symptoms including depression, anxiety, personality disorders, schizophrenia, and alcohol and drug dependency, have involved over 3,000 subjects. Unfortunately, research studies have not been done with specific minority groups or diversity issues. In his summary, Strümpfel makes several cogent points.

- The studies show efficacy for the most serious and widespread disturbances with both in-patient and out-patient populations. (p. 37)

- All the studies that make direct comparison between Gestalt therapy and cognitive behavioral therapy show no significant difference in symptom relief. (p. 28)

- In 11 out of 12 studies that conducted follow-up tests (4 to 12 months posttreatment), stability of treatment goals and therapeutic change could be confirmed. (p. 38)

Historically, the difficulty in doing quantitative research to confirm the effectiveness of Gestalt therapy is that the approach is process oriented and does not follow a standard protocol. Some Gestalt therapists assert that the integrity of the orientation is severely compromised if research is conducted on just a part of the approach.

Perhaps the most promising research on the effectiveness of Gestalt therapy is being conducted by Greenberg and a number of his associates (see, for example, Greenberg & Foerster, 1996; Greenberg & Paivio, 1997; Greenberg & Rice, 1981; Greenberg & Watson, 1998). This research is ongoing and attends to the process of psychotherapy as well as the outcome. This type of process research is essential because Gestalt therapy cannot be captured by its parts, manualized, or conceptualized only as a symptom relief approach. Strümpfel (2004) states, "Greenberg's combination of process and evaluation data for analysis purposes is therefore of great importance for future researchers who want to understand the human interactive element between therapist and client" (p. 25).

Despite the increasing support for the effectiveness of Gestalt therapy, more research must be done (Frew, 2003). There is a need for more studies with a wider range of clinical populations and "disorders" (not a Gestalt-friendly term) and with more sophisticated research designs that include comparisons to the effectiveness of other counseling orientations and enough specificity that the findings can be replicated by additional research. Studies with nonmajority populations are acutely needed.

Another promising and largely unexplored avenue of research for Gestalt therapists is qualitative research. "Qualitative research is an inquiry process of understanding based on distinct methodological traditions of inquiry that explore a social or human problem. The researcher builds a complex, holistic picture, analyzes words, reports detailed views of informants, and conducts the study in the natural setting" (Creswell, 1998, p. 15). Qualitative approaches may be a fertile ground for future research endeavors in Gestalt therapy because the inquiry process is inherently phenomenological, and Gestalt therapy as a whole, not in its parts, could be examined. Qualitative studies typically start by questioning the "how" or "what" rather than the "why" of quantitative research, and these questions mirror the questions asked by Gestalt therapists. Finally, qualitative research explores multiple dimensions of a problem in all its complexity, and that approach may fit well in our efforts to assess the effectiveness of our counseling interventions with nonmajority clients.

Idiographic Evaluation

Gestalt therapists take nomothetic data seriously and utilize information from the results of that kind of research. Central to Gestalt therapy, however, is attending to the process and outcomes of particular client-counselor relationships. The goals of Gestalt therapy are increased awareness and the restoration of contact functions that are necessary in the current field conditions. Shifts in levels of awareness and quality of contact cannot be measured using traditional scales such as the Beck Depression Inventory (although some Gestalt therapists employ standardized measures to track symptom fluctuations). Rather, shifts in awareness and contact are typically tracked utilizing self-report (client) and observation (by the counselor).

Signs of a "successful" Gestalt therapy would be a client's ability to expand present awareness of aspects of self and environment and the maintenance of this increased clarity of perception of self and other over time and across situations. Clients would be able to more quickly identify what they want and move into the environment with energy and confidence to seek the satisfaction of those wants, needs, and interests.

The process of therapy is examined and "evaluated" continuously by Gestalt therapists. Such formative evaluation is essential to Gestalt therapy. A brief case example can illustrate how the process of counseling is attended to and how the effectiveness of the therapist is assessed in an ongoing way. David is a second-generation Japanese American, and this is the second session with a female European-American Gestalt therapist. David entered counseling to deal with the loss of his job as a software engineer.

> C (Client): My father called last night and is flying into town on business and wants to have dinner.
>
> T (Therapist): What perfect timing. I'm sure you are looking forward to telling him about losing your job and getting his advice and support.
>
> C: Yes, I suppose you are right . . . [Client's voice trails off and he looks out the window.] What I would really like to talk to you about today is some problems my son is having in school.
>
> T: David, I noticed that after I made the comment about your looking forward to your father's visit, your energy shifted, you looked away from me and then changed the subject.
>
> C: You're right.
>
> T: Can you tell me what happened for you when I made that comment?
>
> C: I'm not exactly sure, but I will try. Something about your not really understanding my true feelings about his visit.
>
> T: I get it. I realize now that I told you how I thought you would feel and I didn't ask you how you did feel.
>
> C: I would like to tell you how I feel.
>
> T: And I would very much like to hear how you feel.
>
> C: I don't want to see my father because I am humiliated and have lost face by losing this job. I can't look him in the eye because I have dishonored him.

The counselor made a mistake by forgetting to explore the meaning of the father's visit through the eyes of her client. She imposed her meaning rather than proceeding phenomenologically. These kinds of misses occur all the time in counseling. The counselor immediately observed that something shifted with David, in his voice, his energy, and his eye contact, when he changed the subject. She made an intervention, which simply pointed out what she observed without interpretation. That allowed the client to describe two of his experiences, how he felt when she made the first intervention and how he felt about his father's coming to town. This exchange recovered the counseling session and repaired the rupture in the therapeutic contact between the counselor and the client.

Idiographic evaluation is simply attending to the impact of your interventions moment to moment in a counseling session. There is often a vast difference between intention (what we hope to communicate) and impact (how the intervention is actually heard and felt by the client). Gestalt therapists consistently monitor the impact of their words and behaviors with a client. If our words or behaviors (e.g., looking at the clock during a session) seem to result in a change in energy or affect, we usually ask the client, "What happened for you when I said that or looked at my watch?" If clients feel sufficient safety and support to chance honest contact with us, they will tell us about our impact and this becomes the focus of the counseling at that moment. Periodically checking in with clients about the process of counseling allows the Gestalt therapist to make course adjustments along the counseling trail. If counselors don't pursue their impact, the trail can be completely lost and the effectiveness of their work will be diminished.

Compatibility of the Approach with Diverse Clients

I conclude this section on evaluation by commenting on Gestalt therapy and its application with diverse clients. Sue and Sue (2003) make the case that most forms of counseling and psychotherapy are "culture bound" and may even have the agenda of "converting" clients to the dominant society's values (p. 106). They point out that the culture-bound characteristics of traditional Western counseling approaches are a focus on the individual, an emphasis on verbal or emotional expressiveness, a belief in the power of insight, a requirement of self-disclosure, a separation of mental and physical functioning, the ability to tolerate ambiguity, and a protocol in which clients must initiate most of the communication.

If Gestalt therapy is practiced phenomenologically, sensitively, flexibly, and with an adherence to context (field theory), it is not culture-bound in those ways and can be a very useful and effective approach with diverse clients. Of course, it is not perfectly compatible with every client, either majority or minority, but it is a promising orientation in this world of increasing diversity.

Gestalt Therapy: Blind Spots, Limitations, and Challenges

Throughout this chapter, I have argued the case that contemporary Gestalt therapy has evolved as a culturally sensitive and diversity friendly orientation. Now to complete the picture I will point out the blind spots, limitations, and challenges that must be considered as Gestalt therapy continues to evolve and to respond to the context now.

Blind Spots

The blind spots in any orientation to psychotherapy can be identified by closely examining the critical components that define the approach. For Gestalt therapy, the cornerstone concept from which all others are derived is organismic self-regulation. It is assumed that every individual can identify a need and, given sufficient awareness and environmental resources, take action to satisfy that need. Notice, however, that the term is *self-regulation*, not "self-other regulation." Though not well explicated in the Gestalt literature, there is a tacit belief that when individuals self-regulate and attend to their own needs first and foremost, those around them will benefit or at least be able to self-regulate in kind. In other words, when the boat begins to rock, "every person for him- or herself" is the best approach. In Gestalt therapy, this is our blind spot.

It is not uncommon to encounter a client who puts the needs of others ahead of her or his own. The concept of organismic self-regulation may not make any sense to clients from collectivistic cultures in which the family or community takes precedence over the individual. Alfonso, a Latino client, is telling a counselor how much he misses his wife and children, who are in Mexico while he works in the United States. The counselor says, "It is obvious and clear that you want to go home to be with your family." Alfonso's face and tone shift from sadness to firm resignation, and he says, "You are wrong. I want what is best for my family and for the time being that means I keep this job."

Even in the majority culture, there are many situations in which individuals subsume their needs to address the needs of others. A mother who puts the needs of her child ahead of her own, or a husband who walks away from a successful and rewarding career to care for his spouse who is recovering from a stroke would be examples of individuals who suspend self-interest to attend to others.

Limitations

The majority of clients seen by first-generation Gestalt therapists like Fritz and Laura Perls were White, well-educated individuals who were not dealing with severe mental health issues. In the ensuing years, Gestalt therapy has been utilized in a wide range of settings and with a wide range of clients. The theory behind the therapy has also been applied to work with couples, families, groups, and in organizational development efforts. Unfortunately, the information available about the effectiveness of Gestalt therapy as it has branched out from its original form and client base is primarily theoretical or anecdotal. As stated earlier, Gestalt therapy lacks a quantitative research base to verify its effectiveness or to compare it to other approaches with similar client populations. This is a significant shortcoming and limits the approach from receiving the notoriety of other orientations that have supporting empirical research.

A second limitation is related to the training of Gestalt therapists. It takes many years to achieve even a minimal level of competency in Gestalt therapy. Despite the rigorous course of study required to begin to master this approach, there is no national certification process and the level of training completed by those calling themselves Gestalt therapists varies widely. Indeed, in the 1960s and 1970s, it was very common for individuals to attend a weekend workshop or a series of workshops and then to announce that they were Gestalt therapists. Given the nature of the orientation and the instrumental role the therapist plays in translating the therapy to each client and situation, the path to becoming a Gestalt therapist is long and winding, and it involves extensive professional and personal development. A limitation of this approach is formed by the intersection of the extensive training necessary to practice it competently and the lack of a certification process that would define the minimum standards required to be a Gestalt therapist.

A third limitation that can impact the effectiveness of Gestalt therapy is the potential for a therapist's own blind spots to get in the way of attending accurately to what a client presents. A common example would be a therapist who follows his or her own figure of interest during a session rather than the one brought forward by the client. I have participated in workshops with well-known Gestalt therapists who created elaborate and emotionally powerful experiments that had very little to do with what the client was interested in. Because there is no manualized or step-by-step procedure for conducting Gestalt therapy, it is more likely that the personal issues of the therapist can leak into the work with clients. Gestalt therapists are required to pursue their own therapy as part of their training to minimize this limitation.

Challenges

The biggest challenge facing Gestalt therapy is overcoming the perception of those outside the orientation about its very nature and identity. Despite the attempts of many within the Gestalt community to present a more balanced and contemporary picture of the approach, the general therapeutic community still tends to identify Gestalt therapy with the way Fritz Perls practiced and wrote 40 years ago. Fueling the misperceptions are the majority of academic textbooks in the field that continue to depict Gestalt therapy as confrontational and technique driven. This widespread misperception of the essence of Gestalt therapy often results in the orientation being routinely disregarded as a viable approach for a wide range of clients and diversity concerns.

There are two other commonly held perceptions about Gestalt therapy that are also inaccurate and pose a challenge for those of us who practice this orientation. Both of these notions are captured in the following quote by Ivey, D'Andrea, Ivey, and Simek-Morgan (2002): "There are now relatively few individuals who practice Gestalt as a theory in itself" (p. 285). The implication is that Gestalt therapists are going the way of the dinosaur and those who do practice Gestalt combine it with other orientations (e.g., cognitive-behavioral therapy). Certainly the proportion of legitimately trained Gestalt therapists to practitioners of other orientations is less than it was in the 1970s. Nevertheless, there are thousands of psychotherapists around the world who identify themselves as exclusively Gestalt.

Furthermore, most Gestalt theorists today, including this author, believe that combining Gestalt with other orientations cannot be done in a way that maintains the theoretical integrity of the approach. I vividly remember a workshop presented by Arnold Lazarus in 1988 on multimodal therapy, an approach that borrows techniques from a variety of therapy orientations. Several hours into the training he showed the audience a video of his work with a client using the empty chair technique. After the video ended, he declared that he was using Gestalt therapy with this client. His statement about using Gestalt therapy contributed to the myth that you can combine the Gestalt approach with others. It served to perpetuate the idea that Gestalt therapy is a toolbox of handy and powerful exercises any therapist can use. In fact, it is a holistic orientation that cannot be adopted in parts and that requires years of training and supervision to practice effectively. These inaccurate perceptions of Gestalt therapy pose a significant challenge. It is incumbent on the Gestalt therapy community to find ways to educate those outside the orientation about the current status of the theory, how it is practiced, and how clients benefit from this approach.

The final challenge is one I addressed in the limitations section. Gestalt therapists with a few exceptions have been content to promote the effectiveness of the approach without conducting research to support those claims. Despite the fact that the practice of Gestalt therapy with its focus on process is not a perfect marriage with quantitative research methods, there are ways to examine the effectiveness of the approach and to compare it with other psychotherapy orientations. In addition, doing this research with diverse clients will bolster the proposition I have made throughout this chapter, that Gestalt therapy is a viable approach in our increasingly diverse world.

Future Development: Gestalt Therapy in a Diverse World

Gestalt therapy has the theoretical and methodological range to remain a viable and effective psychotherapy orientation in the future. As the world changes, so must Gestalt therapy. We instruct our clients to be aware of the current field conditions. Gestalt therapy must do the same. The future development of Gestalt therapy will require a commitment from the Gestalt community to continually examine the "context now" and to assess the degree to which our theory, values, and intervention methods are congruent with the clients who are seeking our assistance.

The Gestalt community itself must grow to ensure the development of the approach. The pendulum has swung in recent years away from many of the orientations described in this book, including Gestalt therapy. The Gestalt therapy community must find ways to attract the new generation of counselors and therapists who are entering the field. Ultimately, it will be their task to continue to develop the approach and to demonstrate through research and practice that Gestalt therapy has a prominent place in a diverse world.

Summary

1. Gestalt therapy was developed by Fritz and Laura Perls and has roots in psychoanalysis, existentialism, and Gestalt psychology.

2. Fritz Perls popularized the therapy in the 1960s. However, his style of practice, which was confrontive, technique driven, and, at times, insensitive, became widely known as the essence of how to practice Gestalt therapy.

3. Since the 1980s, Gestalt therapy has emerged from the shadow of Fritz Perls and has been practiced with more balance and attention to the client-counselor relationship, the client's subjective experience, and the interpersonal and environmental field.

4. This chapter's author became a Gestalt therapist after realizing that Gestalt therapy could be practiced in a nonconfrontive way and that it was not an

approach developed to identify abnormality or to encourage clients to adjust to their environments.

5. There are many ways to practice Gestalt therapy, but all Gestalt therapists adhere to the philosophical foundation of field theory, phenomenology, and dialogue.

6. The cornerstone concept of Gestalt therapy theory is organismic self-regulation. Clients are viewed as having the capacity to identify their needs and interests and to make contact with the environment in ways to have these needs and interests satisfied. This concept is also outlined in a model called the cycle of awareness and contact.

7. The process of Gestalt therapy involves the restoration of awareness and the increase in the quantity and quality of contact with the environment. Interruptions in the cycle of awareness and contact are examined in the counseling process. Five contact boundary disturbances or phenomena have been identified: introjection, projection, retroflection, confluence, and deflection. They can be healthy processes (phenomena) if they are in the client's awareness and appropriate to the immediate environmental conditions, or unhealthy processes (disturbances) if out of awareness and artifacts of times and conditions past.

8. According to Gestalt therapy, clients change when they become more fully aware of the "what is" and do not attempt to be something different. Staying with the present "what is" requires self and environmental (including the counselor and counseling relationship) support.

9. Gestalt therapists utilize the experiment to shift the focus of counseling from talking to action, which heightens awareness and/or contact in the moment.

10. The client-counselor relationship is at the heart of Gestalt therapy. The relationship becomes the vehicle for change and proceeds collaboratively, examining both the content and process of counseling.

11. Gestalt therapy is compatible with nonmajority clients because it proceeds phenomenologically, validates the client's experience, fosters dialogue, attends to the most present need, and does not prohibit self-disclosure if such disclosure would support the client and the goals of therapy.

12. Gestalt therapy can be utilized in both short-term and longer-term therapies and can therefore accommodate the requirements of different counseling settings.

13. Gestalt therapy is evaluated both nomothetically and idiographically. Research efforts in Gestalt therapy to validate its effectiveness have

intensified in recent years, but more study is necessary, particularly with nonmajority client populations.

14. Gestalt therapy does not have many of the culture-bound dimensions mentioned in the multicultural counseling literature and is therefore a very useful approach in a world of diversity.

15. Gestalt therapy has its blind spots, limitations, and challenges. The primary blind spot is the significance Gestalt therapists place on organismic self-regulation as central to the theory and practice. The emphasis on self, not other, could create difficulty for individuals who put others or the community first. Limitations are the paucity of empirical research supporting the approach, the absence of a certification process to ensure that Gestalt therapists are properly trained, and the potential for Gestalt therapists' unawareness of personal issues to negatively impact their counseling effectiveness. Finally, Gestalt therapists to this day are challenged by widespread misperceptions about the true nature of the approach and the lack of research about how the approach is compatible with diverse clients. The Gestalt therapy community must acknowledge and address these factors to ensure the sustainability of the orientation in the years to come.

Key Terms

assimilation (p. 245)
awareness (p. 244)
closure (p. 244)
confluence (p. 252)
contact (p. 245)
contact boundary (p. 251)
creative adjustment (p. 247)
cycle of awareness and contact
  (p. 245)
deflection (p. 252)
dialogue (p. 241)
empty chair (p. 232)
environment (p. 228)
experiment (p. 253)
field (p. 240)
figure (p. 229)

figure formation and destruction
  (p. 243)
gestalt (p. 229)
ground (p. 229)
holistic (p. 230)
introjection (p. 251)
organismic self-regulation (p. 230)
paradoxical theory of change
  (p. 248)
phenomenological inquiry (p. 238)
phenomenology (p. 241)
process (p. 230)
projection (p. 251)
retroflection (p. 252)
technique (p. 232)
top dog–underdog dialogue (p. 232)

Resources for Further Study

Professional Organizations

Association for the Advancement of Gestalt Therapy (AAGT)
www.aagt.org
Training Centers: New York Institute for Gestalt Therapy (New York City), www.newyorkgestalt.org; Pacific Gestalt Institute (Los Angeles), www.gestalttherapy.org; Gestalt Therapy Training Center Northwest (Portland, Oregon, and Vancouver, Washington, www.gttcnw.org; Gestalt Training Center of San Diego (LaJolla, California), www.gestalt.org/file9.htm; Gestalt International Study Center (South Wellfleet, Cape Cod, Massachusetts), www.gisc.org; Gestalt Center for Psychotherapy and Training (New York City), www.gestaltnyc.org; and Center for the Study of Intimate Systems (Gestalt International Study Center, Cape Cod, Massachusetts), www.gisc.org/csis.html.

Professional Journals

Gestalt Review
www.gestaltreview.com
British Gestalt Journal
www.britishgestaltjournal.com
International Gestalt Journal
www.international-gestalt-journal.org

Suggested Readings

Latner, J. (1986). *The Gestalt therapy book*. Highland, NY: Gestalt Journal Press.

A very thorough review of the theoretical concepts of Gestalt therapy.

Nevis, E. (Ed.). (1992). *Gestalt therapy: Perspectives and applications*. New York: Gardner Press.

This book contains chapters on theory, diagnosis, ethics, and application to working with special populations.

Perls, L. (1992). *Living at the boundary*. Highland, NY: Gestalt Journal Press.

A series of thoughtful essays by the co-founder of Gestalt therapy.

Woldt, A., & Toman, S. (Eds.). (2005). *Gestalt therapy: History, theory and practice*. Thousand Oaks, CA: Sage.

The first book about Gestalt therapy designed as a textbook.

Yontef, G. (1993). *Awareness, dialogue, and process: Essays on Gestalt therapy.* Highland, NY: Gestalt Journal Press.

> An excellent resource for students who want to learn more about field theory, phenomenology, and dialogue.

Zinker, J. (1977). *Creative process in Gestalt therapy.* New York: Brunner/Mazel.

> This book elaborates on the cycle of awareness and contact and on the experiment.

Other Media Resources

Gestalt Archives at Kent State University, Ohio 44240
http://speccoll.library.kent.edu/other/gestalt.html
Gestalt Research Conference
Gestalt International Study Center
Cape Cod, MA 02663
www.gisc.org
Society for Gestalt Theory and Its Applications (GTA)
www.gestalttheory.net

Chapter 8

Behavior Therapy I: Traditional Behavior Therapy

Michael D. Spiegler

What do each of the following case vignettes have in common?

- A second-generation Japanese-American woman was unable to discuss problems she was having at work with her boss. Despite her primary identification with her American culture, her parents had always taught her to show deference toward people in authority. However, she wanted to be able to talk openly with her boss. She learned to express her desires appropriately by observing her counselor demonstrate effective ways of expressing feelings to superiors politely yet forcefully. (*modeling*) She practiced these behaviors—initially with the therapist, later with people less threatening than her boss, and finally with her boss. (*behavior rehearsal*)

- To enhance the self-image of a man whose body was deformed by a birth defect, his counselor instructed him to substitute positive, self-enhancing thoughts (e.g., "I look just fine") for his habitual negative, self-effacing thoughts (e.g., "I look like a freak"). (*cognitive restructuring*)

- A 7-year-old boy frequently bullied smaller children. The frequency of the boy's bullying decreased when he was not allowed to attend recess or gym (his favorite activities at school) each time he was caught fighting. (*response cost*)

- A woman worked hard for wages that were substantially lower than the wages her male co-workers earned. To relieve her frustration, she drank excessively and verbally vented her irritation on her family. The counselor taught the woman coping skills, including muscle relaxation and self-instructions to remind her that her family was not the source of her frustration. In counseling, she role-played being in various frustrating situations and practiced applying the coping skills. Then she used the skills in her everyday life whenever she felt frustrated and had the urge to drink or act abusively. (*stress inoculation training*)

- An 82-year-old woman experienced anxiety about interacting with residents in the nursing home she had recently entered. She was taught muscle relaxation and then, while relaxed, she imagined increasingly more anxiety-evoking situations (beginning with nodding hello to another resident and ending with spending time conversing with a small group of residents). (*systematic desensitization*)

- A young single mother had beaten her 3-year-old son on several occasions when he had had a temper tantrum. The more she tried to get her son to stop crying, the angrier she got. First the counselor taught the mother anger management skills. Then, to directly reduce the boy's temper tantrums and indirectly decrease his mother's anger and physical abuse, the counselor taught the mother to ignore her son during a temper tantrum (*extinction*) and to reinforce him with attention when he was behaving appropriately. (*differential reinforcement*)

- A gay couple who had been together for 11 years sought help because they "fought all the time" and believed that they no longer loved each other. Their counselor taught them communication skills and problem solving for dealing with conflicts. (*social skills training* and *problem-solving therapy*)

- In a predominantly Latino-American junior high school, students were required to speak only English in class. However, a number of first-generation immigrant students often reverted to Spanish because they could express themselves better in their native tongue. They were taught to subvocally say, "Speak only English," to remind themselves each time they raised their hand to speak in class. (*self-instructional training*)

The vignettes you've just read provide just a sample of the therapeutic procedures (named in parentheses) that compose behavior therapy. In contrast to most other counseling approaches that have a basic unitary method of treatment, behavior therapy incorporates many different specific *behavior therapies* (although, as you will learn, they all have the same fundamental purpose). Behavior therapists also refer to specific behavior therapies as *behavior therapy techniques* (the terms are synonymous and I will use them interchangeably). However, unlike the techniques of other approaches that are specific therapeutic tactics (such as free association in psychoanalytic therapy and experiments in Gestalt therapy), a behavior therapy technique is a self-contained, stand-alone therapy.

Because there are so many behavior therapies, covering them requires two chapters. This chapter and the next are meant to be read in sequence. In this chapter, you'll first learn about the history and evolution of behavior therapy and the theory of change that guides all behavior therapies. Then you will be introduced to what I have called *traditional behavior therapy*, which includes stimulus control, reinforcement and punishment, exposure therapies, and modeling therapies. In the next chapter, the discussion will move to *cognitive-behavioral therapy*, which grew out of traditional behavior therapy and employs both traditional behavior techniques and newer cognitive techniques that directly modify clients' thoughts and beliefs. Figure 8.1 (p. 278) shows the two branches of behavior therapy and the specific therapies that compose each branch. The next chapter also will discuss general issues that are relevant for all behavior therapies: an evaluation of the behavior therapy approach, an overview of the problems and client populations for which behavior therapies are applicable, a critique of behavior therapy, and suggestions for future development of behavior therapy in a diverse world. Throughout this chapter and the next, the term *behavior therapy* will be used generically to refer to both traditional behavior therapy and cognitive-behavioral therapy.

Origins and Evolution of Behavior Therapy

The inspiration for traditional behavior therapy came from experimental work on learning at the beginning of the 20th century. While studying salivation in dogs, Russian physiologist Ivan Pavlov (1927) discovered what would come to be called *classical conditioning*—a learning process in which an originally neutral stimulus, by being repeatedly paired with a stimulus that elicits a particular response, comes to elicit the same response. Inspired by Pavlov's work, John Watson (1914), an experimental psychologist at Johns Hopkins University, founded *behaviorism*, the school of psychology on which behavior therapy is largely based. Behaviorism emphasizes the importance of objectively studying behaviors by dealing only with directly observable stimuli and responses. It rejects mentalistic concepts, such as consciousness, thought, and imagery. In 1924, Mary Cover Jones (1924), one of Watson's students, treated Peter, a 3-year-old who was afraid of rabbits, using precursors of modeling therapy and in vivo exposure therapy. First, Jones had Peter watch other children happily playing with a rabbit (modeling); then, she gradually moved a caged rabbit closer to Peter as he was eating a favorite food (in vivo exposure). Following this treatment, Peter was able to comfortably hold and play with rabbits. (All of the behavior therapies alluded to in this section are discussed in detail later.)

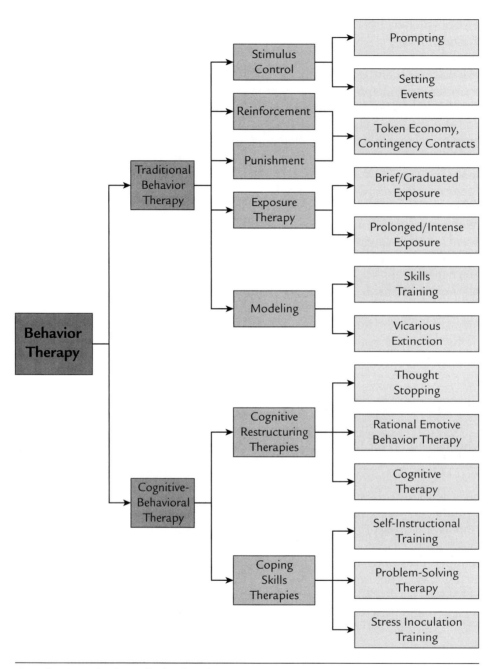

Figure 8.1 The Organization of Behavior Therapies
© 2005 Michael D. Spiegler

Another major influence on the development of behavior therapy came from the investigations of psychologist Edward Thorndike (1911, 1931, 1933) at Columbia University. Thorndike was studying ways to modify behaviors by systematically changing their consequences, which would come to be called *operant* (or *instrumental*) *conditioning*. Subsequently, beginning in the 1930s, psychologist B. F. Skinner at Harvard University "wrote the book" on operant conditioning. Like Pavlov, Skinner (1953) speculated about harnessing learning principles for counseling, but it was Skinner's students and followers who actually did so.

Whereas the study of learning and the founding of behaviorism provided the initial direction behavior therapy would take, the impetus for its development came from a growing discontent with the effectiveness and efficiency of psychoanalytic therapy (e.g., Eysenck, 1952), which was the predominant psychotherapy approach at the end of World War II. Because psychoanalysis was such a lengthy process—frequently requiring years of treatment—it became increasingly clear that it was unsuitable for treating the large number of veterans who required counseling as a result of the war.

Behavior therapy had its formal beginnings in the 1950s, simultaneously in the United States, South Africa, and Great Britain. In the United States, Ogden Lindsley, one of Skinner's graduate students, demonstrated that patients in psychiatric hospitals, whose behaviors appeared to be aimless, would consistently perform simple tasks when given appropriate reinforcers (Lindsley, 1956, 1960, 1963; Skinner, 1954). Lindsley may have been the first to use the term *behavior therapy* to describe the systematic use of learning procedures to treat psychological disorders (Skinner, Solomon, & Lindsley, 1953).

In 1961 at Anna State Hospital (a psychiatric facility in Illinois), Theodoro Ayllon and Nathan Azrin designed a system for changing behaviors through operant conditioning, which they called a *token economy* (Ayllon & Azrin, 1968). Their work paved the way for the widespread application of the token economy with diverse populations, which is described later. Ayllon and Azrin had to obtain patients for their experimental program from existing wards at the hospital. The staff members were reluctant to part with patients whom they were treating successfully, but they were happy to transfer to Ayllon and Azrin's program those patients who had been unresponsive to treatment. As it turned out, the token economy resulted in remarkable changes in the so-called incurable patients, and this outcome strengthened the case for the effectiveness of behavior therapy. Through the mid-1970s, a cycle of resistance from nonbehavioral mental health professionals followed by demonstrations of the effectiveness of behavior therapies under adverse conditions was a common experience for early behavior therapists (Spiegler & Guevremont, 2003).

Also during the 1950s, Joseph Wolpe (1958), a psychiatrist in South Africa who had become disenchanted with psychoanalysis, developed several keystone behavior therapies, most notably *systematic desensitization*, designed for treating problems such as irrational fears and anxiety. Systematic desensitization replaces debilitating anxiety with more adaptive reactions (such as muscle relaxation) to anxiety-inducing events.

Prominent among the professionals Wolpe trained were psychologists Arnold Lazarus and Stanley Rachman. Lazarus (1959, 1961; Lazarus & Abramovitz, 1962) initially made important contributions by adapting systematic desensitization to groups of clients and to children. Lazarus (1976, 1985, 1989a) strongly advocated extending the boundaries of behavior therapy, which eventually led to his developing *multimodal therapy*, an eclectic approach rooted in behavior therapy principles, but using some nonbehavioral techniques. Rachman (1959, 1967) immigrated to Great Britain in 1959, where he introduced systematic desensitization and, working closely with psychologist Hans Eysenck at the University of London's Institute of Psychiatry, spearheaded the development of behavior therapy in Great Britain (Rachman & Eysenck, 1966).

In the 1960s, another major approach to behavior therapy was born. Psychologist Albert Bandura at Stanford University developed a *social learning theory* that included not only principles of classical and operant conditioning but also *observational learning* (Bandura & Walters, 1963)—the process of changing one's behaviors by observing the behaviors of other people. Bandura's (1977) theory, which he now calls *social cognitive theory* (Bandura, 1986, 1997), emphasizes the critical role that cognitions (e.g., thoughts, beliefs, expectations, images) play in psychological functioning, including their role in the development and treatment of psychological disorders.

Making cognitions a legitimate focus of behavior therapy was antithetical to Watson's behaviorism because cognitions are not directly observable. Watson's behaviorism may have been a useful position for early behavior therapists to adopt because it countered the deeply entrenched psychoanalytic perspective that emphasized unobservable, unconscious forces and structures (e.g., id, ego, and superego). Today, however, most behavior therapists believe that dealing only with directly observable behaviors is too restrictive (e.g., Cloitre, 1995). After all, humans think, hold beliefs, have expectations, and imagine. Although cognitive processes cannot be observed directly, they clearly influence how people act and feel.

During the 1960s, *cognitive-behavioral therapy* was created simultaneously but independently by two therapists. Psychiatrist Aaron Beck at the University of Pennsylvania developed *cognitive therapy* (Beck, 1963), and psychologist Albert Ellis (1962) in private practice in New York City designed *rational emotive therapy*, now called *rational emotive behavior therapy* (Ellis, 1993). Both therapies modify the negative and illogical thoughts associated with many psychological disorders, such as depression and anxiety. Later, psychologist Donald Meichenbaum (1974, 1985) at the University of Waterloo in Ontario,

Canada, developed cognitive-behavioral treatment packages, such as *self-instructional training* and *stress inoculation*. Initially, cognitive-behavioral therapies were met with skepticism and served as supplements to traditional behavior therapies, but they rapidly evolved into a major approach in the field. Today a majority of behavior therapists use cognitive-behavioral therapies, which, as you will see in the next chapter, include traditional behavior therapy techniques.

In 1966, the Association for Advancement of Behavior Therapy (AABT) was established in the United States with just 18 members. Psychologist Cyril Franks, who previously had worked with Eysenck and Rachman in London, was its first president. AABT became the major professional organization advocating for behavior therapy and facilitating the field's development. Currently, the organization has some 3,200 members from a variety of disciplines (e.g., counseling, psychology, psychiatry, and social work), publishes behavior therapy journals, and hosts a large annual convention. In 2004, the members of AABT voted to change the name of their organization to the Association for Behavioral and Cognitive Therapies (ABCT), which makes it clear that behavior therapy comprises both traditional behavior therapies and cognitive-behavioral therapies and that it refers to many specific therapeutic procedures.

In the 1970s, behavior therapy emerged as a prominent approach to counseling. Its principles and techniques also were adapted to enhance the everyday functioning of people in areas as diverse as business and industry (e.g., Hermann, de Montes, Dominguez, Montes, & Hopkins, 1973; Pedalino & Gamboa, 1974), childrearing (e.g., Becker, 1971; Christophersen, 1977; Patterson, 1975; Patterson & Gullion, 1976), education (e.g., Keller, 1968; Madsen, Greer, & Madsen, 1975), and ecology (see Spiegler & Guevremont, 1998, chap. 16).

During the 1980s, two important developments spurred an increase in the acceptance and applicability of behavior therapy. First, cognitive-behavioral therapy emerged as a major force in counseling, supplementing traditional techniques with newer approaches. Second, behavior therapy began to make significant contributions to the field of behavioral medicine, a discipline devoted to the psychological treatment and prevention of medical problems (Pinkerton, Hughes, & Wenrich, 1982; Spiegler & Guevremont, 2003, chap. 14).

In the 1990s and continuing into the present, two themes characterized the evolution of behavior therapy. First, new behavior therapies were developed that included components not based on learning principles and not traditionally behavioral (e.g., Forsyth, 1997; Hayes, Strosahl, & Wilson, 1999; Lazarus, 1989a). This is part of a larger movement of psychotherapy integration, which combines treatment procedures from various approaches (e.g., Arkowitz, 1992a, 1992b; Davison, 1995; Goldfried, 1995; Norcross & Goldfried, 2005). As just one example, some behavior therapists have incorporated Gestalt therapy's empty chair technique as part of behavior therapy (Samoilov & Goldfried, 2000). The second theme is recognizing the importance of specifically attending to the needs of diverse clients and testing the applicability of behavior therapies to treating such clients. These efforts will be illustrated as behavior therapy is described in this chapter and the next.

The growth and evolution of behavior therapy can be summarized by likening it to the stages of human development. The theoretical and methodological contributions of early behaviorists such as Pavlov, Watson, Thorndike, and Skinner represent behavior therapy's prenatal stage. Its birth and infancy occurred in the 1950s with the development of early methods for changing the behavior of people with severe psychiatric disorders and the development of systematic desensitization for treating anxiety. This was followed by the proliferation of a variety of behavior therapies in its childhood during the 1960s. In the 1970s, behavior therapy's adolescence was marked by both a growth spurt in its development and a rebellion against the adoption of cognitive factors. Behavior therapy emerged into its adulthood in the 1980s as a firmly established, broad-based approach to counseling and psychotherapy, and since then it has continued to mature (as adults are supposed to do) with a long life expectancy.

Context Then—Context Now

Behavior therapy, like all other approaches to counseling, has been and continues to be context driven. The original driving context involved both a practical necessity and the academic Zeitgeist (German for *spirit of the time*). As I said earlier, the impetus for the development of behavior therapy was the pressing need to treat the many World War II veterans suffering from psychological disorders and the inefficiency of psychoanalysis, the predominant approach to counseling at the time, in helping those veterans. The founders of traditional behavior therapy turned to behaviorism, the school of psychology that stressed the impact of the external environment on directly observable behaviors that were studied empirically through controlled experimental research. In the 1950s, when behavior therapy emerged, behaviorism was a dominant force in psychology and reflected the Western post–World War II enshrinement of science and technology. The resultant new therapy contrasted sharply with psychoanalysis, as you can see in Table 8.1.

The second branch of behavior therapy—cognitive-behavioral therapy— arose in the 1960s in the context of a shifting emphasis in academic psychology from the predominant study of external stimuli and their influence on overt behaviors (i.e., behaviorism) to the study of cognitive processes. The so-called cognitive revolution in psychology (Neisser, 1967) legitimized the empirical study of thought and other mental processes.

The most recent developments in the field of behavior therapy have been in response to two contextual factors, both of which involve underserved clients.

Table 8.1 Basic Comparisons Between Psychoanalysis and Behavior Therapy

	Psychoanalysis	*Behavior Therapy*
Locus of time	Past	Present
Mode of treatment	Verbal	Action-oriented
Treatment strategy	Indirectly explore client's past and unconscious as related to client's problem	Identify and directly change present maintaining conditions of client's problem
How techniques are applied	Same for all clients	Customized for each client
Length of treatment	Lengthy	Brief
Evidence for effectiveness	Uncontrolled, qualitative case studies	Controlled, quantitative experiments

The first factor is the existence of various problems or disorders that behavior therapies and other approaches to counseling have had relatively minimal success in treating (e.g., personality disorders, substance-related disorders, and schizophrenia). The second contextual factor is the changing demographics of our population, which has resulted in an ever-increasing number of culturally diverse clients in need of psychotherapy. Behavior therapists have responded to both contextual factors by modifying existing behavior therapies and developing new ones to meet the needs of these clients.

The Author's Journey as a Behavior Therapist

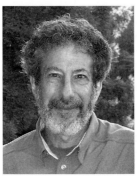
Michael Spiegler

I am fortunate to have been introduced to behavior therapy when it was very young, which means that I have been able to witness much of its growth and evolution. But I did not begin as a behavior therapist.

Like the founders of behavior therapy, my first theoretical orientation was psychoanalytic, which I acquired as an undergraduate at the University of Rochester. I began training as a psychotherapist in graduate school at Vanderbilt University in the mid-1960s by practicing psychoanalytic therapy at the student counseling center. I saw several clients once a week over the 9-month school year. My supervisor,

(*continued*)

Hans Strupp, a noted psychoanalyst, often stressed the importance of taking time to develop a sound therapeutic relationship. But as I was developing a sound relationship with my clients, weeks and months were passing and we were not yet addressing my clients' problems. I became frustrated with the slow pace and even considered it unethical. As part of my graduate training, I also learned and practiced client-centered therapy. There too, I was frustrated—in this case by not being able to make direct, potentially helpful suggestions to my clients.

At the height of my frustration as a novice psychotherapist, I was introduced to behavior therapy by Robert Liebert, a faculty member at Vanderbilt who had recently completed his Ph.D. at Stanford University where he had studied with Albert Bandura. My initial attraction to behavior therapy was that its theory and practice dealt with clients' problems quickly and directly, just the opposite of psychoanalysis and client-centered therapy. Not only did the expedient, direct, problem-focused approach of behavior therapy seem a more ethical and humane strategy for helping people who were in distress, but it clearly was more compatible with my personality.

Throughout my life in various situations, when a problem has arisen, I have immediately shifted into a problem-solving mode, asking, "What is the most effective and efficient way of dealing with this problem?" According to my parents, this aspect of my personality was clearly manifested at an early age. When I was 3 years old, I was at the beach with my family. Nearby, a crowd had gathered. Consistent with the inquisitiveness associated with my age, I went to investigate. Unable to see what the excitement was about with a large crowd of grown-ups blocking my view, I wriggled my way to the front of the crowd. I discovered that a boy about my age was lost. Without hesitation, I authoritatively announced to the assembled crowd, "Let me handle this." Then, approaching my first "client," I inquired, "Sonny, where were you when you last saw your mommy?"

The specific approach to behavior therapy that I adopted as a graduate student was based on Bandura's social learning theory. It employed both traditional and emerging cognitive techniques. In fact, I was a cognitive-behavioral therapist before the term *cognitive-behavioral therapy* had even been coined.

I have had experience with most of the behavior therapies discussed in this chapter and the next—as a clinician, researcher, and scholar. As an academic, I have not only taught and trained students in behavior therapy, but I have also contributed to the development and empirical validation of behavior therapies. For instance, my earliest research efforts involved designing modeling films for alleviating fears (Spiegler, Liebert, McMains, & Fernandez, 1969). As another example, while at the Palo Alto Veterans Administration Hospital, I conceived of the idea of *skills training* as a treatment for chronic psychiatric disorders such as schizophrenia (Spiegler, 1971, 1973; Spiegler & Agigian, 1977), which has since become a widely used intervention for this population (e.g., Liberman et al., 1993).

When I became a behavior therapist, the field was in its childhood, with all the excitement and growth that fits with that period of development. Today, with behavior therapy fully into its adulthood, the excitement still exists (albeit mellowed) as the field continues to grow and maturely reflect on its past, present, and future. What drew me to behavior therapy more than 35 years ago is what I still find most compelling about it today. Behavior therapy is a highly effective and efficient approach to alleviating clients' psychological problems and suffering, which makes it a most worthy and humane endeavor.

Theory of Behavior Therapy

As its name implies, behavior therapy focuses on clients' problem behaviors, including both *overt behaviors* or actions and *covert behaviors*, including feelings, thoughts, and physiological responses. The fundamental theoretical assumption that is the basis for behavior therapy is that *all behaviors*—both adaptive and problematic—*are maintained (or caused) by present events that occur before and after the behaviors have been performed.* **Antecedents** are prerequisites (knowledge, skills, and resources) and environmental cues (e.g., the situational context) that are present or occur *before* a behavior is performed; they "set the stage" for and initiate the behavior. **Consequences** are events that occur *after* and as a result of performing a behavior; they determine whether the person will engage in the specific behavior or similar behaviors again. We are more likely to perform a behavior in the future if the consequences are pleasant or worthwhile and less likely to perform a behavior in the future if the consequences are unpleasant or not worthwhile. The specific antecedents and consequences that maintain or cause an individual to perform a behavior are its **maintaining conditions.**

The **ABC model** depicted in Figure 8.2 shows the functional relationship among antecedents, behavior, and consequences. As an example of this

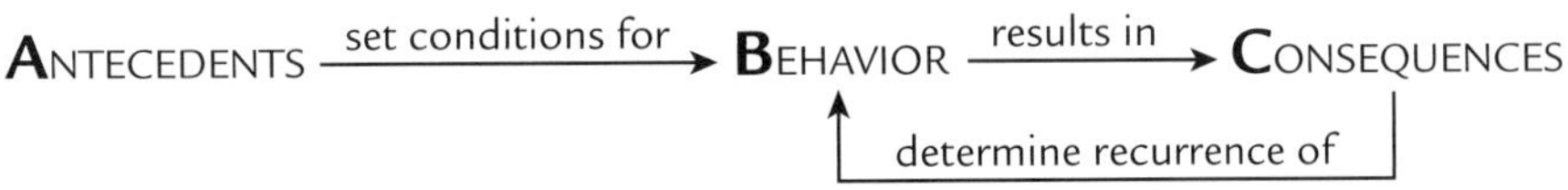

ANTECEDENTS $\xrightarrow{\text{set conditions for}}$ BEHAVIOR $\xrightarrow{\text{results in}}$ CONSEQUENCES

$\uparrow$ determine recurrence of

Figure 8.2 The ABC Model

relationship, consider the behavior you are engaging in right now: reading about the ABC model. Knowing how to read and being assigned this chapter are antecedents for your reading, and they elicit your reading. Learning about the ABC model and using it to conceptualize your clients' problems would be consequences that will influence whether you read similar material in the future. The more useful you find these consequences, the more likely it is that you will read similar material subsequently.

Theory of Change

Behavior therapists distinguish between *present maintaining conditions* and *past originating conditions*. Although a client's problem behavior may have started sometime in the past, because it is occurring presently, it is being maintained by present events (its maintaining conditions). Thus, *behavior therapy treats a client's problem behavior by directly changing the present antecedents and consequences that are causing the problem behavior.* Note that it is the maintaining conditions of the problem behavior that are changed directly, which in turn changes the problem behavior indirectly.

Behavior therapies *accelerate* (increase) adaptive behaviors that clients are not performing sufficiently (e.g., an elderly nursing home resident's eating) or *decelerate* (decrease) maladaptive behaviors that clients are performing in excess (e.g., abusing alcohol). This is done by changing specific antecedents, consequences, or both that are maintaining clients' problem behaviors.

Behavior therapy proceeds in a series of eight interrelated steps that are depicted in Figure 8.3. (1) The client's problem is clarified, and (2) initial treatment goals are formulated. (3) The problem behavior is defined as a **target behavior,** a discrete, measurable aspect of the problem that will be the focus of treatment. (4) The maintaining conditions of the target behavior are identified. (5) A treatment plan is developed to change one or more of the maintaining conditions, and then (6) the plan is implemented. (7) The effectiveness of the treatment plan is evaluated in terms of the treatment goals. If the desired change in the problem behavior has occurred, therapy is terminated, and (8) periodic follow-up assessments are conducted to assure that the change is maintained over time. Measurement of the target behavior begins immediately after the target behavior has been defined in step 3 and continues through the evaluation of therapy in step 7.

If the client's problem has not been alleviated, the step where the process broke down is identified and rectified, and the remaining steps are repeated. For instance, the wrong maintaining conditions may have been identified, the therapy chosen may not have been optimal for the particular client, or the therapy may not have been implemented correctly.

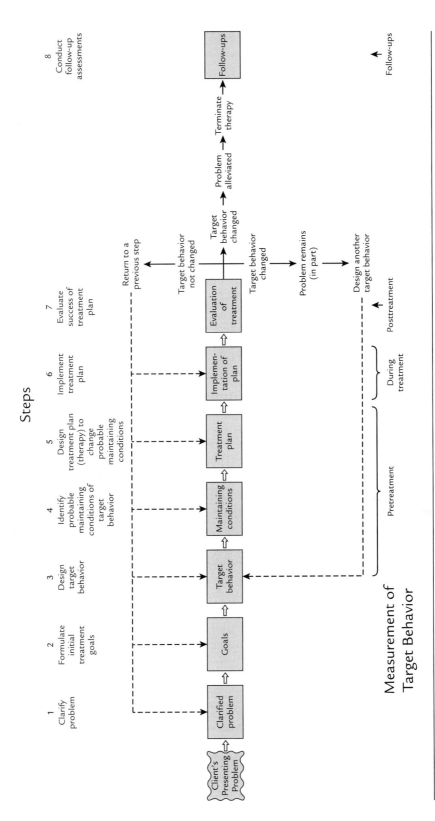

Figure 8.3 The Process of Behavior Therapy

© 2002 Michael D. Speigler and David C. Guevremont

Defining Behavior Therapy

The case vignettes at the very beginning of the chapter gave you an idea of the heterogeneity of behavior therapies. Further discussion about traditional behavior therapies in this chapter and cognitive-behavioral therapies in Chapter 9 will demonstrate just how diverse they can be. What, then, makes each a behavior therapy? All behavior therapies, including traditional behavior therapies and cognitive-behavioral therapies, share common themes and characteristics that distinguish them from other psychotherapies.

Common Themes of Behavior Therapy

Four defining themes—scientific, active, present focus, and learning focus—delimit behavior therapy and distinguish it from other approaches to counseling (Spiegler & Guevremont, 2003).

1. *Scientific.* Behavior therapists are committed to practicing behavior therapy using a scientific approach that involves precision and empirical evaluation (Wilson, 1997). They precisely and unambiguously define the client's behaviors to be changed, the treatment goals, and the therapy procedures that will be employed. Moreover, behavior therapy techniques are validated through controlled, empirical studies that can be replicated (repeated) by other researchers before they are considered acceptable for general use (Chambless & Hollon, 1998; Kendall, 1998; Spiegler & Guevremont, 1994).

The scientific theme of behavior therapy is not surprising, considering that the roots of behavior therapy are in behaviorism and experimental psychology. Further, most of the major figures who originally developed behavior therapy were clinical psychologists, and a scientific approach is a cornerstone of clinical psychology.

2. *Active.* In behavior therapy, clients engage in specific actions to alleviate their problems. In other words, clients *do* something about their problems rather than just talk about them. In contrast with most of the other counseling approaches covered in this book, which are verbal therapies, behavior therapy is an action therapy. In verbal therapies, the dialogue between the client and counselor is the major mode through which therapy techniques are implemented. In action therapies, the therapy techniques involve therapeutic tasks the client does. The primary purpose of the client-counselor dialogue in an action therapy such as behavior therapy is to exchange information, such as when a client describes her or his problem to the therapist, when the counselor explains to a client how to do a **homework assignment** (a between-session therapeutic task), and when the client reports on the homework assignment in the next counseling session.

Behavior therapy is frequently carried out, at least in part, in the client's natural environment. The logic is simple: The client's problem is treated where it is occurring, which obviously is not in the therapist's office (at least I've never had a client whose presenting problem was being anxious in counseling or not getting along with a counselor!). **In vivo** (Latin for *in life*) therapy makes it more likely that the changes that occur during treatment will transfer to the client's everyday life and continue after counseling has ended (e.g., Edelman & Chambless, 1993). To implement in vivo procedures, counselors sometimes work directly with clients in their natural environments. Most often, however, clients serve as their own change agents by carrying out therapy procedures at home, by themselves or with the assistance of people in their lives (such as a parent or spouse).

A final way in which behavior therapy is active is that clients set their own goals for therapy, with advice from their counselor, and often clients are asked to choose the specific therapy procedures to be implemented, after the therapist describes the possible alternatives to the client.

3. *Present focus*. Clients' problems always occur in the present. Thus, the problems are assumed to be caused by current conditions (although they may have begun in the past). After assessing the current factors causing the client's problem, behavior therapists implement procedures to change these current factors, which in turn will alleviate the problem. Note the contrast with other counseling approaches, such as psychoanalytic therapy, which assume that the causes of clients' problems lie in the past.

4. *Learning focus*. There are three ways in which learning is central to behavior therapy. First, the behavioral model holds that all problem behaviors are influenced by learning, even if they have biological roots. Second, in behavior therapy, clients learn new (adaptive) behaviors to replace old (maladaptive) behaviors. There is a strong educational component in behavior therapy, and behavior therapists often are teachers and clients are learners. Third, the development of many behavior therapies was based on basic learning principles, and theories of learning (most notably classical and operant conditioning) often are used to explain how behavior therapies work.

Other Common Characteristics of Behavior Therapy

In addition to the four defining themes, behavior therapies generally share four common characteristics: individualized, stepwise progression, treatment packages, and brevity (Spiegler & Guevremont, 2003).

1. *Individualized*. Standard behavior therapy procedures are tailored to each client's unique problem and personal characteristics. For instance, to

motivate clients to engage in adaptive behaviors, behavior therapists often employ reinforcement, which involves providing the client with a consequence that increases the chances the client will engage in the behavior again. However, the specific reinforcer (the consequence that makes the behavior recur) is likely to vary with the client's age (e.g., stickers can be reinforcers for children, but not for adults) as well as a host of other demographic factors, including cultural identification (e.g., cream cheese might be a reinforcer for a Jewish-American 3-year-old and kimchi—a spicy Korean cabbage dish—for a Korean-American of the same age).

2. *Stepwise progression*. Behavior therapy often proceeds in a stepwise progression—from simple to complex, from easier to harder, or from less threatening to more threatening. For example, a 12-year-old girl refused to eat solid food because she believed she would choke (Donohue, Thevenin, & Runyon, 1997). The behavior therapist had the girl construct a hierarchy of foods based on how difficult they are to swallow (e.g., ice cream at the bottom of the hierarchy and steak at the top). The therapist instructed the girl's mother to give her only foods from the bottom of the hierarchy for a few days and then to gradually move up the hierarchy, slowly introducing foods more difficult to swallow.

3. *Treatment packages*. Two or more behavior therapy procedures frequently are combined in a **treatment package** to increase the effectiveness of the therapy. This practice is analogous to the treatment of cardiovascular disease with medication, diet, and exercise. For instance, the therapist in the previous example might instruct the mother to supplement the technique of progressively introducing foods that are more difficult to chew (shaping) with reinforcement (e.g., giving her daughter a small treat other than food when she successfully eats a new food).

4. *Brevity*. The course of behavior therapy is relatively brief, generally involving fewer counseling sessions and often requiring less overall time than other types of counseling. This is because behavior therapy procedures directly change what is maintaining clients' problems and because clients in behavior therapy engage in therapeutic tasks on their own outside therapy sessions. Of course, the length of counseling varies with the client's specific problem.

Practice of Traditional Behavior Therapy

Now, as you read about the major traditional behavior therapies, remember that all behavior therapies work by changing the maintaining conditions of the client's problems. As you will see, there are many ways to do this.

Changing Antecedents That Elicit Behaviors: Stimulus Control

Sometimes clients' problems are maintained by the absence of antecedents that elicit desirable behaviors or the presence of antecedents that elicit undesirable behaviors. In such cases, **stimulus control** is employed to modify (control) these antecedents (stimuli). This can be done by modifying *prompts* or by modifying *setting events.*

Prompts are cues that remind or instruct us to perform a behavior. We rely on prompts to guide our everyday behaviors, such as a call from a dentist's receptionist to remind us of an appointment or a sign indicating the way out of a parking lot. Different kinds of prompts are used in behavior therapy, as the following examples illustrate.

- An *environmental prompt* was used with an elderly woman suffering from dementia who repeatedly went into other people's rooms in a residential facility (Bird, Alexopoulos, & Adamowicz, 1995). The counselor hung a large red stop sign on the other residents' doorframes, and then taught the woman to stop and walk away whenever she saw the sign. The woman's inappropriate entries dropped from a daily average of 44 to 2 following a single 2-hour counseling session.

- In couple therapy, one partner in a lesbian relationship learned to use her partner's crying as a *behavioral prompt* to respond with sympathy rather than annoyance, which had been her typical response.

- To increase meaningful participation of elderly clients in exercise classes, day care staff used a *verbal prompt* (such as saying, "All together now!") to remind clients when they were not participating (Thompson & Born, 1999). With clients for whom verbal prompts were insufficient, the staff employed a *physical prompt*, such as moving the clients' arms or legs for them.

Setting events are broad conditions in the immediate environment that influence the likelihood that a client will engage in particular behaviors. Consider the setting events for a 76-year-old woman's excessive and debilitating ruminations about her medical condition (Gorenstein, Papp, & Kleber, 1999). Typically, the woman ruminated on days that she was not doing her volunteer work and had no activities scheduled. Her ruminations were decreased by changing the setting events that were maintaining her ruminations—namely, the absence of activities to keep her busy. The treatment consisted of changing her schedule so that she worked at her volunteer job three days a week and had activities scheduled on the other four days.

Insomnia may be maintained by inappropriate setting events. This occurs because one's bed becomes associated with a host of behaviors other than sleeping, such as reading, watching TV, talking on the phone, snacking, and worrying about not being able to fall asleep. A simple yet highly effective treatment developed by Richard Bootzin (1972; Bootzin, Epstein, & Wood, 1991) changes the setting events by having clients follow a set of rules.

As part of one treatment package for late-life insomnia, elderly community residents (mean age 67) were given the following instructions, based on Bootzin's rules (Morin, Kowatch, Barry, & Walton, 1993).

1. Get into bed only when sleepy.

2. Use the bed only for sleeping and sex.

3. When still awake after 15–20 minutes, get out of bed and only return when sleepy.

4. Repeat rule 3 as many times as necessary.

5. Get out of bed at the same time every morning.

The treatment package also included instruction in basic sleep hygiene (e.g., being aware of the effects of stimulants, certain foods, and exercise on sleep) and modifying one's thoughts (cognitive restructuring) to change dysfunctional beliefs about sleep. The treatment package reduced the clients' insomnia, and their improved sleep was maintained over time.

Stimulus control procedures can be implemented easily, with little time and effort required (e.g., instructing a client to do something or posting a sign that reminds the client to perform a particular behavior). The purpose of stimulus control procedures is to get clients to perform a target behavior, but ultimately for the behavior to continue, it must be reinforced.

Changing Consequences to Accelerate Adaptive Behaviors: Reinforcement

Reinforcing people to get them to act in particular ways certainly was not invented by behavior therapists. What behavior therapists have done is discover the basic principles of reinforcement and systematically apply them in order to change clients' problem behaviors effectively and reliably. **Reinforcement** occurs whenever the consequences of a behavior increase the likelihood that a person will engage in the behavior again. The reinforcing consequence is known as a **reinforcer.** Reinforcers usually are pleasant or desirable. They can be *tangible* (e.g., a favorite food), *social* (e.g., praise), *activities* (e.g., listening to music), or *token* (e.g., money). Because what is pleasant for one person may not be for another, behavior therapists identify the specific events that will serve as reinforcers for each client through questioning, observing the client's regular activities, and having the client select personal reinforcers from a large array of potential reinforcers that generally motivate people's behaviors.

One behavioral theory of depression holds that depression is maintained by low rates of positive reinforcement in a person's life (Lewinsohn & Graf, 1973; Teri & Gallagher-Thompson, 1991; Teri & Uomoto, 1991). These conditions certainly hold for many elderly people who are suffering from physical ailments, have lost the ability to engage in regular activities, and are institutionalized, which would account for the high rate of depression in this population (Meeks & Depp, 2002). Increasing pleasant events that are reinforcing consequences has been shown to be effective in reducing depression in the elderly, including those suffering from Alzheimer's disease (e.g., Teri & Gallagher-Thompson, 1991) and dementia (Teri & Uomoto, 1991), and is applicable to elderly clients of various ethnicities (e.g., Lichtenberg, Kimbarrow, Morris, & Vangel, 1996). The elderly certainly are not the only people for whom low rates of positive reinforcement can be a factor in depression, as the following case illustrates.

P. L. was a 34-year-old professional writer who had been in a lesbian relationship for 12 years. She became depressed when her partner ended the relationship 3 months prior to her entering counseling. P. L. and her partner had maintained an active social life, which was a primary source of enjoyment and satisfaction for her. Without her partner, P. L. had withdrawn from social contacts and activities. She was functioning adequately in her work and was filling the time she had previously spent in social activities by taking on additional writing tasks. When her therapist asked her whether she was enjoying her extra work (to find sources of pleasant events and positive reinforcement), P. L. said, "No, but I feel obligated to do it, and it fills up the time."

Because P. L.'s richest source of positive reinforcement had come from social activities, the first goal of therapy was to reinstate some of them. This was accomplished by using extra work to reinforce her engaging in social activities. Although she reported no particular pleasure doing the extra work, she had been doing it frequently. According to the *Premack principle*, a less frequent behavior (in this case, social activities) will increase if it is reinforced by a more frequent behavior (in this case, extra work), regardless of how desirable or enjoyable the more frequent behavior is. The therapist, with P. L.'s input, set up a treatment plan whereby P. L. was permitted to do a specified amount of extra work *only after* she had spent a specified amount of time in a social activity. This intervention not only increased P. L.'s social activities but also, as expected, decreased her depression.

Reinforcement increases the likelihood that a person will engage in a behavior again. But how do you get someone to perform a behavior for the first time? **Shaping** involves reinforcing a person for performing successively closer approximations to or components of a total behavior so that ultimately the person is performing the complete behavior. (It is the "hot" part of the children's game of "hot and cold" that involves one child's directing another to an unknown location by saying "hot" as the child moves closer to the location and "cold" as the child moves farther away from it.) Shaping is used to accelerate behaviors that a client performs infrequently or that a client finds difficult or complex.

Shaping was employed to train a 9-year-old girl with autistic disorder to exit a building in case of a fire (Bigelow, Huynen, & Lutzker, 1993). The behavior was broken down into its logical component parts or steps, and the girl was reinforced when she performed each component. For example, one of the steps was getting down on the floor. The counselor first prompted getting down on the floor (by saying, "When there is smoke, get down on the floor") and then reinforced her for doing so (by praising the girl for complying). Prompting often is combined with shaping to modify clients' behaviors, such as with elderly nursing home residents to increase grooming and social behaviors and to reduce wandering (Carstensen & Fisher, 1991).

Changing Consequences to Decelerate Maladaptive Behaviors

The most desirable strategy for decelerating undesirable behaviors is **differential reinforcement,** which involves reinforcing a client's engaging in a behavior that is a more desirable alternative to the undesirable behavior. The undesirable behavior is called the *deceleration target behavior,* and the more desirable alternative is called the *acceleration target behavior.* For instance, to reduce hitting herself, a young girl with severe mental retardation was reinforced for playing with a puzzle (Nunes, Murphy, & Ruprecht, 1977). Differential reinforcement indirectly decelerated her self-injurious behavior because while she was using her hands to play with the puzzle, she could not hit herself. On the other end of the age spectrum, self-injurious behaviors (Mishara, Robertson, & Kastenbaum, 1974) and repetitive screaming (Cariaga, Burgio, Flynn, & Martin, 1991) of elderly nursing home residents have been reduced by reinforcing desirable behaviors that are incompatible with the undesirable behaviors.

Sometimes differential reinforcement does not decelerate the maladaptive behavior sufficiently or quickly enough. When this is the case, behavior therapists either (1) eliminate reinforcement for the deceleration target behavior or (2) administer undesirable consequences for the deceleration target behavior. Behavior therapists employ a variety of strategies to achieve these aims, and all of them involve changing the consequences of a behavior so that the client is less likely to engage in the behavior again, which is formally known as **punishment.** (The term *punishment* frequently connotes the use of physically aversive consequences. As you will see in the following two sections, most behavior therapy strategies that operate through the principle of punishment do not involve physically aversive consequences.)

Eliminating Reinforcement

All behaviors are maintained by reinforcement. If the reinforcers that are maintaining a behavior are eliminated, the person eventually stops performing the behavior, a process called **extinction.** When social attention is the reinforcer, extinction consists of ignoring the individual when he or she engages in the undesirable behavior. For instance, a treatment package of extinction and reinforcement was used with elderly nursing home residents suffering from osteoarthritis to reduce their *pain behaviors* (such as complaining of pain, taking pain medication, moving gingerly) that were maintained by social attention and to increase participation in physical exercise (Miller & LeLieuvre, 1982). When the residents exhibited pain behaviors, staff members refrained from giving them attention and interacting with them (extinction). When they exhibited *well behaviors* (such as talking about feeling good, refusing pain medication, exercising), the staff gave them attention and praised their well behaviors (reinforcement). Not only did this treatment package increase exercise compliance, but it also resulted in a reduction in the clients' use of pain medication and their reported pain.

Extinction is most often used when the deceleration target behavior is being reinforced by social attention because ignoring is an easy intervention to implement. However, extinction does not always involve withholding social attention; withholding social attention is appropriate only when it is social attention that is maintaining the deceleration target behavior. Extinction involves depriving the client of whatever is reinforcing the deceleration target behavior. Consider the case of a child who starts fights with other children in his class in order to be sent to the principle's office and therefore get out of doing schoolwork. In this instance, not giving the child attention would be an inappropriate intervention. Instead, no longer allowing the child to avoid schoolwork would extinguish his starting fights.

Time out from positive reinforcement (or **time out,** for short) involves temporarily withdrawing a client's access to generalized reinforcers immediately after the client performs the deceleration target behavior. For instance, parents are using a time-out strategy when they have their child stand in a corner for several minutes following a misbehavior. Time out from positive reinforcement can be thought of as time-limited extinction (Spiegler & Guevremont, 2003).

Administering Undesirable Consequences

One method of administering undesirable consequences involves **response cost,** the removal of a valued item or privilege that the client possesses or is entitled to. Examples of response cost in everyday life are parking tickets, loss of points for a late assignment, and loss of TV time for a child's misbehavior. In each case, there is a cost for performing a particular undesirable behavior. Besides being a highly effective intervention, parents from different backgrounds (African-American and White, low and middle-upper socioeconomic class) who use response cost with their children consider it to be a highly acceptable procedure (Heffer & Kelley, 1987). In general, acceptability or palatability of a therapy is important because it allows the procedure to be used; therapies low in acceptability, even if highly effective, may not be used.

In some cases, the response cost may involve clients' forfeiting their own money, as would be the case if a Republican client were to agree to donate $50 to the Democratic party every time she or he got drunk. This can be an effective form of treatment for two reasons. First, clients usually won't forfeit valuables because the mere threat of such a response cost is sufficient incentive to decelerate the maladaptive behavior (e.g., Boudin, 1972; Mann, 1972, 1976). Second, the effects of response cost often endure when the contingency is no longer operative (Armstrong & Drabman, 1998; Sullivan & O'Leary, 1990). In general, clients consider response cost an acceptable deceleration therapy, in part because the client must agree to the terms beforehand (Blampied & Kahan, 1992; Jones, Eyberg, Adams, & Boggs, 1998).

Overcorrection is a second way of administering undesirable consequences. Overcorrection decelerates maladaptive behaviors by having clients correct the effects of their actions (restitution) and then intensively practice an appropriate alternative behavior (positive practice) (MacKenzie-Keating & McDonald, 1990). It was originally developed to treat behaviors that harm or annoy others or that are self-destructive (Foxx & Azrin, 1972).

Overcorrection was used to eliminate a frequent and disruptive behavior of a 50-year-old patient with an estimated IQ of 16 who had been hospitalized for 46 years. Since the age of 13, Ann had frequently overturned chairs, tables, and beds (Foxx & Azrin, 1972). Because Ann was essentially nonverbal, as her restitution the staff asked her to nod her head appropriately to indicate whether she was sorry and whether she intended to do it again. Also as restitution, she was required to put the piece of furniture she had overturned in its proper position and to straighten any disarray (e.g., completely remaking a bed she had overturned). For her positive practice, Ann had to straighten all similar furniture on the ward (e.g., neatening each of the beds on the ward). Initially, Ann failed to comply with the staff's instructions to engage in this positive practice. Consequently, a staff member physically prompted the required movements by guiding her limbs with just as much bodily pressure as was necessary and then faded the prompts by reducing the pressure as Ann began to perform the movements on her own. In an 8-day baseline before overcorrection was implemented, Ann overturned an average of 13 pieces of furniture a day. After 2 weeks of overcorrection, Ann was overturning an average of one per day. After 11 weeks of training, Ann's overturning behavior was completely eliminated.

Overcorrection is also used to treat behaviors that have negative consequences primarily for the client. Examples include self-injurious behaviors of a child with mental retardation (Harris & Romanczyk, 1976); excessive, stereotypic behaviors (Rojahn, Hammer, & Kroeger, 1997); and eating non-nutritive substances, a disorder known as *pica*, which may be seen in clients with developmental disabilities (Ellis et al., 1997).

Administering **physically aversive consequences** that result in unpleasant physical sensations, including pain, is the third way of decelerating maladaptive behaviors with undesirable consequences. Mild electric shock is the most frequently used aversive stimulus. It creates a brief, sharp, stinging sensation that lasts for only a few seconds and results in no tissue damage. Other examples of physically aversive consequences are snapping a rubber band around one's wrist, smelling a noxious odor, tasting a bitter substance, and hearing a loud noise. Physically aversive consequences are used infrequently, mainly because of ethical objections and potential negative side effects such as avoidance of the person administering the consequences and emotional responses such as crying and tantrums (e.g., Carey & Bucher, 1986; Kazdin, 1989). But in a small number of cases, physically aversive consequences may be necessary because alternative behavior therapies for decelerating maladaptive behaviors—differential reinforcement, time out from positive reinforcement, response cost, and overcorrection—often take somewhat longer to work than physically aversive consequences. Thus, when time is of the essence (as when an individual is engaging in self-destructive behaviors or attacking others), physically aversive consequences may be the treatment of choice.

Token Economies

A **token economy** is a system for motivating clients to perform desirable behaviors and to refrain from performing undesirable behaviors. Clients earn tokens—token reinforcers such as poker chips or points—for adaptive behaviors, and they lose tokens for maladaptive behaviors. The tokens are exchanged for actual reinforcers called **backup reinforcers** (which vary considerably with the client population). Detailed, explicit procedures for clients' earning, losing, and spending tokens are a key element of a token economy. The majority of token economies are used with groups of clients (e.g., children in classrooms, elderly nursing home residents, patients in a psychiatric facility), which makes them a highly efficient form of treatment.

Token economies also can be implemented with individual clients, as in the case of Mr. A., an 82-year-old retired longshoreman who had suffered a massive heart attack (Dapcich-Miura & Hovell, 1979). Mr. A. was not following his physician's orders to exercise, eat foods high in potassium, and take his medication. Mr. A.'s granddaughter, who lived with him, agreed to administer the token economy. Mr. A. earned poker chips for walking, drinking potassium-rich orange juice, and taking his medication. He exchanged the poker chips for two backup reinforcers: the privilege of choosing what he wanted for dinner at home and going out to eat at a favorite restaurant. The token economy significantly increased each of the three healthful behaviors. Additionally, instituting the token economy appeared to improve Mr. A.'s relationship with his family by reducing arguments about Mr. A.'s adherence to his medical regimen.

Exposure Therapy

Often the best way to reduce one's anxiety or fear is to expose oneself directly to it—hence the common wisdom of getting back on the horse that has just thrown you. **Exposure therapies** are used to treat anxiety (and other negative emotions, such as fear and anger) by exposing clients—under carefully controlled and safe conditions—to whatever it is that is making them anxious. There are two basic models of exposure therapy: brief/graduated and prolonged/intense (Spiegler & Guevremont, 1993). In both models, clients can either be exposed to anxiety-evoking events in their imagination or in vivo (to the actual event).

Brief/Graduated Exposure Therapies

Brief/graduated exposure therapies expose the client to threatening events (1) for a short period (ranging from 10–15 seconds to a few minutes) and (2) incrementally, beginning with aspects of the events that produce minimal anxiety and progressing to more anxiety-inducing aspects.

Systematic Desensitization   **Systematic desensitization,** developed by Joseph Wolpe (1958), is the prototype of brief/graduated exposure therapies. In systematic desensitization, the client imagines successively more anxiety-arousing situations while engaging in a behavior that competes with anxiety. The client gradually (systematically) becomes less sensitive (desensitized) to the situations. The therapy involves three steps.

1. The therapist teaches the client a response that competes with anxiety. Most often the response is **progressive relaxation,** which involves alternately tensing and relaxing the major groups of skeletal muscles. Clients are trained to differentiate between tension and relaxation, which allows them to purposefully relax in response to tension. Here is an excerpt from the typical instructions clients follow to learn progressive relaxation (if you follow the instructions, you will experience the technique).

Close your eyes, settle back comfortably. . . . Let's start with your left hand. I want you to clench your left hand into a fist, clench it very tightly and study those tensions, hold it . . . [5-second pause] and now release the tension. Relax your left hand and let it rest comfortably. Just let it relax . . . [15-second pause]. Once again now, clench your left hand . . . clench it very tightly, study those tensions . . . [5-second pause] and now release the tension. Relax your hand and once again note the very pleasant contrast between tension and relaxation.

2. The specific events that cause anxiety are ranked in terms of increasing anxiety in an **anxiety hierarchy.** As the example shown in Figure 8.4 makes clear, the specific events and their order is idiosyncratic to the client; you might order them differently.

3. The client repeatedly visualizes the anxiety-evoking events, in order of increasing anxiety, while performing the competing response. The following excerpt from a systematic desensitization session illustrates this process.

Mai Lee was a 38-year-old woman who had immigrated to the United States from Vietnam 5 years previously. Although she had a decent command of English, she became anxious when she needed to convey something important in English, especially to strangers. She also thought that her accent made her appear stupid. Prior to the first session in which the desensitization process was implemented, Mai Lee learned progressive relaxation and developed an anxiety hierarchy with her counselor. During desensitization, Mai Lee was seated in a comfortable reclining chair. After

15. Death of a close relative
14. Thoughts about your own mortality
13. Death of a friend
12. Death of a co-worker
11. Driving by a bad automobile accident
10. Seeing a bad automobile accident on TV
 9. Reading in the newspaper about someone killed
 8. Thoughts of a terrorist attack
 7. Thoughts of an earthquake
 6. Seeing a bad fire
 5. Flying in an airplane
 4. Looking down from a height
 3. Being alone in a strange place at night
 2. Thoughts about witches and ghosts
 1. Hearing a siren

Figure 8.4 One Client's Anxiety Hierarchy for Fear of Death

several minutes, during which time she relaxed her major muscle groups, the counselor began.

> I'm going to ask you to imagine scenes from the anxiety hierarchy we constructed. You'll imagine them clearly, and they generally will interfere little with your state of relaxation. However, if at any time you feel discomfort while imagining a scene, signal me by raising your left index finger. Now, let's begin.
>
> First, I want you to imagine that you are walking up to the customer service desk at a car dealership to explain the problem you are having with your car. You are worried that you won't explain yourself well and that the service rep will discount what you have to say. Visualize that situation and how you are feeling. [20-second pause] Now stop imagining that scene and just concentrate on your relaxed state. If the scene disturbed you, raise your left index finger now. [Client raises her finger.] Just continue relaxing. [10-second pause]
>
> Now imagine the scene again. [Counselor describes scene and pauses for 20 seconds.] Now erase the scene from your mind. Just focus on the calm feeling that comes from a relaxed state. If you experienced anything but slight discomfort while visualizing the scene this time, raise your left index finger now. [Client does not raise her finger.] Good. Just continue soaking up the feelings of relaxation. [15-second pause]
>
> Now, I want you to imagine that the service rep at the car dealership has called over his manager so you can explain the problem with your car to her. You are thinking that you did not express yourself well enough to the service rep and now you have to explain the problem again to another person. [This scene was repeated four times before the client experienced no discomfort.]
>
> Just continue relaxing. In a moment, I am going to count backwards from five and you will open your eyes and feel very calm and refreshed. Okay, five, four, three, two, and one. Open your eyes, sit up, and notice how relaxed you feel.

Systematic desensitization is a highly versatile therapy. When muscle relaxation is not an appropriate competing response (as with young children, adults with arthritis, and people with some physical disabilities), other competing responses can be used, such as thinking pleasant thoughts, eating, or listening to music. Individuals as well as groups of clients can be treated using systematic desensitization (e.g., Anton, 1976; Lazarus, 1961; Paul & Shannon, 1966; Spiegler et al., 1976; Taylor, 1971). Desensitization has been used to treat a variety of problems associated with negative emotional reactions besides anxiety, including anger (e.g., Rimm, deGroot, Board, Heiman, & Dillow, 1971), asthmatic attacks (e.g., Moore, 1965), insomnia (e.g., Steinmark & Borkovec, 1974), motion sickness (e.g., Saunders, 1976), nightmares (e.g., Shorkey & Himle, 1974), sleepwalking (e.g., Meyer, 1975), and racially related emotional responses (Cotharin & Mikulas, 1975).

In the last study just cited, desensitization of racially related emotional responses was used with volunteer White students in a racially integrated high school in the South who reported unwanted prejudicial feelings. The students received 3 months of biweekly desensitization sessions. Following treatment, not only did the students report less racial-related anxiety, but they also acted in ways that indicated that their prejudice declined, such as attending social functions involving predominantly African Americans which they would not have done before treatment.

Relaxation Training   Progressive relaxation also is used without systematic desensitization to reduce anxiety and stress. Relaxation training is suitable for elderly clients because this population often responds well to treatments that are structured and time-limited (Lewinsohn & Teri, 1983). For example, progressive relaxation has helped the elderly deal with stressful situations in general (DeBarry, 1982a, 1982b; DeBarry, Davis, & Reinhard, 1989; Radley, Redston, Bates, & Pontefract, 1997; Wethrell, 1998), reduce anxiety related to engaging in new activities or those they have not done in a long time (Radley et al., 1997; Teri, 1991), alleviate insomnia (Engle-Friedman & Bootzin, 1991) and chronic headaches (Nicholson & Blanchard, 1993), and reduce depression (DeBarry, 1982b; DeBarry et al., 1989; Gonzales, 2001; Smith, 2001; Teri, 1991). In addition, progressive relaxation in conjunction with other relaxing exercises (such as yoga stretching and breathing exercises) has been shown to be effective with diverse clients, for example, in reducing depression with Korean (Smith, 2001) and Puerto Rican clients (Gonzales, 2001).

In Vivo Exposure Therapy   **In vivo exposure therapy** essentially is systematic desensitization in which the client is exposed to the actual anxiety-evoking events (rather than imagining them). **Differential relaxation,** which consists of relaxing all muscles not needed for the behaviors being performed, usually is substituted for progressive relaxation because the muscles the client is using in the in vivo situation (e.g., leg muscles to stand) must have some tension. Sometimes the therapist's presence—which is reassuring and calming to the client—serves as a competing response. The in vivo exposure proceeds up an anxiety hierarchy, and the client has the option of terminating the exposure if it becomes too uncomfortable. The basic procedures of in vivo exposure are illustrated in the case of a 36-year-old man who had been in a psychiatric hospital for 7 years and was intensely afraid of venturing outside the hospital (Weidner, 1970). As Weidner reports:

> After several relaxation sessions in the office, the relaxation sessions were continued while the patient was seated in an automobile. Each week the

automobile was driven by the therapist closer to the gate of the hospital grounds, and then farther and farther away . . . until a five-mile drive took place during the third session in the car. During each trip outside the hospital, the patient was let out of the car for increasing lengths of time, going from one minute to a half-hour in three weeks. Concomitant with therapy sessions outside the hospital grounds, the patient was encouraged to go on trips with other patients. By the seventh week, the patient had been to a country fair in the neighboring state, an art show across the river, a local fireman's carnival, and a fishing trip. The art show was the only trip on which the therapist accompanied the patient, and even then, he was alone for half the two-hour show. After the seventh session it was no longer necessary to encourage the patient to go out on day passes, since he signed up for passes and outside activities on his own. At the end of seven in vivo [exposure] . . . sessions, the patient felt comfortable enough to venture outside the hospital without the support of the therapist [or other patients]. (p. 80)

Prolonged/Intense Exposure Therapies

Prolonged/intense exposure therapies, often called **flooding,** expose the client to threatening events (1) for a lengthy period (typically 10 to 15 minutes at a minimum and sometimes more than an hour) and (2) beginning and continuing with aspects of the events that elicit high anxiety (hence the name *flooding*). Despite the intensity of the exposure, the feared negative consequences do not actually occur—a characteristic of all exposure therapies. The exposure continues until the client's anxiety peaks and then begins to decline. The exposure in flooding can occur in the client's imagination or in vivo.

Imaginal Flooding   One advantage of imaginal flooding is that there are no practical restrictions regarding the types of anxiety-evoking situations that it can be used to treat. Victims of even the most traumatic experiences (e.g., floods, automobile accidents) can be safely exposed to them in imaginal flooding, as is illustrated in the following case.

Six months before his referral for academic and behavioral problems by his school principal, a 14-year-old Lebanese boy had been abducted in Beirut by the Lebanese militia and held for 2 days (Saigh, 1987). The boy was suffering from posttraumatic stress disorder. He avoided going to the area where he had been abducted and was experiencing anxiety related to recollections of the abduction. He also had difficulty concentrating and remembering information, and he was depressed. The client had not experienced these problems before he was abducted.

The therapist described the pros and cons of imaginal flooding and systematic desensitization, and the client and his parents chose flooding. Before treatment, the client's emotional and cognitive functioning was assessed. Also, to assess the client's degree of anxiety, two of the therapist's assistants unobtrusively observed the client as he attempted to perform 12 specific behaviors in a *behavioral avoidance test* (beginning with leaving his home and walking to the area of his abduction, later entering a store in the area and making a purchase, and ending with his walking home by another route).

Each of the six therapy sessions consisted of 60 minutes of flooding, involving four scenes related to his abduction (e.g., "being interrogated, responding, receiving repeated blows to the head and body, and experiencing intermittent periods of isolation" [Saigh, 1987, p. 148]). (It may seem that dealing with the client's recollections of traumatic experiences that occurred in the past is contrary to the present focus of behavior therapy. In fact, memories are present events, and it is those present memories that were maintaining the client's posttraumatic stress symptoms.)

Immediately after treatment, the client's anxiety and depression decreased, and his memory and concentration improved significantly. These treatment gains were maintained at a 4-month follow-up. Immediately after treatment and 4 months later, the client completed all 12 steps of the behavioral avoidance test, compared with only four steps prior to therapy. After the termination of therapy, the client visited the area where he had been abducted several times and reported experiencing no abnormal anxiety on these occasions. Finally, the client expressed satisfaction with the flooding treatment, and he commented that the success of the therapy was adequate compensation for the discomfort he experienced during the flooding sessions.

In Vivo Flooding In vivo flooding—prolonged/intense exposure to the actual anxiety-evoking events—often includes **response prevention,** in which clients are specifically prevented from engaging in their typical anxiety-reducing behaviors. Response prevention is an essential component in the treatment of obsessive-compulsive disorder, in which a person is preoccupied (obsessed) with particular anxiety-evoking events and alleviates the resulting anxiety by performing maladaptive, ritualistic behaviors (compulsions).

Consider the case of R. H., a 36-year-old Catholic man who had a 14-year history of religious-related obsessions and compulsions (Abramowitz, 2001). He obsessed about being "damned to hell" because he had said or done things that he mistakenly believed were against Catholic doctrine (e.g., laughing at a tasteless joke). To alleviate his guilt about his assumed transgressions, R. H. compulsively sought reassurance that he had not sinned, such as by mentally reviewing the events or by talking to a priest. He spent more than 8 hours a day preoccupied with his obsessional doubts and seeking reassurance about his religious failings.

To expose R. H. to events that triggered anxiety, the therapist instructed R. H. to deliberately behave in ways that he considered sinful (e.g., telling a tasteless joke). The response prevention entailed refraining from engaging in any behaviors he had previously used to reduce his uncertainty about the sinfulness

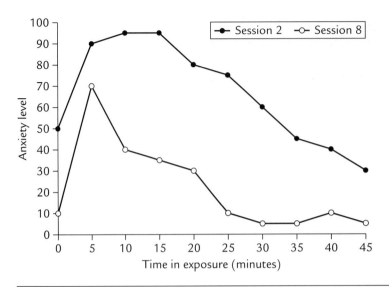

Figure 8.5 Levels During Imaginal Flooding for Religious Obsessions and Compulsions
Adapted from Abramowitz, 2001.

of his deed. Imaginal flooding also was used to expose R. H. to the consequences he feared would occur for his "sinful" acts. Figure 8.5 shows the expected peaking and subsequent decline of anxiety during R. H.'s imaginal flooding.

At home, between treatment sessions, R. H. engaged in daily in vivo and imaginal flooding (using audiotapes of in-session imaginal exposure). At the end of 8 weeks of treatment, R. H.'s obsessions and compulsions decreased significantly and remained at that level at a 6-month follow-up. Additionally, R. H. reported being more hopeful about his life and more interested in engaging in social and recreational activities that had not been part of his life prior to treatment.

In the report of R. H.'s case, the therapist comments on the unique challenges of treating religious obsessions and compulsions, which, in most cases, requires consultation with clergy.

> Differences between normal and pathological religious practices must be clarified and . . . [clients] should understand that the purpose of treatment is to restore normal religiosity. Moreover, a clear explanation of how exposure is consistent with this goal seems crucial for fostering a successful therapeutic relationship and maintaining high motivation. (Abramowitz, 2001, pp. 83–84)

Response prevention has been used to treat obsessive worry, such as in the case of a 76-year-old woman who worried about a minor physical discomfort that she thought might be symptomatic of serious disease but that was in fact not (Gorenstein et al., 1999). The woman reduced her anxiety by compulsively seeking reassurance that she was not ill through reading books and talking to friends and physicians. The response prevention consisted of the woman's delaying her reassurance rituals for 24 hours, at which point she was permitted to reassess her discomfort. Gradually, the delay period was increased to several days. The woman's worry decreased considerably and, for the most part, so did her physical "symptoms."

Flexibility in terms of modifying standard procedures is important in treating the elderly. For example, with clients suffering from cognitive deficits, which often is the case with the elderly (Calamari, Faber, Hitsman, & Poppe, 1994; Colvin & Boddington, 1997) and also people with mental retardation (Hiss & Kozak, 1991), repeating treatment rationales and instructions many times may be required. Supervision may be necessary for treatment compliance, as was the case with a 78-year-old man suffering from obsessive-compulsive disorder (Carmin, Wiegartz, Yunus, & Gillock, 2002). Flooding with response prevention was unsuccessful on an outpatient basis, but it was successful when the man was in the hospital, where the response prevention could be monitored by staff members.

Exposure Therapies and Diverse Clients

Abundant empirical evidence indicates that, in general, exposure therapies are highly effective in reducing anxiety and other negative emotions that are the result of a wide array of disorders, including phobic disorders, obsessive-compulsive disorder, and stress disorders (Spiegler & Guevermont, 2003). Most of the evidence comes from studies in which the clients were from the majority culture. However, the number of studies involving diverse clients has increased significantly in recent years.

For the treatment of anxiety disorders in Latino-American youths, one promising finding is that exposure therapies in both individual and group formats seem to be as effective with them as with European-American youths (Pina, Silverman, Fuentes, Kurtines, & Weems, 2003). This is an important finding not only because Latino Americans are the largest and fastest-growing minority group in the United States but also because anxiety disorders in youths are the most prevalent psychiatric disorders that do not diminish without treatment (e.g., Woodward, & Fergusson, 2001).

A recent study demonstrated the efficacy of flooding for obsessive-compulsive disorder among African Americans and Caribbean Americans (Friedman et al., 2003). However, earlier research had indicated that whereas African Americans suffering from agoraphobia, another anxiety disorder, can benefit from exposure therapy, the decrease in anxiety may not be as great as for

European Americans (Chambless & Williams, 1995; Williams & Chambless, 1994). One possible reason for this difference is that existing racial prejudice may interfere with the process, and hence with the outcome, of exposure therapy. This can be seen in the following reconstructed dialogue between a European-American behavior therapist and her African-American client as they attempted in vivo exposure for anxiety about going to a shopping mall (Williams & Chambless, 1994, p. 159).

> C (Client): I really don't want to do this today.
>
> T (Therapist) [*Thinking anticipatory anxiety was the issue.*]: I know you are anxious about going there, but think of it as a chance to confront and overcome the fear.
>
> C: No, you don't understand. I don't have any money with me. I can't buy anything.
>
> T: That's okay. You can window shop. A lot of people do that. For some people, it's a cheap way to have a good time.
>
> C: That's okay for you. White people can go into a store and just browse. But if a Black person does it, the store security people will watch her like a hawk. If I don't act like I'm really buying something, they'll think I'm stealing.

Another explanation for African Americans' not benefiting as much as European Americans from flooding for agoraphobia might be that stressors in the lives of many African Americans (such as financial hardships and living in high crime areas) may contribute to higher levels of general anxiety. Clearly, factors specific to a particular group of people must be considered in understanding clients' problems and in structuring treatments appropriately.

Reluctance to seek treatment and follow through with it once in therapy is a general problem in the mental health field. It is especially salient with members of certain ethnic populations for whom counseling for personal problems is not an accepted practice in their culture. For instance, young African-American men may be disinclined to seek psychological treatment either because they believe that they will be mistreated in therapy or because of the powerful peer pressure on inner-city youths to take a stoic, tough-guy attitude toward personal problems (Griffith, Ezra, & Baker, 1993). In such cases, behavior therapies that clients find more acceptable are likely to be better choices for them. For example, brief/graduated exposure would be a better choice than prolonged/intense exposure for anxiety disorders because the former involves less distress than the latter (e.g., Greyson, Foa, & Steketee, 1985; Horne & Matson, 1977; Richard, 1995; Smith, Marcus, & Eldredge, 1994).

Behavior therapists also must consider possible diversity factors—including racial, cultural, socioeconomic, gender, sexual orientation, and age factors—that may be relevant to the maintenance and treatment of problem behaviors. The importance of taking into account diversity factors can be seen in the treatment of a 39-year-old African-American female physician suffering from a chronic, severe social phobia (Fink, Turner, & Beidel, 1996). The client reported experiencing anxiety when she interacted with other medical professionals and in social situations, especially with strangers. Consequentially, she avoided such encounters whenever possible. Initially, imaginal and in vivo flooding resulted in a moderate reduction of her anxiety. However, the flooding achieved its greatest effectiveness only after her counselor discovered that interaction with European-American physicians was particularly troublesome for the client. At that point, the counselor introduced racial variables into the situations to which she was exposed, which made a significant difference in the potency of the flooding treatment.

Earlier I mentioned the importance of flexibility in adapting standard treatment methods for the elderly. Flexibility needs to be a general guideline with diverse clients for whom special circumstances and issues may be more the rule than the exception. In working with low-income women, for example, removing structural barriers, such as having limited access to transportation and babysitters, which makes coming to therapy difficult, can be a prerequisite for administering counseling (Feske, 2001; McNair, 1996; Miranda, Azocar, Organista, Munoz, & Lieberman, 1996).

Modeling Therapy

Learning by observing what people do (observational learning) is a pervasive part of human life. People learn language, attitudes and values, preferences, standards for how to act, mannerisms, emotional responses, and countless social skills by observing others. **Modeling therapies** work by exposing a client (an observer) to a person (a model) who is engaging in a behavior from which the client could benefit by imitating. Besides observing a model's behaviors, clients also observe the consequences of the model's behaviors. These *vicarious consequences* tell clients what is likely to happen to them if they imitate the model. Models can be *live*, that is physically present, or *symbolic*, such as people or characters on TV or in books.

Modeling therapy serves four basic functions: (1) teaching behaviors, (2) prompting behaviors, (3) motivating to perform behaviors, and (4) reducing fear or anxiety. Modeling is often part of a treatment package involving other behavior therapies such as prompting, reinforcement, shaping, role playing, and **behavior rehearsal** (practicing performing a behavior).

In contrast to the directive nature of many behavior therapies, modeling therapy has the advantage of being subtle. The client need not be told to perform a particular behavior; just being exposed to a model engaging in the behavior and to the reinforcement the model receives for performing the behavior (vicarious reinforcement) may be sufficient to foster imitation. Because of this feature, modeling therapy is useful with clients from cultures in which subtlety and self-determination are valued (e.g., Cambodian, Native American, and Slavic).

Modeling therapies have been used primarily for two broad classes of problems: skills deficits and fear or anxiety. The next two sections describe a variety of modeling therapy procedures to deal with these problems.

Skills Training

Skills training refers to treatment packages that may consist of modeling, direct instruction, prompting, shaping, reinforcement, corrective feedback, behavior rehearsal, and role playing. The purpose of skills training is to teach clients to cope with skills deficits. Modeling is an essential component of skills training because direct instruction often is insufficient to communicate the subtleties of performing complex skills, and prompting and shaping alone may be insufficient (e.g., Charlop & Milstein, 1989; Gambrill, 1995). The client may need to "see" the behavior performed (e.g., Star, 1986). After skills are learned and practiced in the safety of the therapy session, clients are given homework assignments to use the skills in their daily lives; the homework begins with simple, nonthreatening situations and progresses to more involved and potentially threatening situations.

Skills training has been used for a wide array of skills deficit problems and clients. Examples include teaching language as well as social and daily-living skills to children with autistic disorder (e.g., Charlop & Milstein, 1989; Charlop, Schreibman, & Tryon, 1983; Egel, Richman, & Koegel, 1983; Lovaas, 1977, 1987) and mental retardation (e.g., Goldstein & Mousetis, 1989; Rietveld, 1983), training adults with chronic psychiatric disorders to engage in social and daily living skills (e.g., Spiegler, 1971, 1973; Spiegler & Agigian, 1977), teaching children and adults to avoid being abducted (Miltenberger & Thiesse-Duffy, 1988; Poche, Brouwer, & Swearingen, 1981; Poche, Yoder, & Miltenberger, 1988) and sexually abused (Lumley, Miltenberger, Long, Rapp, & Roberts, 1998; Miltenberger et al., 1999; Wurtele, 1990; Wurtele, Currier, Gillispie, & Franklin, 1991; Wurtele, Marrs, & Miller-Perrin, 1987), increasing peer interaction among children (Ballard & Crooks, 1984; Gumpel & Frank, 1999; O'Connor, 1969; Rao, Moely, & Lockman, 1987), and reducing aggressive behaviors in clients ranging from African-American elementary school children (Middleton & Cartledge, 1995) to institutionalized elderly patients (Vaccaro, 1992).

Similarity between the model and the observer generally enhances imitation (Bandura, 1986), and similarity is maximized by **self-modeling,** which involves clients' serving as their own models of adaptive functioning (Meharg & Woltersdorf, 1990). With **covert self-modeling,** clients imagine themselves performing the target behavior. With **video self-modeling therapy** (Dowrick, 1991, 1994), clients watch videos of themselves performing adaptive behaviors, which often promotes all four functions of modeling (teaching, prompting, motivating, and reducing performance anxiety).

Video self-modeling was one component of a treatment package designed to help elderly patients at a hearing center in Uppsala, Sweden handle problems associated with their hearing deficits (Andersson, Melin, Scott, & Lindberg, 1995). First, skills training was used to teach the patients various tactics for improving their hearing while holding conversations in locations where there is loud background noise (which is especially difficult for people with hearing impairment). Then they were videotaped successfully conversing with one another with loud restaurant noise in the background. Finally, they watched the videotape of themselves and observed their engaging in the difficult behavior. The treatment package resulted in the patients' coping better with their hearing impairments than comparable patients who received no treatment.

All too frequently in nursing homes, psychotropic medications are used to control disruptive behaviors rather than treat clients' disorders (Office of Inspector General, 1996). In a nursing home in New York City, elderly clients suffering from dementia and schizophrenia were exposed to a modeling treatment package—including *cognitive behavior rehearsal* (practicing in one's mind) and reinforcement—to decrease their verbally disruptive and demanding or combative behaviors as well as to improve their overall functioning (Mansdorf, Calapai, Caselli, Burstein, & Dimant, 1999). Not only was the treatment effective in meeting these goals, but it made it possible for the staff to reduce the dosages of psychotropic medication given to the clients as "chemical restraints."

Although skills training has been used to teach clients a wide variety of skills, social skills and assertive behaviors are the most frequent targets of skills training.

Social Skills Training   *Social skills,* the interpersonal competencies necessary to successfully interact with others, are essential for functioning on a daily basis. A deficit in social skills often is related to a variety of adjustment problems throughout life (Frame & Matson, 1987). This is particularly true for bicultural teens who are struggling to develop a sense of identity and social competence in the face of competing cultural values. For instance, whereas Latina adolescents traditionally are socialized to be submissive and passive, they also are exposed to contrasting values of the dominant Western culture, such as individualism, independence, and ambition. "Consequently, the Latina adolescent may feel trapped and in a 'cultural double bind,' meaning, if she tries to assert herself, her family may view this behavior as insolent and disrespectful; on the other hand if she does not, she runs the risk of adversely affecting her sense of self" (Peeks, 1999, p. 142).

Social skills training—skills training specifically for developing social skills—has been used to help Latina adolescents deal with such conflicts (e.g., Peeks, 1999; Planells-Bloom, 1992). Group social skills training may be especially appropriate (Peeks, 1999). In contrast to individual social skills training, a group format has the advantage of enabling clients to share their common cultural background and the cross-cultural conflicts they are experiencing.

Although social skills deficits in children and adolescents are well recognized, they also occur in adults. For example, social skills training has been used to teach elderly clients conversational skills to decrease their feelings of loneliness and to teach them how to reinforce and extinguish the behaviors of people on whom they depend (e.g., relatives and caretakers) (Carstensen & Fisher, 1991). Because adults with schizophrenia have severe social skills deficits, social skills training often is a component of the treatment of schizophrenia (Spiegler, 1971; Spiegler & Agigian, 1977).

Assertion Training   **Assertion training** is a specialized skills training procedure that involves a treatment package to teach people both how and when to behave assertively. *Assertive behaviors*—a particular class of social skills—are actions that secure and maintain what you are entitled to in an interpersonal situation, without violating the rights of others. Assertive behaviors may involve standing up for your rights, refusing unreasonable requests, expressing opinions and feelings, and expressing desires or requests. Such assertive behaviors appear a priori to be both appropriate and adaptive, but that is not always the case, depending on the context or situation (Gambrill, 1995**)**. For example, the appropriateness of acting assertively varies in different cultures. Assertive behaviors generally are considered admirable in many Western cultures in which individualism and independence are valued. In contrast, in cultures that value collectivism and interdependence, such as Japanese and Puerto Rican cultures, assertive behaviors are likely to be seen as socially inappropriate. Even in cultures that consider asserting one's rights to be appropriate, acting assertively may not always be the best choice. Consider an everyday example. Your waiter leaves you the check. You look it over and find that you have been overcharged by a small amount. You can act assertively and wait for your waiter to return and ask for the check to be corrected. However, if you are in a hurry, you may decide to pay the higher amount, which would be an unassertive but appropriate response under the circumstances.

Modeling is a major component in assertion training. Besides its being a generally efficient and effective means of teaching clients assertive behaviors, modeling is particularly useful in teaching clients the stylistic components of assertive behaviors that are difficult to describe verbally, such as appropriate voice volume and expression to show confidence.

Modeling and behavior rehearsal in therapy sessions are followed with homework assignments in which clients practice assertive behaviors in a stepwise progression (from easy to difficult and from less threatening to more threatening) in their everyday lives.

The nature of assertion training is illustrated in the case of Amira, a 33-year-old woman from Yemen who had immigrated to the United States 3 years previously. She worked as an insurance agent in an office where there were only three female agents, and Amira was the youngest and newest. Since the beginning of her employment, the male agents frequently asked Amira to do a variety of stereotypical female tasks, such as bring in coffee and lunch for the office staff. Because Amira had been raised with the traditional Yemenite value that serving men is appropriate, she initially acquiesced to her co-workers' requests. However, as she became increasingly assimilated into the dominant United States culture, she became conflicted about being the "office housewife," and this led her to seek counseling. The following is an excerpt from the initial assertion training session.

C (Client): I know that my traditional upbringing feeds into my complying with my colleagues' requests, but I don't think it is appropriate—this is not Yemen. It's the United States. They are taking advantage of me.

T (Therapist): You know, you can refuse to comply with their unreasonable requests.

C: I'm not sure that I know how to do that. I've never done it before. It's a little scary.

T: What we can do is to teach you appropriate assertive behaviors for the situation and then you can practice them with me. When you feel comfortable enough, you can gradually begin to use them in your office.

C: I guess so, but it goes against all I've known for most of my life.

T: Well, let's just try a simple role play and see how it goes.

C: Okay.

T: For the moment, let's role-play a typical situation for you. You pretend that you are one of your male co-workers, and I'll pretend I am you. You ask me to do something unreasonable, and I'll give you an example of an appropriate assertive response. Let's try it. Ask me to do something unreasonable.

C: All right. Bob might say, "Hey, Amira, you're not doing anything important. How about going to get us some coffee and donuts, like a good little girl." [*role playing*] He said something just like that yesterday.

T: "I'd love some coffee, Bob, but I'm in the middle of working up a quote for a client. So maybe you or someone else could get us all coffee." [*modeling*]

C: I couldn't say that. It goes against my grain. It's scary.

T: Well, you certainly don't have to use my exact words. I'm just giving you an example. What would you feel comfortable saying for a start? Let's switch roles. You be yourself, and I'll be Bob. You respond to what I say. "Amira, some of us would like some coffee. How about getting it for us?" [*role playing*]

C: "Oh, I guess so. But I am busy right now. As soon as I finish, I guess I could." [*behavior rehearsal*]

T: Not bad. [*reinforcement*] It sure isn't totally giving in to the request; and you're not exactly saying that you will. [*feedback*]. Do you think you could go one step further and tell Bob you don't want to get the coffee?

C: What would I say?

T: How about something like, "I'd rather not go for coffee." [*modeling*] Words to that effect make it clear that you don't want to but you aren't actually saying no, which may be hard for you at first. [*direct instruction*] Let's try again. "Amira, some of us would like some coffee. How about getting it for us?" [*role playing*]

C: "I'm really busy, Bob, so this isn't a good time for me to get coffee." [*behavior rehearsal*]

T: Very good. [*reinforcement*] That's much better. [*feedback*] Your first response indicated you probably would get the coffee later. Now you are saying no, albeit indirectly. [*shaping*] Do you see the difference?

C: Yeah, I do.

The modeling and behavior rehearsal continued for several sessions until Amira felt comfortable enough to attempt responding assertively to unreasonable requests her male co-works made.

Typically, the therapist models appropriate assertive behaviors for a client, as in the previous example. Sometimes clients will use people in their everyday environment as models of assertive behavior. This was the case with a 7-year-old girl who had been sexually abused (Krop & Burgess, 1993). Subsequently, whenever she felt taken advantage of she responded with emotional outbursts and sexually inappropriate behaviors. The girl's treatment consisted of her visualizing scenes in which a peer model assertively dealt with negative feelings (e.g., the model told the teacher that she didn't think it was fair to ask her to erase the blackboard because she had done it earlier in the day).

Hundreds of studies have demonstrated the efficacy of assertion training for clients with diverse problems across the age spectrum (Gambrill, 1995). Outside of behavior therapy, assertion training has been used in other approaches to psychotherapy (such as Gestalt therapy). One application of assertion training in health psychology has been to prevent HIV infection by teaching people who are especially vulnerable to contracting HIV to refuse to engage in unsafe sex practices (e.g., Carey et al., 2000; Kalichman, Cherry, & Browne-Sperling, 1999; Weinhardt, Carey, Carey, & Verdecias, 1998). These applications have been effective in reducing the risk of contracting HIV by decreasing the number of sexual partners and sexual contacts with strangers people have and increasing their use of condoms.

Reducing Fear by Modeling: Vicarious Extinction

Fear or anxiety is maintained by two sets of factors: anticipating negative consequences (e.g., expecting to be turned down when asking for a date) and skills deficits (e.g., not knowing how to ask for a date). Modeling treats both sets of maintaining conditions simultaneously. The process is called **vicarious extinction** and involves a model who demonstrates an anxiety-evoking behavior without incurring negative consequences. Modeling can be live (e.g., the therapist engages in the anxiety-evoking behavior) or symbolic (e.g., in a movie). Usually, a **coping model** is employed—that is, someone who is initially fearful and at least somewhat incompetent in performing a behavior but who then, in the course of the modeling sequence, becomes more comfortable and skilled in performing the behavior (Meichenbaum, 1971). Coping models increase model-observer similarity and thus enhance imitation.

In one unusual case, a mother served as a model for her 4-year-old daughter who needed restorative dental work but was intensely afraid of going to the dentist (Klesges, Malott, & Ugland, 1984). The mother also was afraid of dentists (a likely maintaining condition of her daughter's fear), which made her useful as a coping model. In the initial sessions, the daughter and mother watched videos of dental procedures (*symbolic modeling*) and spent time in the dental office (*in vivo exposure*). Later, the mother allowed dental procedures to be done on her with some initial hesitancy (*live modeling*) and commented that it "wasn't all that bad" (*vicarious reinforcement*). After seven therapy sessions, the daughter was able to undergo two dental procedures under local anesthesia without any outward signs of fear. By the end of her daughter's therapy, the mother also had overcome her intense fear of dental procedures, which is what makes this case unusual. This outcome is not surprising because although the mother was not treated directly for her fear of dentistry, she was exposed to the video models, she had participated in the in vivo exposure, and she experienced self-modeling and behavior rehearsal when she served as a model for her daughter.

Participant modeling is a treatment package in which the therapist models the anxiety-evoking behavior for the client, then encourages and guides the client to practice the behavior (Ritter, 1968a, 1968b). The three basic steps are:

1. *Modeling.* The therapist first models the anxiety-evoking behavior for the client.

2. *Prompting, behavior rehearsal,* and *in vivo exposure.* The therapist verbally prompts the client to imitate the behavior she or he has just modeled. Then, to help the client engage in the behavior, the therapist physically prompts the client. For example, with a client who is afraid of riding on elevators, the therapist might take the client's arm and guide the client into an elevator. The physical contact between the therapist and client also reassures and calms the client, and these feelings compete with anxiety (which is a component of in vivo exposure).

3. *Fading prompts.* The therapist gradually withdraws verbal and physical prompts. The client begins to perform the behavior with the therapist present but without physical contact and finally without the therapist present.

The behaviors that are modeled and practiced are arranged in an anxiety hierarchy, and the treatment proceeds from the least to the most threatening behaviors. The basic steps in participant modeling are illustrated in the following case.

Bhagwan M. was a 37-year-old man who had lived all but the last 7 months of his life in a small village in the mountains of northern India. Bhagwan was living with relatives who had brought him to the United States for medical treatment. When Bhagwan recovered from his illness, his relatives asked him to remain with them, which he did. He adjusted well to his new culture and life except that he was intensely afraid of crossing streets, which meant that he had to remain at home except when he was driven someplace by his relatives. Bhagwan was highly motivated to overcome his fear, and a behavior therapist was found who spoke Hindi.

The initial therapy sessions were held in a residential area with narrow streets and little traffic. The therapist first modeled walking across a street a number of times as Bhagwan watched. Then the therapist firmly took Bhagwan's arm and walked with him across the street. This was done repeatedly until Bhagwan reported minimal anxiety. The street crossing was continued as the physical contact gradually was reduced (holding the client's arm lightly, then just touching it) until it was eliminated and the therapist just walked with the client. This too was gradually reduced: first the therapist walked slightly behind Bhagwan, then several feet behind him, and finally the therapist remained on the sidewalk. In later sessions, these procedures were repeated on increasingly wider and busier streets. Between sessions, Bhagwan practiced walking across streets on his own. After 11 sessions, Bhagwan felt comfortable crossing most streets on his own.

Film and video modeling for common fears can be a highly cost-efficient treatment. Standard films or videos depicting coping models gradually overcoming specific fears can be made and then shown to many clients. Frequently, one or two viewings of a brief modeling film is sufficient to vicariously extinguish fears (e.g., Melamed & Siegel, 1975; Spiegler, Liebert, McMains, & Fernandez, 1969; Vernon, 1974). The earliest uses of film and video modeling were for fear of small animals, such as dogs (Bandura & Menlove, 1968) and snakes (Spiegler et al., 1969). Standard modeling videos for treating and preventing fear of medical and dental procedures have been used with thousands of patients (e.g., Allen, Danforth, & Drabman, 1989; Jay, Elliott, Ozolins, Olson, & Pruitt, 1985; Melamed & Siegel, 1975; Shipley, Butt, & Horwitz, 1979; Shipley, Butt, Horwitz, & Farbry, 1978; Vernon, 1974), and many pediatric hospitals use video modeling to prepare children for hospitalization and surgery (Peterson & Ridley-Johnson, 1980).

Storytelling is another variation of symbolic modeling used to treat fear. Parents and teachers frequently use stories, rather than direct instructions, to help children cope with fears (compare with Swaggart et al., 1995). Modeling has the advantage of providing suggestions rather than directives, which puts children in charge of their own behaviors. To reduce children's fears in the wake of major disasters (such as the devastating hurricanes in the southeastern United States in the summer of 2005), parents have been advised to expose their children to stories that depict similar-age models who are coping with fear. In response to the widespread fear among children immediately after the 9/11 disaster, the TV series *Sesame Street* produced a segment depicting Elmo (a fuzzy puppet) as a coping model who deals with his fear after a fire in his neighborhood.

Efficacy of Modeling Therapy

Overall, modeling is highly effective and efficient in reducing skills deficits and treating fear and anxiety-related disorders (Bandura, 1986; Rachman & Wilson, 1980). Modeling simultaneously teaches clients adaptive behaviors, prompts their performance, motivates their practice, and reduces anxiety about performing the behaviors. Modeling often is a component of cognitive restructuring and cognitive coping skills therapies, as you will see in the next chapter. Finally, modeling is an inherent component of many behavior therapies as well as other forms of counseling because counselors serve as positive models for their clients in a variety of ways (e.g., by exhibiting optimism, evaluating problems rationally, and expressing emotions appropriately).

To Be Continued

As I explained at the beginning of this chapter, behavior therapy is too broad an approach to be covered in a single chapter. This chapter has introduced behavior therapy and examined the so-called traditional behavior therapies. The next chapter covers cognitive-behavioral therapies and concludes with general issues that pertain to the entire field of behavior therapy: evaluation, relevant problems and client populations, critique, and future development.

Summary

1. Contemporary behavior therapy consists of two branches: traditional behavior therapy (described in this chapter) and cognitive-behavioral therapy (described in the next chapter). The term *behavior therapy* refers to both branches.

2. The inspiration for traditional behavior therapy came from experimental research on learning conducted in the early 1900s, and its philosophical roots lie in behaviorism. Behavior therapy began in the 1950s, when Wolpe developed systematic desensitization. The impetus for behavior therapy came after World War II with the pressing need for a more effective and efficient means of treating veterans with psychological disorders than psychoanalytic therapy could offer. Early behavior therapy efforts were met with strong resistance from nonbehavioral mental health professionals.

3. In the 1960s, Bandura's social learning theory, Beck's cognitive therapy, and Ellis's rational emotive therapy ushered in cognitive-behavioral therapy. In the 1970s, behavior therapy emerged as a major counseling approach. In the last 15–20 years, there has been increasing integration of nonbehavioral counseling techniques into behavior therapy and attention to applying behavior therapy to diverse client populations.

4. The basic theory of behavior therapy is the ABC model that describes the functional relationship of antecedents, behavior, and consequences.

Antecedents (events that are present before the behavior is performed) "set the stage for" and elicit a behavior, and the consequences of engaging in a behavior determine whether the person will repeat the behavior. Behavior therapies directly change the present antecedents and consequences that are maintaining (causing) a client's problem behaviors.

5. The process of behavior therapy involves eight basic steps: clarifying the client's problem, formulating goals, defining a target behavior, identifying the maintaining conditions of the target behavior, designing a treatment plan to change the maintaining conditions, implementing the treatment plan, evaluating the effectiveness of the plan, and conducting follow-up assessments.

6. All behavior therapies share four defining themes—scientific approach, engagement in specific actions, present focus, and learning focus—and generally share four common characteristics—individualized treatment, stepwise progression, treatment packages, and brevity.

7. Stimulus control procedures change antecedents that elicit behaviors. The antecedents can be prompts that provide cues to remind or instruct clients to perform behaviors and setting events that are environmental conditions in which behaviors occur.

8. Reinforcement (consequences that increase the likelihood that a person will engage in a behavior) motivates clients to engage in adaptive and desirable behaviors. Shaping involves reinforcing components of a behavior in sequence until the full behavior is performed.

9. Differential reinforcement is used to indirectly decrease undesirable behaviors by reinforcing more adaptive alternative behaviors. Direct therapies for decreasing undesirable behaviors include extinction, time out from positive reinforcement, response cost, overcorrection, and physically aversive consequences.

10. A token economy is a system for motivating clients to perform desirable behaviors and to refrain from performing undesirable behaviors. Clients earn token reinforcers for desirable behaviors and lose them for undesirable behaviors. They exchange the tokens for actual reinforcers.

11. Exposure therapies treat anxiety and other negative emotional responses by exposing clients to the events that create the negative emotions. In brief/graduated exposure, the client is exposed for short periods to threatening events in a gradual manner. Systematic desensitization has the client imagine successively more anxiety-arousing situations while the client engages in a response that competes with anxiety, usually progressive relaxation (which by itself is used as a treatment for anxiety). In vivo

exposure therapy involves systematic desensitization with actual exposure to anxiety-inducing events.

12. Prolonged/intense exposure therapies (flooding) expose clients for extended periods to highly anxiety-evoking events. The exposure can be in the client's imagination or to the actual events (in vivo). Flooding often involves response prevention in which clients are prevented from engaging in their typical anxiety-reducing behaviors.

13. Modeling therapies expose a client to a model who performs behaviors from which the client can benefit by imitating. Not only do clients observe a model's behaviors but they also observe the consequences of those behaviors, which influences whether the clients will imitate the model. Models can be live (physically present) or symbolic (as on TV).

14. Modeling therapies serve four functions: teaching behaviors, prompting behaviors, motivating behaviors, and reducing fear or anxiety.

15. Modeling is a key component in skills training, which is a treatment package for treating clients' skills deficits; other components that may be included in skills training are direct instruction, prompting, shaping, reinforcement, corrective feedback, behavior rehearsal, and role playing.

16. Self-modeling, in which clients serve as their own models (in their imagination or on a video), maximizes observer-model similarity, which enhances imitation.

17. Social skills training is used to ameliorate deficits clients have in interpersonal competencies. Assertion training is a specialized social skills training procedure that teaches clients when and how to behave assertively. The appropriateness of assertive behavior varies with the context, which includes specific situations as well as cultural norms.

18. Vicarious extinction involves reducing fear or anxiety by having a client observe a model who performs the feared behavior without the model incurring negative consequences. A coping model who is initially fearful and incompetent and then gradually becomes more comfortable and competent performing the feared behavior is typically used in vicarious extinction.

19. In participant modeling, the therapist models the anxiety-evoking behaviors for the client, then verbally and physically prompts the client to perform the behaviors, and finally fades the prompts.

20. Film/video modeling has been used to treat fear of medical procedures in both children and adults. Storytelling is another form of symbolic modeling used to reduce fear and other negative emotions in children.

21. Modeling therapies are effective and efficient treatments for skills deficits and for anxiety-related disorders. They simultaneously teach clients adaptive behaviors, prompt performance, motivate practice, and reduce anxiety about performing the threatening behaviors.

Key Terms

ABC model (p. 285)
antecedents (p. 285)
anxiety hierarchy (p. 299)
assertion training (p. 310)
backup reinforcers (p. 297)
behavior rehearsal (p. 307)
brief/graduated exposure therapies (p. 298)
consequences (p. 285)
coping model (p. 313)
covert self-modeling (p. 309)
differential reinforcement (p. 294)
differential relaxation (p. 301)
exposure therapies (p. 298)
extinction (p. 295)
flooding (p. 302)
homework assignment (p. 288)
in vivo (p. 289)
in vivo exposure therapy (p. 301)
maintaining conditions (p. 285)
modeling therapies (p. 307)
overcorrection (p. 296)
participant modeling (p. 314)
physically aversive consequences (p. 297)

progressive relaxation (p. 298)
prolonged/intense exposure therapies (p. 302)
prompts (p. 291)
punishment (p. 294)
reinforcement (p. 292)
reinforcer (p. 292)
response cost (p. 295)
response prevention (p. 303)
self-modeling (p. 309)
setting events (p. 291)
shaping (p. 293)
skills training (p. 308)
social skills training (p. 310)
stimulus control (p. 291)
systematic desensitization (p. 298)
target behavior (p. 286)
time out from positive reinforcement (p. 295)
token economy (p. 297)
treatment package (p. 290)
vicarious extinction (p. 313)
video self-modeling therapy (p. 309)

Resources for Further Study

The professional organizations, professional journals, suggested readings, and other media resources for Chapter 8 are listed at the end of Chapter 9.

Chapter 9

Behavior Therapy II: Cognitive-Behavioral Therapy

Michael D. Spiegler

In Chapter 8, you were introduced to traditional behavior therapy, the older branch of behavior therapy. Now you will learn about the other, more recently developed branch of behavior therapy: **cognitive-behavioral therapy,** which consists of interventions that directly or indirectly change clients' cognitions (e.g., thoughts and beliefs) that are maintaining their problem behaviors.

After describing this second branch of behavior therapy, I will discuss some general issues that pertain to both branches. In those sections, and elsewhere in the chapter, remember that the term *behavior therapy* refers to both traditional behavior therapy and cognitive-behavioral therapy.

All behavior therapies—traditional and cognitive-behavioral—are predicated on the same basic theory of change: changing a problem behavior involves changing its maintaining conditions, which are found in the antecedents and consequences of the behavior. Further, all behavior therapies are united by sharing the same defining themes and common characteristics I discussed at the beginning of Chapter 8.

Practice of Cognitive-Behavioral Therapy

The major difference between the traditional behavior therapies and cognitive-behavioral therapies is a shift in focus from changing overt behaviors (observable actions) in the former to changing cognitions (covert behaviors that are not directly observable) in the latter. You should note, however, that cognitive-behavioral therapies often change clients' overt behaviors in order to change maladaptive cognitions that are maintaining psychological disorders and problems. To do so, they employ many traditional behavior therapy techniques—such as prompting, reinforcement, and modeling—which accounts for the hyphenated name *cognitive-behavioral* (where *behavioral* is short for *overt-behavioral*). There are two broad categories of cognitive-behavioral therapy: cognitive restructuring therapies and cognitive-behavioral coping skills therapies.

Cognitive Restructuring Therapies

Cognitive restructuring involves replacing maladaptive cognitions with adaptive cognitions (and thereby restructuring the cognitions). Cognitive restructuring therapies are used to treat a client's excess of maladaptive cognitions. As discussed previously, dealing with concrete, observable phenomena is a hallmark of behavior therapy. How, then, do behavior therapists deal with cognitions that are internal, private behaviors? You may discover the answer by doing the following one-minute exercise before you continue reading.

> Identify a problem that you must solve or deal with in the near future. Then, think about the problem for a minute. As you think about the problem, pay attention to your thinking and note the *form* or *nature* of your thoughts. Then continue reading.

If you were able to pay attention to your thoughts, you probably discovered that you were using words, phrases, and perhaps full sentences to think. Such **self-talk,** what people say to themselves when they are thinking, is the major focus in cognitive restructuring therapies. However, people usually are not aware that they silently talk to themselves. It is only when clients pay attention to their self-talk that they can change the cognitions that are maintaining their problems. Thus, the first step in cognitive restructuring therapies is for clients to become aware of their self-talk—especially before, during, and after their problem behaviors occur.

In cognitive restructuring therapies, clients learn to monitor their self-talk, identify maladaptive self-talk, and substitute adaptive self-talk for maladaptive self-talk. And the general strategy of cognitive restructuring has also been used in novel ways. For example, Goldfried (1988) used the Gestalt empty chair technique for treating anxiety disorders that are maintained by a client's conflicting "sides." The client alternated sitting in two different chairs, each chair representing one of the "sides," and talked to the other chair ("side"). Valdez (2000) proposed using this technique to help bicultural Latino-American clients struggling with the conflicting pulls of their Latino and European-American cultural identities. One chair would be used for the client's Latino identity and the other for the client's European-American identity. Valdez suggested that verbalizing the self-talk based on each cultural identity (perhaps in Spanish and English, depending on the identity "talking") facilitates identifying maladaptive assumptions and beliefs that can then be cognitively restructured. For instance, if a client's Latino self-talk included, "I shouldn't have to always speak in English," the client could restructure this thought to make it more adaptive, such as by thinking, "I can use Spanish whenever I am at home or with family and Latino friends."

In the following sections, three cognitive restructuring therapies are described: thought stopping, rational emotive behavior therapy, and cognitive therapy. In each of these therapies, cognitive restructuring is a primary mechanism of change, but other cognitive and behavioral techniques are used as well.

Thought Stopping

Thought stopping is an elegantly simple technique used to decrease the frequency, duration, and intensity of persistent, disturbing thoughts (e.g., constantly worrying about one's appearance or self-depreciating thoughts such as "I can't do anything right") (Wolpe, 1958; compare with Ellis, 1989b). Thought stopping consists of two phases: (1) interrupting the disturbing thoughts, and then (2) replacing the disturbing thoughts with nondisturbing competing thoughts.

First, when the disturbing thought occurs, the client sharply says, "Stop!" Clients initially say "Stop!" aloud and later say it to themselves silently. This usually eliminates the intrusive thoughts momentarily. (You may be able to observe how this works by thinking for a moment about something upsetting and then deliberately screaming "Stop!" aloud. Obviously, this is best done when you are alone.) However, the thoughts the client has interrupted are likely to reappear if the client does not begin thinking about something else. Accordingly, in the second phase of thought stopping, immediately after saying "Stop!" the client focuses on a prepared thought (e.g., "There are lots of things that I do right") that competes with the disturbing thought (e.g., "I can't do anything right").

Both phases of thought stopping were used in premarital counseling with an Orthodox Jewish couple, Mordecai and Chana, who had recently become engaged. Mordecai became intensely jealous when Chana had even the most innocuous interactions with other men (e.g., at work, in a store). Mordecai used thought stopping to temporarily eliminate his jealous thoughts and then he imagined Chana's being especially attentive toward him.

Thought stopping has even been used for clients with thought disorders, as in the case of a 67-year-old woman who was involuntarily hospitalized for a number of psychotic symptoms, the most prominent and disruptive of which were paranoid delusions about her husband (Dupree, 1993). The woman was taught the two-phase thought-stopping procedure. In her case, simply vocalizing "Stop!" was insufficient to interrupt her intrusive thoughts. Accordingly, she wore a rubber band around her wrist and snapped it in conjunction with saying "Stop!" when she had the intrusive thoughts. The combination of the physically and vocally disruptive stimuli was effective. It also allowed the hospital staff to assess how often she was using thought stopping because, whereas subvocalizing "Stop!" cannot be observed by others, snapping the rubber band can be. For the second phase of thought stopping, the woman was instructed to make positive, assertive self-statements. Her paranoid thoughts diminished in the hospital, and this effect transferred to her home environment when she was discharged. Seven years later, she reported that her paranoid thoughts were minimal, and she attributed this largely to the thought stopping.

Thought stopping is probably the quickest behavior therapy for clients to learn and implement and, like other cognitive-behavioral therapies, it provides clients with self-control skills that they can generalize to other problems (Newman & Haaga, 1995). Because thought stopping usually is part of a treatment package (e.g., Broder, 2000; Lerner, Franklin, Meadows, Hembree, & Foa, 1998), little controlled research on its specific efficacy has been carried out (Tryon, 1979), although it is used relatively frequently.

Rational Emotive Behavior Therapy

Rational emotive behavior therapy (REBT) (Ellis, 1993, 1995, 1999) employs cognitive restructuring to change irrational thoughts that cause psychological problems. Developed more than 40 years ago by psychologist Albert Ellis, REBT follows from Ellis's theory of how psychological disorders develop and are maintained. His theory is based on a simple yet powerful idea. To appreciate this idea, consider the following example. A man is rushing to an appointment and is delighted to find an open parking space. He is about to back into it when another driver who comes "out of nowhere" takes the spot. The man is mad, annoyed, frustrated. If you asked the man what he thinks is responsible for his negative emotions he might reply, "It's not fair; that so-and-so took *my* spot." In saying this, the man implies that the other driver's behavior has caused him to be upset.

This is not so, according to Ellis's theory, which would hold that it is not the event (the other driver pulling into the spot) that causes the man to be upset, but rather his illogical or irrational *interpretation* of the event. Life isn't fair, and the parking space did not actually belong to the man any more than it belonged to the other driver. Ellis acknowledges that this is not an original idea and credits the ancient Greek Stoic philosopher Epictetus, who said that people are disturbed not by things, but by the views they take of them.

Ellis believes that psychological problems are maintained by common irrational beliefs that come from faulty reasoning or logical errors about the world and oneself (Bernard & DiGiuseppe, 1989; Ellis & Bernard, 1985). Examples include

- *Absolute (dichotomous) thinking.* Viewing an event as black-or-white or all-or-none, such as "I always have to succeed"

- *Overgeneralizing.* Concluding that all instances of a situation will turn out a particular way because one or two instances did, as when a student gets a low grade on an exam and then believes that she or he is a poor student

- *Catastrophizing.* Blowing a minor event far out of proportion, as when a man who twists an ankle skiing concludes that he will never be able to ski again.

Ellis has identified two major themes in clients' irrational thoughts. One is a *sense of personal worthlessness*, which generally involves overgeneralization (e.g., "Because I didn't succeed this time, I'll never succeed"). The other is a *sense of duty* that is manifested in self-talk containing words such as *must, should,* and *have to.* Such beliefs are irrational because there are very few things that people absolutely have to do or must do. Ellis coined the colorful term *musterbation* for self-talk that involves this sense of duty (Ellis & Dryden, 1987).

The aim of REBT is to modify irrational beliefs, first by identifying thoughts based on the irrational beliefs, then by challenging the irrational beliefs, and finally by replacing thoughts based on irrational beliefs with thoughts based on rational beliefs.

The dialogue that follows provides the flavor of REBT. It is an excerpt from the second session with a 26-year-old woman who was experiencing anxiety and depression related to her recently having told her mother and stepfather about her lesbian sexual orientation (Wolfe, 1992, pp. 260–261). Her parents were quite disturbed by their daughter's coming out, and since then they have, for all intents and purposes, disowned her.

C (Client): I'm really pissed off at my parents. They're insisting that I go to my cousin's wedding. I said I wouldn't go unless Maggie [the woman the client had been dating for a year] could come with me, and they absolutely blew up. But I'll be damned if I'll drag along some token male. So for two weeks we've barely been speaking to each other. And now I feel *really* guilty!

T (Therapist): No question but that these situations can become sticky, and I can certainly appreciate how frustrating it is to have your partner excluded from a family event. I gather you're feeling pretty angry. Is there anything else you are feeling?

C: Yeah, I'm feeling really bummed out—depressed, I guess. It just seems that whatever I do, I'm never really going to fit in. I'm sick of the constant hassles.

T: When your parents came down on you about forbidding you to bring Maggie to the wedding, what were your thoughts?

C: That they have no right to tell me, at age 26, who I can take to a wedding; and that they should be more supportive . . . .

T: Do you see the "should" behind "they have no right to criticize me"?

C: Well, they shouldn't! Do you mean to tell me that you think it's okay for them to hassle me?

T: It's not okay. It's a pain in the neck! And there is no question it would be *preferable*—in terms of your relationship with your parents and with Maggie—if they didn't give you such a hard time. Let's try an experiment, shall we? If you really believed it would be *preferable* if your parents and society disapproved of your lesbianism, as opposed to believing it was an awful thing they must not do, how do you think you'd feel?

C: Well, I still wouldn't like it.

T: No reason you should like it or feel happy about it. My guess is that you'd still feel some negative feelings—say, disappointment or mild frustration—but not rage and depression. But when you escalate a *preference*—it would be preferable if my family didn't hassle me—to an absolutistic must—they must not—you're generally going to feel fairly emotionally disturbed, angry, enraged, then get into even more difficulties with your family and feel guilty about that.

C: Yeah—every time I get upset, they use it as further proof that I'm emotionally disturbed and that's why I'm a lesbian!

T: So let's see if we can dispute some of these shoulds and awfulizings. First, where is it written that people must not be prejudiced?

C: Well, a hell of a lot of people are; so I guess there's no law. But it's really awful that they cause so much pain to people. Do you know my stepfather calls Maggie "hairy legs"?

T: They do act badly at times and cause hassles. But you have far more control than you allow yourself over the amount of pain and disturbance with which you react to these hassles. Now is it really awful and intolerable, on the same level as being tortured to death or having a child die? Or just a first-class pain in the neck?

C: Well, I guess if you put it that way . . . but I can't *stand* it when they keep pressuring me about Maggie.

T: You obviously don't like it—and there's no reason you should—but you *are standing* it. The trick is to learn to stand it with less upsetness. . . . Now let me suggest two homeworks for you to do this week.

C: Homework! As though I didn't have enough work to do. Why does everything have to be so hard?

T: Are you perchance telling yourself yet again that "it's *too* hard . . . poor me that life is such a grind"?

C: Yeah. [Grinning.] Something like that.

T: And when you think that, how do you feel?

C: Pretty depressed and anxious.

T: Well, one of your homeworks—the cognitive, or self-talk, one—is to continue to dispute the idea that the world shouldn't be so unfair. That I shouldn't have to work so hard to be happy, shouldn't have parents who pressure me to get married, shouldn't have to work at my therapy. Your behavioral assignment is to assertively, rather than aggressively, let your parents know that while you understand their concern over your sexual orientation, you feel frustrated and sad at their nonacceptance of Maggie into their life. [Talking to her parents was rehearsed in the session using role playing, with therapist coaching and feedback, to prepare the client for actually talking to her parents.]

Many of the characteristics of REBT are illustrated in this client-therapist dialogue. The therapist openly challenges the client's illogical self-talk and beliefs and models this process for her. *Active disputing* of irrational beliefs, which is confrontational in nature, is a key element that distinguishes REBT from similar cognitive restructuring therapies (Ellis & Bernard, 1985). Once the therapist has an understanding of the client's core irrational beliefs, as much as 90% of the session may involve the therapist's challenging the rationality of the client's thoughts and debunking the client's myths about how the world "should be" (Ellis, 1989a; Kopec, Beal, & DiGiuseppe, 1994; Lazarus, 1989b). The client's task is to learn to identify and dispute irrational thoughts and beliefs and then to replace them with rational thoughts. The client first rehearses these skills in the therapy sessions and then practices them at home. Clients are also given homework assignments that involve overt behaviors, such as the client's assertively confronting her parents in the previous case.

Potentially, REBT could treat any problem maintained by irrational beliefs (e.g., Dryden & Hill, 1993; Ellis, 1994a, 1994b, 1994c, 1994d), and it has been used to treat a wide array of problems, including anxiety disorders, anger, depression, antisocial behaviors, stuttering, and sexual dysfunctions (Abrams & Ellis, 1994; Alvarez, 1997; Balter & Unger, 1997; Greaves, 1997; Haaga & Davison, 1989; Rieckert & Moller, 2000; Scholing & Emmelkamp, 1993a, 1993b). REBT has been applied to diverse client populations. Self-defeating beliefs among African-American high school students about their mathematical abilities have been changed by REBT (Shannon & Allen, 1998). Components of REBT have been successfully employed in the treatment of Puerto Rican adolescents with depression (Rossello & Bernal, 1999). REBT has been used with the elderly who are vulnerable to irrational thoughts and beliefs related to aging (Dryden & Ellis, 2001; Ellis, 1999) and may have an increased risk of suicide (McIntosh, Santos, Hubbard, & Overholser, 1994). Common irrational beliefs in the elderly include "I must do as well as I did when I was younger," "Other people must treat me kindly and fairly because of my age," and "I should have the good health I used to have and not be ill and disabled." For clients with strong religious convictions, REBT can capitalize on those convictions to challenge clients' irrational beliefs and reinforce the use of adaptive thoughts (Nielsen, 2001; Robb, 2001). For example, a client who is thinking, "I must get my job back" might be reminded of Ecclesiastes' reflections, "For everything there is a season. . . . a time to keep, and a time to cast away."

Based on the belief that African Americans with strong racial consciousness are less likely to use and abuse substances, REBT was used in the service of developing a positive racial identity in a 30-year-old African-American man with a history of crack cocaine and alcohol abuse (Fudge, 1996). The man sought counseling because he was anxious and depressed. His irrational beliefs about his African heritage were manifested in statements such as, "Being Black means I'll never be good enough" and "Black men don't do school; therefore doing well in school means that I'm not a Black man" (Fudge, 1996, p. 328). The REBT treatment focused on challenging these thoughts and replacing them with more rational thoughts that would bolster his positive racial identity.

The emphasis on challenging and confronting clients in REBT may be especially suited for African Americans and Latino Americans who tend to prefer active and directive counseling (Sapp, McNeely, & Torres, 1998). This preference may be related to the finding that African Americans are prone to an external locus of control (the belief that they are controlled by external factors and do not have control over their own lives) (Sapp, 1996, 1997). In contrast, REBT may be less effective with clients from cultures (such as Native American, Japanese, and Southeast Asian) that eschew direct confrontation. However, these conjectures have not been empirically verified.

Cognitive Therapy

Cognitive therapy, another cognitive restructuring therapy, was conceived by psychiatrist Aaron Beck (Beck, 1963, 1976) at the same time (the early 1960s) that Ellis was developing REBT, but Beck and Ellis appear to have created their theories and techniques independently (Bernard & DiGiuseppe, 1989). Although both therapies challenge irrational beliefs, they use different approaches. In Beck's cognitive therapy, clients are taught to view their beliefs as tentative *hypotheses* to be tested by gathering evidence that refutes (or supports) them (Hollon & Beck, 1986); in contrast, Ellis's REBT relies on logical disputation to challenge distorted beliefs. The major differences between REBT and cognitive therapy are summarized in Table 9.1.

Beck's theory of the development and maintenance of psychological disorders shares the same fundamental premises as Ellis's theory, although there are some conceptual differences. For instance, Beck refers to irrational, maladaptive cognitions as **automatic thoughts,** viewing distorted thoughts as if they were reflexes that do not involve prior reflection or reasoning (Beck, 1976). In Beck's view, clients consider their automatic thoughts to be totally plausible, which, in part, accounts for the powerful influence these thoughts have on clients' emotions and actions.

According to Beck's theory, psychological disorders occur when people perceive the world as threatening. This perception impairs normal cognitive functioning because "perceptions and interpretations of events become highly

Table 9.1 Major Differences Between REBT and Cognitive Therapy

	Rational Emotive Behavior Therapy	*Cognitive Therapy*
Basis of approach	Rationality	Empirical evidence
Techniques	Instruction, persuasion, disputation	Empirical hypothesis testing
Change mechanisms	Primarily cognitive restructuring	Combination of cognitive restructuring and overt behavioral interventions
Role of therapist	Model of rational thinking (recognizing and disputing irrational beliefs)	Co-investigator seeking to empirically test client's irrational beliefs
Therapist style	Confrontational	Collaborative
Role of homework	Practice disputing irrational beliefs and cognitive restructuring	Gather evidence to establish validity of beliefs

Adapted from Spiegler & Guevremont, 2003.

Table 9.2 Common Cognitive Distortions Made by Clients

Cognitive Distortion	Definition	Example
Arbitrary inference	Drawing conclusions without adequate or any evidence	Thinking that you were not hired for a job because of your gender when, in fact, the person hired was clearly more qualified
Personalization	Erroneously believing that an external event is related to you	Believing that two strangers you walk past are talking about you
Selective abstraction	Focusing on part of something while ignoring the total context	Concluding that your clothes look bad because there is a small stain on one of your shoes
Overgeneralization	Drawing a broad conclusion based on only one or two examples	Believing that you'll never get a date because one person turned you down
Dichotomous thinking	All-or-none, either-or thinking with no room for any middle ground	Believing that because you were late for your first appointment, the entire day will go badly

Adapted from Beck & Weishaar, 1989.

selective, egocentric and rigid" (Beck & Weishaar, 1989, p. 23), which results in systematic errors in reasoning. For example, children who are anxious may view friendly gestures as hostile (Bell-Dolan, 1995), and adults suffering from panic disorder tend to interpret physical sensations catastrophically (such as increased heart rate meaning a heart attack) (Otto & Gould, 1995). Table 9.2 presents some of the common (and sometimes overlapping) cognitive distortions that clients make; often clients' irrational beliefs are based on combinations of cognitive distortions.

The goals of cognitive therapy are (1) to correct clients' faulty information processing, (2) to modify the irrational beliefs that maintain clients' maladaptive actions and emotions, and (3) to provide clients with skills and experiences that foster adaptive thinking (Beck & Weishaar, 1989). These goals are accomplished in the context of a close client-counselor collaboration, in which the client is an active participant. To establish this collaboration, counselors must develop empathic understanding of clients' views of the world, which includes their cognitive distortions (Burns & Nolen-Hoeksema, 1992). For example, many elderly clients come to counseling with beliefs such as, "Therapy is for crazy people," "The counselor will fix my problems," "I'm too old to change," or "Depression is a normal part of aging" (Dick-Siskin, 2002). Clearly it is important for counselors to recognize that an elderly client may hold one or more of these erroneous beliefs. Similarly, counselors sometimes hold irrational beliefs about the elderly (e.g., "They are too old to change" or "It is impolite to challenge an elderly client") that must be corrected if there is to be an effective client-counselor collaboration (Dick-Siskin, 2002).

Cognitive therapists help clients recognize their automatic thoughts and the dysfunctional beliefs on which they are based. They do this by asking clients to become aware of and to verbalize their self-talk when they are emotionally distressed. Cognitive therapists then use the *Socratic method* (also called *guided discovery*), which involves asking clients questions to guide them toward discovering their maladaptive cognitions. This process is illustrated in the following excerpt from a cognitive therapy session with a college senior who was seriously abusing alcohol (based on Beck, Wright, Newman, & Liese, 1993.)

> T (Therapist): How are you going to deal with all the drinking that will occur at the party you and your roommates are throwing this weekend?
>
> C (Client): There's no way I am going to not drink! I'll just have to deal with it afterwards.
>
> T: What bothers you about not drinking at the party?
>
> C: I wouldn't be fun if I didn't drink.
>
> T: So, if you weren't fun, what would be so bad about that?
>
> C: People would ignore me.
>
> T: If they ignored you, what would that mean?
>
> C: They didn't like me?
>
> T: So suppose people ignored you and that meant they didn't like you. What would be the consequences for you?
>
> C: Well, I guess word would get out on campus, and I'd be a social outcast. I'd have no friends; no one to hang out with; no girl would want to date me.
>
> T: And all of that would happen just because you weren't drinking at your own party?
>
> C: Well, I guess that's a bit of an exaggeration.
>
> T: It sure is. I think it is important for you to see how one irrational belief builds on another and leads you to assume that the worst will happen—just because on this one instance you didn't drink.
>
> C: I didn't realize that was what I was doing. Without analyzing it, it did seem catastrophic; but maybe it's not.

Becoming aware of their automatic thoughts is a crucial initial step for clients in cognitive therapy. But clients typically are reluctant to get rid of their automatic thoughts because they believe they are accurate. To convince a client that her or his automatic thoughts are not necessarily true, the therapist invites the client to view the automatic thoughts as hypotheses that can be empirically verified rather than viewing them as proven facts (i.e., "the way things are"). Working together, the therapist and client develop "experiments" that the client can implement to test these hypotheses, a process Beck calls **collaborative empiricism** (Beck & Weishaar, 1989). For instance, an African-American man believed that his boss ignored him because he was Black. His counselor suggested that the man check out the validity of this hypothesis by observing how frequently his boss interacted with other workers in the office, including other African Americans. To his surprise, the man discovered that his boss rarely spoke to any of the workers. Thus, his dysfunctional belief, which was based on arbitrary inference and personalization, was refuted with empirical evidence. He was then able to see his boss as someone who was "generally disinterested in his employees irrespective of the color of their skin." Not only was this perspective accurate, but it also was more adaptive because the client was no longer disturbed by what he had perceived as racial prejudice.

Sometimes testing the validity of a seemingly irrational belief reveals that the belief is valid—that it is consistent with what actually is occurring. This would have been the case if the man had discovered that his boss mainly ignored African-American employees. In such instances, the therapist would help the client to construe the situation in a way that fits the data but does not result in maladaptive reactions. For example, the man might have changed his thoughts to: "My boss appears to ignore his Black employees. Well, that's his loss, not mine, because we are an asset to the company."

In addition to the basic procedures just described, there are a number of specialized techniques used in cognitive therapy that fall into two categories: cognitive interventions and overt behavioral interventions.

Cognitive Interventions   A variety of cognitive interventions, which are rooted in cognitive restructuring, are used to change clients' cognitions *directly*. Here are a few examples.

- Counselors provide relevant information, such as the reasons that a fear is irrational (e.g., people rarely are injured on escalators).

- Clients keep a *thought diary* in which, over the course of a day, they record such information as their automatic thoughts, the situations in which the automatic thoughts occur, their emotions at the time, the logical errors they are making, and possible rational responses to the situation

Automatic Thoughts	Situation	Emotions	Logical Error
No one is going to listen to me.	Preparing to give a talk	Anxious, angry	No evidence
She didn't have a good time and doesn't like me.	Arlene shook my hand after second date	Depressed	Arbitrary inference
I just can't do well in French	Got a B on a French exam	Hopeless	Dichotomous thinking
I turned the wrong way. I'll never find the theater.	Turning left when I should have turned right going to the play	Helpless	Overgeneralizing
I'll never be able to go to school again.	Walking into class with my fly open	Anxious	Catastrophizing

Figure 9.1 Part of One Client's Thought Diary

(e.g., Beck et al., 1993; Foa & Rothbaum, 1998). Figure 9.1 shows an excerpt from one client's thought diary.

- Clients are taught to *generate alternative interpretations* of situations that result in automatic thoughts. First they listen to the therapist model appropriate alternatives, and then they practice the process modeled by the therapist. For example, a man believed a co-worker he was attracted to did not like him because the co-worker never made eye contact with him when they were in the same room. His therapist guided the man to develop the alternative interpretation that the co-worker was shy.

- *Reattribution of responsibility* is used when clients believe that they have more control over potentially negative outcomes than they actually do. For instance, a college student was worried that her parents would not have a good time when they visited for Parents' Weekend. The counselor used Socratic questioning to get the student to realize that she could take her parents to a variety of activities that might be enjoyable, but she had no control over her parents' enjoyment of the activities.

- *Decatastrophizing* is employed when clients anticipate worst-case scenarios, which is common in anxiety disorders. Through Socratic questioning, the client comes to see the absurdity of highly unlikely consequences and to consider more probable, noncatastrophic outcomes. For example, losing one's wallet is not likely to make someone destitute.

Overt Behavioral Interventions   Clients also can change their irrational thoughts *indirectly* by changing their overt behaviors. Overt behavioral interventions are especially helpful with clients who are apathetic and have difficulty thinking clearly, as is often the case with clients who suffer from major depression. At least initially, it is difficult to engage such clients in cognitive interventions because they are not thinking clearly, and cognitive interventions are less effective with such clients (Bowers, 1989). Overt behavioral interventions can provide alternative strategies. Three overt behavioral interventions that are often used in cognitive therapy are activity scheduling, mastery and pleasure ratings, and graded task assignments.

Generating an **activity schedule**—a written, hour-by-hour plan of what a client will do on a given day—is useful when clients are inactive and have difficulty motivating themselves to do even the most mundane tasks (e.g., such as getting dressed), which is characteristic of clients who are severely depressed. Activity scheduling also is helpful for clients who are anxious and feeling disorganized and overwhelmed by daily tasks. The activity schedule gives clients a structure to prompt, guide, and encourage them to engage in active behaviors during the day.

Clients suffering from depression, anxiety, and other problems frequently report that they experience little or no sense of accomplishment or pleasure in their lives. Often, this is a distorted perception. **Mastery and pleasure ratings** provide clients with feedback about their actual accomplishments and pleasure. Clients rate each activity on their activity schedule for mastery (sense of accomplishment) and for pleasure (feelings of enjoyment) using a 6-point rating scale (Beck, Rush, Shaw, & Emery, 1979). Using a rating scale encourages clients to relinquish their dichotomous thinking and recognize partial successes and small pleasures.

Graded task assignments are a shaping technique in which clients are encouraged to engage in small, sequential steps that lead to a therapeutic goal. This technique was part of cognitive therapy for a 42-year-old Japanese-American man, Makoto S., who had been admitted to a hospital with multiple physical complaints. The hospital physicians found no physical basis for his complaints. Somatic complaints often are key symptoms of depression in Japanese clients, which made depression the most likely diagnosis.

Because nonverbal communication is valued in Japanese culture, the therapist primarily used overt behavioral interventions. A series of graded task assignments were employed to get Makoto to walk. He claimed that he could not walk, and he was taken to his counseling sessions in a wheelchair. In the following client-therapist dialogue, you will see how the therapist implements the initial graded task assignment.

T (Therapist): Why is it that you can't walk?

C (Client): I don't have the strength.

T: What would happen if you tried?

C: I'd fall.

T: Are you sure of that?

C: Yes.

T: Well, you could be right. But you also might be mistaken. How about our testing that out?

C: I know I can't walk.

T: You may be right. People who are depressed often think that way, but they find that when they try to walk, they can. Do you think you could take just a few steps to the sofa?

C: Suppose I fall.

T: I'll walk with you and catch you if you fall.

At this point the therapist took Makoto's arm, and Makoto was able to walk to the sofa. The therapist pointed out that Makoto had done better than he had thought he could and suggested that Makoto try to walk to the office door. With much skepticism, Makoto attempted this and succeeded. Over the course of the next three sessions, increasingly longer walks were achieved, which provided evidence to refute Makoto's automatic thought that he could not walk. More-over, as is typically found with clients who are depressed (Beck et al., 1979), Makoto's mood became more positive for a short time, and this provided the motivation to attempt increasingly more active behaviors. The more Makoto was able to do, the harder it was to tell himself that he was unable to engage in normal, everyday activities and the more positive his mood became.

Uses of Cognitive Therapy   Beck originally developed cognitive therapy to treat depression, which he found was associated with distorting thinking. However, distorted thinking is also found to accompany many psychological disorders. Cognitive therapy has been adapted to and found to be effective in treating a wide array of psychological problems (e.g., Salkovskis, 1996), including anxiety (e.g., Hollon & Beck, 1994; Otto & Gould, 1995), obsessive-compulsive disorder (e.g., van Oppen & Arntz, 1994; van Oppen et al., 1995), marital distress (e.g., Abrahms, 1983; Baucom & Epstein, 1990; Beck, 1988; Dattilio & Padesky, 1990; Epstein, 1983), schizophrenic delusions and hallucinations (e.g., Alford & Beck, 1994; Alford & Correia, 1994; Kingdon & Turkington, 2005; Morrison, Renton, Williams, & Dunn, 1999), substance abuse (e.g., Beck et al., 1993), stress in women being treated for breast cancer (Antoni et al., 2001), and coping with an HIV diagnosis among gay men (Antoni et al., 2000).

Consider how cognitive therapy has been useful in treating clients suffering from posttraumatic stress disorders (e.g., Chemtob, Novaco, Hamada, & Gross, 1997; Foa & Rothbaum, 1998). With victims of sexual assault, for example, cognitive therapy has helped clients change their automatic thoughts related to anger (e.g., "Why did he choose me?"), shame and guilt (e.g., "I should have fought harder"), and hopelessness (e.g., "I'm permanently damaged").

Besides being a treatment of choice for depression (e.g., Lewinsohn, Clarke, & Rohde, 1994; Pace & Dixon, 1993; Scott, Scott, Tacchi, & Jones, 1994; Shapiro et al., 1995; Teasdale, Segal, & Williams, 1995), cognitive therapy also may prevent the recurrence of depression to a greater degree than other therapies (Elkin et al., 1989; Hollon & Beck, 1986; Hollon, Shelton, & Davis, 1993; Shea, 1990; Teasdale et al., 1995; compare with Otto, Pava, & Sprich-Buckminster, 1995). This effect may be due to the fact that cognitive therapy makes clients aware of how thinking is associated with depression and provides them with generalizable skills (such as cognitive restructuring and mastery and pleasure ratings) to cope with a variety of events that may trigger depression in the future (Spiegler & Guevremont, 2003). Cognitive therapy might also prove useful in preventing relapse in other disorders for the same reasons. Another benefit of cognitive therapy related to depression is that it appears to decrease the risk of suicide (Brown et al., 2005).

Schema-based cognitive therapy identifies and modifies clients' schemas that are maintaining their problem behaviors. A **schema** is a broad, pervasive, and rigid cognitive theme about oneself, others, or the world that a person uses to interpret particular events. Personality disorders (e.g., borderline personality disorder) often are maintained by maladaptive schemas rather than by automatic thoughts (Beck & Freeman, 1989). Abandonment/instability and mistrust/abuse are two examples of broad-based schemas that people with personality disorders are likely to hold (Young, 1994). For instance, a woman with an abandonment/instability schema asked her boyfriend to go out to dinner. He told her, "I'd love to, but I had a really hard day and am tired. How about a rain check?" The woman took this as an indication that their relationship was deteriorating and that her boyfriend did not want to be with her. Similarly, when a man who held a mistrust/abuse schema brought his car to a dealership for repair, he fully expected that mechanics would not do the work adequately and that he would be overcharged.

Generally, schemas begin in childhood and continue to be held into adulthood without the person's ever questioning the validity or usefulness of the perspective the schemas provide. Schema-based cognitive therapy (e.g., McGinn & Young, 1996) involves identifying a client's schemas and then activating them through imagery and role playing to assess the significance of these schemas for the client. The client's critical maladaptive schemas are modified using the same basic cognitive therapy techniques used to change automatic thoughts. For instance, clients may be asked to provide evidence from their lives that supports or contradicts their schemas and to perform graded task assignments involving behaviors that contradict the schemas.

Cognitive therapy is being used increasingly with clients from diverse populations, often with modifications that are tailored to the clients' ethnic backgrounds. For instance, a treatment program for depression in African-American adolescents used ethnically related cartoon characters to illustrate how negative thoughts contribute to depression and how positive thoughts can improve mood (Lewinsohn et al., 1994). Similarly, an adaptation for Turkish children involved listening to stories in which culturally relevant characters learned to replace negative thoughts with positive thoughts about test anxiety (Aydin & Yerin, 1994). With religious clients, using religious rationales for treatment and religious arguments to counter the clients' irrational beliefs (similar to those used in the REBT treatment for religious clients described on page 329) has been found to be more effective than standard cognitive therapy for that population (Propst, Ostrom, Watkins, Dean, & Mashburn, 1992).

Cognitive therapy that involves examining and correcting negatively biased, maladaptive beliefs may be useful for gay clients who are having difficulty accepting their homosexual orientation (Kuehlwein, 1992). Examples of such beliefs are "A gay life-style means forgoing experiences that are only for heterosexuals" (e.g., stable relationships and childrearing), and "Being gay requires acting in certain ways that fit with mainstream stereotypes" (e.g., going to art galleries instead of sporting events). Through collaborative empiricism, gay clients can learn about the lives and habits of other gay men and collect data that refute their false assumptions. For instance, clients can discover that many homosexual couples have long-term stable relationships and that many gay men enjoy sports.

For the elderly, cognitive therapy has been found to be an effective treatment for depression (Koder, Brodaty, & Anstey, 1996) and for reducing suicide risk (McIntosh et al., 1994). Additionally, cognitive therapy has been used in the treatment of late-life insomnia (Morin, Colecchi, Stone, Sood, & Brink, 1999) and generalized anxiety (worry) (Gorenstein, Papp, & Kleber, 1999). Modifications for treating elderly clients with cognitive therapy may require taking into account age-related cognitive deficits (Wetherell, 2002) by slowing the pace; frequently repeating information; emphasizing concrete, overt behavioral change strategies over more abstract cognitive strategies (Church, 1983); and using idiomatic terms for technical terms (e.g., "loopy conclusions" for overgeneralizations or arbitrary inferences) (Tanner & Ball, 1989). Cognitive therapy also has been used efficiently and effectively to treat depression in elderly clients with physical disabilities (e.g., Thompson, Gallagher-Thompson, & Breckenridge, 1987).

Cognitive-Behavioral Coping Skills Therapies

As you have seen, cognitive restructuring therapies deal with a client's *excess of maladaptive thoughts*. In contrast, cognitive-behavioral coping skills therapies are used to treat clients' problems that are maintained by a *deficit of adaptive cognitions*. The focus shifts from what clients are thinking to what they are *not* thinking. As with cognitive restructuring therapies, coping skills therapies change both cognitions and overt behaviors. Let's look at three cognitive-behavioral coping skills therapies: self-instructional training, problem-solving therapy, and stress inoculation.

Self-Instructional Training

Many times each day we tell ourselves what to do, what to think, and how to feel. "Left at the next corner." "Don't forget to pick up milk." "It's not the end of the world; I'll get another chance." "Cheer up; you have only 5 minutes left on the treadmill." Such self-talk, which is known as *self-instruction*, serves five functions: (1) focusing attention, (2) guiding behavior, (3) evaluating performance, (4) providing encouragement, and (5) reducing anxiety. Psychologist Donald Meichenbaum developed **self-instructional training** to teach people to instruct themselves to cope effectively with difficult situations (Meichenbaum & Goodman, 1971). Self-instructional training consists of the following five steps, each of which is illustrated with an example of a teenager who completes schoolwork with little or no thought.

Step 1: Cognitive modeling. **Cognitive modeling** involves a model demonstrating for a client the process of talking aloud about what he or she is thinking. The model may be the counselor or someone the counselor brings into the session for this specific purpose. In self-instructional training, the model verbalizes aloud self-instructions for performing a desired behavior as well as for staying focused, evaluating one's performance, and providing self-reinforcement. For example, with a geometry problem, the model might say aloud:

> Read the problem carefully. [Model slowly reads the problem aloud.] What is the problem asking me to do? Okay, bisect the line on the page. I need my compass. Okay, now carefully put the point at one end and scribe a wide arc across the line. Just go slow. That's good. Now, carefully do the same thing from the other end of the line. Did it. Okay, now take my ruler and connect the two points where the arcs meet. I've done it. The line that connects the two arcs cuts the original line in half. Good work.

Step 2: Cognitive participant modeling. The client performs the behavior while the model verbalizes the self-instructions aloud.

Step 3: Overt self-instructions. The client performs the behavior while verbalizing the self-instructions aloud.

Step 4: Fading of overt self-instructions. The client performs the behavior while whispering the self-instructions.

Step 5: Covert self-instructions. Finally, the client performs the behavior while saying the self-instructions subvocally.

Clients first practice the steps with brief, simple tasks and then with lengthier, more complex tasks. For young children, the self-instructional training may be presented as a game using pictorial prompts to remind the child to self-instruct.

Self-instructional training has been used for more than 35 years to treat diverse problems, ranging from impulsive behaviors (e.g., Guevremont, Tishelman, & Hull, 1985; Kendall & Finch, 1978; Meichenbaum & Goodman, 1971) and specific fears (Kendall, 1994; Ollendick, Hagopian, & King, 1997) to the bizarre thoughts and speech of clients with schizophrenia (e.g., Meichenbaum & Cameron, 1973; Meyers, Mercatoris, & Sirota, 1976) and cognitive and motor performance deficits of children and adults with brain injuries (O'Callaghan & Couvadelli, 1998; Suzman, Morris, Morris, & Milan, 1997). Although self-instructional training is employed more often with children, it also is used with adolescents and adults, including the elderly (Meichenbaum, 1974). Even individuals with significant intellectual impairment can benefit from self-instructional training, as evidenced by its use to guide job-related tasks of adults with all levels of mental retardation (Rusch, Hughes, & Wilson, 1995). Examples of self-instructions that might be used on the job would be "I have to just look at what I am doing," "Check my work," and "Finish this one before moving to the next one." This training has resulted in significant improvements in work-related on-task behaviors (e.g., Rusch, Morgan, Martin, Riva, & Agran, 1985), accuracy of performance (e.g., Hughes & Rusch, 1989), completion of tasks (e.g., Rusch, Martin, Lagomarcino, & White, 1987), and punctuality (e.g., Sowers, Rusch, Connis, & Cummings, 1980).

Problem-Solving Therapy

Because problems are an inevitable part of living, problem solving is useful in numerous contexts for coping with many of life's difficulties (e.g., D'Zurilla & Chang, 1995). Indeed, inadequate problem solving is associated with a host of difficulties throughout the life span. For example, adolescents who have poor problem-solving skills are likely to have interpersonal difficulties, be depressed, and be victimized by bullies (e.g., Asarnow & Callan, 1985; Biggam & Power, 1999; D'Zurilla, Chang, Nottingham, & Faccini, 1998; Frye & Goodman, 2000; Kant, D'Zurilla, & Maydeu-Olivares, 1997; Lochman & Curry, 1986).

Problem solving and the basic components of problem-solving therapy are not new, of course. What was new 35 years ago was psychologist Thomas D'Zurilla's realization that problem-solving strategies could be used not only to solve everyday, practical problems, but also to treat and prevent psychological problems (D'Zurilla & Goldfried, 1971). Additionally, problem-solving therapy can be employed to deal with the practical problems that are related to a client's psychological problems. Consider the earlier example of the African-American man who believed that his boss didn't talk to him because he is Black. If in his "research" he had discovered that his boss does indeed talk to White workers much more than to Black workers, problem-solving therapy could have been used to help the client deal with this situation.

In **problem-solving therapy,** clients sequentially follow a series of seven interrelated steps or stages to treat a specific psychological problem for which they have sought treatment (Spiegler & Guevremont, 2003).

Stage 1: Adopting a problem-solving orientation. First, clients must recognize that they have a problem, and then they must view it as potentially solvable. Counselors describe the problem-solving orientation to clients and then describe how it works to alleviate problems. One of the advantages of problem-solving therapy is that it allows clients to conceive of psychological troubles as problems, rather than illnesses, which removes some of the sting and stigma often associated with psychological problems. This is especially important for clients whose cultural mores stigmatize mental illness (e.g., with Portuguese, Pakistani, and ultra-Orthodox Jewish clients).

Stage 2: Defining the problem. The counselor works with the client to define the problem precisely and in detail, which is crucial for the succeeding stages.

Stage 3: Setting goals. To set goals, the counselor essentially asks the client: "What must happen so that you no longer have the problem?" The counselor works with the client's answer to ensure that the resulting goals are specific, unambiguous, and achievable. The goals can be (1) *situation focused*—that is, aimed at changing the problem situation itself (e.g., finding a job); (2) *reaction focused*—that is, aimed at changing the client's emotional, cognitive, and overt behavioral reactions to the problem situation (e.g., feeling competent rather than incompetent when unemployed); or (3) both (Nezu, Nezu, D'Zurilla, & Rothenberg, 1996). Although the counselor guides the client in making the goals explicit and obtainable, it is the client who has the final say about the basic goals (which is a fundamental tenet of behavior therapy).

Stage 4: Generating alternative solutions. In this stage, the client generates as many solutions as possible to maximize the chances of finding a successful one. Brainstorming—in which any possible solution is entertained, no matter how impractical or outlandish it might appear—helps the client do this.

Stage 5: Choosing the best solution. From the alternatives generated, the client then chooses the best solution, using an overall evaluation of the potential consequences (to the client and others, in the short and long term) of each alternative as the criterion.

Stage 6: Implementing the solution. The client implements the chosen solution. For effective implementation to occur, the client must (1) possess the requisite skills to carry out the solution, (2) have an opportunity to implement the solution, and (3) be sufficiently motivated to implement the solution. This may involve teaching the client the necessary skills, changing conditions in the client's everyday environment, and establishing reinforcement contingencies, respectively.

Stage 7: Evaluating the effectiveness of the solution. Finally, when the solution has had time to take effect, the client evaluates its success in terms of the client's previously established goals. If the problem has been solved, therapy is terminated. If it has not, then the client repeats one or more of the previous stages, depending on the stage where the process faltered.

Clients are taught problem solving through cognitive modeling, prompting, self-instructions, shaping, and reinforcement (Nezu et al., 1996; Nezu, Nezu, & Houts, 1993; Watson & Kramer, 1995). The procedures are essentially the same for both adults and children (Braswell & Kendall, 2001). Problem-solving therapy is particularly useful in the treatment of adult depression (D'Zurilla & Nezu, 2001), including depressed mood in the elderly (Arean et al., 1993; Levendusky & Hufford, 1997), but it also has been applied to a wide array of problems including eating disorders (Black, 1987; Johnson, Corrigan, & Mayo, 1987), smoking (Shaffer, Beck, & Boothroyd, 1983), habitual gambling (Bujold, Ladouceur, Sylvain, & Boisvert, 1994), marital discord (Jacobson, 1991; Jacobson & Margolin, 1979; O'Leary & Turkewitz, 1978), child abuse (Dawson, de Armas, McGrath, & Kelly, 1986; MacMillan, Guevremont, & Hansen, 1989), and adherence to HIV medication regimens (Safren, Otto, & Worth, 1999).

In the last example, problem-solving therapy was used to overcome a major obstacle to significantly prolonging life in people with HIV—namely, failing to take highly effective medications. The intervention focused on difficulties HIV patients typically have, such as getting to appointments, communicating with health care providers, obtaining medications, and coping with medication side effects, all of which affect adherence to medication regimens. Although the general efficacy of this program has not yet been evaluated, there are a number of successful case examples. For instance, problem solving was effective with a gay man in his 30s who had to deal with both a complex and frequently changing medication regimen and a demanding work schedule that sometimes interfered with his taking his medication on time (Safren et al., 1999).

Any life difficulty that can be viewed as a problem is potentially amenable to problem-solving therapy. Problem-solving therapy can help clients solve immediate problems as well as provide them with the coping skills needed to solve and prevent future problems (e.g., Kendall & Gerow, 1995). Another advantage of problem-solving therapy is that although it is a form of psychotherapy, it does not have the same negative connotations that psychotherapy has because it is viewed as solving a problem rather than treatment. This may make it a more acceptable form of help, not only for clients who are from cultures that stigmatize mental illness itself, but also for clients from cultures that stigmatize psychotherapy (e.g., German and French Canadian).

Stress Inoculation Training

Stress-evoking events, both large and small, are part and parcel of living. Although we often cannot control these events, we can control how we view and cope with them to minimize the array of negative reactions commonly labeled stress (e.g., anxiety, anger, depression, hypertension) (Lazarus & Folkman, 1984). In **stress inoculation training,** another intervention developed by Meichenbaum (1977, 1985), clients learn coping skills and then practice using them while being exposed to stress-evoking events. The goal is for clients to be prepared to deal with stressors when they encounter them in their daily lives, thereby reducing the stress they experience. Stress inoculation is analogous to biological immunization, which prepares the body's immune system to deal with disease-causing microorganisms (Poser, 1970; Poser & King, 1975; Spiegler, 1980). Stress inoculation training consists of three phases: conceptualization, coping skills acquisition, and application.

Phase 1: Conceptualization. In the first phase, the counselor explains to the client how negative reactions to stressful events emanate from one's perception of the events, rather than from the events themselves (which is consistent with Ellis's theory discussed earlier), and how the client can learn coping skills to reconstrue and deal with potentially stress-evoking events in order to minimize their negative consequences.

Phase 2: Coping skills acquisition. Next, clients learn and rehearse cognitive and overt-behavioral coping skills, such as differential relaxation, cognitive restructuring, and problem-solving self-instructions. The specific coping skills are customized for the client and for the presenting problem. If the problem is fear, the client might learn to gather accurate information about threatening events. For chronic pain, the client might learn to use self-distracting thoughts.

Phase 3: Application. In the final phase, clients rehearse applying their new ways of viewing and coping with stress-evoking events. Application involves five steps: (1) *preparing* for an event, (2) *confronting and coping* with the event, (3) *dealing with temporary difficulties* in coping with the event, (4) *assessing one's performance* in coping with the event, and (5) *reinforcing oneself* for successfully coping with the event. Initially, clients engage in these steps during therapy sessions with simulated stress-evoking events. Later, they perform homework assignments involving the actual stress-invoking events encountered in their lives.

Finally, clients are trained in *relapse prevention*, which provides a strategy for dealing with the inevitable setbacks that occur in coping with real-life events (Marlatt & Gordon, 1985). Clients are taught to reconstrue failures and temporary reversals as "learning experiences." The client and the therapist identify high-risk situations—those in which relapses are most likely—and then the client rehearses coping with the high-risk situations.

A stress inoculation training program that helped African-American preteens with sickle cell anemia (a disease that occurs almost exclusively in the African-American community) to cope with the pain associated with the disease illustrates the application phase of stress inoculation (Gil et al., 1997). In the program, the patients were taught specific coping skills: to relax their muscles, to think pleasant thoughts, and to subvocalize calming self-instructions. First, they rehearsed using these coping skills while low-intensity pain was induced in the therapy session. Then the patients were given homework assignments to practice these coping skills on a daily basis. This one-session treatment lowered the patients' reported pain along with negative thinking about their illness.

Stress inoculation has been used to treat and prevent a wide array of problems in adults, the three most common being anxiety (e.g., Meichenbaum & Cameron, 1972; Suinn, 2001), anger (e.g., Novaco, 1975, 1977a, 1977b; Suinn, 2001), and pain (e.g., Turk, 1975, 1976). It has been used to treat posttraumatic stress disorder in adults—for instance, with women who have been sexually and physically assaulted (Foa & Rothbaum, 1998; Rothbaum, Meadows, Resick, & Foy, 2000) and with children ages 8 to 10 who were sexually abused (Farrell, Hains, & Davies, 1998).

Stress inoculation training has the potential to prepare people to deal with almost any stress-inducing event. For example, it might help adolescents with gay, lesbian, and bisexual orientations cope with the significant stress they experience related to such issues as homophobia, accepting their sexual identity, disclosing their sexual orientation to others, and developing both sexual and platonic relationships (Safren, Hollander, Hart, & Heimberg, 2001). Stress inoculation with gay men who are HIV positive has been shown to decrease their dysphoria, anxiety, and overall mood disturbance as well as heighten their immune systems (Lutgendorf et al., 1997). It has also improved their cognitive coping strategies and social support needed to deal with HIV-related stress (Lutgendorf et al., 1998).

Most of the controlled research studies that have evaluated stress inoculation training have indicated that it is an effective treatment (Meichenbaum, 1985; Meichenbaum & Deffenbacher, 1988), and 3- to 4-year follow-up studies have demonstrated long-term maintenance of treatment gains (Liddell, Di Fazio, Blackwood, & Ackerman, 1994; Meichenbaum & Deffenbacher, 1988). Like problem-solving therapy, stress inoculation training is useful for dealing with both current and future problems.

One advantage of stress inoculation training for diverse clients is that the specific coping skills taught can be individualized for clients, as has been done with elderly individuals (Lopez & Silber, 1991). Another advantage, shared with problem-solving therapy, is that learning skills may be a more acceptable form of help for clients from ethnic backgrounds in which self-help rather than psychological treatment is the socially acceptable way to deal with problems. However, the effectiveness of stress inoculation training may be limited with clients who have difficulty learning specific skills, such as clients with severe mental retardation or brain damage.

* * *

This completes my discussion of cognitive-behavioral therapy. In the remainder of the chapter, I'll address a number of general issues that pertain to all behavior therapies (i.e., both traditional behavior therapies covered in Chapter 8 and cognitive-behavioral therapies).

The Client-Counselor Relationship in Behavior Therapy

In behavior therapy, the client-counselor relationship is considered a *necessary but not sufficient* condition for successful treatment (e.g., Fleece, 1995; Lazarus, 1996; Raue, Castonguay, & Goldfried, 1993; Raue & Goldfried, 1994; Schaap, Bennun, Schindler, & Hoogduin, 1993). The client-counselor relationship is analogous to the role of anesthesia in surgery (Gaston et al., 1995). Anesthesia is necessary for surgery to take place; without it the most skillful surgical procedures cannot be done. Yet the crucial factor in the success of the surgery is the surgical procedure itself, not the anesthesia. Similarly, a good client-counselor relationship improves the effectiveness of behavior therapy, but the crucial elements for the success of the therapy are the therapeutic techniques.

That the client-counselor relationship is not the primary modus operandi of change in behavior therapy does not mean that it is unimportant. Because behavior therapy is a collaborative effort between the client and the counselor throughout the course of treatment and because behavior therapy involves joint decisions and work, a sound client-counselor relationship is necessary. In addition, a good client-counselor relationship facilitates the implementation of specific therapy procedures in a variety of ways. It increases the client's positive expectations and hopes for success; it encourages the client to complete homework assignments that may involve risk-taking; it helps to overcome obstacles that arise in therapy, including noncompliance; and it increases the potency of the counselor's praise and approval (Gaston et al., 1995; Keijsers, Schaap, & Hoogduin, 2000; Kohlenberg & Tsai, 1991, 1994, 1995; Raue & Goldfried, 1994).

Trust is the basic ingredient of a good client-counselor relationship. The client-counselor relationship is especially important with diverse clients because there are two potential sources of mistrust when dealing with such clients. First, clients who are outside mainstream Western culture may be less trusting of the counseling process. For example, cultural norms may dictate that one should handle one's psychological problems without involving "outsiders." Even though behavior therapy is an action therapy, clients often view therapy stereotypically as a verbal therapy, and in many cultures talking about one's problems is not an acceptable means of dealing with them. The second potential source of mistrust may occur when the client and counselor do not share diversity characteristics, such as race or sexual orientation. Clients may not trust that their counselor can understand their worldview and can appreciate how their worldview influences their presenting problem. And the flip side is that just as minority culture clients may not believe that their majority culture counselor understands their perspective, majority culture clients may not think that their minority culture counselor understands their view.

To counter such mistrust, the counselor must pay special attention to building rapport with the client in a manner that is appropriate for the particular client. For instance, with Latino clients, beginning counseling sessions with more extensive small talk than usual before launching into the nitty-gritty work of counseling is likely to generate rapport, because prolonged small talk is the mode of initiating interactions in many Latino cultures.

Respect for clients and their diversity is essential. The counselor must accept the client's presentation of her or his problem—in other words, embrace how the client perceives the problem rather than how the therapist might view it (Hays, 1995). Allowing clients to decide what they need and what will work for them in counseling is empowering. This may be particularly important with clients whose perspectives often have been dismissed or ignored by the majority culture, as with Native Americans (Hays, 2006).

Evaluation of Behavior Therapy

Throughout the presentation of behavior therapy in this and the previous chapter, the evaluation of this approach to counseling has been interwoven into the general discussion with an emphasis on three crucial issues: the effectiveness of behavior therapy, the problems and clients for which behavior therapy is suitable, and the compatibility of behavior therapy with diverse clients. The following section summarizes the current status of these three crucial issues.

Effectiveness of Behavior Therapy

Effectiveness—how well a method of psychotherapy works in alleviating client problems—has to be the bottom line for any psychotherapy. Behavior therapy rests on a foundation of commitment to a scientific approach to therapy, which includes validating its therapy procedures empirically. In other words, the evidence for the effectiveness of behavior therapies must come from scientific research rather than from therapist impressions, client testimonials, or the popularity of the therapeutic approach. Thousands of studies have been carried out to determine the effectiveness of behavior therapies. The overall verdict is clear: as a group of therapy procedures, behavior therapy has a strong and broad empirical base. Moreover, compared with all of the other approaches to psychotherapy, it has the broadest and the strongest empirical base (e.g., Chambless & Ollendick, 1996, 2001).[1]

In an effort to promote the use of effective psychological treatments, *empirically supported treatments* have been identified for the most prevalent psychological disorders (American Psychological Association, 1995; Crits-Christoph, Wilson, & Hollon, 2005; Sanderson, 2003; Weisz, Weersing, & Henggeler, 2005). Traditional behavior therapies and cognitive-behavioral therapies are by far the most frequently listed empirically supported psychotherapies. Two prime examples are exposure therapies (for various anxiety disorders including phobias and obsessive-compulsive disorder) and cognitive therapy (for depression).

The effectiveness of behavior therapy is determined, both nomothetically, across a range of clients and presenting problems, and idiographically, for individual clients.

The nomothetic evidence supporting the effectiveness of behavior therapies comes from controlled experiments, which are the most valid form of evidence. In experiments, groups of clients receive a particular behavior therapy and are compared with groups of similar clients who do not receive the therapy. The latter clients are included in the experiments to control for factors other than the treatment that might cause changes in the clients' problems. These factors might include being on a waiting list and expecting treatment, receiving the attention and caring of a therapist, and experiencing various placebo effects associated with psychotherapy (e.g., clients' beliefs that the treatment will alleviate their problems). Experiments whose primary focus is assessing the

---

[1] This is not to say that other approaches for which there has been little empirical research are not effective therapies. There just is little scientific evidence for their effectiveness in most cases. This state of affairs is due, in large part, to the fact that most other counseling approaches do not have the strong scientific ethic that characterizes behavior therapy.

relative effectiveness of two or more therapies (behavior therapies or other forms of therapy) may not include such control groups.

Effectiveness in these controlled investigations is assessed through four outcome measures: meaningfulness of change, transfer and generalization, long-term maintenance, and acceptability of the treatment (Spiegler & Guevremont, 2003).

1. *Meaningfulness of change.* Meaningfulness of change is the degree to which the changes that occur as a result of therapy make a genuine difference in clients' lives. Meaningfulness of change is determined by comparing the change to relevant norms or making clinical judgments about how adaptive the changes have been for clients. Consider the example of clients who on average compulsively wash their hands 20 times a day. Reducing hand washing to 5 times a day clearly demonstrates a meaningful change (closer to the norm as well as adaptive). However, reducing hand washing to 17 times a day, although an improvement, would not make a significant difference for clients (the frequency of hand washing would still be well above the norm and it would still interfere with their daily lives).

2. *Transfer and generalization.* If a therapy is effective, clients must *transfer* the new, adaptive behaviors they developed in therapy to their everyday environments, where the behaviors are relevant. Further, in many cases it is appropriate and desirable for the changes to *generalize* to aspects of clients' lives other than those that were the specific focus of counseling. For instance, suppose a man had learned assertive behaviors in his therapy sessions in order to appropriately refuse his wife's unreasonable demands. He should be able to use these assertive behaviors with friends and co-workers (generalization) as well as use them with his wife (transfer).

3. *Long-term maintenance.* Effective therapy also requires that the beneficial changes that result from therapy will endure over time, which is known as *long-term maintenance.* This is measured in periodic follow-up assessments, which can involve face-to-face or telephone interviews with clients and significant others, mailed questionnaires, or behavioral observations. Nomothetic outcome studies of behavior therapies now typically include follow-ups continuing at least 2 years beyond the completion of the therapy.

4. *Acceptability of the treatment.* Obviously, effective therapy can be useful only if it is employed to treat clients. Whether it is used depends, in part, on the degree to which clients find a therapy's procedures acceptable or palatable. Acceptability is an individual matter for each client. However, some behavior therapies generally are more acceptable (e.g., reinforcement and modeling therapies) and some less acceptable (e.g., punishment and flooding) to clients.

In nomothetic outcome experiments, the effectiveness of therapy is assessed for a group of clients. Inevitably, some clients in a study will benefit more than others, and some may not improve at all. Effectiveness of the therapy is based on the average benefit to the clients receiving the treatment.

Therapists must evaluate the effectiveness of generally effective behavior therapies for individual clients, which involves idiographic evaluation. In behavior therapy, the success of treatment for a particular client is measured by the degree to which the client's therapeutic goals have been met. Although this could be said for any psychotherapy, in behavior therapy success can be determined more reliably than in many other therapy approaches because clients' goals are defined specifically, unambiguously, and measurably. For example, the goal of "feeling better enough to return to work full-time" is specific, clear, and measurable, whereas the goal of "feeling better" is general and vague.

In behavior therapy, idiographic evaluation is not done just to determine if termination is appropriate. Collecting data to assess clients' progress toward meeting their goals during the course of treatment is an integral part of behavior therapy practice. As soon as the client's problem is defined as a concrete target behavior, assessment of the target behavior begins. Before the therapy is chosen and implemented, measurement of the target behavior provides a baseline to which changes during and following the intervention can be compared. As in nomothetic evaluation, successful idiographic evaluation requires that there be meaningful change that transfers to the client's everyday life and that the change is maintained over time.

Problems and Clients Treated by Behavior Therapy

Behavior therapy has been used to treat the gamut of client problems—including problems that are acknowledged to be very difficult to treat, such as autistic disorders, schizophrenia, and substance-related disorders. Behavior therapy treats clients of all ages, ranging from infants to the elderly, and it is the most successful approach for clients with very limited intellectual abilities. Further, traditional behavior therapy is especially suited to client populations for which verbal psychotherapies cannot work, such as infants, toddlers, and other groups who have limited or no verbal communication. Behavior therapy is regularly implemented outside the counselor's office in the actual settings where clients' problems occur, such as in homes, schools, institutions, work places, and the client's community (e.g., on public transportation, in shopping malls).

Behavior therapy arguably has the broadest scope of all counseling approaches. In my experience as a behavior therapist, I have never encountered a client who *potentially* could not be treated by one or more behavior therapies.

Nonetheless, behavior therapy is not a panacea. Certainly, behavior therapy does not have equal success with all client problems and disorders. And the approach or style of behavior therapy is not for everyone—an issue I will address in a section on the limitations of behavior therapy later.

Compatibility of Behavior Therapy for Diverse Clients

Behavior therapy (like most other counseling approaches) was developed in the context of Western cultures and primarily with White, middle-class heterosexual clients. As the number of diverse clients treated by behavior therapy has increased, behavior therapists have been adapting their techniques to better serve these new populations, as has been discussed throughout this chapter. In fact, the basic nature of behavior therapy and the way it is practiced make behavior therapy inherently suited and adaptable to treating diverse clients.

Behavior therapy is individualized for each client and her or his unique problem. Behavior therapists are attuned to considering clients' differences, both between diversity groups and within diversity groups (Neal-Barnett & Smith, 1996). Put another way, behavior therapists do not conform to the uniformity myth, which holds that all people from a particular diversity group are the same. For instance, in treating a Chicana teenager living in Los Angeles, a behavior therapist might begin by assessing the degree to which the girl identifies with her Mexican heritage versus the degree to which she identifies with urban American teen culture.

Behavior therapy's emphasis on the external environment includes factors such as cultural and ethnic identification. Both its active nature and reliance on empirical evidence makes behavior therapy well suited for clients from cultures that value a "doing" and "show me" approach rather than a "talking about" and "tell me" approach (e.g., Native Americans). Focusing on the present, rather than delving into the past, may be attractive to certain cultural and ethnic groups, such as Alaska Natives for whom the present is the salient time frame (Reimer, 1999).

The brevity of behavior therapy is advantageous to economically disadvantaged clients who can ill afford either to pay for longer-term therapy or to take much time away from their jobs and family obligations (e.g., they may have no access to daycare for children). Behavior therapies, by virtue of both their brevity and their empirical support, are more likely to be approved for health insurance coverage, which makes behavior therapies more accessible than other therapies for those lower-income clients.

Short-term therapy also may be more palatable than long-term therapy to people from cultures in which psychotherapy is viewed with skepticism or even disdain. This is true, for example, among some Asian Americans and Latinos, who believe that personal problems should not be shared with others, especially people outside one's immediate family. The emphasis on learning, in contrast to treating, also makes behavior therapy more acceptable to clients from cultures that stigmatize psychotherapy (as may be true for clients of Irish or French Canadian descent).

Behavior Therapy: Blind Spots, Limitations, and Challenges

Despite its many strengths, behavior therapy—like all approaches to counseling—is far from perfect. In the tradition of behavior therapists' acting as their own strongest critics, it is now time to acknowledge some of behavior therapy's blind spots, limitations, and challenges.

Blind Spots

Behavior therapy has three major blind spots: its present focus, its narrow focus, and its emphasis on the external environment.

By focusing on the present, behavior therapists give little credence to the influences of a client's past on his or her problem. Although behavior therapists believe that the maintaining conditions (or direct causes) of client problems are in the present, knowing about a client's past history may elucidate present circumstances and maintaining conditions. In addition to not focusing on the past, behavior therapists generally do not attend to the present momentary experiences of clients in therapy sessions. In contrast, Gestalt and person-centered therapists, for example, focus on here-and-now reactions and interactions that occur in the therapy session and use these reactions and interactions for assessment and treatment purposes (compare with Kohlenberg, Tsai, Parker, Bolling, & Kanter, 1999).

The narrow focus in behavior therapy on treating specific target behaviors is another potential blind spot. People are more than the sum of their behaviors. Thus, by dealing with specific behaviors rather than with the whole individual, important issues may be overlooked. Further, behavior therapists rely on precise measurement rather than detailed qualitative description of client problems. However, qualitative descriptions can provide a rich, in-depth understanding that measures of frequency, duration, and intensity cannot provide.

The third blind spot stems from the fact that behavior therapists consider external factors to be the major source of the maintaining conditions of client problems. In doing so, behavior therapists ignore thoughts and feelings that clients are unaware of—that is, what psychoanalysts and others refer to as the unconscious realm. Indeed, the unconscious has always been anathema to behavior therapists. The result of this neglect of the unconscious is that factors that might have relevance are overlooked.

Limitations

The two major limitations of behavior therapy are its difficulty treating some disorders and problems that are especially recalcitrant and dealing with the fact that the basic style of behavior therapy is not conducive for some clients.

Although behavior therapies have been demonstrated to be highly effective in treating a number of disorders (such as anxiety and mood disorders), they have been less successful in treating some other disorders, such as substance-related disorders and personality disorders. The intense physiological reinforcement of habit-forming drugs and the longstanding and pervasive nature of personality disorders make these problems highly resistant to change. Consequently, behavior therapy—along with every other approach to counseling—has had limited success in treating these disorders. Consequently, behavior therapists have been developing and testing innovative treatments specifically for these disorders. Two examples are Alan Marlatt's relapse prevention for substance-related disorders (Marlatt & Donovan, 2005) and Marsha Linehan's (1993) dialectical behavior therapy for borderline personality disorder.

A second limitation of behavior therapy is that its basic style and procedures do not fit well with some clients. For example, some clients would rather solve their problems by talking about them with a therapist rather than by engaging in the active, therapeutic tasks required in behavior therapy. Additionally, the personal style of some clients may not fit with behavior therapy's close collaboration of therapist and client in the design and implementation of treatment as well as the hands-on direction that behavior therapists offer; such clients may prefer to solve problems on their own and at their own pace, relying on a therapist only to facilitate and encourage this process. Further, the direct, straightforward nature of behavior therapy can be incongruent with clients from some cultural backgrounds, such as Japanese Americans and Native Americans, who may prefer to communicate indirectly about their problems. Finally, behavior therapy is a no-nonsense approach, getting straight to the business of dealing with clients' problems quickly and efficiently. This could be a problem for some Latino clients, whose cultural norms stress the importance of small talk as a prerequisite for engaging in any business with others.

Challenges

Among the challenges facing behavior therapy are enhancing long-term maintenance of treatment gains, preventing problems and disorders, and developing empirically supported treatments for diverse clients.

It is well known that losing weight is easy compared to keeping it off. Similarly, providing behavioral interventions that result in maintenance of changes that occur in therapy long after the therapy is terminated is a major challenge (e.g., Chorpita, 1995; Kendall, 1989). One strategy behavior therapists use to facilitate long-term maintenance of treatment gains is to teach clients self-control coping skills that will transfer to their natural environment and generalize to other life problems that occur in the future. However, this is not always effective because clients may forget to apply the skills or they may lose their proficiency in implementing the skills over time. A second approach is to provide clients with posttherapy interventions, such as periodic booster sessions or maintenance sessions. These regular check-ups may be required for years (e.g., Jacobson, 1989; Wolf, Braukmann, & Ramp, 1987). Developing, refining, and empirically validating such interventions are important challenges for behavior therapists.

The old adage, "An ounce of prevention is worth a pound of cure," is certainly germane to behavior therapy. Some behavior therapies have preventive strategies built in, such as problem-solving therapy and stress inoculation training, both of which provide clients with generalized coping skills. Using behavior therapy principles and procedures for primary prevention was first proposed in the 1970s (Poser, 1970). In the ensuing years, however, behavior therapists have done relatively little to meet the challenge of prevention; treatment always seems to take precedence. Behavioral prevention could prove particularly useful for those disorders that have been most resistant to treatment with behavior therapy (e.g., substance-related disorders). Given the personal and societal advantages of prevention over treatment, behavioral prevention is a worthwhile challenge.

A last noteworthy challenge to behavior therapy is to determine how behavior therapy can be more compatible with the ever-increasing diversity of the clients it serves. As I will discuss in the next section, there are three primary initiatives facing behavior therapists regarding diversity issues. First, the practice of adapting behavior therapy for the treatment of diverse clients needs to be based on empirical findings (i.e., what will actually work with the client population) rather than speculations gleaned from cultural norms and prevailing stereotypes. Second, some of the underlying assumptions of behavior therapy that were developed outside the context of treating diverse clients need to be changed to be more compatible with new client populations. Third, efforts need to be made to recruit and train behavior therapists who themselves are culturally diverse.

Future Development: Behavior Therapy in a Diverse World

As I discussed earlier, the basic nature of behavior therapy makes it inherently suited to treating diverse clients. Behavior therapy has been used with clients who vary in age, gender, culture, ethnicity, race, sexual orientation, religion, and intellectual and physical capabilities. Still, behavior therapists believe that serving widely diverse clients can be further refined, and they are actively engaged in efforts to make behavior therapies more informed and sensitive to issues of diversity (e.g., Hays, 2001; Hays & Iwamasa, 2006; Hinton, 2006; Hoffman, 2006).

Standard behavior therapy procedures have been modified to be more compatible with the diverse clients now being treated. The problem is that most of these modifications have been made ad hoc—that is, they emanate from what one would expect to be useful or appropriate based on norms or stereotypes of the diversity group (e.g., the inclusion of humor in therapy *should be* useful for Jewish clients whose culture values humor) (e.g., Hatch, Friedman, & Paradis, 1996; McNair, 1996; Organista & Muñoz, 1996; Preciado, 1999). Recommendations for adapting behavior therapies to diverse clients need to be empirically based, which is an important task for future research.

Because the restricted cultural context in which behavior therapy was developed influenced some of its underlying theoretical assumptions, these assumptions may need to be modified to facilitate working with more diverse clients. For example, behavior therapy often takes for granted that Western logic and rationality reflect universal truths. However, that is not so; logic and rationality are culture specific. This means that cognitive restructuring therapies with clients other than White, middle-class European Americans may require a redefinition of rationality or, more precisely, an identification of what is considered rational in the client's culture. For instance, suppose a client said that she was distressed because she wanted to marry a man outside her religious faith and that would mean that she would never have contact with her family again. A therapist might be tempted to point to the irrationality of that conclusion because the client jumped to the conclusion and blew things out of proportion. However, in some religious faiths, such as ultra-Orthodox Judaism, the custom is that if someone marries out of the faith, the person is no longer considered a member of the family and the family will no longer make any contact with or recognize the existence of the person (e.g., pictures of the individual are removed from the home and family members never speak about the person). Thus, if the woman were a member of such a religious group, her concern that she would lose her family if she married outside her faith would not be irrational. Cognitive-behavioral therapy for this woman's distress would not involve substituting a rational belief for an irrational one, but instead would help her cope with the reality of her situation.

Finally, although the U.S. population is becoming increasingly diverse, the demographics of graduate students and faculty at the universities that train behavior therapists have remained relatively stable (Neal-Barnett & Smith, 1996; Safren, 2001). Thus, recruiting behavior therapists representing diverse groups is an important initiative for the future of behavior therapy.

Summary

1. Cognitive-behavioral therapy changes cognitions that are the maintaining conditions of clients' problems. Cognitive-behavioral therapies fit into two categories. Cognitive restructuring therapies teach clients to change maladaptive cognitions (self-talk) that maintain their problem behaviors and to substitute more adaptive cognitions. Cognitive-behavioral coping skills therapies teach clients adaptive responses—both cognitive and overt behavioral—to deal effectively with the difficult situations they encounter.

2. Thought stopping decreases the frequency, duration, and intensity of disturbing thoughts by interrupting them and substituting competing thoughts.

3. Rational emotive behavior therapy (REBT) employs cognitive restructuring to change irrational thoughts. REBT is based on the principle that it is beliefs about events in our lives, rather than the events themselves, that maintain psychological problems. Maladaptive thoughts result from logical errors in thinking, including absolute thinking, overgeneralizing, and catastrophizing. Two themes are common in irrational ideas that lead to psychological problems: personal worthlessness and a sense of duty.

4. REBT therapists teach clients to identify their irrational thoughts, challenge the irrational beliefs on which the thoughts are based, and substitute thoughts based on rational beliefs for their irrational thoughts.

5. Cognitive therapy is similar to REBT. Both assume that psychological disorders are maintained by distorted cognitions, and both use cognitive restructuring. However, cognitive therapy uses the Socratic method to help clients identify their automatic thoughts and empirical hypothesis testing as a means of changing existing beliefs—rather than directly challenging the beliefs, as in REBT.

6. Cognitive therapy involves a collaborative effort of the client and therapist. Clients are taught to view automatic thoughts (maladaptive cognitions) as hypotheses subject to empirical validation, rather than as established facts. Clients test out the hypotheses through homework assignments in which they make observations to refute the hypotheses.

7. Cognitive therapy procedures that directly change clients' cognitions include analyzing faulty logic, obtaining accurate information, self-recording automatic thoughts, generating alternative interpretations of events, reattributing responsibility about negative outcomes, and decatastrophizing.

8. Cognitive therapy procedures that indirectly change clients' cognitions by changing overt behaviors include generating activity schedules, making mastery and pleasure ratings, and engaging in graded task assignments.

9. Originally developed to treat depression, cognitive therapy is now used to treat many different psychological disorders with a wide spectrum of diverse client populations.

10. Cognitive-behavioral coping skills therapies treat problems that are maintained by a deficit of adaptive cognitions by changing both cognitions and overt behaviors.

11. In self-instructional training, clients learn to instruct themselves to cope effectively with difficult situations. Self-instructions serve four functions: focusing attention, guiding behavior, providing encouragement, and evaluating performance. The five steps of self-instructional training are cognitive modeling, cognitive participant modeling, overt self-instructions, fading of overt self-instructions, and covert self-instructions.

12. Problem-solving therapy teaches clients a systematic strategy for approaching psychological problems and serves the dual purpose of treating clients' immediate problems and preparing clients to deal with future problems on their own. The seven stages of problem solving are adopting a problem-solving orientation, defining the problem, selecting goals, generating alternative solutions, choosing the best solution, implementing the best solution, and evaluating the effects of the solution. Problem-solving skills are taught to clients through cognitive modeling, prompting, self-instructions, and reinforcement.

13. Stress inoculation training helps clients cope with stress by teaching them coping skills and then having clients practice the skills while they are exposed to stress-evoking events. Stress inoculation training consists of three phases: conceptualization, coping skills acquisition, and application. Anxiety, anger, and pain are the most frequently treated problems.

14. In behavior therapy, the client-counselor relationship is considered necessary but not sufficient for successful treatment. Clients are presumed to be helped primarily by the specific behavior therapy techniques. However, a trusting relationship facilitates the counseling process and is especially important in working with diverse clients.

15. The evidence to support the effectiveness of behavior therapies comes from controlled experiments that use four outcome measures: meaningfulness of change, transfer and generalization, long-term maintenance, and acceptability of the treatment. This nomothetic research has demonstrated that, as a group of therapy procedures, behavior therapy has a strong and broad empirical base.

16. The progress and success of treatment for a particular client (idiographic evaluation) is measured by the degree to which the client's goals for therapy have been met, which, in behavior therapy, can be determined more reliably than in many other therapy approaches because client goals are defined specifically, unambiguously, and measurably.

17. Behavior therapy has been used to treat the gamut of client problems and a wide range of client populations, including those for whom verbal psychotherapies cannot work.

18. The major blind spots of behavior therapy are its present focus, its narrow focus, and its emphasis on the external environment. Its major limitations are treating some especially recalcitrant disorders and problems and dealing with the fact that its basic nature is not conducive for some clients. Behavior therapy's challenges include enhancing long-term maintenance of treatment gains, preventing problems and disorders, and developing empirically supported treatments for diverse clients.

19. Because of its basic nature and the way it is practiced, behavior therapy is inherently suited to treating diverse clients. These factors include individualized treatment, emphasis on the external environment, active nature, emphasis on learning, reliance on empirical evidence, present focus, and brevity. Still, behavior therapists are interested in enhancing their treatment of diverse clients, which includes generating empirically supported modifications for existing treatments to serve specific populations, adjusting some of their underlying theoretical assumptions to fit with diverse worldviews, and encouraging more people from diverse backgrounds to become behavior therapists.

Key Terms

activity schedule (p. 333)
automatic thoughts (p. 328)
cognitive-behavioral therapy (p. 320)
cognitive modeling (p. 337)
cognitive restructuring (p. 321)
cognitive therapy (p. 328)
collaborative empiricism (p. 331)
graded task assignments (p. 333)
mastery and pleasure ratings (p. 333)

problem-solving therapy (p. 339)
rational emotive behavior therapy (REBT) (p. 323)
schema (p. 335)
schema-based cognitive therapy (p. 335)
self-instructional training (p. 337)
self-talk (p. 321)
stress inoculation training (p. 341)
thought stopping (p. 322)

Resources for Further Study

Professional Organizations

Association for Behavioral and Cognitive Therapies (ABCT)
http://www.aabt.org/
305 7th Avenue, 16th Floor
New York, NY 10001
800-685-2228

National Association of Cognitive-Behavioral Therapists (NACBT)
http://www.nacbt.org/
P.O. Box 2195
Weirton, WV 26062
800-853-1135

Academy of Cognitive Therapy (ACT)
http://www.academyofct.org/
One Belmont Avenue, Suite 700
Bala Cynwyd, PA 19004-1610
610-664-1273

International Association for Cognitive Psychotherapy (IACP)
http://www.cognitivetherapyassociation.org/

Professional Journals

Behavior Modification
http://bmo.sagepub.com/
Behavior Therapy
http://www.elsevier.com/locate/bt
Behaviour Research and Therapy
http://www.elsevier.com/locate/bt
Behavioural and Cognitive Psychotherapy
http://www.cambridge.org/journals/journal_catalogue.asp?mnemonic=BCP
Child and Family Behavior Therapy
http://www.haworthpress.com/store/find.asp
Cognitive and Behavioral Practice
http://www.elsevier.com/locate/bt
Cognitive Behaviour Therapy
http://journalsonline.tandf.co.uk/(50l1d42nw0rsh045mhh2obml)/app/home/journal.asp?
referrer=parent&backto=linkingpublicationresults,1:300302,1&linkin=

Cognitive Therapy and Research
http://www.springer.com/west/home/generic/search/results?SGWID=
4-40109-70-35753187-0
Journal of Applied Behavior Analysis
http://seab.envmed.rochester.edu/jaba/
Journal of Behavior Therapy and Experimental Psychiatry
http://www.elsevier.com/locate/bt
Journal of Behavioral Education
http://www.ovid.com/site/catalog/Journal/1521.jsp?top=2&mid=3&bottom=
7&subsection=12
Journal of Cognitive Psychotherapy: An International Journal
http://www.cognitivetherapyassociation.org/journal/default1.aspx?pagename=jcp.aspx
Journal of Psychopathology and Behavioral Assessment
http://www.springer.com/west/home/generic/search/results?SGWID=
4-40109-70-35608747-0
Journal of Rational-Emotive and Cognitive-Behavioral Therapy
http://www.rebt.org/journal.htm
the Behavior Therapist
http://www.abct.org/mentalhealth/journals/?fa=tBT

Suggested Readings in Traditional Behavior Therapy

Alberti, R., & Emmons, M. (2001). *Your perfect right: Assertiveness and equality in your life and relationships* (8th ed.). San Luis Obispo, CA: Impact.

A self-help primer to assertion training. This book comes out in a new edition every few years, so check for the latest edition.

Bernstein, D. A., Borkovec, T. D., & Hazlett-Stevens, H. (2000). *New directions in progressive relaxation training: A guidebook for helping professionals.* Westport, CT: Praeger.

A practical guide for teaching clients progressive relaxation.

Kazdin, A. E. (1977). *The token economy: A review and evaluation.* New York: Plenum.

A comprehensive review of token economies through the mid-1970s.

Kazdin, A. E. (1978). *History of behavior modification: Experimental foundations of contemporary research.* Baltimore: University Park Press.

An in-depth discussion of the history of behavior therapy (despite the term used in the title).

Spiegler, M. D., & Guevremont, D. C. (2003). *Contemporary behavior therapy* (4th ed.). Pacific Grove, CA: Wadsworth.

A comprehensive textbook that provides details of all the behavior therapy procedures you've read about in this chapter.

Wysocki, P. A. (Ed.). (1991). *Handbook of clinical behavior therapy with the elderly client.* New York: Plenum Press.

> The title describes this book written by experts in various aspects of treating a major diverse population—the elderly.

Wolpe, J. (1990). *The practice of behavior therapy* (4th ed.). New York: Pergamon.

> Wolpe's last revision of his classic book that details the practice of brief/graduated exposure therapy and other behavior therapy techniques.

The following seven volumes in the *How to Manage Behavior Series* are 30-page pamphlets providing the nuts and bolts of specific behavior therapy techniques.

Ayllon, T. (1999). *How to use token economy and point systems* (2nd ed.). Austin TX: Pro-ed.

Hall, R. V., & Hall, M .L. (1998). *How to select reinforcers* (2nd ed.). Austin, TX: Pro-ed.

Hall, R. V., & Hall, M .L. (1998). *How to use planned ignoring (extinction)* (2nd ed.). Austin, TX: Pro-ed.

Hall, R. V., & Hall, M .L. (1998). *How to use systematic attention and approval* (2nd ed.). Austin, TX: Pro-ed.

Hall, R. V., & Hall, M .L. (1998). *How to use time out* (2nd ed.). Austin, TX: Pro-ed.

Thibadeau, S. F. (1998). *How to use response cost.* Austin TX: Pro-ed.

Van Houten, R. (1998). *How to use prompts to initiate behaviors* (2nd ed.). Austin TX: Pro-ed.

Suggested Readings in Cognitive-Behavioral Therapy

Beck, A. T. (1989). *Love is never enough.* New York: Harper & Row (Perennial Library).

> A practical guide to better relationships from a cognitive therapy perspective, by the originator of cognitive therapy.

Burns, D. (1980). *Feeling good.* New York: Morrow.

> A do-it-yourself cognitive therapy guide for mild depression; extremely helpful and provides a good understanding of cognitive therapy as applied to depression.

D'Zurilla, T. J., & Nezu, A. M. (1999). *Problem-solving therapy: A social competence approach to clinical intervention* (2nd ed.). New York: Springer.

> Perhaps the best single book on problem-solving therapy.

Ellis, A. (1962). *Reason and emotion in psychotherapy.* New York: Lyle Stuart.

> The classic introduction to rational emotive behavior therapy, by its originator.

Meichenbaum, D. (1985). *Stress inoculation training.* Elmsford, NY: Pergamon Press.

> The nuts-and-bolts of stress inoculation training, by the psychologist who developed this treatment.

Other Media Resources

The Association for Behavioral and Cognitive Therapies (http://www.aabt.org/) has a series of videotapes and audiotapes that provide demonstrations of behavior therapies and interviews with the innovators and leaders in the field.

The American Psychological Association's (http://www.apa.org/) Psychotherapy Videotape Series includes demonstrations of a variety of behavior therapies.

Chapter 10

Reality Therapy

ROBERT E. WUBBOLDING

Reality therapy began in the 1960s in a mental hospital and a correctional institution and has spread to populations far removed from severe emotional disturbance and criminal behavior. It is based on the two interrelated premises that people should be held responsible for their behavior and that people choose how they behave. Formulated by psychiatrist William Glasser, reality therapy and its underlying theory—choice theory—have been applied to a wide variety of problem behaviors and human endeavors.

Origins and Evolution of Reality Therapy

The two settings in which Glasser developed reality therapy—the psychiatric ward of a Veterans Administration hospital in Los Angeles and a correctional institution for delinquent girls in Ventura, California—offered diverse populations and a wide array of problems. As with many counseling methods, Glasser formulated his system based on his personal experience with his patients. Trained in conventional psychoanalytical theory, he rebelled against his formal training when he made an interesting observation: although the therapy practiced by his teachers seemed to be effective, it was very different from what they taught. Their strategy from the outset of therapy was to hold patients responsible for their own behavior, which seemed to result in the patients improving. The strategy provided the basis for the future counseling system we now call *reality therapy*. The notion of holding clients responsible for how they behave, which ran counter to theories of psychotherapy in the 1960s, is in many ways a basic principle by which people have always lived. In the world outside that of counseling and psychotherapy, people are, in fact, held responsible for their behavior. Glasser's reality therapy incorporated this real-world principle.

"Reality therapy is one of the newest of man's formal attempts to explain mankind, to set rules for behavior, and to map out how one person can help another to achieve happiness and success; but at the same time, paradoxically, it represents one of the oldest sets of maxims referring to human conduct" (Glasser & Zunin, 1973, p. 287). For example, in the second century CE, Marcus Aurelius wrote about the primacy of personal responsibility in the following ways: "If anything is within the powers and province of man, believe that it is within your own compass also"; "Men's actions cannot agitate us, but our own views regarding them [can arouse our emotions]"; and "The agitations that beset you are superfluous and depend wholly on judgments that are your own" (Antoninus, 1944, p. 21).

In the late 19th and early 20th century, Paul Dubois, a Swiss physician whom Glasser thought of as his spiritual ancestor, had assisted his patients by helping them replace destructive thoughts with helpful thinking (Glasser & Zunin, 1973), and William James, often called the father of American psychology, stated that one of the greatest discoveries in history is the fact that we can change the circumstances of our lives by changing our attitudes. He summarized this simple yet profound thought, "We do not sing because we are happy, we are happy because we sing."

Helmut Kaiser, a psychoanalyst at the Menninger Foundation, was a more proximate influence in the development of reality therapy. He said, "It is the analyst's task to make the patient feel responsible for his own words and his own actions" (Kaiser, 1965/1955, p. 4). He carried this thought even further by emphasizing that anything that makes clients feel responsible for their behavior helps to cure them. G. L. Harrington built upon Kaiser's ideas, adding that a more democratic doctor-patient relationship promotes healing more effectively than an authoritative relationship (Glasser & Wubbolding, 1995). Harrington, who was Glasser's supervisor during his psychiatric training, deviated from the traditional psychoanalytic curriculum and taught Glasser the basic principles of an approach that became reality therapy.

Glasser once told me about a session that he conducted with a woman at the beginning of his psychiatric training. Previously, she had spent most of her 3 years in therapy talking about her grandfather and blaming him for her nervousness and depression. When she began treatment with Dr. Glasser, he asked her how often she had contact with her grandfather. She replied that her grandfather had died many years before. Glasser told her that her grandfather now had no influence in her life unless she chose to remain oppressed by him. Therefore, he would not discuss her grandfather with her in their sessions. After a few months of using this early and inelegant form of reality therapy, which focused on the present, the client stopped the depressed and anxious behavior. (As you will soon learn, in reality therapy feelings such as depression or anxiety are considered behaviors.) Instead of reprimanding Glasser for deviating from conventional therapy, Harrington told Glasser, "Join the club." Emboldened by this success, Glasser continued to expand his techniques into a more sophisticated methodology. Based on what he learned from Harrington, Glasser later developed the specific procedures used in reality therapy as well as adopted and extended a theory of brain functioning known as *control theory* that he later renamed **choice theory,** which, in a nutshell, posits that behavior originates from within and that most behaviors are chosen.

Upon board certification as a psychiatrist in 1961, Glasser began lecturing on reality therapy, emphasizing personal responsibility and choice as its essential elements. In 1965, he published *Reality Therapy,* a book that was widely read by counselors, social workers, and teachers. Because of therapists' interest in further training in reality therapy, Glasser founded the Institute for Reality Therapy in 1967, now named the William Glasser Institute.

When it was first developed, a major criticism of reality therapy was that it was a methodology without a theory. Glasser (1985) resolved this shortcoming by developing a new theory based on Powers's (1973) control theory, which posits that the brain functions as a control system. A thermostat reads the temperature in a room and sends a signal to the furnace or air conditioning unit to take action to achieve the desired temperature. Likewise, the human brain, determining that it does not have what it needs, sends a signal to the behavioral system to take action to fulfill the need in question. Building on Power's concept of the brain as a needs thermostat, Glasser added five basic human needs as the motivational system and emphasized that behavior is chosen, naming his new theory *choice theory* in 1996 (Glasser, 1998).

In the decades since Glasser worked alone, many people have collaborated with him to help expand his ideas. To this day, he has continued to creatively and passionately teach others about choice theory and reality therapy. And interest in reality therapy is widespread, as evidenced by people coming from all over the world to the 2004 conference at the William Glasser Institute in Schaumburg, Illinois. In response to this interest, the William Glasser Institute sponsors an intensive certification program over 18 months. Training sessions take place throughout North America, South America, Europe, Australia, Asia, and the Middle East.

Originally a system of clinical interventions, reality therapy evolved as well into an educational philosophy and delivery system. Because of Glasser's emphasis on personal responsibility, educators have found reality therapy useful. Applied to schools, reality therapy formed the basis of an educational program called Schools Without Failure (Glasser, 1968). This program gradually expanded and eventually incorporated W. Edwards Deming's (1986) concept of quality, which meant that teachers accept only excellent work, aim at continuous improvement, establish an environment satisfying the internal needs of students, and maintain school as a joyful place.

Reality therapy has also been applied to management and supervision. "The world of employment, in which most people spend a high percentage of their time, has surpassed other institutions in affirming the fallacious theory that people can be controlled from above. . . . When the inner sources of human motivation are satisfied on the job, the worker feels the 'joy of work' described by W. Edwards Deming. These innate needs underlie the behavior of all workers" (Wubbolding, 1996, pp. 3–4).

Evolution of Reality Therapy for a Diverse World

Reality therapists believe that the principles of personal responsibility and behavior as a choice are universally applicable. Regardless of race, ethnicity, cultural differences, gender, age, or any other human differences, we are all motivated by the same internal drives and needs. Though human beings around the world may generate different behaviors aimed at satisfying these needs, the needs themselves are universal. This sameness is the basis for Maya Angelou's oft-repeated plea that we be mindful that "there is more that unites us than what separates us."

At the same time, reality therapists recognize the reality of an unbalanced playing field regarding human choices. Many people do not have as many choices as other people have. Because of race, because of gender, because of age, because of ability—there are many cultural barriers hindering effective need satisfaction. However, reality therapists work within clients' contexts, assisting them in diminishing their internal restraints and sidestepping external or environmental obstacles. In counseling minority clients who perceive themselves as victims of prejudice, the reality therapist helps them to see that despite prejudice and discrimination against them, they have choices available to them that perhaps they did not previously see (including systemic change). Reality therapists help clients evaluate and focus on what they can control and work on, including helping them evaluate their perception of being a victim and how this may be helping or hindering them. Further, although people's wants and needs tend to be shaped by the boundaries of their cultures, in our increasingly multicultural society an individual's wants may conflict with his or her culture of origin. Reality therapists help clients examine their wants and needs and make satisfying life choices related to them whether or not these choices take them outside their culture.

Context Then—Context Now

When reality therapy made its first significant appearance in 1965 with the publication of Glasser's *Reality Therapy*, the dominant mode of treatment was psychoanalysis, emphasizing insight into the unconscious and resolving childhood conflicts. Additionally, in opposition to this longstanding and widely accepted method, client-centered therapy was rapidly gaining acceptance. Client-centered therapy stressed the current affective part of the human psyche.

When reality therapy arrived on the scene, it was not greeted with enthusiasm or wide acceptance by the psychological or psychiatric communities. Reality therapy emphasized neither discussion of past conflicts nor feelings as obstacles to self-actualization. However, its emphasis on current actions and consequent personal responsibility made it appealing to educators, correctional workers, social workers, and counselors who worked with troubled youths. Glasser (1972) noted that in the wider society young people seemed to be searching for identity, for roles rather than goals. With its emphasis on satisfying personal needs, reality therapy addressed this legitimate but sometimes excessive hunger of people to "find" themselves. By using reality therapy principles, they could formulate assertive and altruistic behaviors for satisfying their needs and thus determine their role in life, which Glasser believed revolved around how they might connect with others.

Since that time, reality therapy has gained wider acceptance in academia and in the helping professions, as evidenced by its frequent representation in psychotherapy and counseling texts. However, lacking historical hindsight, conclusions about current context must be tentative and perhaps temporary. Still, some observations are useful. Practitioners of reality therapy see clients as responsible for their behavior, which may account for its grassroots popularity and acceptance. Reality therapy offers an antidote to the popular and academic tendency to see problem behaviors as culturally determined and therefore excusable. On a superficial level, the accusation could be made that reality therapy blames victims. Quite the contrary is true. From the perspective of reality therapy, clients liberate themselves from blame and oppression when they realize that they have at least some choice to deal with their plights, dreadful as they might be, in a positive and hopeful manner. The foundational principle for the success of reality therapy is that accusing, blaming, criticizing, demeaning, and colluding with excuses are toxic behaviors that are destructive to the counseling relationship and thus are not tolerated in counseling.

Also, with its emphasis on promoting healthy human relationship as an alternative to the excessive use of medication for treating mental disorders, reality therapy offers a clear path to improving mental health. The current emphasis in reality therapy includes defining mental health as an identifiable entity, not merely the absence of mental illness. The key component of mental health from this perspective is healthy human relationships that satisfy basic human needs, especially the need for belonging—at home, at work, and in the community.

The Author's Journey as a Reality Therapist

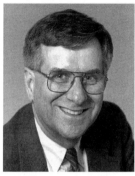

Robert Wubbolding

The principles of reality therapy appealed to me even before I encountered them as underlying tenets of a counseling method. In my view, personal responsibility and the art of making satisfying, ethical, and altruistic choices embody a personal, elusive, and imperfectly attained ideal.

After completing my doctorate in counseling at the University of Cincinnati in 1971, I became an adjunct professor at Xavier University in Cincinnati. At the time I was practicing client-centered therapy. However, I wanted to learn more about various counseling methods so that I could more effec-tively counsel, consult, and teach on the university level. I attended behavior therapy workshops, Adlerian training programs, and rational emotive therapy conferences (including the first international conference on rational emotive therapy in 1975). But it was the reality therapy seminars I attended that had a lasting impact on me. I thought that reality therapy best reflected how people truly live their lives, and it most suited my personal philosophy.

My decision to practice reality therapy had been prompted by my attendance at a workshop on reality therapy conducted by Ed Ford and sponsored by the Case Western Reserve Department of Social Work. What I learned in this workshop was consistent with my belief that in the endeavor to solve one's present problems, it is of little value to excavate one's past and spend an inordinate amount of time examining it. Moreover, the reality therapy approach addressed an issue that I was having regarding my practice of client-centered therapy. Although client-centered therapy embraces personal responsibility and applies to virtually any human being, helping clients "get in touch with their feelings" seemed to me an endless process, impractical in the school settings where I had worked and in the settings where many master's or doctoral counseling students would be working. As I was searching for another system, I began to encourage clients to take action, and I became less corrective in my supervision of graduate students who pushed their clients "to get off dead center" and do something about their problems. In reality therapy, I found an action-oriented delivery system that accommodated, validated, and extended my own values and belief system.

Ford's reality therapy workshop kindled my desire to learn more about this practical approach. So I went to Los Angeles to attend a 4-day training session

(*continued*)

conducted by Glasser, and later that year I attended three other training sessions. My commitment to the principles of reality therapy reached fruition after my first role-play with Dr. Glasser. Even now I remember the session as though it were yesterday. Within 30 minutes, I simulated every type of client I had encountered at the halfway house for female ex-offenders where I was working at the time. With unmatched finesse, Glasser disarmed my manipulations without attacking, demeaning, or rejecting me. I became convinced that there was something to this system that was extremely valuable, even though I did not quite grasp its profundity or subtlety at the time. Eventually Glasser's institute developed the certification process, and I successfully completed the first certification week in 1975. I was especially proud when Dr. Glasser appointed me to teach reality therapy in 1979, which I did in the United States and abroad, and later when he asked me to be the director of training for his institute in 1987, a position I hold to this day.

Theory of Reality Therapy

Reality therapy rests on the principles of choice theory. When I give a lecture on choice theory, I begin by asking students if they believe that their jobs cause them stress. Usually around 95% of them answer yes. I then ask them if being stuck in traffic causes them aggravation. Yes, they agree, yes. Finally I ask if driving in freezing rain down an icy road would cause them anxiety. Almost invariably a high percentage of them state that yes, driving under such conditions would make them anxious. I then explain that according to choice theory, how we act, what we think, and what we feel, both emotionally and physiologically, are behaviors. Our behaviors are not caused by the outside world; our behaviors are our own choices. Skeptical but curious, my students then accompany me on an excursion into human motivation and the origins of human behavior. We consider a variety of examples, such as the fact that skiers would find 2 feet of snow on the ground very satisfying whereas a bus driver might have quite different feelings about encountering these conditions. By reflecting on such examples, my students come to realize that their behaviors, including feelings, originate from within. In other words, how we perceive the world and what we want from the world is the source of human behavior.

Choice theory is a comprehensive explanation of human motivation and behavior based on the concept of inner control. Popular belief has held that we can make people do what we think they should do and that in some ways we can control them. Parents attempt to coerce their children to do the right thing, to avoid trouble, and to be successful. Managers and supervisors in companies and institutions often use fear in a futile attempt to increase motivation and the quality of work output. In education, administrators and classroom teachers sometimes develop a severe case of burnout in their frustrated and doomed efforts to control students, parents, voters, and the public in general. Choice theory offers an alternative to this philosophy of coercion, or as Kohn (1993) called it, "pop behaviorism."

Philosophical Foundations

Vaudeville gave us a classic joke, "Why did the chicken cross the road?" The answer, "To get to the other side," illustrates an ancient and profound truth. As the Roman emperor Marcus Aurelius said, "Nature has an aim in everything." Reality therapy embraces this teleological philosophy of nature and perceives all human behavior as having a purpose. Further, reality therapy focuses on the choices involved in human behavior and posits that these choices are much more extensive than is recognized in conventional wisdom.

   The underlying principles of reality therapy and choice theory posit a system of internal controls through the exercise of which human beings can effectively modify victimization by external forces. We need not remain in the thrall of the past, of our childhood experiences. We need not be bound by societal expectations or restrictions. We need not be paralyzed by oppression. Even in the direst circumstances imaginable, choices exist. The experiences of the existential therapist Victor Frankl provides a perfect example of avoiding the paralysis of external restrictions. Imprisoned in a Nazi concentration camp, Frankl (1984) knew that he had very few choices about his actions, yet he chose to focus on his priorities and the options he did have. For him survival was everything, and all his choices were aimed at staying alive. He also chose to look beyond the dark and diabolical brutality of the concentration camp to a dawn of hope and fulfillment. Most people in the world today have more choices than Frankl had, but life is still not fair. Some people—because of prejudice and life circumstances—have fewer choices than others, but all people have choices. What we do in reality therapy is help clients focus on the possible choices they have.

Theoretical Concepts

Glasser developed choice theory and made it a clinical model and an educational model. Choice theory, which grew out of the cybernetic control theory, is based on the idea that we are not driven to act by past history or by external stimuli from the world around us. Instead, we are driven by our needs and our wants.

Reality therapy's explanation of human needs and wants and the behaviors that are aimed at achieving them are codified in the four principles of choice theory.

Four Principles of Choice Theory

Principle 1. All human beings are motivated by five genetically encoded primary **needs:**

1. *Survival, self-preservation, and physiological needs.* Built into human beings is the biological need or genetic instruction to continue to live, to maintain health, and to preserve individual life as well as the life of the human species. Some survival behaviors are automatic or involuntary, such as digesting food, circulating blood, or developing hunger and thirst. Many other behaviors that fulfill this need are voluntary, such as growing and hunting for food or shopping in a supermarket, sewing a piece of clothing, building a house, and having a baby.

2. *Belonging and love needs.* Inherent in all human beings is a need to connect with other humans, to give and receive love. Reality therapy considers the needs to belong and to love and be loved as having prime importance, second only to the need for survival, because human beings are social creatures. Many diverse human behaviors spring from the need for belonging and love, from infants' crying when they want to be held to people of all ages joining clubs. The need has long been recognized as playing a dominant role in mental health, and failure to fulfill the need for belonging is associated with mental disorders. For example, "A number of studies report that family adversity, parental discord, and friendship difficulties all exert direct provoking effects on the risk of depression" (Hammond & Romney, 1995, p. 668).

3. *Power, achievement, and inner control needs.* As defined in choice theory, *power* refers to the need to feel in charge of our own lives and to feel a sense of accomplishment and inner control. Individuals may seek to satisfy their need for power by exploiting others, and historical examples of such abuse prompted Lord Acton in the 19th century to utter his famous axiom, "Power corrupts and absolute power corrupts absolutely." However, fulfilling this need does not have to be a zero sum game of "I win, you lose." In choice theory, power is seen as the drive for enhanced inner control, competence, self-esteem, and self-worth.

4. *Freedom and independence needs.* One of the most satisfying feelings a person gains from making choices, even minuscule choices, is a sense of autonomy or self-determination that is essential to the integrity of human life.

5. *Fun and enjoyment needs.* The literal meaning of the word *recreation*— to re-create—explains the importance of satisfying the need for fun and

enjoyment. Recreation provides refreshment of body or mind; it is renewal by some form of play, amusement, or relaxation. Aristotle defined a human being as a creature that is risible, able or inclined to laugh, which is one characteristic that separates human beings from most other animals. Certainly, laughter binds people together.

Our basic needs overlap with one another. Humans are social creatures because other humans are necessarily involved in the satisfaction of most needs. We work together to grow, or make, or earn the basics we need for survival. We have fun with other people in order to strengthen our relationships. In deciding to learn a new skill such as golf, painting, or counseling, one learns with other people, thereby fulfilling the need for belonging as well as for achievement and power. And so a reality therapist's answer to the question, "Why did the chicken cross the road?" might be, "He saw another chicken on the other side of the road and chose to get some exercise that was fun and at the same time achieve something, which gave him a sense of freedom."

Principle 2.   The five universal needs engender wants. **Wants** are unique to each individual and develop from choices designed to satisfy needs within the context of a person's family and cultural environment. As we interact with the world around us, we develop specific wants or pictures of what is important to us, what will satisfy our basic needs. This vision of our personal wants is called our **quality world.**

Within each human being there is at least one picture related to survival, belonging, power, freedom, and fun. In describing the importance of the quality world, Glasser (1998) wrote, "Throughout our lives we will be in closer contact with this [quality] world than with anything else we know. Most of us know what's in it to the minutest detail but very few of us know that it, itself, exists. . . . If we knew it existed and understood the vital role it plays in our lives, we would be able to get along much better with each other than most of us do now" (pp. 46–47). Several attributes characterize the pictures or wants that comprise our quality world.

- *Wants are specific:* Whereas needs are general, wants are specific images of people, activities, things, and even core beliefs related to one or more of our basic needs. Our experiences within our culture influence these specific wants. For example, a person born and raised in Beijing forms a quality world culturally different from that of someone born and raised in Bahrain or in St. Louis. Even within a single culture there is great diversity among individuals' wants. At the same time, there is sufficient commonality among individuals' quality worlds to enable societies to function if a majority of the people in the society agree about what they want for their society.

- *Wants may be realistic or unrealistic:* Wants range from being unattainable to being easily attainable. A person wants to go to work in the morning and have a productive day. That is an attainable want. Or someone wants to get in better physical condition. This want is attainable with effort (sacrificing other activities and replacing them with exercise). In contrast, a desire to win a lottery with odds of 5 million to 1 is unrealistic. Yet some people attain even seemingly unrealistic goals, as when an author's first novel becomes a best seller or a wrestler with only one leg becomes a national champion.

- *Wants may be blurred:* When asked what they want from the world around them or from themselves, many clients answer, "I don't know." This is especially likely with minority clients, who may feel that there is no point in clarifying their wants because they have little chance of attaining them.

- *Wants vary in their priority:* Some wants are more important and more pressing than others. Eating lunch is likely to have higher priority than shopping for a wind chime. Wanting career advancement and recognition might override wanting to take a vacation. The motivation behind many cruel jokes is that wanting to be liked for one's sense of humor has a higher priority for many people than wanting to be considered a kind person.

- *Wants may conflict:* A person's wants may conflict with one another. Wanting to enjoy a late night movie is likely to conflict with wanting to get enough sleep to be rested the next day. And one person's wants may be in conflict with other people's wants. A person from a culture that values education may wish to drop out of school, which may create conflict in the family and damage familial relationships.

Principle 3. When our quality worlds are unfulfilled—that is, when we are not getting what we want—we *choose* behaviors that are intended to attain unfulfilled wants. Reality therapists view actions, cognitions or thoughts, emotions or feelings, and physiological functions as four distinct but *inseparable* components of **total behavior.** Action is the most controllable aspect of total behavior, and cognitions are the second most controllable. Emotions are viewed as behaviors that accompany thinking and acting and are considered the third most controllable aspect. Physiology is the least controllable aspect of total behavior.

The causes of actions, thoughts, and feelings—the aspects of total behavior counselors work with—lie in unfulfilled needs and wants. Consequently, viewed from the principles of choice theory, thoughts and feelings are not the causes of actions, but rather thoughts and feelings are actions themselves.

Instead of expressing clients' problems as things that are victimizing them, reality therapists express them as behaviors. With clients who complain of "having back pain," "being depressed," "experiencing anxiety," or "being angry," reality therapists use the verb forms of such words. Clients are *paining, depressing, anxietying, or angering.* Although no one directly chooses to suffer, suffering is often an inevitable consequence of chosen behavior. For example, a man who does not go to work, stays in bed much of the day, and avoids interacting with others is likely to be depressing himself (rather than being depressed). Using verbs to describe clients' complaints emphasizes that what clients are experiencing are their own behaviors, behaviors they have chosen to engage in. If they behave differently, they can change their experience.

Principle 4. Behavior has a purpose, which is to gain the perception of satisfying wants and fulfilling needs. Behavior is not random or aimless. Every component of one's behavioral repertoire, or total behavior, is an attempt to fulfill some aspect of one's quality world and therefore one or more of the human needs. Many behaviors may seem to lack intelligent purpose. Indeed, as the agent of our own behavior, we often ascribe little meaning to our behaviors. And yet from the perspective of choice theory, every action, thought, or feeling is goal centered even if the behavior is ineffective, harmful, or destructive.

Earlier I said that the purpose of behavior was to achieve the *perception* of satisfying wants and fulfilling needs. In most cases, it is the perception that wants and needs have been satisfied—rather than their actually having been satisfied—that influences our behavior. In other words, if we believe (perceive) that a want is satisfied, then we will not be motivated to behave in ways that fulfill the want and its underlying need, and we can move on to fulfilling other wants and needs. As just one example, a classic experiment examined undergraduate students' behavior under conditions in which they believed or did not believe that they had some control over terminating high-intensity noise they were exposed to (Glass & Singer, 1971). Students who had the perception of control over the noise performed more efficiently than those who did not believe they had any control.

The desire to perceive that our wants have been satisfied is strong. We want to perceive ourselves as being capable and competent, as being a loyal friend and good student. In fact, we want such perceptions so much that we will even deny ourselves information that contradicts a perception, as the following example illustrates.

Perception: I can eat all I want and not gain weight.

Information: All my pants are getting tighter.

Denial rationale: My laundry detergent is shrinking my clothes.

As a broader example, consider that prejudice involves obstructing incoming information that might have the effect of changing our perception of another person or a group of people.

Theory of Change

The four components of total behavior occur on four levels of consciousness. Proceeding from the least to the most conscious level: physiological behaviors (e.g., breathing and sensing) are least conscious, then feelings or emotions, next thinking or cognitions, and, at the most conscious level, actions. As we ascend this hierarchy, we gain more explicit control and therefore our behavior becomes more clearly chosen. We do not choose our physiology directly. It is difficult to change our feelings; deciding to feel differently isn't very effective. We have more control over our thinking in that we can change what we say to ourselves (i.e., our self-talk). And we have the most control over our actions. I have found it helpful to view total behavior as a suitcase packed in four layers, with physiological behaviors at the bottom, then feelings, then thinking, and finally actions at the top. Lying in the top layer, actions are the components easiest to access when we reach into the suitcase seeking a behavior to fulfill a want. And indeed, in daily life, most of our behaviors are actions we engage in without thinking. There is an axiom in 12-step programs that is congruent with the behavioral suitcase: "You can act your way to a new way of thinking easier than you can think your way to a new way of acting."

Although actions may seem at times to be automatic, perhaps inevitable, and not chosen, there is always a level at which some choice is available relative to a given action. For example, while no one chooses to have all the symptoms of ADHD (or any psychological disorder), nevertheless some choices remain available about specific actions that can influence the course of the disorder. For example, people with ADHD can frequently remind themselves to stay on task and can select jobs and activities that are stimulating.

Human beings make behavioral changes only after they evaluate the attainability of their wants and the potential efficacy of their plans for satisfying their wants. Whereas many counseling approaches suggest that clients do more of what works and less of what doesn't work, reality therapy explicitly focuses on this indispensable component of counseling. Without self-evaluation, behavioral change is far less likely. Reality therapists assist clients in their self-evaluation by having them describe their wants, their level of commitment to achieving their wants, and their plans for achieving them. They then help clients make a judgment about whether their plans are likely to be effective. In reality therapy, self-evaluation functions like a mirror: clients are asked to look at their total behavior and assess whether it serves them effectively and efficiently.

A popular definition of insanity (which some have attributed to Albert Einstein) is *doing the same thing over and over and expecting a different outcome.* Expecting a different result by repeating the same actions is especially characteristic of drug-dependent individuals and codependent persons raised in addicted families. With many clients confounded and entangled in the drug culture, self-evaluation becomes especially important.

Practice of Reality Therapy

The delivery system for choice theory is reality therapy. Reality therapists have two major objectives: (1) to establish a firm, fair, and friendly counseling atmosphere, and (2) to apply the basic procedures of reality therapy in an artful, creative, and culturally sensitive way.

Establishing the Counseling Environment

The optimal counseling environment is an atmosphere in which the client feels safe, secure, and motivated (Wubbolding, 2002). To create a healthy counseling atmosphere, reality therapists engage in tonic (healthy) behaviors and avoid engaging in toxic (unhealthy) behaviors. Specifically, **tonic behaviors** are healthy counselor behaviors that enable the client to feel safe, secure, and motivated. Here are some examples.

- Using attending behaviors such as forward-leaning body posture, paraphrasing, reflective listening, eye contact, and strategic silence.

- Showing accurate empathy in the typical sense of attempting to see the world as the client sees it. Additionally, in reality therapy empathy means accepting clients not only as they are but also as they can be if they make more effective choices.

- Communicating a sense of hope. The reality therapist maintains and communicates the belief that clients' lives can be better.

- Doing the unexpected; finding creative and innovative ways to connect with clients.

- Reframing negatives as positives; finding a silver lining in past experiences that clients or others see as negative.

- Discussing problems in the past tense and solutions in the present or future tenses, which communicates to clients that they have more control over their lives than they had previously thought.

- Acknowledging clients' feelings without dwelling on them.

- Practicing ethical professional behavior and maintaining updated knowledge of current legal and ethical issues as they apply to counseling.

In contrast to these tonic behaviors, **toxic behaviors** are unhealthy counselor behaviors that cast a negative pall on the counseling process and result in client resistance rather than change. Here are examples of toxic behaviors (beginning with the letters A-G to help you remember to avoid them).

- *Arguing* with clients, as in attempting to persuade them to make particular choices.

- *Blaming* clients or encouraging them to blame outside forces for their behaviors.

- *Criticizing* the outcomes of clients' choices. Many people do not foresee the consequences of their choices. Encouraging clients to make self-evaluations of their behavior and the consequences of their choices is an alternative to criticizing.

- *Demeaning* clients. Although therapists are not likely to intentionally demean clients, they may do so unintentionally.

- *Encouraging excuses.* Many clients see their control as lying outside themselves, do not see that they have need-satisfying choices, and construct explanations that may function as excuses based on such perceptions. The reality therapist, while empathic, does not collude with excuses.

- *Finding fault* with behaviors or circumstances that cannot be changed. Whether or not people were culpable or situations in a client's past were damaging, there is little value to lengthy discussions about past misery.

- *Giving up.* Reality therapists do not give up on the basic procedures of reality therapy and demonstrate a willingness to go the extra mile with clients who feel that they are not respected by the rest of society. They teach clients the value of making a firm commitment to change while acknowledging that achieving a happier life takes hard work, practice, and time.

The Client–Counselor Relationship

Creating an optimal psychological atmosphere is an ongoing process and is fostered by the counselor's empathy and regard for the client, but the counselor must also be firm in keeping the relationship focused on the essentials of identifying what the client wants and how to get it. The counselor seeks to maintain her or his own comfortable identity and style, but at the same time is sensitive and to some degree responsive to the client's identity and style. Other strategies that also contribute to the desired environment include active listening with special attention to the client's use of metaphor, which the therapists can enlarge upon; appropriate use of humor; and facilitative self-disclosure.

In working with clients, it is important that in our efforts to connect with them we understand that their hostility, surliness, anger, and other forms of resistance are the behaviors they are currently generating to get their needs met. One approach to working with resistant clients is to validate their behavior by approaching the resistive behavior with an indirect and less threatening question. Rather than ask, "What are you doing?" a counselor could ask, "What do other people think you're doing?" or, "What do they say you are doing?" As an example, at a halfway house for women who had encounters with the law, a prevalent attitude the women had was that they had not done anything the judge thought they had done. In such a case, it would be judicious to ask, "What did the judge say you did?" Instead of confrontation, this style of questioning involves first accepting the client's denial and then using it to get a foot inside the door of the client's inner, mental house.

An effective client-counselor relationship is the foundation of reality therapy. Reality therapists function as mentors. Once a productive relationship with the client has been established, reality therapists teach the client choice theory and its relevance to, and applications in, their lives. In addition, participation in the client-counselor relationship is itself a vehicle for teaching clients how to improve other relationships in their lives.

The WDEP System

The second objective in reality therapy is application of the basic procedures of reality therapy, and this is facilitated by my **WDEP system** (Wubbolding, 2000). The WDEP system is a set of procedures based on choice theory. Each of the letters represents an essential component of reality therapy.

W = wants and needs that must be identified

D = doing (actions) and direction, the direction in which clients' behaviors are sending them

E = evaluation by clients—that is, *self*-evaluation—of their wants and the effectiveness of the behaviors aimed at obtaining them

P = planning, the course of action clients will take to fulfill their wants and needs

In the following case example, you will see the application of the WDEP system and how tonic behaviors are fostered and toxic behaviors are avoided.

Jamal, a 22-year-old African American, was on probation after being released from prison and was court ordered for counseling to a community agency. He had a history of sexual imposition, armed robbery, and selling drugs.

A high school dropout, Jamal had been diagnosed as having a learning disability, exhibiting oppositionally defiant behavior, and having a conduct disorder. At age 13, he first encountered the legal system because of serious acting out and violent behaviors. Jamal sees himself as a victim of an oppressive society conspiring to discriminate against him and prevent him from succeeding. His mother is reputed in the community to be a "troublemaker" who is enabling her son to avoid responsibility for his behavior. His recent rearrest for street fighting is a pending case because six witnesses failed to answer their subpoenas and appear in court. He has been assigned to a counselor who is European American and in his 40s. In many ways, no two people could be racially and culturally further apart. The counselor knows that to effectively establish a healthy client-counselor relationship with Jamal, he will need to use diversity-sensitive tonic behaviors and avoid toxic behaviors.

The counselor is careful not to argue about the "social justice" issues that Jamal insists on discussing. As legitimate as such issues may be, they are diversions from Jamal's more immediate issues and their implications for his future. Jamal's perception of the world around him is based on his experience and what he perceives as unfair treatment. Especially in the beginning of the relationship, the counselor makes an effort to appreciate Jamal's experience and acknowledge Jamal's perceptions without agreeing with them. The counselor avoids the toxic relationship behaviors of blaming and criticizing, as tempting as they are. The counselor realizes that counseling for Jamal needs to focus on Jamal's responsibility for *his* future, on *his* behavior, on *his* possible choices, and not on how the world has arrayed itself against him. The counselor's goal is to help Jamal look at his own life with the hope that he will "change what he can change, accept what he cannot change, and reach the wisdom to know the difference." This is not a veiled pacification of Jamal, nor is it an attempt to lure him into a kind of blind conformity. Rather, it is based on the principle that the only person whose behavior Jamal can realistically change is his own.

In the interest of clarity and full disclosure, the counselor does not hesitate to verbalize his thoughts and beliefs about personal responsibility, violence, theft, and sexual imposition, all of which are part of Jamal's past destructive behaviors. Jamal challenges the counselor and tests his sincerity, as shown in the following exchange.

> C (Client): How can you help me? You've never been in my shoes. You don't know what it's like. You've never been in prison. You're not my kind.

[The counselor's response is firm, clear, empathic, and sincere.]

> T (Therapist): Jamal, I can't know everything about your life. But my job is not to help you continue on the pathway you've chosen up to now. My job is to help you find another pathway. It's true that I've never been in

prison and that I don't take drugs. But that is one very good reason why I *can* help you. I am an expert at being drug free, staying out of prison, keeping a legal job, and living a life without the law in my face.

Jamal's counselor is not put off by what he might at first perceive as belligerence and avoidance of responsibility, both of which are encouraged by Jamal's family members and friends (gang members). Focusing on each component of the WDEP system, Jamal's counselor proceeds, using the following strategy.

1. *Help Jamal identify and define what he wants from the world around him.* Emphasis is placed on what Jamal wants, not on what he perceives the world is doing to him. When Jamal attempts to sidetrack this aim by shifting the discussion from the personal to the political, the counselor continues to steer the conversation to what Jamal can control and what is most empowering for him. The counselor asks Jamal to define what he wants from the court, from his mother, from his friends, from society, and, not least, what he might hope to gain from the counseling itself.

2. *Explore Jamal's actions.* While some acknowledgement of his resentment and rage fits with the dialogue about Jamal's total behavior, the emphasis is placed on his actions and to some extent on his self-talk (e.g., "They're all against me" and "They won't let me") The counselor engages Jamal in an extensive conversation regarding how Jamal spends his time. In particular, it is important to identify what he does each day that does *not* get him in trouble.

3. *Lead Jamal to conduct a gradually less fearful but relentless self-evaluation centering on the attainability of his wants and the effectiveness of his actions in satisfying his needs, especially belonging and power.* When Jamal attempts to sidetrack the discussion from realistically achievable actions, the counselor continues to focus on what is genuinely helpful by asking such questions as, "How realistic is it to expect the police to stop watching for you?" "How helpful is it to you in the long run if you choose to break the law?" Focusing Jamal's energy on self-evaluation questions, the counselor is gently but firmly helping Jamal examine his life and evaluate the attainability of his wants and the effectiveness of his choices.

4. *In each session, formulate some plan of action.* Throughout the counseling process, the counselor helps Jamal formulate positive plans of action (e.g., to improve his relationship with his mother, apply for a legal job, and investigate a GED program) with the accompanying unspoken message that Jamal has control of his life and can gain more effective control by taking one step at a time. It is critical that the counselor have faith in the reality therapy process and firmly believe in Jamal's underlying goodness and his ability to have a more satisfying life.

Applying the WDEP system to Jamal or to any client of similar or dissimilar backgrounds and cultural experiences requires that reality therapists self-monitor and remain aware of their own biases, social status, and cultural values so they can feel comfortable and unapologetic about themselves.

W: Exploring the Client's Quality World: Wants, Level of Commitment, and Locus of Control

The W component of the WDEP system involves exploring clients' quality worlds, which is a three-part exercise that consists of determining (1) what they want; (2) their level of commitment, or how hard they are willing to work to achieve their wants; and (3) their locus of control—how much control over their own lives they believe they have.

Exploring What Clients Want   The general concept represented by the W component of the WDEP system can be explored by asking any number of questions. Using the grid in Table 10.1, 132 questions can be formulated based on the generic question, "What do you want?" A counselor can adapt the "What do you want" question to any individual. For example, for high school students a counselor might ask what they want from their family, friends, school, and job as well as what they want from themselves. With most high school students, a counselor could ask the question directly by inquiring, "What do you want to do when you graduate?" "What do your parents want you to do after you graduate?" "Do you see a difference between what you want and what your parents want for you?"

The basic question "What do you want" can be adapted for any individual depending on the context. For example, in some cultures it is appropriate to employ a more circuitous manner of communication than the direct manner typically used in psychotherapy based on European-American values. My friend and colleague Masaki Kakitani (professor at the School of Psychology, Rissho University, Japan, and director of the William Glasser Institute, Japan), translates, "What do you want?" into "What are you looking for?" These two questions might appear very similar, but in a culture in which direct communication and assertiveness are not virtues, the second question sounds softer and more acceptable.

A case provided by Dr. Kakitani offers a glimpse at how a Japanese counselor uses reality therapy with a reluctant adolescent client. The Japanese application of reality therapy is not radically different from its use in Western society. One significant difference is that there is more emphasis on the authority role of the counselor, as is evident in the distilled dialogue that follows.

Takao was a 14-year-old Japanese boy in junior high school. He was an only child who lived with his mother and father. He occasionally skipped school, and

Table 10.1 Exploring the Quality World: 132 Ways to Ask W Questions

Fundamental Generic Question: What do you want?	1. What do you want that you are getting?	2. What do you want that you're *not* getting?	3. How much do you want it?	4. How much effort or energy are you willing to exert to get what you want?	5. What will you settle for?	6. What are you getting that you don't want?	7. What are the priorities in what you want?	8. What is your level of commitment regarding categories A–L?	9. How do you perceive categories A–L?	10. What do you have to give up to get what you want?	11. What needs to be done regardless of whether you want to do it?
A. From your family											
B. From your spouse											
C. From your children											
D. From your friends											
E. From your job											
F. From your manager											
G. From your subordinates											
H. From the organization											
I. From your co-workers											
J. From your recreational activities											
K. From yourself											
L. From your counselor/ teacher											

his grades had recently fallen. His mother sent him to a counseling center. Takao was unhappy about being coerced into seeing a counselor and did not appear to be ready for help.

> T (Therapist): Takao, you seem to be unhappy about being here.
>
> C (Client): Yes, my mother made me come.
>
> T: She made you come? You seem to be a strong man. Your mother could hardly make you come unless you chose to come. There is no way for her to drag you here by force. Right?
>
> C: If I wouldn't come, she would be mean and nagging.
>
> T: You don't like being nagged, do you?
>
> C: Of course not!
>
> T: Suppose she stops nagging you, what will you have that you don't have now?
>
> C: I will be happy.
>
> T: Happy, because . . . ?
>
> C: I will be happy because I will be free!
>
> T: Then you must be interested in being free and happy.
>
> C: Sure.
>
> T: Since you don't like being here, you could waste your time with me. But suppose I am able to help you so that you will be freer and happier than you are now. If that were true, would you be interested in working together with me?
>
> C: Sure. I am interested in being free and happy.
>
> T: Then is it true that you are willing to work with me rather than waste time?
>
> C: Sure.

At this point Takao has become a willing client.

> T: Suppose 10 out of 10 equals a good relationship and 1 out of 10 is not a good relationship. What number between 1 and 10 indicates your relationship with your mother?
>
> C: Two or three.

T: Wow! It's better than zero! Suppose you are able to improve your relation-ship with your mother. Would you be happier then than you are now?

C: I guess so.

T: I guess so, too. Do you think you could make your relationship with your mother worse?

C: What do you mean? Make it worse?

T: Yes. Make it worse than now.

C: Surely I could make it worse, if I wanted to.

T: If you could make it worse, then you could also make it better. Right?

C: I guess so.

T: I guess so, too. Could you think of anything you could do differently today when you go back home so that your relationship with your mother might improve?

C: I guess I could stop criticizing my mother.

T: That's a good idea. Would she notice the difference?

C: Yes, she will notice it immediately.

T: I hope she doesn't have a heart problem? Is giving such a shock to her all right? I hope she would not suffer from a heart attack. [Smile.]

C: There is no problem. She grows hair on her heart. [This means that she has a rather strong heart.] [Smile.]

T: I would like to offer you some advice. Don't do too much to surprise her. [Smile.] What do you think about improving just one number on the scale per week? Is that too much improvement?

C: No. I don't think so.

T: Suppose you improve one number on the scale per week. What percent do you think will be improved at the end of the year?

C: I guess more than 50%.

T: Exactly. So improving just a little bit each week adds up! Now let's switch the subject to school. Do you want to go to senior high school after graduating junior high school?

C: Yeah. If they let me go.

T: Which school do you want to go to?

C: Oiso Senior High School.

T: It must be a difficult school to get into.

C: Yes, it is.

T: What is your second choice of school?

C: Ninomiya is my second choice.

Because the student was an unwilling client, the counselor was cautious about the initial contact with him. Accordingly, the counselor began by focusing on relationship building and attempted to uncover Jamal's basic unmet need—namely, the relationship with his mother. The client was interested in being free. He was also interested in being happier. He gradually accepted that a better relationship with his mother would help him become freer and happier (W: want). The counselor asked him to evaluate his relationship with his mother by scaling (E: self-evaluation). The counselor did not emphasize his current behavior (D: doing, thinking, feeling) that was problematic but asked him to make a plan (P: plan) to behave differently (not criticize his mother). The counselor then moved the discussion to school matters in an attempt to find out if his quality world related to school. Because Takao lacked close friends in school, future sessions would focus on his interpersonal relationships with peers as well as teachers and on plans for improving school attendance and grades.

Consider another case that focuses on the client's wants. Christine, who is Japanese American, is an 18-year-old senior at a suburban high school that serves many students of diverse backgrounds. Her father works for a biotech company and her mother is a university professor. Christine's parents have high academic and professional expectations for their daughter. Her counselor is male and European-American.

T (Therapist): Christine, what are your thoughts about what you will do after graduation?

C (Client): My parents think I should go to a prestigious Ivy League premed school.

T: So they would like to see you become a doctor because of the grades and talent you've shown here at school.

C: That about sums it up.

T: And they really want the best for you, don't they?

C: Yes, they definitely want me to have a successful future.

T: If they were sitting here, what do you think they would say about the word *success*?

C: They would probably say that I should become a high-level professional person and make a lot of money.

T: I'm wondering if a major part of your success would be the amount of income you have. Many, but not all, people measure their success by their income.

C: That would be a big part of it. At least that's what my older brother says.

T: Have you talked to him about what you want to do after high school? Sometimes an older brother can be a big help.

C: Yes, both he and I have a lot of friends whose parents are very different from ours.

T: What does he think about your future plans?

C: He has told me that he disagrees with my parents. He doesn't say anything to them, however. He thinks I should do what would make me happy.

T: What do you think would make you happy?

C: I'm not sure right now. I know what I don't want. I don't want to be a doctor.

T: So you have a different idea about your future than what your parents have.

C: I've never said it to them before, but it does seem that way.

T: As you sit here right now, let's talk about this one part at a time. Tell me, what do you think about the fact that even though you haven't discussed it with your parents, you have a different idea about what would make you happy in the future?

C: I seem to be fitting in with a lot of people my age. From what my friends say, they also want something different from what their parents want for them.

In this dialogue we see a young woman respectful of her parents' wishes yet experiencing the same struggles faced by many teenagers in Western society. The counselor is respectful of the client's strong family ties and parental expectations while acknowledging her struggle to find a balance between a culture that values authority and a culture that values self-direction.

Exploring Clients' Level of Commitment   Exploring the level of commitment to achieving one's goals plays a central role in the application of the W component. To that end, an important follow-up question to "What do you want?" is "How hard do you want to work on achieving what you want?" Let us consider prototypic responses to that question that correspond to five possible levels of commitment in order of increasing commitment.

1. "I don't want to be here. Leave me alone." This response represents a commitment of the lowest order; in fact, it is no commitment at all.

2. "I would like the outcome but not the effort." This slightly higher level of commitment is not likely to result in change.

3. "I'll try," "I might," or "I could." Clients at this level have moved above the lowest two levels, but they retain an escape hatch that is likely to lead to failure.

4. "I will do my best." This is higher than the previous level but still incorporates a reserve measure of ambivalence.

5. "I will do whatever it takes." This is firm commitment. (Wubbolding, 2000)

In listening to clients' expression of commitment, reality therapists pay attention to the music or meaning of the words as well as their content. Uncovering the meaning of a client's description of her or his level of commitment requires effort, experience, and, often, outside consultation on the part of the counselor because people use the same words to mean different things. For some clients "I'll try" does represent a firm commitment, while for others it does not.

Exploring Clients' Locus of Control   The third aspect of the W component is helping clients identify their locus of control—that is, how they perceive the causes of their behavior. An *external locus of control*—the belief that what one gets is influenced by others or external situations—reinforces a self-defeating "I can't because they won't let me" worldview, especially in oppressed minority clients. Reality therapists respect clients' feelings of unhappiness, rejection, and oppression but also help clients move toward an *internal locus of control*—the belief that what one gets is influenced by one's own efforts and ability—and view themselves as choice makers in their lives.

D: Discussing the Client's Behavior (Doing) and Resulting Direction

The D component of the WDEP system represents doing and direction. *Doing* encompasses the three components of total behavior over which we have some modicum of control: actions, thoughts, and feelings.

Clients' overall *direction* is the accumulation of where their current choices of behavior are taking them. A typical D question a reality therapist asks is, "If you continue in the same direction you are going, where will you be in a month, a year, two years?" Authentic feelings provide an evaluation of the client's direction. Feelings of anger, shame, resentment, and guilt send a message that a client is not headed in a positive direction. On the other hand, feelings of joy, altruism, comfort, and compassion often indicate that the client is headed in a healthy direction. The reality therapist acknowledges and accepts clients' feelings in a nonjudgmental manner. However, in contrast to therapies in which there is a focus on feelings (e.g., person-centered therapy), in reality therapy feelings are given minimal attention and considered less important than actions and cognitions.

In implementing the D component, reality therapists encourage clients to discuss their action choices. They ask questions such as, "What did you do yesterday when you felt lonely?" "Tell me about the last time you chose a behavior enjoyable to you and others, one that was within the law and that would be acceptable to society." An emphasis on action choices is essential to the effective use of reality therapy because this aspect of human behavior is the most controllable.

Part of the exploration of the D component can be a discussion of the internal self-talk that is related to the choices a client has made. Ineffective or destructive behavior is generally accompanied by self-talk focusing on defeatism and powerlessness. Such beliefs never work to one's advantage. As Powell (2004) put it, "If we internalize the belief that something outside ourselves will change us, we have painted ourselves into the corner of helplessness. If we internalize this belief to the extreme, we become painted into the corner of hopelessness" (p. 27). For example, when clients believe that there is little hope of success because they are oppressed, they sometimes develop self-talk focusing on "I can't," or "Nobody's going to tell me what to do," or even "I have a right to control other people in order to get what I want." Reality therapists help such clients formulate more constructive and potentially self-actualizing self-talk, such as "I can evaluate the merits of what others tell me to do," and "I can control my own behavior," and "my own behavior is the only behavior I can control."

E: Questioning the Client to Stimulate Self-Evaluation

Self-evaluation is the key component of the WDEP system and in behavioral change. The use of self-evaluation questions occupies a central place in reality therapy. Table 10.2 lists examples of self-evaluative concepts—presented as continuums—designed to help clients conduct a searching self-evaluation that results in internal judgments and decisions about their wants, behaviors, and perceptions, which is the crucial ingredient in self-evaluation. Examples of questions derived from the continuums are: "Is what you're doing helping or hurting you?" "To what degree is it helping you?" "What are the consequences of your current direction?" "Will they be pleasant or unpleasant?" "Is the positive

Table 10.2 Continuums for Self-Evaluation

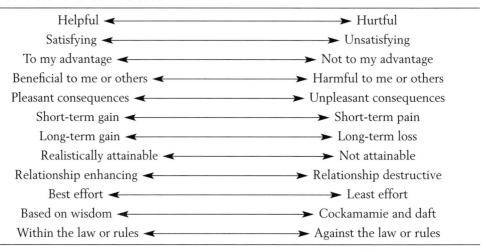

Helpful ◄————————————►	Hurtful
Satisfying ◄————————————►	Unsatisfying
To my advantage ◄————————————►	Not to my advantage
Beneficial to me or others ◄————————————►	Harmful to me or others
Pleasant consequences ◄————————————►	Unpleasant consequences
Short-term gain ◄————————————►	Short-term pain
Long-term gain ◄————————————►	Long-term loss
Realistically attainable ◄————————————►	Not attainable
Relationship enhancing ◄————————————►	Relationship destructive
Best effort ◄————————————►	Least effort
Based on wisdom ◄————————————►	Cockamamie and daft
Within the law or rules ◄————————————►	Against the law or rules

consequence worth the unpleasant side effects of your behavior?" You may find it helpful to formulate additional self-evaluation questions related to the words and phrases in the table.

To illustrate how a reality therapist helps stimulate a client's self-evaluation, let's return to the case of Christine, the Japanese-American high-school student. Christine realized that her career wants (goals) were different from those of her parents. In the following dialogue the counselor continues to help her examine her wants and her actions and make a self-evaluation of them.

T (Therapist): Tell me again your thoughts about a career that interests you.

C (Client): After watching television, I believe I would be good at fashion design.

T: And yet you said last time that your parents are hoping that you would take premed courses in college. There seems to be a difference in the family about your future.

C: I didn't realize it before we talked about it last week, but you are right.

T: So how realistic is it that there will be 100% agreement about your career goals?

C: It doesn't seem likely at this point.

T: And have you let your parents know what your hopes are for your future training?

C: No, it's very hard to say anything to them even though I have drawn many [fashion] sketches and shown them to my parents.

T: So they probably have some idea, but it is hard for you to bring it up in conversation.

C: It is. I don't want to disappoint them.

T: I know you're very close to your parents. Yet, is it going to be satisfactory to you to continue to refrain from discussing this with them?

C: Probably not. I think about it, but I have not brought it up to them.

T: Would it be disrespectful to them if you mentioned that you would like a career in fashion design?

C: Based on the conversations we've had about their relationship with my grandparents, they were very traditional in their behavior toward their parents. So they are influenced by that tradition, but they seem to recognize that young people today like to make up their own minds about such things. I don't think it would be easy for them, but I think they would understand.

T: You seem to be a little nervous about this. It's kind of risky?

C: Yes, it would be a challenge.

T: Are you okay with accepting the challenge and mentioning it to them? Or do you want to continue to not say anything to them? A third choice is to do what you think they expect of you without expressing yourself.

C: I think the best thing would be to mention it to them.

T: I'm not trying to push you to do something you don't want to do, Christine, but these are the choices as I see them. You seem to agree that these are three possibilities.

In this dialogue, the counselor adapts the self-evaluation component to the client whose cultural values are different from his. And yet the counselor is faithful to the principles of reality therapy. He makes a special effort to acknowledge the intrafamily relationships while helping Christine self-evaluate. Clearly there is a delicate balance between the counselor's responsibility to Christine's living in a Western society and maintaining his respect and consideration of traditional Japanese family values. He also does not presume that because the family is Japanese they automatically subscribe to strong family values. He attempts to elicit from Christine a description of intrafamily behaviors, perceptions, and values.

P: Planning a Course of Action to Fulfill the Client's Wants and Needs

Creating a realistic, doable, and measurable plan is certainly not unique to reality therapy. Most counselors are quite familiar with planning. In the age of managed care, planning is a necessity. Choice theory offers counselors specific pathways for planning. Because dysfunctional relationships form the basis of many psychological disorders and create intense pain, making plans to satisfy the need for belonging is an important place to start. Specific plans should also focus on gaining a sense of achievement as well as enjoyment. And because effective planning is a choice, the planning process itself addresses the need for freedom.

As guideline for planning, I have created the acronym *SAMIC*[3] that covers the characteristics of an effective plan and that is useful in counseling, consultation, and parenting.

> S = *Simple.* The plan should be only as complicated as necessary (remember *KIS* for "keep it simple").
>
> A = *Attainable.* A realistically doable plan, though not a guarantee, provides some assurance of successful completion.
>
> M = *Measurable.* A key to successful planning is concreteness. An ideal plan addresses such questions as where? when? how often? with whom?
>
> I = *Immediate.* It is best to rehearse the plan during the counseling session, and the client should implement the plan as soon after it has been formulated as possible.
>
> C = *Controlled by the planner.* The plan is not contingent on others' actions. "I'll get a job" is not as effective as "I will spend 3 hours applying for jobs."
>
> C = *Committed to.* Handshakes, written plans, and follow-up phone calls are techniques that help elicit a firm commitment from clients.
>
> C = *Consistently implemented.* The plan is carried out on a regular basis.

Planning is central to reality therapy as it is for many counseling approaches. Clients readily learn the acronym SAMIC[3] and often teach it to their children and others. However, not every plan contains all the SAMIC[3] characteristics, as they are ideals to be aimed at but they are not always achieved.

Long-Term Versus Short-Term Applications

The length of reality therapy is flexible. In particular, it is well suited to short-term application with beneficial long-term results. While it is very effective for problem solving, the ultimate goal of reality therapy is to provide clients with the understanding and skills necessary to make judicious choices about their life in the future. The underlying message that clients should take away from counseling is: "I have control of my life, and I can make better choices."

Evaluation of Reality Therapy

Studies of reality therapy conducted in different parts of the world have supported the effectiveness of the approach as it applies to individuals and groups from a wide range of cultures with many problem behaviors. Okonji, Ososkie, and Pulos (1996) concluded, "If agencies or counseling programs need to train people to serve ethnically minority clients, they need to consider various treatment modalities, especially directive approaches such as reality therapy" (p. 337). Studies conducted at Sogang University in Korea have indicated a significant increase in a sense of inner control both for male and female students participating in reality therapy (Woo, 1998). M. S. Kim (2001) found that elementary school children in reality therapy group counseling reported a significant increase in internal locus of control as well as personal responsibility for their actions. Lee (2001) studied the effectiveness of reality therapy for treating the aggressive behavior of 16 high school students. He found that assault, irritability, and verbal aggression significantly decreased and recommended that the program be applied to youth in rehabilitation centers and in schools. Prenzlau (2006) found that reality therapy reduced problem behaviors associated with posttraumatic stress disorder (PTSD). The symptoms reduced were somatization (e.g., exaggerated focus on health problems) and rumination (e.g., continuously worrying about injuries incurred in an accident 10 years previously). Comparing reality therapy group counseling with a mutual support group, Lawrence (2004) found a significant difference in factors associated with self-determination for persons with developmental disabilities. Peterson, Chang, and Collins (1997, 1998) conducted studies of reality therapy with Taiwanese college students that found significant increases in perceived internal locus of control and effective need satisfaction.

In summary, there is evidence that reality therapy can be useful in helping clients increase their inner sense of control, self-determination, and effective need satisfaction, as well as reduce antisocial behavior and symptoms of PTSD. Reality therapy has been used in diverse cultures. The best cultural adaptations of reality therapy are made by counselors who are both skilled in the practice of reality therapy and steeped in the values of their own cultures.[1]

---

[1] Examples include Masaki Kakitani in Japan, In-za Kim in Korea, Elizabeth Tham and Kwee Ong in Singapore, Leon Lojk in Slovenia and Croatia, Basheer Al-Rashidi in Kuwait, Maher Omar throughout the Persian Gulf area, Farida Dias in India, Sergei Bogolepov in Russia, Mitchel Messina in South Africa, John Brickell in the United Kingdom, Lothar Imhof in Germany, Liv Thorhild Undheim in Norway, Juan Pablo Aljure in Colombia, Brian Lennon in Ireland, Michael Harel-Hochfeld in Israel, and reality therapists in Australia and New Zealand.

While reality therapy has been shown to be helpful with different problems and in different settings, several improvements in research are necessary (Wubbolding, 2000). The use of genuine reality therapy by well-trained and skilled clinicians and more tightly controlled studies would add to the credibility of the research base for reality therapy. Outcome research is needed on such targets as recidivism in the corrections system and academic achievement in schools as well as change in behaviors related to mental health.

The idiographic evaluation of success for particular clients in reality therapy is accomplished in two ways: (1) by the repeated self-evaluation of clients as they follow their plans of action and (2) by the clients' assessment of how well their goals have been met. Goals that are realistic, doable, and measurable are most likely to be achieved.

Reality Therapy: Blind Spots, Limitations, and Challenges

As with all the therapies, reality therapy has blind spots and limitations and faces critical challenges.

Blind Spots

Reality therapy is a here-and-now system based on principles such as the following: psychological problems are rooted in current dysfunctional human relationships; behaviors are chosen; alternative choices made now and in the future on an habitual basis result in a more need satisfying life (happiness). A rigid adherence to these principles, however, can limit the perceptions of counselors or even blind them to significant influences in the past or present lives of clients. Reality therapy does not take into account, for example, the influence of the unconscious on behavior and on the choices people make. Consequently, reality therapists ignore the use of therapeutic tools that probe the unconscious, such as dream analysis, and that assist clients in gaining insight into the unconscious reasons for their current behaviors. Dismissing the influence of other factors gives the counselor tunnel vision and may result in therapy being less successful than it would have been with a wider purview.

Some critics charge that reality therapy ignores social or environmental influences. Murdock (2004) states, "Reality therapy does not seem to take these phenomena into account. Glasser would probably say that going along with the crowd is more a result of a failure to wake up and make choices than to any magical power of social forces" (p. 273).

Limitations

Because reality therapy is a clear delivery system, it lends itself to the human tendency of wanting to "fix the problem," to correct other people's behavior and to impose one's own values on them (Wubbolding, 2003). Reality therapists are not immune to this tendency. While acknowledging that human beings have more control over actions than cognitions and feelings, they apply the concept of *choice* to phobias, depression, and other *DSM* diagnoses involving emotions as well as to everyday emotions such as sorrow and guilt. However, there may be limitations to the choices people have. Thus, changing actions, especially in relationships, might be insufficient for eliminating pain caused by some past events such as early childhood trauma or by current environmental restraints such as discrimination and other forms of social rejection.

Challenges

Reality therapy's view of how human behavior is generated requires much explanation and clarification. To contend that choice applies to behaviors that are both clearly controllable and to those over which human beings have little direct control confounds someone learning about the approach as well as oversimplifies the theory. Therefore, the main challenge for reality therapy is to train counselors to acknowledge their own limitations and the limitations of the theory and practice of reality therapy. Despite the successes counselors have had using reality therapy, counselors are well advised to help clients set realistic goals characterized by such phrases as "improvement," "better coping skills," and "alleviation" rather than "cure," "total need satisfaction," and "a life free of pain and stress."

Future Development: Reality Therapy in a Diverse World

Reality therapy has been successful with diverse clients within the United States and has been used with clients in other parts of the world. Still, much work remains. Teaching and practicing reality therapy around the world is in its initial stages. My personal goals have been to make reality therapy respected in academia and to promote it cross-culturally. Because making this relatively young therapy acceptable and respected in university training programs requires scientific research, more studies are needed to further this endeavor. Research investigations have already supported its use in Asia and additional studies are under way.

Enthusiasm for the use of reality therapy in a world of diversity is at an all-time high, as evidenced by attendance at the international reality therapy conference each summer. For example, people from every continent in the world except Antarctica were present at the 2004 William Glasser Institute conference in Chicago. It is our hope that the system will be used on an even more widespread basis with minorities in North America and in other cultures around the world.

William Glasser, a controversial figure from the very beginning, continues to expand his ideas. Most recently, he has challenged counselors and therapists to examine the use of psychiatric drugs in therapy (Glasser, 2003, 2004). His most controversial thesis is that psychiatric drugs do more harm than good. He states, "What the present psychiatric establishment has done that can harm your mental health extends far beyond the psychiatrist's office. Now almost all health professionals are caught in this neurochemical 'web.' Brain drugs dominate the entire mental health landscape" (2003, p. 2). Glasser suggests that the concept *unhappiness* be substituted for the widely used term *mental illness.* People who wear diagnostic labels are best treated as unhappy and capable of happiness rather than as mentally ill. He considers choice theory an alternative to the excessive drugging of society that applies to all people regardless of their race, culture, ethnicity, gender, or age. Finally, he believes that better human relationships are more curative than any artificial substance.

Although I totally agree with him regarding the curative potential of human relationships, I think that Glasser's campaign about psychiatric drugs is peripheral to the practice of reality therapy. Not every practitioner of reality therapy is his eager recruit in this endeavor. Some practitioners believe that it is necessary to refer some clients for medication. And so, whether or not you subscribe to Glasser's campaign against the use of psychiatric drugs, you can feel comfortable practicing the principles of reality therapy.

Summary

1. Reality therapy was developed in a mental hospital and a correctional institution in the 1960s by psychiatrist William Glasser who rebelled against the traditional psychoanalytic training he received during his residency. It is based on two interrelated premises: that people choose how they behave and that people should be held responsible for their behavior.

2. Glasser's choice theory, the basis for reality therapy, emphasizes individual choice and moving away from the conventional wisdom that external forces control us and that we are victims of them.

3. All people are motivated by the same internal drives or needs, although they may generate different behaviors aimed at satisfying these universal needs depending on their circumstances.

4. The five basic human needs that drive our behaviors are: (1) survival, self-preservation, and physiological needs; (2) belonging and love needs; (3) power, achievement, and inner control needs; (4) freedom and independence needs; and (5) fun and enjoyment needs.

5. People have specific wants that they believe will satisfy their basic needs. Wants are unique to each individual, may be realistic or unrealistic, may be blurred, may exist in priority, and may conflict with one another.

6. When our quality world—our vision of our personal wants—is unfulfilled, we choose behaviors that are intended to attain the perception that we have attained these wants. Our total behavior consists of four aspects that exist at four levels of consciousness. The four aspects are, from most to least conscious: actions, cognitions, emotions, and physiological functions.

7. The more conscious a behavior is, the more explicit control we can gain over it and the more clearly it can be chosen. Because we have the most control over our actions, reality therapy focuses on changing actions to better achieve our wants and satisfy our needs.

8. In practice, reality therapists begin a relationship with a client by establishing a firm, fair, and friendly counseling atmosphere, engaging in tonic (healthy) counselor behaviors such as communicating a sense of hope and avoiding toxic (unhealthy) counselor behaviors such as blaming and criticizing.

9. Reality therapy can be enacted through the WDEP system, which consists of W = wants and needs that must be identified; D = doing (behaving) and direction, the direction in which clients' behaviors are sending them; E = evaluation by clients (i.e., self-evaluation) of their wants and effectiveness of their behaviors; and P = planning, the course of action clients will take to fulfill their wants and needs.

10. Studies indicate that reality therapy can be useful in helping clients increase their inner sense of control, self-determination, and effective need satisfaction, as well as reduce antisocial behavior and symptoms of PTSD. Reality therapy has been used in diverse cultures.

11. Idiographic evaluation of success for particular clients is accomplished by the repeated self-evaluation by clients as they follow their plans of action and by clients' assessment of how well their goals have been met.

12. Blind spots of reality therapy include the potential that rigid adherence to its here-and-now approach may blind counselors to significant past influences

and ignore social and environmental influences. The therapy is limited in that it considers all problems to be choices when in fact they may not be, which makes reality therapy ineffective with some problems. The challenge for reality therapy is to explain how human behavior is generated more clearly than it has done thus far.

13. Reality therapy has been successful with diverse clients within the United States and has been used by therapists in other parts of the world, but much work remains to make it truly cross-cultural.

Key Terms

choice theory (p. 362)
needs (p. 368)
quality world (p. 369)
tonic behaviors (p. 373)

total behavior (p. 370)
toxic behaviors (p. 374)
wants (p. 369)
WDEP system (p. 375)

Resources for Further Study

Professional Organizations

The William Glasser Institute
22024 Lassen Street, #118
Chatsworth, CA 91311
818-700-8000
www.wglasser.com

Formerly the Institute for Reality Therapy, the William Glasser Institute offers training in choice theory and reality therapy, culminating in a certificate of completion. This 18-month training program is open to mental health professionals, educators, correctional workers, business managers, and others seeking to integrate choice theory and reality therapy into their work.

Center for Reality Therapy
7672 Montgomery Road, #383
Cincinnati, OH 45236
513-561-1911
www.realitytherapywub.com
wubsrt@fuse.net

A branch of the William Glasser Institute, the center provides training for certification and brief workshops on applying reality therapy in areas such as mental health, classroom teaching, probation and parole, youth work, addictions, and supervision/management.

Professional Journals

International Journal of Reality Therapy
Editor: Lawrence Litwack, Ed.D.
650 Laurel Ave, #402
Highland Park, IL 60035

> An independent publication directed to concepts of internal control psychology including reality therapy. Published semiannually.

International Journal of Choice Theory
Editor: Jeff Tirengel, Psy.D.
The William Glasser Institute
22024 Lassen Street, #118
Chatsworth, CA 91311

> The official journal of the William Glasser Institute directed toward enhancing choice theory scholarship and its applications, inaugurated in the summer of 2006. Published semiannually.

Suggested Readings

Glasser, W. (1998). *Choice theory*. New York: HarperCollins.

> A detailed exposition of choice theory, the basis of reality therapy; a foundational book for students of reality therapy.

Glasser, W. (2003). *Warning: Psychiatry can be hazardous to your mental health*. New York: HarperCollins.

> A controversial treatise that suggests that psychiatric drugs are hazardous to mental health. Glasser suggests incorporating choice theory into daily living as a more effective alternative path to happiness and better human relationships.

Wubbolding, R. (2000). *Reality therapy for the 21st century*. Philadelphia: Brunner/Routledge.

> This comprehensive and detailed treatment of reality therapy offers an overview of choice theory along with several extensions of the theory, including amplifications of the procedures summarized in the WDEP system and a summary of studies demonstrating the effectiveness of reality therapy applied to addictions, education, delinquency, residential programs, and other areas.

Wubbolding, R., & Brickell, J. (2001). *Counselling with reality therapy*. Bicester, UK: Speechmark.

> Extends reality therapy to relationship counseling, stages of group counseling, and addictions counseling. Intended for international use, covers paradoxical techniques applied to resistance, use of metaphors, listening for themes, use of silence, creating client anticipation, and communicating hope.

Wubbolding, R., & Brickell, J. (2001). *A set of directions for putting and keeping yourself together*. Minneapolis, MN: Educational Media.

Practical, usable, hands-on source of self-help and tools for use with individual clients, students, families, and groups.

Other Media Resources

Wubbolding, R. (2005). *Dealing with blaming, resisting, whining, avoiding, and excuse making: A group reality therapy approach* (DVD). Cincinnati, OH: Center for Reality Therapy.

A role-play demonstration of group counseling that illustrates the use of the WDEP system with a resistant group of mental health clients who present with varying issues: addiction, drug abuse, and dysfunctional relationships.

Wubbolding, R. (2007). *Reality therapy* (DVD). Washington, DC: American Psychological Association.

The WDEP system applied to a 40-year-old client who moves from his initial unawareness of the impact of his abrupt manner of problem solving with his girlfriend to an awareness that he needs to consider how she receives his communications.

Chapter 11

Feminist Therapy

PAMELA REMER

Attending to diversity perspectives in counseling requires more than learning about and accepting a wide range of cultural values and practices. In contemporary U.S. society, multiple forms of oppression (e.g., sexism, racism, ethnocentrism, classism, heterosexism, ableism, ageism) restrict the potential and full participation of subordinate group members. (See Table 11.1 for the definitions of these forms of oppression.) Thus, from a feminist and diversity perspective, the institutionalization of oppression and privilege, discrimination, cultural values, and cultural socialization processes that constitute individuals' sociocultural contexts must be understood and often challenged in order to effectively counsel a diverse range of clients.

Traditional therapies and psychological diagnostic systems emphasize an **intrapsychic** approach to counseling that views the source of clients' problems as internal/individual, and thus, counseling is aimed at changing clients' dysfunctional thoughts, feelings, and behaviors (Worell & Remer, 2003). This intrapsychic focus ignores clients' sociocultural contexts and disregards the impact of societal oppression on subordinate, disadvantaged individuals. Effective counseling of individuals from disadvantaged or oppressed groups requires methods that attend to external, social sources of pathology and how those toxic sociocultural elements are internalized, which is known as an **interactionist** approach (Remer, Rostosky, & Comer-Wright, 2001; Worell & Remer, 2003).

This chapter focuses on feminist approaches to counseling diverse groups of people. Feminist counseling is especially appropriate for subordinate or oppressed groups because of its interactionist approach and its emphasis on the need for social change to end oppressive societal structures. One feminist approach, *empowerment feminist therapy* (Worell & Remer, 1992, 2003), will be emphasized because of its structural integration of both feminist and diversity perspectives.

Table 11.1 Definitions of Forms of Oppression

Form of Oppression	Definition
Sexism	A form of oppression that subordinates girls and women
Racism	A form of oppression that subordinates certain racial groups in a society; in the United States people of Color are subordinated
Ethnocentrism	A form of oppression in which people from subordinate ethnic groups are devalued and viewed as inferior to the dominant ethnic culture
Classism	A form of oppression in which lower socioeconomic levels are devalued
Heterosexism	A form of oppression in which sexual orientations other than heterosexuality are viewed as unhealthy, abnormal, and inferior
Ableism	A form of oppression in which people with a variety of physical and mental disabilities are devalued and subordinated
Ageism	A form of oppression in which certain age groups are devalued and subordinated

Origins and Evolution of Feminist Therapy

Feminist therapy grew out of the U.S. women's movement of the 1960s and 1970s. The women's movement identified the negative impact of stereotyped gender-role socialization and societal sexism on women. Feminists noted that White, heterosexual males whose cultural contexts were Western and Eurocentric created most existing therapeutic modalities. Thus, these theories were **androcentric** (based on male values and norms) and **ethnocentric** (based on one cultural perspective and set of values). Further, feminist therapists challenged traditional therapies' focus on the internal or intrapsychic causes of problems and their disregard for the role of the cultural context of these problems. Instead, feminist therapists emphasized the social and political sources of women's counseling issues and asserted that social change, rather than individual change, was necessary to alleviate women's distress.

Problems in Specifying the History of Feminist Counseling

Detailing a history of feminist counseling is difficult for several reasons. First and foremost, feminist counseling approaches are rooted in a variety of feminist philosophies, each with its own social and political history (Enns, 1997). Thus, many approaches to feminist counseling currently exist. Second, within each of these feminist approaches to counseling, no single feminist therapy theoretician or "mother" can be credited for developing the approach. Indeed, most of the feminist approaches have had multiple contributors over time. Thus, the life and significant dates of one theoretician/founder cannot be described.

Third, as previously mentioned, feminist counseling approaches emerged out of and intertwined with a variety of grassroots women's movements (e.g., the consciousness-raising groups of the 1960s and 1970s, and the focus on the detrimental effects of violence against women, which led to the development of rape crisis centers and domestic violence shelters in the 1970s). A full history of feminist counseling would need to chronicle the major events of the women's movement. Fourth, feminist therapies are relatively recent phenomena. Thus, this account of the history of feminist therapy and counseling focuses on the general development of feminist counseling and highlights its common threads.

The Women's Movement Critique of Traditional Therapies

In the 1960s and 1970s, women's social ills began to be identified and addressed. Women began to speak out about rape and domestic violence/wife battering. Grassroots social action groups helped establish rape crisis centers, domestic violence shelters, and the like. Women challenged previous "women-caused" views of issues like rape and wife battering and asserted instead that these issues were caused by the societal devaluation of women and societal **sexism.** Those involved in these movements attacked traditional therapies, accusing them of focusing on facilitating psychological adjustment to toxic social environments, engaging in victim blame, and ignoring how society and its institutions oppress women. Leaderless **consciousness-raising** (CR) groups developed as an alternative to therapy. In these CR groups, women were encouraged to identify the commonalities of their personal issues as a means of becoming aware of the social roots of these issues. These groups also focused on societal change and social action. Some traditionally trained mental health professionals participated in these groups and brought these perspectives into their professional practice and writing.

First Publications About Feminist Approaches to Counseling

Articles and books focusing on feminist approaches to counseling women began to appear in the late 1970s and early 1980s (e.g., Brodsky & Hare-Mustin, 1980; Greenspan, 1983; Harway, 1979; Rawlings & Carter, 1977; Sturdivant, 1980; Worell, 1980). These works criticized traditional therapies for their sexist constructs and their focus on intrapsychic psychological adaptation to sexist societal expectations. In this first wave of feminist therapy, authors began to define the foundational elements of feminist counseling and to apply feminist constructs and techniques to issues common in women's lives (e.g., depression, rape, domestic violence, eating disorders). By the 1980s, in the second wave of feminist therapy, several feminist therapy approaches based on different feminist philosophies had been developed and feminist psychologists began to revise traditional theoretical orientations to counseling to make them more compatible with feminist values and perspectives (Enns, 1997; Worell & Remer, 1992, 2003).

Parallel developments in research on women's issues using feminist perspectives provided a foundation for the further development of feminist psychological practice. In addition, professional organizations like the Association for Women in Psychology (AWP) and Division 35 of the American Psychological Association (now known as the Society for the Psychology of Women) were created to support further development of feminist perspectives in therapy, teaching, and research.

Feminist Counseling Milestones

Several feminist counseling projects and documents, which grew out of this new attention to feminist perspectives, serve as the first milestone in the historical development of feminist therapy and counseling. In the early 1970s, an American Psychological Association (1975) task force conducted research on sex bias in counseling and therapy. Its report documented the pervasiveness of gender-role bias and stereotyping in the conduct of therapy. In 1978, the Counseling Psychology Division (17) of the American Psychological Association (APA) created 13 "Principles Concerning the Counseling/Psychotherapy of Women" (Fitzgerald & Nutt, 1986). In these principles, the knowledge, attitude, and skills needed for the competent counseling of women were outlined. The principles asserted that counselors and therapists needed to be knowledgeable about how women are affected by biological, psychological, and social issues; by all forms of oppression; and by inequities in power in relationships (including therapeutic relationships). According to these principles, counselors must be aware of their own values, biases, and attitudes that may discriminate against or limit the potential of women. Counselors must also have specialized skills for working with diverse women, including skills for eliminating institutional and personal gender bias. In 2002, a joint task force of APA Divisions 35 and 17 began revising the 1978 principles into a set of guidelines, Guidelines for Psychological Practice with Girls and Women. These guidelines are now (2006) in the process of being readied for submission to the APA's Council of Representatives for approval. They emphasize the diversity of women's lives and expand the original focus on women to women and girls. If approved, they will serve as aspirational practice guidelines for all psychologists and counselors.

A third feminist historical project, by APA Division 35, was the First National Conference on Education and Training in Feminist Practice held in Boston in 1993 (Worell & Johnson, 1997). Seventy-seven feminist psychologists and 13 graduate psychology students met to discuss the past, present, and future of feminist practice. There were several important outcomes of this conference. First, *feminist psychological practice* was defined as including therapy/counseling, supervision, consultation, writing, assessment and diagnosis, forensics, research, teaching, training, social action, administration, public service, and prevention. This focus on a broader range of psychological practices replaced the narrower one on *feminist therapy* and acknowledged that feminist perspectives were being applied in a variety of practice arenas. Second, using a feminist collaborative process that distributes leadership and responsibility, values diverse voices, and makes decisions by consensus, conference participants identified 14 "Common Themes" of feminist practice. To be included, a theme had to be endorsed by *unanimous consensus* of all participants. Thus, these feminist practice themes represented the common threads of feminist practice and included: (a) "Promotes social change; (b) Assumes the personal is political; (c) Embraces diversity as a requirement and foundation for practice; (d) Includes an analysis of power and the multiple ways in which people can be oppressed and oppressing; (e) Promotes collaboration; (f) Promotes self-reflection on a variety of levels including personal and professional as a life-long process; and (g) Asserts that misogyny and other inequalities are damaging" (Worell & Johnson, 1997, p. 249). Women of Color, lesbian women, and women with disabilities who participated in the conference challenged all participants to give increased attention to the diverse lives of women. For many of us who attended this conference, witnessing feminist process in action was inspiring. The challenges related to diversity motivated many participants to consider how to more effectively integrate multicultural/ diversity perspectives into our models and practice. Meeting the challenge of integrating diversity and feminist approaches constitutes the third wave of feminist practice.

Range of Feminist Counseling Approaches

In response to feminist critiques of traditional therapies, a range of feminist counseling theories has been developed. These counseling theories emerged out of a variety of feminist philosophies (Enns, 1997). While many feminist counseling approaches now exist, the four central ones described here are based on the work of Carolyn Enns (1997).

1. *Liberal feminist counselors* believe the main problems in living are caused by traditional gender-role socializations that constrict the development of both men and women. They believe that change will occur by altering this socialization, ending gender bias, and providing equal opportunities for women and men. They emphasize helping clients to challenge their internalized gender-role messages.

2. *Radical feminist counselors* believe societal institutions oppress women via their sexist, heterosexist, racist, classist, ableist, and ageist structures. *Personal* issues are viewed as arising from social or *political* pathology (i.e., from toxic social environments). Radical feminist counselors emphasize the need to alter **patriarchal** (male-dominated) and other oppressive institutional structures, and thus, they embrace a social justice agenda. Consciousness-raising about the existence of these oppressions and their negative impact on individuals is also an important focus for radical feminist counselors.

3. *Cultural feminist counselors* believe women's problems in living arise because their traits, experiences, values, and abilities are not valued as highly as men's are. Compared to liberal and radical feminist counselors, cultural feminists deemphasize gender-role socializations by viewing women and men as being biologically different. They believe healthier individuals and societies will be achieved by positively revaluing women's traits, behaviors, and perspectives (e.g., subjective ways of knowing, intuition, interdependence, cooperation). Further, this revaluing process results in identifying and honoring women's strengths. Cultural feminist counselors believe empathy and mutual connectedness are important in all relationships, including therapeutic ones.

4. *Women of Color feminist counselors* criticize other forms of feminist counseling for failing to acknowledge that White women's perspectives do not universally apply to all women and for giving sexism too central a focus. Women of Color feminists emphasize the impact of all oppressions, especially racism, ethnocentrism, and classism, on diverse women's lives. They view multiple oppressions (e.g., a poor Latina) as having interacting negative impacts. They also emphasize the importance of honoring a full range of cultural values including harmony and interdependence. Women of Color feminists focus on helping clients identify societal oppressions and their impacts on individuals. They facilitate clients' challenging internalized negative societal messages about their groups and advocate for social change.

All of these feminist counseling approaches assert that societies contribute to people's problems, although they vary in their explanations of societal pathology

Table 11.2 Feminist Counseling Orientations

Orientation	Perspective on Cause of Problems	Focus of Interventions
Liberal	Traditional gender-role socialization	Changing internalized, traditional gender-role messages; creating equal societal opportunities for both women and men
Radical	Oppressive, especially sexist, societal structures	Social change aimed at reducing/eliminating all forms of societal oppression
Cultural	Societal devaluation of women's strengths, values, roles, and perspectives	Identifying and honoring women's strengths, values, and perspectives; emphasizing importance of connected, empathic therapeutic relationships
Women of Color	Oppressive, especially racist and ethnocentric, societal structures	Social change aimed at eliminating all forms of oppression; consciousness raising about negative impact of societal oppression on psychological well-being of people; honoring and celebrating diverse sets of cultural values

and of how social change should be accomplished. They all concur that counselors must be aware of their own values and attitudes and that examination of these attitudes should be a lifelong process accomplished via self-reflection and feedback from others (Enns, 1997; Johnson & Remer, 1997; Wyche & Rice, 1997). Counselors' acknowledgment of their seats of privilege and oppression is also critical to this examination process (Goodman, 2001). Although distinct from each other, these types of feminist counseling also overlap with each other and are mutually influencing (Enns, 1997). See Table 11.2 for a summary of the four types of feminist counseling approaches.

Context Then—Context Now

Feminist counseling approaches are relatively contemporary phenomena originally devised to challenge the intrapsychic focus of traditional counseling approaches and to confront societal sexism and its impact on the lives of women. Feminist practitioners rejected the androcentric and patriarchal worldviews that permeated psychological practice in the 1970s. Indeed, many feminists viewed mental health practitioners as encouraging women to adopt traditional roles, and some feminists believed that no form of psychotherapy could be healthy for women. This critique and challenge of mainstream psychology reflected the women's rights movement in the United States. Feminist approaches brought a radical view to treatment in asserting that sexism was a major contributor to women's problems in living and that social change should be a focus for psychologists. However, most early feminist counseling approaches did not adequately reflect the civil rights movement in the United States that was also occurring during the 1960s and 1970s. That is, feminist practitioners often assumed that all women's experiences were similar to those of White, heterosexual women.

Modern psychologists acknowledge the importance of understanding and embracing a diversity of cultural worldviews and values representing a variety of social positions (e.g., gender, sexual orientation, ethnicity, race, class). To a lesser extent, psychologists also recognize the existence of stereotyping and discrimination of subordinate groups in U.S. society and the impact of that oppression on the mental health of subordinate groups. However, most theoretical orientations do not have specific methods for accomplishing social change and continue to focus primarily on intrapsychic client change.

Feminist psychological approaches in general and feminist approaches to counseling more specifically are clearly still actively evolving. Asserting the detrimental effects of sexism and other oppressive societal elements and working to change oppressive societal institutions remain central, unifying foci of feminist approaches (Enns, 1997). More recently, the focus of feminist therapy has expanded to confront all forms of societal oppression and their impacts on the lives of all subordinate group members. This attention to cultural contexts and focus on social change to end all forms of oppression reflect the concerns of modern psychological diversity perspectives. Indeed, feminist psychological approaches have been congratulated for pioneering social justice pathways for psychology (Goodman et al., 2004).

At least five challenges are currently at the center of feminist psychological practices' evolving history. First, despite strides related to the recognition of the impact of multiple forms of oppression on diverse women, a continuing challenge for all feminist approaches is to integrate the diverse values, perspectives, and concerns of all girls and women into feminist constructs and techniques. Second, feminist psychological practitioners are involved in efforts to bring feminist and diversity perspectives to mainstream psychology and counseling. The previously described Guidelines for Psychological Practice with Girls and Women is an example of endeavors to meet this second challenge. A third current challenge for feminist practitioners is to conduct more research on the effectiveness of feminist counseling interventions. A fourth challenge is to develop further the application of feminist perspectives to men's issues and to treating individuals from other privileged groups. A fifth challenge is actually a continuing one that has always been present for feminist practitioners—that is, transforming society to end all oppressions. Working to meet these challenges will continue to transform feminist psychological practice.

The Author's Journey as a Feminist Therapist

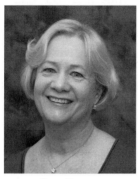

Pam Remer

I grew up learning fairly traditional gender-role messages (e.g., be pretty, let men win, do not be athletic, do not outshine men, be a virgin, be responsible for men's sexual behaviors), yet I also received some nontraditional messages (e.g., women can be and do anything, achieving academically is important). I coped with these mixed messages by trying to follow the traditional ones and camouflaging my nontraditional behaviors. For example, I achieved in school but regretted that I was the high school salutatorian because that meant I had to give a graduation address. Graduating third in my class would have called less attention to my gender nonconformity of appearing intelligent. Similarly, in college I struggled with being too visible as a campus leader. I loved being in leadership positions, yet worried that it would affect my attractiveness to men. Ongoing messages from men on campus about "not wanting to take orders from a woman" fueled my internal battles.

My graduate training occurred from 1969 to 1972 in a traditional program in counseling housed in the University of Colorado College of Education. From my own life experiences, I was drawn to women's issues in counseling. However, feminist counseling approaches were in their embryonic stages when I was in graduate school. As a result, I had no exposure to alternative methods to traditional therapies for counseling women, nor did I learn about women's issues. I now realize that my training (as was everyone else's at the time) was primarily from a White, heterosexual male perspective about White, heterosexual male-defined issues. I struggled to find a theoretical orientation that fit for me. Eventually I took a psychodrama seminar class and fell in love with its role playing and emphasis on creativity and spontaneity. In subsequent psychodrama training, I would learn more about psychodrama's attention to cultural contexts and their often limiting effects on human potential, a construct that became key in my eventual integration of feminist therapy and psychodrama (see Worell & Remer, 2003). Because my formal graduate training occurred at a time when feminist perspectives were just beginning, my journey to becoming a feminist therapist, like that of many of my age cohorts, would become one of self-education via readings, informal mentoring, participation in consciousness-raising (CR) groups, and self-reflection on my own personal and professional experiences.

(continued)

I was hired for my first post-Ph.D. position at the University of Wyoming's counseling center, in part because they wanted to add a woman to their all-male staff. The director encouraged me to address women's counseling issues, so I sought out books that would help me understand specific women's issues (e.g., unwanted pregnancy) and women's socialization. I was excited to discover the concept of **androgyny** as a standard of mental health that encouraged the development of both female and male traits. Androgyny made sense of my internal gender-role message struggles and supported the decisions I had made to achieve and be a leader. I had read about and was intrigued by CR groups for women, so I co-led (with a male psychologist) a CR group for undergraduate women and organized and joined a leaderless CR group for "older" women. I learned a lot from the undergraduate women, who at the time were probably more aware of societal sexism than I was. For example, they confronted me about sexist material in the center's career library. My participation in the other CR group was a major source of personal and professional development for me. I was in awe as I witnessed the power of women sharing their life stories with one another. Although I became known among students and staff as someone who knew about women's issues, I was discouraged from labeling myself "feminist" by several student affairs staff members. Although I outwardly followed their recommendations, my internal path to becoming a feminist counselor was taking form.

After two years at the counseling center, I moved to an academic position in the counseling psychology program at the University of Kentucky, where I have remained for the past 31 years. Here, I had the good fortune to be mentored by Dr. Judith Worell, who was one of the significant early (and ongoing) contributors to the development of feminist psychological practice. As a part of her mentoring, Judy invited me to co-present a workshop on gender-role issues in counseling (definitely a learn-by-doing experience for me). I began to read the articles and books about feminist practice that were emerging in the mid- to late 1970s. I continued to learn about feminist counseling by experimenting with its application in both my counseling and teaching. I began to publicly identify myself as a feminist teacher and clinician. Over the next couple of years, Judy and I developed courses in gender-role development and counseling women and gradually built a specialty area in women's issues within our counseling psychology program.

I believe that through these early experiences at the University of Kentucky my professional path was forever forged by feminist psychological practice. For example, feminist perspectives helped me identify, understand, and challenge the sexist experiences I was having as a female academician in a traditionally male arena. However, my commitment to feminist counseling was significantly deepened by one particular personal life event. After I had been at the University of Kentucky for about three years, I began having flashbacks to a rape I had experienced in my early twenties. As I struggled to heal from this experience, I sought out feminist-oriented readings about rape and applied feminist counseling strategies to myself. By examining what I had been socialized to believe about rape and comparing those beliefs to the realities of my own and others' rapes, I was able to challenge the self-blame I had internalized from society. I began to understand from a deeply emotional place how the *personal* pieces of my rape were indeed *political*. In a very real sense, these feminist perspectives helped save my psychological well-being. I understood firsthand how ignoring the cultural context of what appears to be intrapsychic issues could further harm clients instead of helping them. From this experience, I became interested professionally in helping other sexual assault survivors. I developed a feminist counseling model for rape survivors (Worell & Remer, 2003) and have spent the last five years leading a date rape prevention research team.

Eventually, Judy and I applied our cumulative experience with feminist counseling to the development of empowerment feminist therapy (EFT). Our first rendition of this model was a book that represented our integration of most of the existing feminist counseling approaches (Worell & Remer, 1992). Writing this book helped me to integrate all the different threads of my learning about feminist approaches and to create with Judy our own view of feminist therapy with its focus on empowering women. Following publication of the book and as a result of several professional and personal experiences (many of them painful), Judy and I became aware of the need for greater integration of diversity perspectives into feminist counseling approaches. We decided that we wanted to structurally revise EFT to include attention to all the social positions people hold. This revised version of EFT (Worell & Remer, 2003) gave a central focus to these social positions and the detrimental effects of all oppressions.

Feminist perspectives and feminist psychological practice continue to be the major defining elements in both my personal and professional lives. I am drawn to the concepts of not pathologizing individuals' responses to toxic environments and of emphasizing clients' strengths and coping strategies. I continue to be awed by the strength and resiliency of my clients who have experienced oppression and trauma. I enjoy engaging my clients in consciousness-raising interventions and witnessing the powerful and empowering impacts of their new awareness. I am energized and challenged to address my own seats of privilege as a White, middle-class, educated heterosexual.

Theory of Feminist Therapy

The main goal of this book is to describe the major traditional and modern approaches to counseling and psychotherapy and present the ways in which they are applied contemporarily to a culturally diverse range of clients. In accordance with that goal, I have focused this chapter on empowerment feminist therapy (EFT), an approach that was initially created to integrate the four major feminist approaches (Worell & Remer, 1992) and was later revised to structurally integrate diversity perspectives (Worell & Remer, 2003).

Feminist mental health practitioners assert that *all* counselors hold personal and cultural values and attitudes that affect the counseling process. Value-free counselors, theories, and counseling processes are not possible. Feminist counselors believe that clients have the right to know about these values and attitudes in order to make informed choices about therapists and their therapeutic methods. It is important for counselors to specify and disclose the values underlying their theoretical orientation because these theories guide the therapeutic process. Therefore I begin my discussion of the theoretical concepts of empowerment feminist therapy with full disclosure of its underlying values and worldviews.

Foundational Values and Worldviews

Many of the foundational values and worldviews underlying the constructs of empowerment feminist therapy are shared by the feminist counseling approaches described earlier. EFT values and perspectives include the following propositions that Judy Worell and I have synthesized from a range of feminist approaches. As you read each statement, take time to reflect on how your values and perspectives fit or do not fit. If you are considering integrating a feminist approach to counseling with another theoretical orientation, the constructs and techniques of that theory need to be compatible with these assumptions as well. EFT counselors believe:

1. "Women have individual problems because of living in societies that devalue them, limit their access to resources, and discriminate against them economically, legally, and socially. Thus, sexism is institutionalized in all areas of society—families, religion, education, recreation, the workplace, and laws—and is a major source of problems" (Worell & Remer, 2003, p. 65).

2. Other forms of oppression (racism, ethnocentrism, ageism, ableism, classism, and heterosexism) are also societal realities that negatively impact members of subordinate groups. **Oppression** is the subordination and devaluing of certain social positions in a society.

3. Because societal oppression negatively affects the mental health of all individuals, all forms of oppression need to be eliminated. Thus, social change is crucial to mental health. Individual change is not sufficient. Social change includes altering how people are socialized (e.g., gender-role socialization) and how social institutions are structured.

4. "Psychopathology, which is defined by the dominant culture, is primarily environmentally induced. Likewise, what is considered 'normal' is defined and maintained by the dominant culture" (Worell & Remer, 2003, p. 65).

5. Most gender differences are primarily the result of culturally based gender-role stereotyped constructions, not biology. Both men and women are negatively affected by the gender-role socialization that limits their potential by restricting the range of traits and behaviors that are culturally acceptable.

6. Hierarchal relationships have detrimental effects on subordinate groups.

7. A culturally diverse range of values and perspectives need to be understood and respected. Individuals cannot be understood outside of their cultural contexts.

8. "Non-feminist, non-multicultural therapeutic approaches have been developed primarily from Western, White, male, heterosexual perspectives and value systems. Without transformation, these therapeutic approaches can be detrimental to oppressed and culturally diverse populations" (Worell & Remer, 2003, p. 65).

Theoretical Concepts

Empowerment feminist therapy was built on the previously described assumptions and strove to integrate the unique strengths of liberal, radical, cultural and women of Color approaches to feminist counseling. While the 1992 version of EFT included attention to all forms of oppression, sexism was emphasized. More recently, the EFT model was revised to *structurally* integrate diversity and feminist perspectives. A central goal of EFT is the **empowerment** of clients using feminist perspectives. "Empowerment is a broad goal of feminist intervention that enables individuals, families, and communities to exert influence over the personal, interpersonal, and institutional factors that impact their health and well-being" (Worell & Remer, 2003, p. 24). The following overarching four principles guide the work of EFT counselors.

I. Personal and social identities are interdependent.

II. The personal is political.

III. Relationships are egalitarian.

IV. Women's perspectives are valued.

Principle I: Personal and Social Identities Are Interdependent

Because EFT counselors view societal oppression and socialization as major sources of people's problems, understanding clients' sociocultural contexts is crucial. Every culture is comprised of a variety of social groups that EFT counselors refer to as **social locations,** which are "the identity categories constructed by a given culture that place individuals into discrete social groups. These categories and their positive or negative characteristics are socially constructed by dominant, privileged groups in that culture" (Remer, Worell, & Remer, 2005). These social categories include, but are not limited to, gender, race/ethnicity, sexual orientation, social class status, religious/spiritual orientation, age, educational level, immigration/citizenship status, and physical and mental abilities and disabilities.

In every culture or society, these social locations occupy seats of relative privilege/advantage or oppression/disadvantage. That is, every culture socially constructs each social location, which falls on a continuum ranging from privileged to oppressed. Privileged groups benefit from having access to community resources, being seen by society as having desirable characteristics and qualities, and fitting the norms of the culture. These privileges often are invisible to those who have them (McIntosh, 1986). On the other hand, oppressed social location groups suffer from being denied access to valued societal resources, being discriminated against and devalued, and being judged deficient by comparison to dominant group norms (Goodman, 2001).

Although these social locations and their privileged and oppressed statuses can be viewed as objectively existing in a given culture (Diller, Houston, Morgan, & Ayim, 1996), individuals within a culture vary in their identification with each social location and in their awareness of and perception of the privileged and oppressed status of each location. Individuals' perceptions of their social locations constitute **social identities.** Thus, an individual's sense of self is composed of intersecting and interacting social identities.

Ultimately, to effectively understand our clients' sociocultural environments, counselors must get a picture of both their clients' social locations and social identities. An appraisal of their social locations is important for understanding how their culture and others in their culture perceive and interact with them. An appraisal of their social identities is important for understanding how they perceive themselves and how they have internalized societal treatment of their groups.

As a way of grasping experientially the meaning of social locations and social identities and their interactive nature, I would like you to complete the exercise found in Table 11.3. For each social location given (for an expanded list,

Table 11.3 A Social Locations Exercise

In the spaces to the right, briefly in your own words state who you are or how you define yourself. For example, for the space marked *nationality*, you might write "American" or "Chinese." Then, on the continuum beside each statement, mark an X representing where you see this location on the oppressed-to-privileged continuum.

Gender _____   O--------------------|--------------------P

Age _____   O--------------------|--------------------P

Education
Level _____   O--------------------|--------------------P

Sexual
Orientation _____   O--------------------|--------------------P

Race/Ethnicity _____   O--------------------|--------------------P

Religious/
Spiritual Orientation _____   O--------------------|--------------------P

Social Class Status _____   O--------------------|--------------------P

Nationality _____   O--------------------|--------------------P

Immigration/
Citizenship Status _____   O--------------------|--------------------P

Primary/Secondary
Language(s) _____   O--------------------|--------------------P

Physical Characteristics/
Body Image _____   O--------------------|--------------------P

Physical Ability/
Disability _____   O--------------------|--------------------P

Other _____   O--------------------|--------------------P

Source: Adapted from Remer, Worell, & Remer (2005).

see Worell and Remer, 2003), enter a label that reflects how you identify yourself (your social identity label). For example, for the social location of gender, I label myself as a "feminist woman" and for age, I use the label "nearing retirement." Please be creative in identifying a label that fits the way you see yourself. After you have labeled each location, reflect on whether you see this location as being privileged or oppressed by society and mark an "X" on the oppressed-to-privileged continuum to the right of your label. After you have completed the exercise, take time to reflect on what doing the exercise was like for you. For example, what labels were easy or difficult to specify? How did you reach decisions about where to locate each identity on the oppressed-to-privileged continuum?

As you can already tell, Principle I, *personal and social identities are interdependent*, is a complex process to implement. Several additional considerations, social identity development and saliency, further increase its complexity. **Identity development models** describe the processes by which individuals' social identities are impacted by the advantaged or disadvantaged social positions of their social locations. Specific identity development models have been created for oppressed groups [e.g., Cross's (1980) Black identity, Downing and Roush's (1985) feminist identity, Cass's (1979) homosexual identity] and for privileged groups [e.g., Helms's (1995) White identity]. These models are helpful for understanding identity development for a specific social location but are too specific for understanding the full range of intersecting social identities.

Worell and Remer (2003) generalized and synthesized existing specific identity development models to create a social identity development model that addresses both privileged and oppressed groups. The more general model allows for increased flexibility in identity development comparisons across intersecting social identities and reflects the dynamic nature of privilege and oppression. In this model, individuals can have a mix of both privileged and oppressed statuses and can be at different identity development levels for each social identity.

In Worell and Remer's model (2003), the individual progresses through four levels of social identity development.

1. *Pre-awareness*. The person is not aware of the privilege and oppression associated with a particular social identity.

2. *Encounter*. The individual experiences increased awareness of privilege and oppression.

3. *Immersion*. The individual rejects the oppressing dominant culture.

4. *Integration and activism*. The person comes to appreciate the strengths of both subordinate and dominant groups and commits to working for social change.

A goal of EFT counseling is to facilitate clients' movement in identity development levels for all of their social identities.

In addition to development of social identities, *saliency* also must be addressed. For any given issue that clients bring to counseling, some of their social locations will be more relevant or salient to them. For example, for an Asian-American man who is experiencing racial discrimination at work, race/ethnicity will likely be the most salient social location/identity. For an African-American lesbian who has come out recently to her family and has been rejected by them, both her sexual orientation and race/ethnicity are likely to be salient, and sexual orientation the more salient of the two. Saliency is client determined, and EFT counselors begin by addressing the social locations and identities the client determines are the most salient. Later, the counselor and client explore the full range of the client's social identities and examine the interacting nature and impact of all of the client's identities. For example, the aforementioned African-American lesbian client experiences discrimination in at least three of her social locations—gender, sexual orientation, and ethnicity/race. These three sources of oppression interact to place her in triple jeopardy (Greene, 1994). Further, she may experience racial discrimination in the lesbian community and sexual-orientation discrimination in the African-American community, resulting in her fitting into neither community.

EFT counselors do not assume gender to be the most salient location, but they do believe gender will be relevant for most clients, especially for women because of their subordinate status. That is, gender is just one social identity category to be considered. Most women experience sexism, and gender is socially constructed in all cultures. EFT counselors understand that the meaning of gender and gender socialization processes will vary by ethnicity and other social locations. EFT counselors learn about these different cultural manifestations from reading and by exploring the meaning of gender with their clients.

The *personal and social identities are interdependent* principle is the primary structure for integration of diversity and feminist perspectives. EFT counselors facilitate their clients' identification of their interacting social identities. Explorations of social locations and social identities can also include an assessment for acculturation levels of racial and ethnic groups and assessment for identity development levels for each social identity. By assessing for social identities, EFT counselors begin to construct a picture of their clients' cultural contexts and of how they have internalized these contexts. While this picture will continue to evolve over the course of counseling, beginning with social identities integrates diversity into the counseling process and honors the centrality of diverse social identities in people's lives. Social identity exploration starts the process of mapping the impact of social realities on personal issues for both counselors and clients. That is, the assessment for and mapping of social identities raise the awareness or consciousness of both counselors and clients about the cultural context and ensures that the role of cultural context in client issues will remain central to the counseling process. This attention to intersecting social identities further ensures that counselors will not fall back into the traditional intrapsychic perspectives of most other counseling approaches.

The primary goals of counseling related to Principle I are to help clients become more aware of all their social locations/social identities, how these identities intersect in their lives, and how the privileged and oppressed status of each identity impacts upon their lives. Related goals include facilitating clients' initial understanding of how external, cultural elements are creating or impacting their internal struggles and increasing clients' prizing of their social location groups and themselves. All of these goals will be further enhanced by work related to the next three principles. Finally, the *personal and social identities are interdependent* principle provides a structure for counselors and clients to address the similarities and differences in their respective locations. That is, a part of the social identities exploration involves clients and counselors discussing their respective social identities and the potential impact their similarities and differences may have on their counseling relationship.

Principle I is illustrated in the following counseling dialogue between a White female counselor and a Latina client who sought counseling for depression related to a divorce.

> T (Therapist): You have identified being a Latina and a woman as the two social identities most connected to your distress about your divorce. In your culture, what is the meaning of divorce for a woman?
>
> C (Client): Women are supposed to take care of their families and husbands. Divorce means I have failed as a woman. I have failed my husband, my children, and my community.
>
> T: I hear how deeply you have been affected by your culture's view of divorce. Given the sense of failure you have, your being depressed makes sense.

Principle II: The Personal Is Political

The central theme of most feminist counseling approaches is that *the personal is political* (Enns, 1997; Worell & Johnson, 1997). Given that stereotypes for social groups and socializing messages related to social locations and institutionalized discrimination of subordinate, oppressed social locations restrict the development of all individuals' potential, external societal contexts are viewed as the main sources of individual problems in living. Thus, *what appears to be an internal/personal issue is really an external social or political problem* (Gilbert, 1980; Wyche & Rice, 1997). The idea of pathology is moved from being located in individuals to being located in social environments. This social pathology framework for EFT and other feminist approaches (especially for radical and women of Color feminist approaches) necessitates moving from traditional therapies' primary focus on changing clients' internal feelings, thoughts, and behaviors to changing external social contexts, including altering how people are socialized and how social institutions are structured. Thus, social action/change is a crucial focus for EFT counselors. Principle II qualifies EFT as a social justice approach (Goodman et al., 2004). Further, working in tandem, Principles I and II illustrate how the oppression and privilege associated with all "social locations interact and influence the development of problems in living" (Worell & Remer, 2003, p. 68).

In accordance with Principle II, counselors help clients identify and separate the internal and external sources of their problems. Key to this process is increasing clients' awareness (consciousness raising) about the existence of societal oppression and privilege and increasing their awareness about how these phenomena are intertwined with how people are socialized (e.g., to be racially prejudiced) and how societal structures are constructed (e.g., the U.S. economic structure that results in women and minorities earning less than their White male counterparts) (Fassinger, 2001). Next, EFT counselors help clients discover how cultural socialization and institutionalized oppression have contributed and are still contributing to the "personal" issues that motivated them to seek counseling. This shift from internal to external causes of problems is a major source of empowerment for clients because the burden of their self-blame and self-insufficiency is lifted. This shift is also an important step in healing the inner wounds of oppression inflicted by society.

Next, counselors help clients from both oppressed and privileged social locations explore how they have internalized toxic social perspectives. For example, using *gender-role analysis*, counselors facilitate clients' identification of gender-role socialization messages they have learned about how to be a female or male. Given the new awarenesses that emerge from these explorations, clients must then decide what changes they want to make in themselves to challenge and replace these internalized messages, which is a feminist form of cognitive restructuring (replacing negative thoughts with positive ones). Clients must also decide whether to work to change the sociocultural environments that spawned their issues. "The focus is on changing the unhealthy external situation and the internalized effects of that external situation, rather than on helping the client adapt to a dysfunctional environment" (Worell & Remer, 2003, p. 68).

Given that the internalization of societal pathology is seen as normal, subordinate group clients are not blamed for internalizing or for their responses made to cope with these toxic environments. Thus, what other therapy modalities view as "symptoms" are relabeled as "coping strategies" to deal with unhealthy environments (Greenspan, 1983; Wyche & Rice, 1997). For example, depression in a person of Color might be viewed as a consequence of being discriminated against rather than a personal deficit. However, clients are also challenged to take responsibility to work toward change both in themselves (e.g., to expand their behavioral repertoire beyond prescribed gender roles) and their environments (e.g., working to change laws or institutional policies that discriminate). EFT counselors assess both the internal and external dimensions of clients' lives. Similar to most therapeutic modalities, feminist counselors assess intrapsychic dimensions related to psychological and physical health. Feminist counselors do not adhere to the symptom-driven perspectives of most therapeutic modalities whose diagnostic categories primarily locate the origins of dysfunction in individuals. Because feminist counselors view assessment and diagnosis very differently, mainstream diagnostic and assessment approaches are problematic for feminist practitioners. For example, Worell and Remer (2003) identified several unique feminist assessment perspectives. Feminist counselors assess for social locations and social identities. They focus assessments on clients' cultural contexts, and if they use traditional diagnostic labels they view clients' reactions as occurring within and influenced by these cultural contexts. Feminist counselors assess for client strengths and coping abilities. For example, a lesbian woman who keeps her sexual identity a secret from family and co-workers is not judged to be lacking assertiveness or self-esteem, but rather is perceived as coping with a society that oppresses and often harms gays and lesbians.

An assessment of external factors requires different tools than those used in most traditional, intrapsychic-focused therapies. Feminist therapists have developed some unique tools and borrowed others for assessing the external dimensions of clients' lives. EFT therapists examine how a culture defines a particular counseling issue (cultural analysis), how societal hierarchical relationships contribute to the problem (power analysis), and how socialization processes support privilege and oppression (e.g., gender-role analysis).

The ultimate goal of most feminist practitioners is to end all oppressions (Wyche & Rice, 1997). The social change dimension of feminist counseling applies to both counselors and clients. Most feminist practitioners incorporate working for social justice into their professional endeavors. EFT counselors support clients' working for social change, but they do not script or push for it. In fact, clients often naturally gravitate to participating in social change projects as a result of their new awareness about the social sources of their problems. Their efforts may range from macro levels of change (e.g., changing stalker laws) to micro levels (e.g., confronting friends and family about their heterosexist statements). For example, after several sessions to resolve a trauma of being physically assaulted, a White female client related to her feminist counselor that she had stopped making racist remarks and had been confronting family and friends about their racism. The following is an excerpt from one of their sessions.

C (Client): Lately something weird has been happening.

T (Therapist): Something "weird"?

C: Yes. I hate to admit this, but prior to my assault, I treated Black people poorly. I saw them as inferior to me and I often put them down and even called them names behind their backs. Now, I'm different.

T: Prior to your attack, you discriminated against African Americans, but now that has changed. How are you different now?

C: Now I understand what being targeted and treated as an object by another human being feels like. I see that what my friends and I did was very hurtful. In fact, I identify with Black people's pain. I no longer make racist remarks and I will not tolerate discriminatory behavior by others in my presence. I confront my friends and family when they put Blacks down. I'm looking for a different job because I don't want to be around several co-workers who constantly make racist remarks.

Principle III: Relationships Are Egalitarian

Most contemporary societies are arranged hierarchically, and people in subordinate positions in those societies are often discriminated against and oppressed. Feminist counselors see these patriarchal, hierarchical relationships as part of social pathology. Thus, they value egalitarian relationships among people both in society and between client and counselor. The egalitarian relationship aspects of feminist approaches reflect three philosophical underpinnings and goals. First, feminist counselors strive toward building egalitarian therapeutic relationships to not recreate or mirror destructive societal hierarchical relationships and to serve as an antidote to oppressive, hierarchical relationship structures. Second, building egalitarian therapeutic relationships makes empowerment of clients a central focus and reduces the chances that counselors will impose their own values on clients (Worell & Remer, 2003). Third, egalitarian, collaborative relationships create therapeutic environments where clients are safe enough to express their own "truths." As therapists accept and honor these phenomenological truths, clients increase their trust in themselves and their experiences.

Principle III, *relationships are egalitarian*, has several implications for the therapeutic process. Collaborative feminist therapeutic relationships help empower clients. Feminist counselors do not pathologize their clients. Feminist counselors do not view themselves as healthy and their clients as unhealthy. Two types of expertise are honored. Clients are treated as experts on themselves and their life experiences. Counselors' expertise is based on their professional knowledge and skills as well as their lived experiences.

Feminist practitioners use several strategies to balance the power differentials between themselves and their clients. First, counselors demystify the counseling process for clients by informing them about the counseling process, client rights, and counselor responsibilities. Second, feminist counselors disclose their relevant values which allows clients to make informed choices about continuing counseling with a particular therapist. Feminist counselors also support their clients in deciding on their own values rather than adopting without examination the values of society, family, or their counselors. Third, feminist counselors and clients jointly develop counseling goals (Remer & Rostosky, 2002).

Fourth, contrary to many traditional therapies, feminist counselors self-disclose about their relevant life experiences. For example, I usually tell my clients who have been sexually assaulted that I am a rape survivor. When appropriate, I also share some of the struggles I encountered during my healing process. By disclosing, I help my clients identify our common experiences as women. These disclosures often result in their perceiving that the *personal is political.* Counselor self-disclosure can also be used to explore differences with their clients. For example, if I am counseling an African-American rape survivor, some of our experiences may be similar (e.g., experiencing victim blame). However, our gender-role socialization messages as well as some of the specific ethnic messages we received about rape are likely to be different. A fifth strategy for establishing more egalitarian therapeutic relationships is to treat clients' reactions to therapists as real, here-and-now responses rather than viewing them as transference (Greenspan, 1983).

Principle III is illustrated by the following example of my interaction with a White male client who sought counseling for depression and communication difficulties. In this session, the client says that he thinks he may have raped his previous girlfriend and wants to explore whether he did or not. He has never mentioned this incident previously.

> T (Therapist): Before we take a look at what happened between you and your girlfriend, I want to share something about myself that I have not mentioned because it didn't seem relevant to what you have been working on, but now it is. When I was in my early 20s, I was date-raped. I'm worried that this experience might negatively affect my ability to help you accurately assess what took place. You might want to talk about this experience with a different therapist.

> C (Client): Whew! You were raped. [Long silence, client thinking.] I trust you. I think that your experience may help me understand what happened between my girlfriend and me. Would you be willing to share some of your experience with me?

> T: As we explore what happened in your situation, I would be willing to answer specific questions you have.

Principle IV: Women's Perspectives Are Valued

The fourth principle of EFT, *women's perspectives are valued*, is representative of cultural feminist counseling perspectives. In most cultures, the characteristics, roles, and values associated with female-related traits are devalued compared to those associated with male-related traits. So while women are rewarded for behaving in accordance with female gender-role socialization messages, they are also devalued for doing so (Broverman, Broverman, Clarkson, Rosenkrantz, & Vogel, 1970). Many feminist counselors, especially cultural feminists, view this devaluation of female-related characteristics as a type of social pathology that is then internalized by women and men. For example, Latinas, Asian-American women, and European-American women in the United States are socialized to put others' needs before their own and then may be criticized for being enmeshed with their families or dependent on their husbands. Feminist counselors also believe that many of these female qualities and values (e.g., empathy, cooperation, interdependence, intuition/subjective ways of knowing) are strengths that if revalued would make social structures healthier. Thus, both female and male clients are encouraged to try seeing these traits as valuable. If female clients decide to embrace this value transformation, their appreciation of themselves and of their strengths are increased. The impact for male clients can be an expansion of their role repertories. According to feminist counselor beliefs, societies would be positively transformed by embracing female-related qualities and values. For example, cooperative, interdependent relationships could result in fewer wars and lower incidences of domestic violence.

The fourth principle has another set of implications. The phrasing *women's perspectives are valued* highlights that multiple and diverse women's perspectives and values exist and that all women's voices and perspectives need to be honored. Feminist counselors value clients' subjective ways of knowing, and their feelings and emotions are honored. Feminist counselors appreciate the power of empathy in therapeutic relationships. They also focus on clients' strengths rather than on their deficits, problems, and pathologies.

In summary, in accordance with the fourth principle of EFT, female clients and clients from other subordinate groups are introduced to the idea of relabeling socially devalued traits as strengths, to validate their inner truths and perspectives, and to self-define themselves (Sturdivant, 1980). They also may be encouraged to join appropriate CR groups and to work with others to accomplish social change. They are challenged to recognize and appreciate the value of the diverse perspectives of all women and other subordinate groups.

The following counseling excerpt illustrates Principle IV. The interaction occurs between a European-American female counselor and Latina client struggling with a recent divorce. This case scenario is a continuation of the one introduced at the end of Principle I.

> C (Client): I now understand that the divorce was not entirely my responsibility. I was not a perfect wife, but my husband also made a decision to have an affair. Yet I still believe that it is important for women to take care of their families.

> T (Therapist): You realize that the divorce was not primarily your fault. We have explored how the cultural messages you received as a Latina may have contributed to your depression about the divorce. After looking at the benefits and costs of those messages, you believe the cultural messages fit for you. You value meeting the needs of your family. You see this nurturing ability as a strength. Am I understanding you correctly?

> C: Yes.

Practice of Feminist Therapy

The four principles of empowerment feminist therapy are accomplished through employing a variety of techniques. Some of these interventions (e.g., gender-role analysis, power analysis) are original and unique feminist creations, and some are adapted from other approaches (e.g., reframing, bibliotherapy) and given a unique feminist focus or twist.

Feminist Therapy Interventions

In this section, the following feminist interventions are described: cultural analysis, social identities analysis, gender-role analysis, power analysis, consciousness-raising groups, counselor self-disclosing and self-involving responses, bibliotherapy, reframing and relabeling.

Cultural Analysis

In general, all strategies for examining the cultural contexts of clients' lives fall under the umbrella of *cultural analysis* (Worell & Remer, 2003). Thus, social identities analysis, gender-role analysis, and power analysis, three techniques that will be described subsequently, are all forms of cultural analysis. In addition to these specific examinations, the general cultural contexts of clients' lives and issues need to be examined using feminist and diversity lenses. The following questions illustrate the application of these lenses to analyze clients' cultural contexts.

- How is the client's issue (e.g., sexual harassment) defined by the dominant culture, and how does this definition reflect the values of privileged groups within the culture?

- What societal myths or beliefs are related to the issue?

- How are clients' social locations, social identities, and identity development levels related to the issue?

- How do diagnostic categories used by the mental health system relate to the issue, and how do they locate the problem in individuals?

To be competent to do cultural analyses, feminist counselors educate themselves about the cultural contexts of common client issues. Using cultural analysis questions and feminist/diversity critiques, feminist counselors and their clients collaboratively examine the cultural contexts of the clients' issues. Information giving, clients' self-reflection on their lived experiences, and bibliotherapy enhance the cultural analysis process (Worell & Remer, 2003). For example, an EFT counselor of a European-American female who was abused by her ex-husband would assess that domestic violence is generally condoned in U.S. dominant culture and is supported by patriarchal structures where men occupy the majority of positions of power in society. Further, the female victim is often held responsible for her own abuse and blamed for not being an adequate wife. If this client is at the *preawareness* level of her gender identity development, she will probably have internalized these societal beliefs and think she was abused because she provoked her husband. The EFT counselor will give information to the client about how domestic violence is supported by patriarchal structures and help the client replace her beliefs based on societal myths about domestic violence with knowledge based on accurate information.

Social Identities Analysis

Earlier in this chapter, you completed a social identities exercise in which you described some of your own social locations and then indicated where each of them fit on an oppression-to-privilege continuum. The process used in this exercise is the central element in an analysis of social identities. A second component of social identities analysis is to collaboratively assess the identity development level of each social location that is salient to a client's issues. One strategy for accomplishing this identity development assessment is to examine where clients place each of their social identities on the oppression-to-privilege continuum. For example, if a person of Color places her or his race/ethnicity location on the privileged end of the continuum, it is likely that the individual is not aware of societal racism and is in Level 1, *preawareness*, of racial identity development. This assessment yields data about how aware clients are of privilege and oppression and to what degree they have internalized these external phenomena. Clients' level of identity development has implications for the counseling process. For example, clients at Level 1 will particularly benefit from consciousness raising, that is, learning about the existence of privilege and oppression and connecting their own lived experiences to these phenomena.

Gender-Role Analysis

Gender-role analysis is a uniquely feminist counseling strategy that serves two functions: assessment and promotion of client change. Gender-role analysis begins with clients identifying the societal messages they have received through-out their lives about how women and men should be (i.e., acceptable traits) and act (societally desirable behaviors) (Worell & Remer, 2003). Next, feminist counselors help clients identify both the sources of these messages (e.g., family, peers, media, religious institutions, and educational institutions) and the positive and negative impact of these messages both on clients' lives and on society in general. This aspect of the analysis increases the likelihood that clients will begin to recognize the need for social change. For those internalized messages clients judge to be negatively impacting their lives and society, clients must next decide if they want to change (cognitively restructure) the messages. If they decide to alter an internalized message, they construct a new, more self-enhancing one to replace the old one.

The following interaction occurred during a gender-role analysis for a client who was sexually abused as a child by her uncle. The client reported that one of her gender-role messages was that women should be able to control men's sexual behavior. For example, "a female should not get a male too sexually worked up if she doesn't want to have sex" and "if a male gets sufficiently aroused, he can't stop himself." Through gender-role analysis, the client determined that it is impossible for one person to control another person's sexual behavior. She also recognized that these messages had contributed to blaming herself for the abuse.

> T (Therapist): So you can see how inaccurate and unfair these messages are and how they have led to your blaming yourself for what your uncle did to you. What alternate message would you like to construct for yourself?

> C (Client): Both women and men are responsible for their behaviors and decisions. Children are not capable of controlling the behavior of adults in their lives.

For clients from diverse ethnic or immigrant groups, at least two sources of gender-role messages are possible—those messages conveyed by the dominant European-American culture via societal institutions and the media and those messages conveyed by clients' ethnic communities. Thus, multiple sources and multiple messages often create conflicts for these clients. By exploring the mixed gender-role messages they have received, clients with subordinate social locations reach a clearer understanding of how their internal conflicts mirror and are created by their external environments.

Power Analysis

Power is the "ability to access personal and environmental resources to effect personal and/or external change" (Worell & Remer, 2003, p. 78). Individuals' use of power is influenced by the privileged or oppressed statuses of intersecting social locations. That is, access to environmental resources will be supported by society if individuals have social locations of privilege or will be thwarted if they occupy oppressed social locations. Given these perspectives on power, a third uniquely feminist assessment and intervention strategy is *power analysis*. Power analysis helps clients become more aware of their valued (privileged) or devalued (oppressed) societal status and about how those statuses affect their responses in their personal and professional relationships. Power analysis also helps highlight the existence of power differentials between advantaged and disadvantaged groups.

Power analysis, as described by Worell and Remer (2003), has several steps. First, EFT counselors teach clients about different kinds of power. These include role (e.g., employer, employee), resource, legal, institutional, normative (e.g., having the behavior and traits valued by society), physical, referent (e.g., being associated with someone else who is powerful), and reward (e.g., being in a position to reward others for acceptable behavior) power. Second, clients learn about the variety of ways that power can be enacted (e.g., direct vs. indirect, personal vs. concrete resources, competence vs. helplessness) (Johnson, 1976). Third, clients learn how access to different kinds of power is influenced by subordinate or dominant group statuses. For example, dominant group individuals have institutional power via their access to leadership positions in societal institutions and are allowed more direct means of exerting power in general. Both subordinate and dominant group power perspectives are analyzed. Oppression cannot exist without **privilege** and vice versa. The effects of too little power on disadvantaged groups and of too much power on advantaged groups must both be examined (Brickman, 1984).

The fourth step in power analysis involves clients' identifying the sources of power to which they have access in each of their social locations. Fifth, clients examine how their internalized gender-role messages and internalized socialization messages associated with their different social identities impact their past and current uses of power. They also identify how environmental barriers, such as sexism, racism, and ethnocentrism, are affecting their use of power. Challenging and changing internalized messages that limit use of a variety of kinds of power is crucial to clients' expanding the ways they use power. However, EFT counselors also acknowledge the role of environmental barriers and thus help clients assess the costs and benefits to them of using alternate kinds of power. EFT counselors (and clients) often work to change social institutions to reduce the environmental barriers. Finally, clients try out alternate kinds of power in their lives (Enns, 1997).

Consciousness-Raising Groups

As described earlier, leaderless consciousness-raising groups where women meet to discuss their common issues were an important part of the women's movement in the United States. Feminist counselors have adapted CR groups for counseling. These adapted versions may be leaderless but are often led by feminist counselors. In these groups, members share their life experiences and examine how these experiences have been affected by their socialization and by their external sociocultural environments. These groups may be focused on a particular issue (e.g., a battered women's group) or on a particular social location (e.g., a men's group, a group for lesbians), or they may be more general in nature. CR groups have several advantages over individual counseling. First, multiple individuals sharing their experiences intensifies the identification of common social roots of issues and vividly illustrates the *personal is political* principle. Second, the group members have the opportunity to contribute to each other's growth, which in turn aids them in identifying and applying their strengths. Finally, if group members are motivated to work for social change, they are likely to be more effective working together than individually.

Counselor Self-Disclosing and Self-Involving Responses

Many traditional approaches to counseling emphasize the importance of counselor expertise and objectivity and value a hierarchical therapeutic relationship. Counselor self-disclosure, counselors sharing about themselves and their life experiences, is discouraged or prohibited by these approaches. Contrary to these traditional theoretical perspectives, feminist counselors value egalitarian counselor-client relationships, treat the clients as experts on themselves, challenge the possibility of value-free counselors and counseling, and value the subjective knowledge derived from the lived experiences of both clients and counselors. Thus, *counselor self-disclosing* is permitted and valued because it helps equalize therapeutic power and can contribute to identifying the common external conditions related to client issues. For example, if I am counseling a rape survivor who says she now feels from different than most women, I can share that I, too, am a rape survivor. The client's view of being an outlier will be challenged and she will also develop hope about the possibility of her healing.

Counselor self-involving responses, the here-and-now reactions of the therapist to client disclosures, model expression of feelings and make similar contributions to the therapeutic process. As an example, an EFT counselor who is listening to the story of a battered woman who is minimizing the severity of her partner's physical and emotional abuse would share how afraid he or she is about the client's safety. Often this type of self-involving response will break through the client's denial that her partner's behavior "is not that bad." While feminist counselors value self-disclosure and self-involvement, they still recommend making careful decisions about when to use these interventions so that they foster client growth and the therapeutic relationship. For example, I would probably not disclose about being a rape survivor to a client who comes to me for career counseling because it would have no relevancy to the client's issues.

Bibliotherapy

The knowledge most members of subordinate groups possess about their worlds and their own group(s) has been filtered through White, male, heterosexual, and able-bodied lenses. The result is that both subordinate and dominant group individuals are misinformed about subordinate groups and have narrow perspectives about their own strengths and problem areas. Bibliotherapy, reading books and articles that counter these misperceptions or employ alternate lenses, is crucial to increasing awareness about privilege and oppression, to challenging dominant worldviews, and to promoting subordinate clients' positive view of themselves and their groups. Further, reading about feminist perspectives on issues common in women's lives (e.g., incest, rape, sexual harassment, wife battering) may challenge a woman's inclination toward self-blame.

Reframing and Relabeling

Reframing and relabeling are techniques common in family counseling approaches (Grunebaum & Chasin, 1978). When making a reframing response, a counselor uses a different perspective, or change of reference, for viewing an individual's behavior. In family therapy, the reframe shifts from an intrapersonal definition of clients' issues to an interpersonal one. For example, a family counselor might point out that a positive result of a teenager having a drug problem (individual problem focus) is that it motivated the whole family to seek counseling (family problem focus). Feminist counselors use reframing to shift the focus from an individual-centered (intrapsychic) problem to a society-centered one (toxic cultural context). For example, in the case of a European-American female client who was depressed about not performing adequately at work and who also revealed being sexually harassed at work, the EFT counselor suggested that she reframe the source of her problem as a sexist and woman-devaluing cultural context and helped the client understand how she had introjected society's devaluation of her when she labeled herself "inadequate."

In making a relabeling response, counselors change the evaluative label of clients' responses or qualities from a negative one to a positive one. Consistent with both Principle II, *the personal is political*, and Principle IV, *women's perspectives are valued*, feminist counselors relabel societally devalued characteristics as positive. The depression of the sexually harassed woman is not viewed as a pathological symptom (a negative evaluation) but rather as a natural outcome of being sexually harassed and a way of coping (a positive evaluation) with that harassment.

Theory of Change

A theory of change for empowerment feminist therapy is embedded in two perspectives. First, EFT counselors believe that if social oppression of subordinate groups is decreased and eventually eliminated, many problems in living experienced by subordinate group members will be alleviated. Because these social changes will also alter stereotyped myths and messages and the hierarchical relationships between oppressed and privileged groups, the mental health of privileged group members will be improved as well. Thus, the first basic tenet of change for feminist counseling approaches is that changing toxic social structures will positively impact the mental health of individuals. Thus, feminist counselors commit themselves to working for social change in their communities and professional arenas and support social change efforts by their clients.

Because social change is complex, difficult, and slow to accomplish, an additional theory of change is needed. EFT counselors believe that individual (and to some extent social) change is also accomplished when clients gain awareness (have their consciousness raised) about the existence of privilege and oppression and about how those phenomena have impacted and continue to impact their lives. Most clients come to counseling with an intrapsychic view of their problems. That is, they either believe the problem is located in themselves (e.g., "I'm inadequate") or in someone else ("She is too emotional"). Feminist counselors educate clients about the cultural contexts that surround and contribute to their counseling issues. Collaboratively, they explore clients' life experiences with oppression and privilege. Clients identify the socialized messages they have received related to each of their social locations, how they have internalized those messages, and the impact of those messages on their lives. This consciousness-raising process lets clients separate the external from the internal sources of their issues and facilitates their movement in their social identity development levels. This new awareness leads clients to begin working to undo the internalized negative effects and to alter their social contexts. Thus, empowerment and change is accomplished via consciousness raising that makes the invisible external realities more visible.

Long-Term Versus Short-Term Therapy

Feminist counselors do not apply any a priori assumptions about the length of counseling for a particular client. Instead, they make those decisions collaboratively, with the client's taking into account the nature of her or his issue and perceived needs. In general, feminist counseling may be longer than a symptom reduction–directed therapy because feminist approaches attend to facilitating the integration of new perceptions gained and to the development of expanded role repertoires and strengths.

Application of the Four Principles of EFT

Janice is a 20-year-old, second-generation, Asian-American college junior majoring in electrical engineering. She sought counseling for depression and anxiety.

Her counselor, Paul, is a 50-year-old Asian-American male who professionally identifies himself as a "multicultural feminist" counselor. The description of their counseling sessions, which follows, does not detail their total interactions, but rather highlights how Paul applied the four empowerment feminist therapy principles and related techniques.

Application of Principle I: Personal and Social Locations Are Interdependent

During the first several counseling sessions, Paul attended to understanding Janice's depression, anxiety, and life situation from her perspective and to building a collaborative, mutually trusting relationship. During this early stage of counseling, Paul assessed Janice's social locations and identities. Janice identified her Asian-American ethnicity as most important to her and as most relevant to her counseling issues. She explained that she is one of only four Asian-American students in her program and the only woman. As a result, she feels isolated and alone. Despite performing well in the program, she doubts her abilities and questions her career choice.

Paul estimated that Janice was in Level 2, *encounter*, of racial identity development because Janice perceived that being an Asian American put her in the slightly oppressed area of the oppression-to-privilege continuum. Because she had some awareness of racial discrimination in U.S. society in general but little awareness of how racism might be impacting her experience in her professional training program, Janice attributed her problems to internal stress and to "not measuring up."

Paul and Janice also explored her gender social location. Janice marked this location in the middle of the oppressed-to-privileged continuum, and her verbal accounts led Paul to estimate she was in Level 1, preawareness, in her gender-identity development. He knew from his experiences at the university that the engineering department had a long history of being White, male dominant, and criticized for being both racist and sexist. He hypothesized that Janice's depression and anxiety might be a result of her internalizing her hostile and toxic academic environment.

Paul and Janice also engaged in a dialogue about their respective social locations. Janice disclosed that she had requested Paul because he was an Asian American. He noted that they were different on gender, and they discussed how their similarities and differences might affect their therapeutic relationship.

Application of Principle II: The Personal Is Political

Because Janice said her racial social identity was most salient to her situation and because she was in a higher level of racial identity compared to gender identity development, Paul began his counseling exploration related to Principle II by having her identify the messages she learned growing up about being an Asian American. Paul began with her higher level of social identity development because he could build on her greater awareness of oppression with racial social location to help her become more aware of sexism. She remembered being teased about her eyes and skin color in her primarily White elementary school, hearing that Asians were supposed to be good at math and science, and receiving encouragement in high school for her academic performance in the sciences. In high school, she had several close friends—a couple of White friends from school and a couple of Asian-American friends from the Asian-American community. She also recounted several direct experiences with racial discrimination, including being followed by security guards while shopping in a major department store.

Paul asked Janice to reflect on how the messages she received and her past experiences related to race might be impacting her current academic situation. As a result of the cultural analysis they had just completed, she was able to see how the faculty might be discriminating against the students of Color in the program and eventually was able to see how this contributed to her feeling isolated.

In later counseling sessions, Paul gave Janice information about the intersection of racism and sexism for women of Color, especially in White, male-dominated professions. They then performed a gender-role analysis. First, Paul had Janice list the gender-role messages she had learned from her Asian-American community, and second, they explored the dominant cultural gender-role messages she had received. From her ethnic community, Janice had learned that girls were not as valuable as boys (e.g., her father conveyed his disappointment that she was not a boy), that women were supposed to be wives and mothers and take care of others, be polite and deferential, be pretty, and be protected by men. She also had learned that she could gain her parents' approval by excelling in school. But now that she had entered her twenties, she was also receiving strong messages about needing to marry and have children, especially sons. Her "academic achievement redemption" for being a girl was now turning into a liability as she was supposed to be turning her attention away from career aspirations to getting married and becoming a mother. Many of the dominant White, European-American gender-role messages were reinforcing her ethnic cultural messages.

The gender-role analysis helped Janice be aware of the mixed gender-role messages (e.g., achieve, but then give up your career to be a mother) she had received and how her internal conflict mirrored these messages. She also realized how sexism pervaded her program's structure (e.g., despite being near the top of her class, she had difficulty securing a summer internship), the faculty's behavior (e.g., sexist remarks and jokes made in class), and her peers' responses to her (e.g., not being invited to join study groups composed primarily of White males). She made connections between the sexism and racism in the program and her self-doubts about her abilities, depression, and anxiety. She became more aware of the similar oppressive elements of the racism and sexism she had experienced and of how they were interacting in her current situation. With Paul's support, Janice made connections with other women in the other engineering programs in her college. As a result of sharing their common oppressive experiences in the program, they decided as a group to approach the academic ombudsman to file a complaint. This challenging was outside Janice's cultural comfort zone and gender-role socialization, but taking this social action as a part of a group made it more achievable for her.

Application of Principle III: Relationships Are Egalitarian

Paul worked on building an egalitarian relationship throughout his work with Janice. He was aware that although he shared Janice's subordinate status as a person of Color, he also had gender-role privilege as a man. As a part of his ongoing development as a multicultural feminist therapist, he had focused on learning about his unearned, invisible privileges as a man and a heterosexual. He was also aware that his identity development in each of his social locations would affect how he conceptualized and intervened with his clients. Thus, he made a commitment to being mindful in every aspect of his life of how these privileged positions might be influencing his behavior and relationships with others.

When he and Janice explored her race discrimination experiences, he self-disclosed similar encounters from his own life. When they discussed sexism, he shared some of his privileged gender experiences. Both of these types of self-disclosures helped validate Janice's perspectives and make connections to the *personal is political*.

Application of Principle IV: Women's Perspectives Are Valued

Paul helped Janice relabel her depression, anxiety, and lack of confidence as natural outcomes of being devalued and discriminated against and as important signs that her external environment was harmful to her well-being. He had Janice identify the positive strategies she used to cope with the racism and sexism that she encountered and expand her coping repertoire.

General Strengths and Weaknesses of Feminist Counseling Approaches

Feminist psychological practice was given birth by the women's movement, and so its primary focus initially was on the detrimental effects of societal sexism on the lives of women. As feminist approaches evolved, increased attention was given to the diversity of all women's lives and to multiple forms of oppression.

Because feminist counseling approaches were developed to examine and challenge the effects of multiple sources of oppression in clients' lives, they are naturally designed for clients from subordinate social locations. At a macro level, these approaches advocate for social change designed to reduce and eliminate all forms of oppression. On a micro level, they help clients to become aware of and examine their cultural contexts and the impacts of those contexts on their lives and issues.

For many oppressed clients, both the contexts and their effects have previously been invisible. Thus, the internal and external sources of clients' problems have been entangled, with clients frequently and inappropriately blaming themselves for their situations. The main strength of feminist counseling approaches is that they empower clients by making the invisible visible and shifting internalized oppression from self to the socialization processes and oppressive institutional structures that have frequently given birth to or contributed to clients' problems.

Focus on Oppression and Social Change

The strengths and weaknesses of any counseling approach are often flip sides of the same coin. While a strength of feminist counseling approaches lies in their focus on oppression and on empowering individuals from oppressed groups, one corresponding weakness is their applicability to individuals from privileged social locations. That is, individuals in privileged locations do not suffer from oppression. However, the principles of feminist therapies can also be applied to White, heterosexual males and other individuals who have primarily privileged positions in society. Feminist techniques can generally be applied in a somewhat similar fashion to both privileged and oppressed individuals. For example, gender-role messages often have a restrictive, negative impact for both women and men. Thus, gender-role analysis can be used with male clients to raise awareness about the restrictive impact of adhering to male gender-role socialized proscriptions.

However, an additional focus is needed for working with privileged positions, as opposed to oppressed ones. Feminist counselors raise privileged clients' awareness about both privilege and oppression and, when appropriate, explore with these clients how their heretofore invisible privileges and their exercising of these privileges may be contributing to the problems they brought to counseling. For example, a feminist counselor working with a White male client who is having difficulty being an effective administrator to his primarily female staff would ask the client to identify the male gender-role messages he has learned. This gender-role analysis would help the client see how his male socialization has resulted in his relying on a limited and stereotyped set of behaviors for relating to his staff. The counselor would also have this White male client examine how his use of privilege and power (e.g., making sexist comments to the staff) might be contributing to his problems as a manager. Helping privileged individuals to understand their impact on others, especially subordinate group members, creates new alternative solutions to interpersonal conflicts at home and at work. This owning of privilege facilitates identity development and opens possibilities for privileged group members to become allies in the battles to end oppression of subordinate groups.

Role of Values

Because feminist counselors use feminist lenses to critique societal institutions for their hierarchical structures and for their stereotyping that limits the potential of all social groups, feminist therapy has been criticized for imposing its values and beliefs on clients. Generally speaking, feminist counselors' strongest values and beliefs are grounded in a desire to eliminate all types of oppression. However, differentiating between judgments about what is oppressive and what are variations in cultural values and practices is a value-laden process. Indeed, it has been said that one difference between multicultural and feminist therapies is that multiculturalists "honor" culture while feminists "challenge" culture. Thus, a potential danger inherent in feminist counseling is that counselors' values will too strongly influence clients or will conflict with clients' values.

Feminist counselors employ a number of strategies to reduce this potential danger. First, they become acquainted with the clients' social identities and the values clients hold related to these identities. Second, they build collaborative therapeutic relationships and treat clients as experts on themselves. While feminist counselors do raise awareness about cultural norms, stereotypes, and forms of discrimination, they invite clients to decide whether to challenge or change particular values or practices. For example, in the gender-role analysis intervention one of the final steps is for clients to decide if they want to change their internalized messages. Feminist therapists value clients' making informed decisions. As long as societal oppression and privilege and socialization processes that emanate from these hierarchical arrangements are invisible, informed choice is not possible. Using consciousness-raising interventions, feminist counselors aim to enhance individuals' abilities to make real choices for their lives.

A third way that feminist counselors minimize imposition of their values on clients is to state and own their relevant values to clients early in the counseling relationship so that clients can make an informed choice about whether to continue with the counselor. Feminist counseling approaches also stress the importance of feminist counselors' awareness of their intersecting social identities and of their values and worldviews.

While I believe that feminist counselors must guard against imposing their values on clients, I do not believe potential imposition of counseling values is unique to feminist therapy. Instead, I see it as a potential hazard for counselors from all theoretical orientations. Indeed, a greater danger exists for practitioners who assume their approaches are free of values and are apolitical. All counseling approaches are based on a set of values. Worell and Remer (2003) assert, "both challenging social structures (feminist therapy) and supporting social structures (traditional theories) are 'political acts'" (p. 70).

Deemphasis of Intrapsychic Sources of Client Problems

As previously described, feminist approaches to counseling are interactionist, viewing the sources of clients' problems as resulting from the interaction of internal and external factors. Feminist approaches tend to highlight the external sources, but do not ignore intrapsychic or biological sources. Nevertheless, another potential weakness of feminist counseling approaches is that internal sources of client problems may be minimized or missed. One can argue that many problems have a clear biological basis (e.g., ADHD, schizophrenia, OCD). Most feminist counselors agree that underlying physical and biological factors must be identified and treated. But they also argue that even these problems occur in a cultural context. These cultural contexts define mental health and influence how a culture reacts to individuals with a particular problem. Further, the problems in living with biologically based phenomena are often created by cultures. Physical disabilities are an excellent example of this latter phenomenon. A person who is having difficulty adjusting to the loss of physical mobility following an auto accident may be viewed as primarily having a biologically based problem (i.e., a spinal cord injury). Feminist counselors would view the problem primarily as a societal-based one, occurring because our society does not provide adequate services to people with disabilities, constructs physical building structures that create barriers to wheelchairs, and discriminates against and stereotypes individuals who are not "able bodied."

Evaluation of Feminist Therapy

Although feminist therapists have created treatments for a variety of client issues and client populations, they have often not researched the effectiveness of these treatments. To a large degree, most of the paradigms used for determining the efficacy of psychotherapies are incompatible with feminist principles and perspectives. Worell (2001) delineated five levels of feminist interventions—prevention, education, remediation, empowerment, and community change—and she identified several problems associated with evaluating the outcome of feminist psychological practice. Most counseling interventions involve remediation, so only one level or aspect of feminist psychological practice is relevant.

Further, the mainstream view of reducing symptoms conflicts with the main constructs of feminist approaches that focus on empowerment, resiliency, coping strategies, and social change. That is, even with respect to the remediation level of practice, feminist approaches need entirely different outcome targets and measures that focus on well-being and thriving in oppressive environments. Additional feminist-appropriate outcomes include expansion of individuals' role repertoires, reduced self-blame, heightened awareness of harmful social contexts including privilege and oppression, and increased self-trust. Because feminists advocate for social change, appropriate outcomes for social change and prevention levels could include reduction in negative life events (e.g., reduction in sexual assault rates), change in individuals' discriminatory attitudes and change in societal structures (e.g., more women and subordinate group members in leadership positions).

Another challenge to doing traditional empirical outcome research is that many feminist counselors combine feminist theory and interventions with other theoretical orientations. Thus, questions arise about whether to evaluate the outcomes of feminist practice solely or in combination with other approaches. Yet another challenge to evaluating feminist practice outcomes is that even when feminist tenets are used to construct treatment interventions and the outcomes of the treatment are assessed, these treatments are not always clearly labeled "feminist." Thus, these programs are not counted as feminist interventions in reviews of the research literature (Remer & Rostosky, 2001).

Despite these challenges, some feminist treatment outcome studies have been conducted. For instance, Cook (1999) created a feminist Gestalt-based group treatment for adolescent girls who had elevated depression and anxiety scores. Treatment participants had significantly higher self-esteem scores and significantly lower depression and anxiety scores than wait-list control participants at posttest. D'Haene (1995) investigated the effectiveness of a cultural feminist-based group intervention designed to individually and collectively empower adolescent girls. A feminist–process driven qualitative research approach was used to evaluate outcomes. The qualitative analyses lent support to the effectiveness of this feminist approach to increasing empowerment in adolescent girls. Westbury and Tutty (1998) researched the effectiveness of a body-focused feminist treatment for women who had been sexually abused as children. Compared to wait-list control participants, treatment group participants were significantly less depressed and anxious at posttest.

On the prevention level, several researchers have investigated the efficacy of feminist-based date rape prevention programs. Medley (2000) designed and evaluated the effectiveness of a feminist-cognitive date rape prevention program for university undergraduate students. Treatment group participants were significantly less accepting of rape myths at posttest than were wait-list control participants. Members of a Counseling Psychology Date Rape Prevention Team

(Remer et al., 2004) created an interactive date rape prevention program based on empowerment feminist therapy for university resident advisors. On posttests, participants were significantly less accepting of rape myths and had significantly fewer misperceptions about sexual interest in target behaviors than on pretest.

Worell (2001) proposed a series of unique approaches to address the challenges to feminist treatment outcome research described earlier in this section. She and her colleagues developed the Therapy with Women scale (TWS), (Robinson & Worell, 1991) to measure whether therapists used feminist techniques and the Client Therapy with Women Scale (CTWS) (Worell, Chandler, Robinson, & Blount, 1996) to measure clients' perceptions about their therapists' use of feminist interventions. Worell and Chandler (1999) also developed the Personal Power Scale (PPS) to measure feminist empowerment outcomes. Across several studies using these instruments, common feminist therapy interventions were identified and validated. Specifically, clients perceived that their feminist therapists used these feminist interventions, and clients of feminist therapists were found to have high empowerment scores at therapy termination (Chandler, Worell, Johnson, Blount, & Lusk, 1999).

Feminist clinicians and researchers have begun to lay a good foundation for researching the efficacy of feminist interventions. This foundation includes both treatment outcome research, which follows paradigms being used to investigate the efficacy of other therapeutic modalities (e.g., demonstrating reduction in client symptoms), and research that challenges these existing paradigms (e.g., Worell, 2001). Evaluating the outcomes of feminist models and interventions remains a major challenge for feminist practitioners. In doing this research, we must challenge existing paradigms that are symptom driven. Using feminist principles, we also must develop more treatment models for a variety of client issues and for diverse client groups, label these treatments as "feminist," and research their effectiveness.

Feminist Therapy: Blind Spots, Limitations, and Challenges

While EFT and feminist counseling approaches in general have many strengths, especially for counseling people from oppressed groups, they also have blind spots, limitations, and challenges. In the next section, these blind spots, limitations, and challenges will be described. Because many were discussed in detail earlier, they are only briefly summarized here.

Blind Spots and Limitations

Feminist counseling approaches have at least five blind spots or limitations: focus on subordinate, oppressed groups; challenging of societal values; deemphasis of internal sources of clients' issues; emphasis on the role of cultural contexts; and changing societal structures to address individual problems.

Feminist counseling approaches were developed for individuals from subordinate, oppressed groups. Feminists have not given much attention to applying feminist perspectives and interventions to counseling people from privileged groups. Further, given that most clients have intersecting social identities that are a mix of privileged and oppressed statuses, complete exploration of clients' social identities requires addressing privileged positions.

A second blind spot/limitation is a result of feminist therapies' challenging of societal values and structures that subordinate certain groups. Feminist practitioners walk a fine line between honoring diverse cultural perspectives and challenging them. If feminist counselors fail to fully understand the cultural values of clients from diverse cultural groups, they run the risk of imposing their own values and minimizing the potential negative effects on clients of challenging social rules and norms.

A third blind spot or limitation emerges from feminist counseling approaches' deemphasis on the internal sources of clients' issues. While feminist approaches do have important safeguards for critiquing traditional intrapsychic diagnostic conceptualizations, feminist interventions for treating biologically based mental health problems (e.g., schizophrenia, autism) are very limited. However, it is important to remember that all diagnostic categories are influenced by the cultures in which they exist. Feminist counselors have made major contributions to our understanding of these cultural contexts and their influence on what is diagnosed, in whom it is diagnosed, and on how diagnosed individuals will be treated.

Feminist counseling approaches in general, and EFT specifically, emphasize the role of the cultural context in creating many of the problems clients bring to counseling. A potential blind spot of this emphasis is overlooking or minimizing individuals' contributions to their problems. This lack of emphasis on the internal aspects of problems can lead to clients' failing to take responsibility for making needed changes in themselves.

A fifth blind spot or limitation of feminist counseling is that changing detrimental societal institutions and socialization processes is often time consuming. Further, while these social changes are necessary and are good prevention interventions, they may not result in direct or timely change for individuals in distress.

Challenges

Given these blind spots and limitations, feminist practitioners face at least five challenges: integration of diverse perspectives, creating counseling interventions for working with individuals from privileged groups, mainstreaming of feminist psychological perspectives, researching the effectiveness of feminist interventions, and ending all types of societal oppression.

Over the last 15 years or so, feminist practitioners have been giving more attention to integrating diverse cultural perspectives into their theories and interventions. However, the integration of feminist and diversity perspectives remains an ongoing challenge that cannot be neglected.

Although a case has been made in this chapter for how feminist therapy does apply to dominant group members, more attention needs to be given to detailing this application. Thus, a second challenge for feminist practitioners is to expand feminist theoretical constructs and interventions to addressing privileged clients and issues that emerge from privilege.

A third challenge for feminist counselors is to mainstream feminist psychological perspectives and theory. Feminist approaches have a lot to offer related to counseling a range of diverse clients, and thus we can no longer be content to be dissenting or contrasting voices on the fringe of psychological therapies. Inclusions of feminist chapters in books on theories of counseling (such as this text) suggest that progress on this challenge is already being made.

Fourth, research on the effectiveness of feminist counseling approaches and interventions is sorely needed. In meeting this challenge, we will also have to expand and confront psychology's existing paradigms for validating clinical interventions. For example, therapeutic change cannot focus solely on symptom reduction and intrapsychic change. All theories should be challenged to address toxic societal conditions.

Finally, ending all types of societal oppression remains the most daunting challenge for feminist practitioners. Although this challenge is central to feminist psychological approaches, it must be addressed by all mental health counselors.

Future Development: Feminist Therapy in a Diverse World

Feminist approaches to counseling were originally developed to address women's issues and their subordinate, oppressed status in U.S. society. More recently, feminist approaches have incorporated a more inclusive focus on all diverse and oppressed groups including people of Color; lesbian, gay, and bisexual people; people living in poverty; and people with a variety of disabilities.

Our priorities for the future include continuing our effort to incorporate diversity guidelines such as the American Psychological Association's Guidelines for Psychotherapy with Lesbian, Gay, and Bisexual Clients (2000) and Guidelines on Multicultural Education, Training, Research, Practice, and Organizational Change for Psychologists (2002) and continuing to expand feminist theory and practice to more effectively counsel privileged clients.

Summary

1. In contemporary American society, multiple forms of oppression (e.g., sexism, racism, ethnocentrism, classism, heterosexism, ableism, ageism) restrict the potential and full participation of subordinate group members. Thus, from a feminist and diversity perspective, the institutionalization of oppression and privilege, discrimination, cultural values, and cultural socialization processes that constitute individuals' sociocultural contexts must be understood and often challenged in order to effectively counsel a diverse range of clients.

2. The intrapsychic focus of traditional psychotherapies ignores clients' sociocultural contexts and disregards the impact of societal oppression on subordinate, disadvantaged individuals. Therefore, effective counseling of individuals from disadvantaged or oppressed groups requires interactionist methods that attend to external, social sources of pathology and to the ways those toxic sociocultural elements are internalized.

3. Feminist therapy grew out of the U.S. women's movement of the 1960s and 1970s. Traditional therapeutic models were criticized for being androcentric (based on male values and norms) and ethnocentric (based on one cultural perspective and set of values). Feminists asserted that social change was necessary to alleviate women's distress.

4. A detailed history of the development of feminist therapy is difficult to track because feminist counseling approaches are rooted in a variety of feminist philosophies, no single feminist therapy theoretician can be credited for developing the approach, feminist counseling approaches emerged out of and intertwined with a variety of grassroots women's movements, and feminist therapies are relatively recent phenomena.

5. Four examples of feminist counseling approaches are liberal (which focuses on the harmful effect of traditional gender-role socializations constricting the development of both men and women), radical (which concentrates on the sexist, heterosexist, racist, classist, ableist, and ageist patriarchal social structures that harm women), cultural (which emphasizes how women's traits, experiences, values, and abilities are not valued as highly as men's and

deemphasizes gender-role socializations by viewing women and men as being biologically different), and women of Color (emphasizes the impact of all oppressions, especially racism, ethnocentrism, and classism, on diverse women's lives). The unifying foci of these approaches are the harmful effects on individuals of negative societal conditions and the need to work for social change.

6. Most early feminist counseling approaches often assumed that all women's experiences were similar to those of White, heterosexual women. Modern feminist psychologists acknowledge the importance of understanding and embracing a diversity of cultural worldviews and values representing a variety of social positions (e.g., gender, sexual orientation, ethnicity, race, class).

7. Empowerment feminist therapy (EFT) was created to integrate the unique strengths of liberal, radical, cultural, and women of Color feminist counseling approaches. The four guiding principles of EFT are (I) personal and social identities are interdependent; (II) the personal is political; (III) relationships are egalitarian; and (IV) women's perspectives are valued.

8. Principal I: Social groups are referred to as social locations, each of which occupies a seat of relative privilege/advantage or oppression/disadvantage. Individuals within social locations each have their own perceptions of social identities. To understand clients effectively, counselors must get a picture of both the clients' social locations and social identities. The primary goals of counseling related to Principle I are to help clients become more aware of all their social locations/social identities, of how these identities intersect in their lives, and of how the privileged and oppressed status of each identity impacts their lives.

9. Principle II: The personal is political principle reflects feminist counselors' beliefs that personal issues are created by social and political conditions. Pathology is moved from being located in individuals to being located in social environments. In accordance with Principle II, counselors help clients identify and separate the internal and external sources of their problems via consciousness raising, and without pushing, support work toward social change.

10. Principle III: EFT counselors build collaborative, egalitarian relationships with clients so as not to recreate the destructive, hierarchical relationship structures of society. Contrary to many traditional therapies, feminist counselors often self-disclose about their relevant life experiences in order to foster egalitarian relationships.

11. Principle IV: Qualities and values stereotypically associated with being female or with being a member of a societally subordinated group are valued and viewed as strengths by feminist counselors.

12. Feminist counselors use a variety of counseling techniques. Some of these are uniquely feminist (e.g., cultural analysis, social identities analysis, gender-role analysis, power analysis, and consciousness-raising groups) and some are adapted from other theories (e.g., self-disclosing and self-involving counselor responses, bibliotherapy, and reframing and relabeling).

13. The feminist therapy theory of change holds that changing toxic social structures will positively impact the mental health of individuals. However, because social change is complex, difficult, and slow to accomplish, feminist therapists also focus on individual change via consciousness raising.

14. Treatment outcome research is still in its infancy, in part because the efficacy of most treatments is usually measured by demonstrating reduction in client symptoms. This intrapsychic client dysfunction focus is incompatible with feminist therapy. Innovative feminist approaches that measure client strengths and resiliency have been proposed as an alternative to traditional outcome studies.

15. The blind spots and limitations of feminist therapy include its focus on subordinate, oppressed groups (thus, little attention has been paid to its potential with privileged groups), challenging of societal values (which may sometimes result in imposition of values on clients), deemphasis of internal sources of clients' issues (which may result in important internal factors being minimized or missed), emphasis on the role of cultural contexts (which may result in missing clients' own contributions to their problems), and changing societal structures to address individual problems (which is time consuming and may not immediately address individuals' problems as needed).

16. The challenges facing feminist therapy are integrating diverse perspectives, creating counseling interventions to fit clients from priviledged groups, mainstreaming feminist psychological perspectives, resourcing the effectiveness of feminist interventions, and ending societal oppression.

Key Terms

androcentric (p. 398)
androgyny (p. 406)
consciousness raising (p. 399)
empowerment (p. 409)
ethnocentric (p. 398)
identity development models (p. 412)
interactionist (p. 397)

intrapsychic (p. 397)
oppression (p. 408)
patriarchal (p. 402)
power (p. 422)
privilege (p. 423)
sexism (p. 399)
social identities (p. 410)
social locations (p. 410)

Resources for Further Study

Professional Organizations

American Psychological Association, Division 35, Society for the Psychology of Women
Website: www.apa.org/divison/div35

American Psychological Association, Division 51: Society for the Psychological Study of Men and Masculinity
Website: www.apa.org/divisions/div51

Professional Journals

Psychology of Women Quarterly
Subscriptions available from www.blackwellpublishing.com/journal

A publication of APA Division 35.

Psychology of Men and Masculinity
Subscriptions available from: www.apa.org/journals/men

A quarterly publication of APA Division 51.

Sex Roles: A Journal of Research
Subscriptions available from www.ovid.com/site/catalog/journal

An interdisciplinary, behavioral science journal with a feminist perspective.

Suggested Readings

American Psychological Association. (2002). *Guidelines on multicultural education, training, research, practice, and organizational change for psychologists.* Retrieved June 2005 from www.apa.org.

Guidelines for psychological practice with racial and ethnic minority individuals, including suggestions for knowledge, attitudes, and skills needed for effective multicultural psychological practice.

Enns, C. Z. (1997). *Feminist theories and feminist psychotherapies: Origins, themes, and variations.* Binghamton, NY: Harrington Park Press.

Carolyn Enns defines a variety of feminist philosophical perspectives and how they are reflected in major feminist therapy approaches.

Goodman, D. J. (2001). *Promoting diversity and social justice: Educating people from privileged groups.* Thousand Oaks, CA: Sage.

Diane Goodman defines social justice and outlines how to do social justice training with members of privileged social locations so that they can be allies for oppressed groups in working for social change.

Goodman, L. A., Liang, B., Helms, J. E., Latta, R. E., Sparks, E., & Weintraub, S. R. (2004). Training counseling psychologists as social justice agents: Feminist and multicultural principles in action. *The Counseling Psychologist, 32,* 793–837.

The issues involved in training counseling psychologists to accomplish social change in communities, focusing on a social justice–oriented counseling psychology program at Boston College.

Worell, J., & Johnson, N. G. (1997). *Shaping the future of feminist psychology: Education, research, and practice.* Washington, DC: American Psychological Association.

Summaries of the working groups from the First National Conference on Education and Training in Feminist Psychological Practice, reflecting the commonalities and the challenges faced by feminist practitioners in integrating more effectively perspectives of women from diverse social locations.

Worell, J., & Remer, P. (2003). *Feminist perspectives in therapy: Empowering diverse women.* Hoboken, NJ: Wiley.

EFT and its structural integration of diversity perspectives, applied in depth to four common counseling issues for women—depression, wife battering, rape, and career choice—plus integration with other therapeutic orientations, feminist ethical practice, and training issues.

Other Media Resources

American Psychological Association. (1994). *APA psychotherapy series: Feminist therapy* [Video]. Washington DC: American Psychological Association.

Walker, L. (1994). *The abused woman: A survivor therapy approach* [Video]. New York: Newbridge Communications.

Chapter 12

Family Therapy

SANDRA A. RIGAZIO-DIGILIO AND TERESA MCDOWELL

Family therapy has enjoyed great popularity since its introduction in the middle of the last century and has proved to be effective for a wide range of psychological and relational disorders. Because of its effectiveness, many counselors and therapists develop skills in both individual and family modalities. You have most likely already read the chapters in this book on the traditional models of individual therapy. In this chapter, we discuss the traditional models of family therapy that have their origins in each of three classic orientations: the psychoanalytic, cognitive-behavioral, and existential-humanistic approaches. We then look at the contemporary postmodern, ecological, and integrative approaches that have emerged as part of the increasing awareness, across mental health professions, that the nature of human and systemic differences and of changing contexts requires multiple theoretical perspectives and approaches so practitioners can provide effective counseling and therapy in the modern world of diversity.

Origins and Evolution of Family Therapy

Family therapy emerged as a distinctive mode of treatment in the mid-20th century. It began as an alternative to traditional individually oriented treatments and included all members of the family in the same treatment room working with one clinician. In the 1950s, John Bowlby began seeing whole families for treatment at the Tavistock Clinic in England. During that same time, Vojin Matic, a psychoanalyst in Yugoslavia, was including families in the child treatment process (Kaslow, 2000). In the United States, John Bell of Worcester, Massachusetts, was one of the first therapists to begin seeing intact families. Mary Richmond wrote about the importance of treating the family as the unit as early as 1917.

The rationale for treating whole families was based on significant changes in perceptions about health and distress. Building on the ideas of Adler (1931), who believed "that psychological problems began in childhood and early intervention was the best way to prevent future occurrence of mental illness" (Green, 2003, p. 50), early practitioners and researchers began breaking with tradition and working with intact family units. In the 1930s and 1940s, Harry Stack Sullivan advanced interpersonal dynamics in psychiatry and Karen Horney addressed the significance of social and cultural factors in the development of mental disorders. Many new models of family treatment began to appear based on the general systems theory of Ludwig von Bertalanffy (1950). The groundbreaking work of anthropologist Gregory Bateson and his colleagues in the early 1950s concerning the role of communication patterns in families with schizophrenic members energized other professionals to begin seeing intact families. On the U.S. east coast, practitioners/researchers Theodore Lidz, Nathan Ackerman, Emily Mudd, Lyman Wynne, Murray Bowen, and Ivan Boszormenyi-Nagy were all charting new applications of family therapy methods. On the west coast, Virginia Satir, John Weakland, and Paul Watzlawick, to name but a few, also were treating families and theorizing about work with family clients.

Emergence of Traditional Family Therapy Models

In 1961, the influential journal *Family Process* was launched. It provided a forum for family-oriented researchers and practitioners, regardless of their professional discipline, to begin sharing findings and conceptualizations about work with families. By the mid-1970s, six approaches, each with its own charismatic leaders (denoted in parentheses), dominated the family therapy landscape: communication/validation family therapy (Virginia Satir), structural family therapy (Salvador Minuchin), intergenerational family therapy (Murray Bowen), strategic family therapy (Jay Haley), symbolic-experiential family therapy (Carl Whitaker), and MRI brief family therapy (John Weakland and Richard Fisch).

Each of these family therapy models used a systemic framework to broaden the concepts and methods associated with one of the traditional approaches to individual counseling and therapy. This shift from an individualistic to a systemic framework offered extended ways to look at health and disorder. For example, traditional approaches focused on the individual as the primary actor, while the influence of family members was relegated to noncritical background data. Conversely, the systemic perspective viewed the family as the primary unit and held that all members of the family were important contributors to clients' psychological functioning and development.

Models that originated from the psychodynamic tradition emphasize intrapsychic and intergenerational phenomena and rely heavily on Freudian concepts and theories. For example, Bowen's multigenerational model of family therapy (1960) had its roots in the psychoanalytic tradition of working with the client's past to resolve issues in the present. Cognitive-behavioral/interactional approaches, as typified by structural (Minuchin, 1974) and strategic (Haley, 1963) family therapies, focus on effective learning processes that expand organizational structures, communication, and interactional processes. Existential-humanistic approaches, such as Virginia Satir's communication/validation theory (1964) and Carl Whitaker's symbolic-experiential therapy (1967), are typical of family models that focus on understanding and expanding an individual's subjective experience. Note that then, and still today, various theory-specific models of family work have emerged, including Adlerian family therapy (Sherman & Dinkmeyer, 1987), behavioral family therapy (Jacobson, 1981), Gestalt family therapy (Kempler, 1981), object relations family therapy (Slipp, 1984), contextual family therapy (Boszormenyi-Nagy, 1987), and the Milan approach to family therapy (Selvini-Palazzoli, Boscolo, Cecchin, & Prata, 1978), to name a few. Although we think it is important for students to be aware of them, discussion of these models is beyond the scope of this chapter.

The decade from 1975 to 1985 was one of expansion and domination for the six systemic approaches to family therapy (Beels, 2002). Research in each school coupled with further elaboration of theory and practice solidified the influence these models had on the field. While there was some attempt to integrate strategies and conceptualizations across these schools (e.g., Lebow, 1987; Stanton, 1981), the power of the original schools did not change, and these integrative attempts, while foreshadowing advances to come, received little attention.

Emergence of Contemporary Family Therapy Models and Approaches

Beginning in the early 1980s, the basic assumptions and strategies associated with the original models underwent a series of reevaluations generated by trends in the social sciences in general, and in the field of family therapy in particular. We will consider four of the trends that led to the development of contemporary family therapy models and approaches: feminism, multiculturalism, social constructionism, and evidence-based practice.

First, the feminist branch of the field, led by Goldner, Hare-Mustin, Luepnitz, Ault-Riche, James, Avis, Walters, Carter, Papp, and Silverstein, accused the proponents of the predominant forms of family therapy of minimizing the role of gender, power, and privilege. This group strongly objected to the idea that males and females are equally to blame for spousal violence. Further,

Hare-Mustin (1978) noted that the stereotypical way therapists relate to their clients reinforces paternalistic patterns of control and disempowerment. "Moreover, they reminded the field that, perhaps unlike in the nonhuman sciences, the act of theorizing and 'therapizing' occurs within a moral context, and that our choice of a theoretical explanation must be determined both by careful observation as well as by moral sensibilities and implications" (Gurman & Fraenkel, 2002). In other words, the way family therapy was conducted was just as important as the results.

Following feminist critiques, multiculturalists (Boyd-Franklin, 1989a; Carter & McGoldrick, 1988; Falicov, 1988; Ibrahim, 1991; Pinderhughes, 1989) helped the field take a broader look at the social and cultural influences experienced by clients and therapists. No longer was it acceptable to assume that a therapist enters the family free of cultural baggage. Therapist and client systems are part of wider cultural and social groups that have norms governing both public and private interaction. Multiculturalists charged that these sociocultural influences must be accounted for in treatment. Further, the act of treating a family also reflects social, cultural, and political values of the organizations sponsoring the treatment. Church-related programs, freestanding community clinics, private practice groups, hospital settings, and university programs all reflect different values about the nature of service and those served. Multiculturalists stressed that the deeper, culturally embedded aspects of the therapeutic relationship must also be acknowledged (e.g., Aponte, 1987; Locke, 1998) and that the wider social and cultural groups with which the family identifies need to be considered in the diagnosis, treatment, and outcome evaluation of family work (Imber-Black, 1988; Walsh, 1998).

In the mid-1980s family therapy was critiqued through the lens of post-modernism, a perspective which had been gaining substantial momentum in the field of philosophy, sociology, and psychology for more than 30 years. At first, questions about the philosophical and conceptual foundations of the dominant forms of family therapy were posed. These questions asked where and how predominant ideas originated, but also addressed in general the nature of knowing. Up to that point, social science—including family therapy—had been dominated by modern scientific notions that a single reality existed and laws governing human behavior could be discovered, measured, and predicted. Now the argument about whether or not a tangible hard reality exists, independent of the knower, came to center stage. The postmodern view acknowledges the *social constructions* humans use to order and influence their world. This argument caused family therapists to reexamine their beliefs regarding one "ideal" **family structure** and to consider multiple images of productive family life.

The three preceding trends can be viewed within the broader umbrella of the postmodern revolution. At the same time, a practical demand was being made of all areas of psychotherapy, including family therapy: the requirement to comply with managed health care expectations to provide evidence-based treatment. This focus on treatment efficacy and client outcomes dictated that family therapy be applied in consistent treatment protocols to promote continuity across providers. The value of evidence-supported models is that they create a certain standard of care for all families seeking treatment for a particular issue. The downside of these models is that they may be viewed as more artificial and removed from the family's lived experience and the therapist's professional judgment and could have serious consequences for the survival of family therapy as a unique discipline within the mental health field.

These four trends were influential in moving the field toward contemporary models of family therapy that can be classified within three broad approaches: postmodern, ecological, and integrative. Postmodern approaches (e.g., Anderson, 1995; Anderson & Goolishian, 1988; McNamee & Gergen, 2000; Neimeyer & Neimeyer, 1994) reflect a rejection of assessment practices that pathologize clients and treatment practices intended to change dysfunction assumed to reside within individuals. These models advance multidimensional, nonpathological, and contextual practices that provide ways to understand client differences in context and to directly influence the variety of individual, relational, social, and cultural factors that contribute to how disorder is defined and managed by mental health professionals. Ecological approaches (e.g., Becvar & Becvar, 1994; Imber-Black, 1988) provide frameworks that make it possible for clinicians to address the primary elements of a client's wider ecology (i.e., her or his immediate and extended family, associates, and wider historical, sociocultural, and political contexts). These models offer guidelines for weighing the importance of individual, family, and wider contextual variables when assessing and treating each client or client system. Integrative approaches (e.g., Anderson & Bagarozzi, 1983; Breunlin, Schwartz, & MacKune-Karrer, 1992; Pinsof, 1994; Rigazio-DiGilio, 2000) offer frameworks to help clinicians organize theories, therapies, and strategies into broader models of practice. Practitioners are introduced to different models and can select strategies and techniques to expand their clinical repertory so that they can better tailor their interventions to the unique needs of each client.

Context Then—Context Now

Traditional family therapy developed in the post–World War II context of large-scale social and cultural changes that increased the need for treating families, not just individuals. A key change was improved transportation systems, which made it possible for corporations to open plants and factories anywhere in the United States. This required a mobile family unit to follow the wage earner's job. If a textile plant closed down in one state and opened up in another and the workers wanted to maintain their jobs, these employees and their dependents would have to move. This uprooting of certain family members from within a network of **extended family** placed in high relief the significance of the **nuclear family.** Owning a house in the suburbs, replete with supermarkets and shopping malls and far from cities and relatives, became the goal of American newlyweds. Television reflected this trend of glorifying the nuclear family. Popular shows both standardized the two-parents/two-children nuclear family and turned infrequent visits with grandparents and other relatives into a comedic theme. In the real world, however, the stresses on those forming isolated nuclear families and those left behind became more and more evident.

Contemporary family therapy models and approaches developed in the context of instantaneous worldwide communication, technological advances, and the infusion of racially, culturally, and ethnically diverse individuals, partners, and families, all of which impacted even our most remote communities during the last 30 years of the 20th century. At work, we were confronted with the issue of managing a diverse labor force. In education, the tensions and opportunities created by shifts in demographics prompted teachers and professors to search for curricula that were both accurate in subject matter and multiculturally sensitive. Even at home, media news became increasingly international as world leaders attempted to define a new world order. As a result, mental health professionals became increasingly aware of the need to be equipped to work with diverse individuals, families, and larger cultural groups within an intercultural context because they would be centrally responsible for attending to emotional, human, and systemic reactions to cultural integration and differentiation (Rigazio-DiGilio & Ivey, 1995).

The Authors' Journeys as Family Therapists

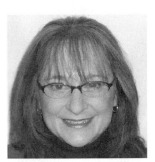

Sandra Rigazio-DiGilio

Sandra Rigazio-DiGilio

I am a second-generation Italian American. My family, community, and cultural heritage taught me the importance of being a boundary spanner. The front yard of my childhood home was situated within a developing Italian neighborhood. The back yard opened to a thriving Irish community. Over the years, my parents played a significant role in bringing together these two fractious groups. From the many stories of their union and from my childhood experiences, I learned about the differences in attitudes

(*continued*)

and beliefs that can exist within one's own family, culture, and community, and I learned ways to enter and respect the culture of others while not relinquishing my own.

In 1977, with a master's degree in rehabilitation counseling in hand, I became a child protective service worker in a city with a large Latino population, and a large deinstitutionalized "chronically ill" population that had no adequate housing or outpatient services. As was true across our nation, the decentralization of promised federal funding left this city without the resources necessary to manage either situation. I vividly recall one telling incident. After testifying with colleagues that state-funded residential care must continue for an 11-year-old boy who was verbalizing homicidal thoughts toward his mother, the judge, identifying us as "well-meaning but ill-informed social workers," terminated the services. Shortly thereafter, the mother died by her son's hand.

My husband and I were in the midst of training at the Bristol Hospital Post Degree Program, which trained professionals from various mental health disciplines in the specialty of marriage and family therapy (MFT). MFT training at that time was theoretically specific and had a competitive culture, each program vying for disciples and funding. To survive, each program staked out its theoretical territory at the expense of broader formulations. Finding the way out of this state of affairs was a bit difficult, because noticing commonalities across models was perceived as being disloyal to one's program.

For me, the idea of breaking loyalties was akin to breaking family rules, and quite a difficult transition, given my Italian heritage. My move toward integration did not emerge from the profession's knowledge or from mentors but rather from my practice as an inpatient and outpatient clinician at Bristol Hospital. In that real world setting, I found my services of little value to many who came to me for help; what I knew from my training was not sufficient. At the same time, my life experiences in the wider community began to speak to me of the limits of our therapy models, which were not just limiting but actually exclusionary and biased.

In my doctoral work at the University of Massachusetts, I began my professional collaboration with Dr. Allen Ivey, a longtime mentor, colleague, and friend. My work with him broadened my vision. At his "table," I was invited to sit among multidisciplinary professionals, joined together for a common purpose. I became active in publications and presentations geared toward varying disciplines and speaking with a common voice. Since joining the faculty at the University of Connecticut in 1990, my scholarship agenda has focused on advancing integrative and alternative models of family therapy. Throughout this time, my private practice work has enriched my cross-cultural education. I regularly receive referrals to work with children and families in the inner-city

Jamaican community. Also growing is my work with children and families living through the dying process—and I have helped develop a community of professionals and families facing this very intimate and unique experience.

At this time in my journey, I am most drawn to moments of interdisciplinary collaboration. Given my background and experience, this just seems logical to me. And this is part of what you will gain from this book. The idea is to learn from each of the authors, knowing each frame of reference is part of a broader whole—a wider territory that you must navigate in your career.

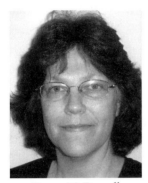

Teresa McDowell

Teresa McDowell

I grew up in the culturally diverse region of the southwest United States. I was the third of four children in a robust, intense household filled with conflict, chaos, joy, warmth, and deep connection. We were part of a group of privileged European-American families who played central roles in our town economy and politics. Inside the family, however, we played out daily struggles of class differences and gender oppression. I still vividly recall how the complete tone of the family shifted when my father came home. We went from relaxed and playful to being quiet and paying close attention to making sure everything was in the order my father preferred. My father clearly protected and cared for us, but he existed in a class above that of my mother and all of us children. Even more obvious were the gender discrepancies, having their roots in my parents' backgrounds. My father's parents were English/Swedish farmers who lost their place in the world via the Great Depression. My mother's were well-educated English/Irish Southerners who became dispersed through alcoholism and chronic illness. These differences were demonstrated through my father's focus on pragmatism and learning the value of hard work while my mother focused on our learning language skills and music. My father's work ethic, although a positive force in our lives, was enforced through his absolute and, at times, abusive authority. My mother's aesthetic ethic was transmitted through her unwaveringly gentle spirit and creativity as a caregiver and musician. Thus I grew to adulthood benefiting from my family's privileged location in the broader society while experiencing gender oppression and other misuses of power inside my family. Both influences have significantly shaped my work as a family therapist.

I entered a master's program in marriage and family therapy in the early 1980s. I was trained primarily in brief therapy models. These approaches were a

(*continued*)

great fit for me. Systems theory helped me make sense of the world in a whole new way because it allowed me to put together the many pieces of family life I had experienced. For example, I began to see how my mother's relaxed nature and passive resistance to my father's authority further prompted his attempts to control her, which in turn increased my mother's resistance. Brief, strategic models came naturally, tapping into both the playful and pragmatic themes in my family of origin. During this period of development in the field, feminist critiques were on the horizon but had not impacted upon mainstream family therapy. Culture was treated as an "add-on" and considered primarily through readings about groups that were outside the European-American, middle-class norm. Diversity was offered as something to "celebrate" without critical analysis of power, privilege, and oppression. Likewise, spirituality and religion were to be kept out of the secular therapy room.

I have been deeply influenced by the work of popular educators (e.g., Paulo Freire, 1970) and social activists (e.g., Phyllis Cunningham, 2000), who have shaped my work on racial equity and cultural democracy in family therapy (e.g., McDowell, 2004; McDowell, Fang, Brownlee, Gomez Young, & Khanna, 2002; McDowell et al., 2003; McDowell & Jeris, 2004). I have been personally and professionally challenged to inspect the influences of my social identities and my White, middle-class, heterosexual privilege and to learn fundamentals of multicultural work that were not in my original training.

Family Therapy: Basic Assumptions

All family therapists view families as systems and take the following into consideration in their case conceptualizations: family development, family structure, family culture, and family functioning.

Families as Systems

In order to understand family interactions, it is important for family practitioners to know key concepts associated with family systems thinking. These concepts are based on systems theory developed in the field of biology and emphasized in the work of Ludwig von Bertalanffy (1968). Here are some of the basic tenets of general systems theory.

1. *The whole of a system is greater than the sum of its parts.* The family is not just a group of individuals. The family system has a collective identity that is different from the individual identities held by each of its members.

For example, you may know a family that appears to be very outgoing, yet some members may not fit into that collective identity.

2. *Individual parts within a system relate to one another in some consistent fashion.* Within families are smaller units of relationships. For example, there are individual members, parent units, parent-child units, and sibling units. How members come together to form smaller units, and what opportunities they have to influence the family as a whole, evolve over time. For example, the degree of autonomy parents foster in their young children will be evident in the family interactions when those children are adolescents.

3. *A system is structured by the relationships among its parts.* How members of the family form relationships within the family contributes to how families function. Sometimes the relationships are clear and working for all members. At other times the relationships are not clear, and confusion arises. For example, consider how relationships in a family might be upended when the primary caregiver becomes ill and all other members need to decide how to fill in that role.

4. ***Boundaries*** *among a system's parts and between the system and the external environment regulate the flow of information among parts of the system and between the system and the external environment.* Families are open systems that receive information from both individual members and units within themselves and from wider systems outside themselves such as schools and media. Families create boundaries to mediate their relationships with each of their members and with significant community and cultural groups.

5. *Systems tend to be self-regulating and exhibit both stability and the capacity to change.* Families work to balance the need to change and adapt to new demands and the need to maintain stability for their members. Families find unique ways to balance these needs for change and consistency. Sometimes families are unable to reach a balance and enter into a state of disequilibrium. It is during this time that relationships may be renegotiated and structures may be altered. In general, families maintain this balance by modifying the rules and relationships as their members grow and change over time.

6. ***Feedback loops*** *help maintain the structure of the system.* Negative feedback limits change and helps to maintain equilibrium. Positive feedback encourages change. Family systems theory requires counselors to be aware of the cycles of interaction that happen between and among the members of the family. In counseling, it is not unusual that parents will complain that one child is a problem while another child is viewed as perfect. The reality is that the positive and negative feedback loops operating within the family have been established to perpetuate the image of the "good" child and the "bad" child. Family therapists work to redirect and rebalance the negative and positive feedbacks loops within the family to provide space for all individuals to grow and develop.

7. *Changes in one part of a system impact all other parts of the system.* Because of the intricate network of feedback loops within a family, any change in one part of the family system will affect all other members. If a child is diagnosed with a life-shortening illness, all members of the family are affected. If a grandparent comes to live with a family, again all members are affected. As children naturally progress from childhood to adolescence to young adulthood, the internal relationships are altered and new arrangements are required for all members of the family. When events affect the wider community, such as natural disasters, economic changes, and environmental catastrophes, families will be affected and this, in turn, will cause the internal familial relationships to be disrupted, thereby causing change for all members of the family, whether they were directly involved with the precipitating event or not.

Family Development

In counseling families, therapists need to know what is going on in the family members' lives from a developmental perspective. Consider, for example the Elder family, who entered treatment because of the increasingly defiant behaviors of their 18-year-old son, Matthew. Although from a developmental perspective it is important to recognize that Matt may be dealing with issues of identity and intimacy, it is equally important to know what developmental issues each family member and subgroup, as well as the family system as a whole, is facing. In this case, the mother had recently remarried, and she and her second husband were working towards building a new sense of family that included Matt and his 5-year-old stepsister, Juliana. Such *bonding* experiences were in fact counter to Matt's goal of leaving home. This example indicates the need to understand the presenting problem in the context of family development. Family therapists use developmental models to help them understand individual development as well as the changes in the configuration of families as a whole as they move through the life cycle.

When the first models of family development were developed, family scientists assumed that families moved through predictable stages of development and reached increasing levels of differentiation, organizational complexity, and hierarchical integration over time. As a result, family life cycle theories put forward by Duvall (1977), Hill and Rodgers (1964), Barnhill and Longo (1978), Haley (1973), and others came to rely on stage-specific formulations that centered on the changing constellation of family groups over time—usually following a couple through a traditional pattern of marriage, childbearing, childrearing, child launching, and later life.

Table 12.1 Family Developmental Stages and Tasks

Developmental Stage	Illustrative Developmental Tasks
Young adults	Developing financial, functional, and psychological independence
New couple	Being committed to new partnerships and system formation
Childbirth and childrearing	Accepting into the system new dependents who require guidance and nurturance
Middle marriage	Opening boundaries and increasing role responsibilities to include children's independence and grandparents' frailties
Leaving home	Accepting multiple avenues of entry to and exit from the family system
Families in later life	Accepting the shifting of generational roles

Adapted from Carter, B., & McGoldrick, M. (1988). *The changing family life-cycle.* Boston: Allyn & Bacon. Adapted with permission.

Today's mainstream models still tend to rely on stage-specific formulations and offer different ways to understand how each member's developmental stages influence how members interact with one another and the overall tasks that families need to address (see Table 12.1).

These models provide an explanatory context for the tasks families must master and stress the value of knowing key developmental tasks and life stages of the family, a special group of people comprising individuals who are experiencing their own individual and collective challenges in life. However, while these frameworks suggest key points in the family life cycle that may promote treatment, practioners of contemporary approaches are careful to use a cultural and contextual lens when using these theories to understand the families they work with. The reason is that most of the mainstream models were built on traditional, North American/European frames of reference and during a time when cultural diversity and alternative family forms were considered more as background data (Lewis, Lewis, Daniels, & D'Andrea, 2002; McGoldrick, 2002). The idea is for counselors to use general knowledge of developmental stages and tasks, as well as nonnormative circumstances (e.g., the death of a young child), as a backdrop with which to *begin* rather than conclude a clinical inquiry and treatment.

Family Structure

Family structure is a very fluid concept and can apply to a wide variety of constellations of individuals as long as they identify themselves as a family. There are legal definitions of family membership, but there are also social definitions that go beyond civil statutes. For example, an uncle who lives in a child's home may be as influential as the child's parents. The rigid focus on the nuclear family, prevalent in the early days of family therapy, has loosened to include a wide variety of family types and structures in order to meet the shifting configurations found in real families, such as blended families, adoptive families, families including gay/lesbian parents, extended families, and single-parent families.

Family Culture

Family culture has two meanings. First, we can look inward at the way the family thinks, feels, and behaves. The rituals, beliefs, values, and customs it develops can be traced to larger groups that have significantly influenced one or more family members. Sometimes the adults establish the family customs, and sometimes the children inspire new ways of behaving based on their interaction with others outside the family. The second meaning of family culture pertains to the ethnic, social, political, religious, educational, and professional communities with which the family identifies. Mental health professionals must be competent in understanding and using the family's internal culture, as well as the external cultural resources, to promote family development and growth.

The thoughts, feelings, and actions of family members are often beyond our vision. Even when they are visible, the reasons behind them are not always evident. Beliefs are the rules and regulations imposed on the family. Sometimes these are self-imposed; sometimes they come from influential elements of the wider community. Many times these beliefs are not shared openly among family members, and each "believes" he or she knows what's going on. The same point can be made about the therapist's relationship with the family. Sometimes the therapist holds tacit beliefs about why the family is doing what it's doing and does not share these with the family. The existence of different views and beliefs about what is happening and why, needs to be understood and, in many cases, discussed across various levels of the therapeutic alliance.

One way to pass on family culture and beliefs is through rituals and traditions. Rituals and traditions provide continuity for families. Members know what's expected, how to act, and what is valued. Often meaning is attached through special foods, clothing, activities, music, and humor. Rituals help the family feel connected to other groups and reinforce its sense of active membership. Sometimes the family's rituals and traditions can impede healthy development; at other times these activities intensify the positive aspect of family life. A major focus for family practitioners is to help the family evolve rituals and traditions that will support its growth and development. Rituals go beyond the celebrations and festivals; they include the everyday rituals families go through. For example, there are family rituals about how emotions are to be expressed. These rituals often reflect cultural expectations and mores. For example, while many people in Italian and Jewish families may use emotional expressiveness to share their sense of suffering, those from Scandinavian, Asian, and Native American backgrounds may tend to withdraw into themselves, not discussing their feelings with others, or letting their feelings be known only indirectly.

Family Functioning

The primary function of families is to provide stability for their members while at the same time providing support to manage new life situations. According to Anderson and Sabatelli (1999), five characteristics of family systems positively influence this central function. Their research indicates that families function most effectively when members (1) have common purposes and tasks, (2) share a sense of family history, (3) experience emotional bonding with one another, (4) devise strategies for meeting the needs of individuals and the collective, and (5) maintain firm yet flexible boundaries within and between family subsystems. A key concept within this framework is that families need to recognize the interdependence of their members and strive to provide support for individual as well as family growth. Remember, the family unit is the culture bearer, and as such, the concepts of healthy family functioning vary widely among cultures and family types.

When power differentials exist between the family and the wider community, the nature of family functioning is altered. Issues of social and economic oppression negatively influence the development of individual and familial competencies. This is especially true when the environment labels a family's familiar ways of perceiving and acting as substandard or deviant (Miller, 1976). For example, consider gay couples who grapple daily with a wide variety of financial obstacles because of the lack of legal sanction for their partnerships. Family clinicians working with this specific population often provide relational therapy to help couples while also spending a portion of their time in advocacy functions aimed at broader systems change toward more egalitarian treatment of domestic partners.

Traditional Family Therapy: Theory and Practice

In this section, we highlight one model within each of the three classic traditions in order to offer examples of family therapy approaches. To help illustrate the approaches and their differences, each will be applied to the following case study. As you read this brief sketch, consider the first thoughts that come to your mind about this family. Who would you want to talk to first and why? What information would you want to gather?

Rita Olsen was a 15-year-old girl who had stayed away from home for several days without parental permission. On that occasion, her father, Oscar, called the police and reported Rita as a runaway. According to Ina, Rita's mother, there were "no problems" for several months after this incident. Then Rita left home again without parental permission—this time while Oscar was working away from home. Ina did not report Rita as a runaway but got into a verbal altercation with her when Rita finally returned home. Rita's 12-year-old sister, Diana, became frightened and called the police. After these incidents, the Olsens sought the help of a family therapist. The therapist learned that Oscar's extended family was of primarily Scandinavian decent. They had lived and worked for five generations as fishermen and oyster farmers in the same community, a small town on the Northwest coast. Ina emigrated to the United States from Sweden when she was 19. She left all of her family in Sweden and had limited contact with them. Although she and Oscar had been married for 16 years, Ina felt isolated and somewhat marginalized in the Olsen family's community because of her "foreign" status and accent. Oscar owned a commercial fishing boat and worked on the ocean, often for months at a time. Ina was a stay-at-home parent.

Psychodynamic/Historical Approaches

Psychodynamic and historical family systems approaches emphasize individuals in relationships across generations and over time. There have been several highly influential theorists whose works are most closely associated with family-of-origin dynamics. Among these are Murray Bowen, Nathan Ackerman, James Framo, Ivan Boszormenyi-Nagy, and Jill and David Scharff. For these theorists, present-day experiences of individuals and families are shaped by historical relationships, forces, and events. While they share a common belief that historical relationships are highly influential in the present, these theorists differ considerably in their explanations of how intergenerational dynamics occur, what deserves our greatest attention in families, and how to intervene.

Theory of Change

Psychodynamic/historical approaches emphasize the need for individuals to work out issues from past relationships that are interfering with current functioning and emotional maturity. By identifying family-of-origin patterns and childhood experiences, therapists working from these models can encourage curative encounters via the therapy process itself as well as through planned contact with family members outside of therapy.

Bowen's Family Systems Approach

Murray Bowen is perhaps the most influential contributor to present-day family systems theory. Along with others who pioneered the field of family therapy, Bowen moved from individual psychoanalytic perspectives into viewing individuals as inseparable from their social contexts and relationships and was among the first to consider the family as an emotional unit. Bowen's family systems theory focuses heavily on understanding the emotional forces in families of origin (Bowen, 1978). This approach assumes that each individual has his or her own emotional system and each family has a collective emotional system. The construct of **differentiation of self** from the family of origin is central to this theory. Therapists working from this perspective are interested in each family member's ability to respond to periods of heightened family anxiety without becoming emotionally fused or *triangulating* tension between two family members to ensnare a third member. There are eight major concepts in Bowen's family systems approach.

1. *Differentiation of self.* Differentiation of self refers to the degree of fusion between our emotional and intellectual functioning. Bowen believed that the better able we are to maintain a sense of self while simultaneously maintaining connection to others and the better able we are to think in the presence of emotion, the less symptomatic we become under stress. Interdependence, rather than dependence or independence, is the ultimate relational goal.

2. *The nuclear family emotional system.* This is a developmental concept dealing with patterns throughout courtship and marriage/commitment. The level of differentiation of self plays a key role in this system because it determines the degree of emotional fusion between partners. The degree of fusion of a couple depends on the level of differentiation from family of origin each partner maintained prior to marriage. When both partners are highly differentiated, they can be close and supportive without losing their individuality. Less differentiated individuals are more likely to become fused, losing their sense of self (Bowen, 1972). Bowen termed the results of this fusion the *undifferentiated ego mass* or *family ego mass.*

3. *Family projection process.* In this process, parents project part of their immaturity and dysfunction onto one or more of the children. This projection usually focuses on one child, leaving the other children relatively uninvolved. The selection of the child for projection is influenced by such factors as circumstances surrounding pregnancy and birth, special

relationships with sons or daughters, and parent's lifestyle. The child who is the object of parental projection is the most poorly differentiated and emotionally attached to the parents. Children who are outside the projection process can actually become more differentiated in adulthood than their parents (Bowen, 1972).

4. *Triangles and triangulation.* Bowen (1972) also noted that unstable, two-person systems under stress seek to regain balance by bringing in another person. This new triangle is the basic building block in a family's emotional system. Triangles are not limited to three separate individuals. The third side of a triangle can be made up of an entity such as work or substance abuse, or a group of people such as friends, relatives, or children. **Triangulation,** the process of extending a two-person system to include a third person or entity, allows the couple to project their anxiety onto another, thus relieving the twosome of the unwelcome stress. The role of scapegoat is often played by the third member of a family triangle, and it is not uncommon to see a parent triangulated by two siblings. The patterns and intensity of the triangle relationships within the family is one of the significant factors in Bowen's multigenerational transmission process.

5. *The multigenerational transmission process.* Bowen used this term to describe the way in which patterns of differentiation are transmitted from generation to generation (Bowen, 1972, 1974). Depending on their emotional involvement with parents, children from the same family may emerge with varying degrees of differentiation of self. If a child grew up outside the emotional field of the family, she or he will develop a higher level of differentiation than either parent. Those children who are somewhat involved with parents are likely to establish a degree of differentiation similar to that of the parents. Children who are in the most significant, intense triangles with parents—those who are the objects of the projection process—emerge with lower levels of differentiation than their parents. Through the multigenerational transmission process, poorly differentiated children will cause their own children to be even more poorly differentiated than they are, while highly differentiated children will raise their own children to be even more highly differentiated than they are, and so on.

6. *Sibling position.* Bowen (1976) borrowed this concept from Toman's studies of sibling position personality profiles. Toman (1976) assessed children in normal families, noting their position and characteristics. He was able to assign a group of traits to each of ten positions. This provided a scale of normality by which to compare the development of children. Bowen believed that through comparison with this scale, children could be identified who were the objects of the projection process. The more intense the projection process, the more infantile the child becomes regardless of his or her true position. For example, if an oldest child develops a personality profile equivalent to Toman's youngest child, it supports the hypothesis that

this is the most triangulated child. Bowen felt that by using sibling position, differentiation, and projection, it is possible to assemble personality profiles for individuals in the past and present generations. In assessing couples, a partner's comparative sibling position is also predictive of some aspects of their marital functioning.

7. *Emotional cutoff.* The process of children distancing themselves emotionally from their parents is referred to as emotional cutoff (Bowen, 1974; 1976). The pattern of cutoffs depends on how unresolved emotional attachment to parents is handled. Bowen argued that everyone has some degree of unresolved emotional attachment. Lower levels of differentiation indicate greater attachment and more significant unresolved issues. How an individual separates himself or herself from the past, affects not only his or her relationship with parents but also influences emotional attachment and separation in current relationships. Emotional cutoff may be accomplished by either physical or emotional methods. The type of mechanism used to distance does not reflect the degree of differentiation. The person who runs away by physically moving from parents is just as attached as the one who remains close but distances psychologically.

An open relationship with extended family is the opposite of emotional cutoff (Bowen, 1974). In an open system, members have a reasonable degree of emotional contact with one another. Openness is an effective mechanism for reducing overall anxiety. A continued low level of anxiety allows family members to slowly differentiate. Nuclear families that are relatively cut off from their families of origin are more vulnerable to marital problems, difficulty with children, and so on. Bowen believed, therefore, that the nuclear family remains healthier and more symptom free when it remains in emotional contact with families of origin.

8. *Societal regression.* This concept draws a correlation between family systems and greater societal systems. Bowen's family systems theory assumes that when a family is under continual extreme stress, its members will increasingly rely on emotional rather than intellectual decisions. This results in symptoms that lead to a lower level of functioning. Bowen suggests that this same process is occurring in societies. Worldwide, societies are experiencing greater and greater stress as a result of such factors as over-population, food and resource shortage, and pollution. We are responding to this stress with increasingly emotional decisions. This results in a rise of symptoms, which in turn increases stress, the pattern being repeated in circular fashion.

Practice of Bowen's Family Systems Approach   Bowen (1975) believed the progress of therapy is based on the therapist's emotional functioning, ability to remain neutral, and knowledge of triangles. It is necessary for the therapist to relate meaningfully to each person without becoming entangled in the family emotional system. Bowen believed that a proper emotional distance is reached when the therapist is able to see both humorous and serious sides of family issues. He encouraged therapists to remain calm by focusing on facts rather than emotions. The therapist often functions as a coach, encouraging family members to articulate thoughts in the midst of emotion and speak using "I" statements.

Bowen's family systems theory focused more on explaining family functioning and goals than on specific intervention techniques. In general, family systems therapists are process rather than content oriented as they prompt family members to speak calmly and directly to the therapist from "I" positions. Partners and/or other family members are encouraged to talk about emotional processes and are discouraged from talking directly to each other. A typical intervention pattern would be for one partner to make a comment to the therapist, who intentionally would not make a comment in order to avoid triangulation. Instead, the therapist would then ask the other partner to respond. As the process continued, the therapist would ask questions that center on thoughts, ideas, and opinions. Subjective feelings are, in fact, avoided in this approach. If a member of the couple or family became emotional, the therapist would respond by asking the person to express the thought behind the feeling. According to Bowen, it is essential for the therapist to maintain her or his neutrality.

Family genograms are also a hallmark of this approach (McGoldrick, Gerson, & Shellenberger, 1999). The family genogram is a graphic representation of the multigenerational family tree. Used effectively, it can make covert family patterns overt. Genograms can help families see the intergenerational transmission process at work and identify existing triangles. By using focusing skills, the therapist can make visible the recurring themes and behaviors that flow from one generation to the next. Genograms can be effectively integrated with individual or family counseling to help clients concentrate on family and cultural influences. Several efforts have been made to expand the family genogram. Some versions focus on intergenerational assessment (DeMaria, Weeks, & Hof, 1999). Others focus on cultural awareness and identity (Congress, 1994; Hardy & Laszloffy, 1995) or examine specific dimensions of cultural identity, such as religion and spirituality (Frame, 2000). Still others help explore pertinent historical, contextual, and cultural dimensions of client and client experience, over time and across contexts (Hartmann, 1988; Rigazio-DiGilio, Ivey, Kunkler-Peck, & Grady, 2005).

In working with the Olsens, a therapist taking a family systems approach would talk with Ina and Oscar about their families of origin while assessing the family's current level of emotional differentiation. In this case, Ina divulged that she left Sweden in part because of an abusive relationship with her own father, now deceased. Angry with her mother for failing to protect her, she had communicated with her only a few times over the past 20 years. While she had some contact with extended family in Sweden, she tended to cut off emotionally from her past. Oscar, on the other hand, had no experience living away from his family and often felt pulled between the requests of his parents and siblings and those of his wife. Ina was frustrated by what she saw as Oscar's over-responsiveness to his family and underresponsiveness to her and the children. As Ina and Oscar described these relationships to the therapist, their daughters reacted differently. Diana became visibly distressed and tearful, whereas Rita became increasingly angry and withdrawn.

From this perspective, the family might be encouraged to recognize patterns of emotional fusion and cutoff across generations. The therapist could encourage Ina to take steps to write, call, and eventually visit her extended family in Sweden, carefully considering patterns and emotions that emerged at each juncture of the process. Likewise, Oscar might be helped to identify patterns in his family of origin that interfered with his being adequately involved with his wife and children. Sessions with Oscar and his family of origin could be helpful in developing alternative, less reactive connections. While working with Ina and Oscar, the therapist would assume the triangulated position that once belonged to Rita in order to help the couple manage anxiety while differentiating thoughts and emotions within their relationship.

Cognitive-Behavioral/Interactional Approaches

Influential family theorists reflective of this orientation include Salvador Minuchin, Jay Haley, Cloé Madanes, and James Alexander. In their writing, these theorists pay close attention to cognitive processes, behavioral sequences, organizational structures, rules, and communication. Cognitive-behavioral/interactional approaches tend to be brief, focus on the here and now, and offer specific interventions to help families develop new perspectives and interactional patterns. For example, therapists working from a *strategic family therapy* (Madanes, 1981) approach include a structural analysis but focus on the dynamics of overt and covert power in relationship to presenting problems. From this perspective, problems often indicate incongruent hierarchies. Therapists attempt to identify these problems and then develop specific, targeted interventions to correct ineffective interactions. Consider a couple in which one partner suffers from chronic anxiety. In this hierarchy, he or she as the "sick one" may be "one down," yet because of the symptom maintains significant power or influence in the family. Likewise, the "healthy" partner is "one up" yet helpless to influence the anxiety.

Theory of Change

Those therapists working from the cognitive-behavioral/interactional orientation are interested in creating here-and-now change in family interactional patterns.

This often starts with helping the family reconsider, or **reframe,** the problem in a way that allows them to explore new ways of relating. While symptom removal is important, shifts in basic underlying conceptions and relational patterns are the focus of enduring change. Therapists working from these models are typically very active in the change process as they attempt to bring about new sequences of behavior in the therapy room and via between-session tasks. Interventions may be direct or indirect. Therapy is planned in stages in which specific goals are targeted.

Minuchin's Structural Family Therapy

Salvador Minuchin is well known for his innovative and active approach to working with families in poverty. Nearly a half a century has passed since Minuchin began working with families, yet his ideas about family structure and normative family functioning continue to impact the field. *Structural family therapy* (Minuchin, 1974) emphasizes using metaphors of family structure and hierarchy. Therapists working from a structural perspective think in terms of how families are organized into multiple **subsystems** based on interactional patterns. Spousal, parental, and sibling subsystems are considered particularly germane to family functioning. Assessment of families often includes drawing a **family map** that indicates interactional processes between family members and boundaries between subsystems. This approach is normative in that it is assumed that although many family structures (e.g., single-parent families, grandparent-headed families) can work well, the hierarchy within families and boundaries between their subsystems need to be clear and promote the development of all members. Symptoms are more likely to appear when this is not occurring. We now consider five family systems concepts described by Minuchin.

1. *Boundaries.* Boundaries are a way of talking about who is involved in various subsystems and how. The permeability of boundaries can be thought of as existing along a continuum from rigid and impermeable to diffuse and highly permeable. Boundaries vary over time according to context, culture, family developmental stage, and preferred relationship styles. For example, when a couple first comes together, they may form a tightly knit dyad that temporarily excludes friends and extended family. Later on, when a child is born, the couple's extended family and friends may become more connected and involved. Boundaries become problematic when they are established in ways that interfere with family and individual development/functioning. For example, when a father and daughter continually exclude the mother (rigid boundary around father-daughter subsystem), it may interfere with the functioning of spouses and be maintained at the expense of the mother-daughter relationship.

2. *Subsystems.* All members of the family belong to multiple groupings, or subsystems. These are based on commonalities of many kinds, including gender (all the females in the family), interests (all baseball players), position in the family (the youngest cousins), and so on. Structural family therapists are particularly interested in three subsystems: parental, spousal, and sibling. The parental subsystem may include mother and father, same-sex parents, mother and grandmother, or many other groupings of those who see themselves as responsible for the care of the children in the family. Spousal subsystems include primary partners. Those in the spousal system are often the same family members who are in the parental system (e.g., same-sex partners with a child, husband and wife). The sibling subsystem includes all related children in the family. Minuchin argued that one's membership in one subsystem should not affect one's membership in another subsystem. Thus, parental concerns should not interfere with the partners' intimate relationship, and so on.

3. *Hierarchy.* Family hierarchy refers to the degree and type of influence each member has to carry out a specific role. Parents need to have the necessary status and authority in a family to oversee the well-being and offer supportive and corrective direction to their children. Some families are organized so that grandparents maintain the greatest influence. Others believe parents should be primary or that fathers should have the final say in major family decisions. Minuchin argued that many family hierarchies can work well as long as they are clear and meet the needs of all family members.

4. *Alliances and coalitions.* Family members who maintain particularly close relationships, sometimes to the exclusion of others, are described as in alliance. If members join an alliance in reaction to a third family member, they are described as a coalition. For example, a father and son may be in coalition against an alcoholic mother, habitually sharing with each other their unhappiness about her behavior. If this situation remains "stuck," the coalition can contribute to the problem. On the other hand, if this is a temporary arrangement that causes family members to seek treatment, then the coalition has been useful.

5. *Family maps.* Family mapping is a tool structural family therapists use to describe family relationships, including subsystems, boundaries, and hierarchies. Maps are visual representations of repetitive family interactional patterns, most often in the here and now. Maps are also used to set structural goals and to assess change. Using a structural map allows therapists a guiding conceptual framework to understand and treat families.

Practice of Minuchin's Structural Family Therapy   Structural therapists take a very active role in the family change process in order to create here-and-now change in family interactions. They attempt to create this change during therapy sessions and through between-session tasks. All interactions with clients are guided by steps toward overall structural goals. For example, when initially meeting with a client system, a therapist might respect an imbalanced hierarchy by first addressing whoever is most in charge, yet challenge the imbalance later in therapy after the therapeutic relationship is well developed. Structural therapists are interested in helping families create new interactional patterns that meet the developmental needs of each family member and the family as a whole within its social context. For example, families may be guided and challenged to decrease conflict avoidance and increase direct, resolvable expressions of difference. Structural therapists often engage clients in **enactments,** in which family members are encouraged to speak directly in new ways, often about avoided topics. Enactments allow for new interactional patterns to emerge in the therapy process that can then be reinforced between sessions to create lasting structural change. Structural therapists are concerned throughout the therapy process about shifting relationships in the family. For example, it is common that structural therapists look for ways to encourage parents to act as a team in guiding their children, to increase partner communication, to enhance the connections between disengaged family members, and to clarify boundaries between families and outside systems to ensure families get adequate support.

Working from a structural family therapy perspective, the Olsens's therapist would be careful to connect with each member of the family, listening and watching carefully to assess family interaction. She or he would develop a structural map or diagram of the family subsystems and consider how to take steps toward structural goals. In this case, Rita reported that she was very close with her mother and, in fact, felt they were nearly equals because Ina relied on Rita to help run the household whenever Oscar was away. Ina saw Oscar as underinvolved in both parenting and the marriage when he was home. Oscar felt that when he returned from being gone for months at a time, the family did not seem to need him. The therapist facilitated enactments in the family by asking that members talk directly to each other about these important issues. The therapist noticed that Diana stood up for her father throughout the conversation and interrupted when tension grew between her parents. Diana and Rita said very little to each other, explaining to the therapist that they had little in common.

Interventions from this structural perspective might include finding creative ways for parents to work as a team even when Oscar was away; asking the couple to spend time together to strengthen their marriage; encouraging extended family and community support for Ina during months in which she was acting as a single parent; encouraging Oscar to spend time connecting more with Rita while Ina enjoyed time with Diana; helping Ina and Oscar develop a supportive parenting network in the community; and clarifying how Rita and Diana can still be sisters even when it is helpful to the family for Rita to take on some parental duties.

Existential-Humanistic Approaches

Existential-humanistic family therapy models rely less on theorizing and more on the experience of the therapeutic encounter. Therapists working from these perspectives are interested in offering families opportunities for personal and family growth through therapeutic experiences that act as catalysts for change. By encouraging emotional expression, expanding possibilities for connection, and unblocking barriers to communication, the therapist facilitates unique, idiosyncratic, personal, and relational growth. Symbolic-experiential family therapy (Napier & Whitaker, 1972) and communication/validation therapy (Satir, 1964) are enduring examples of these approaches. These models encourage pragmatism over theory and spontaneity over planned techniques/interventions, relying on the unique experiences, expressions, and potentials of all individuals and families. The focus is on identifying and expressing emotions as well as clarifying patterns of communication. Clinicians working from this perspective often engage multiple generations in the process as they attend to both present and past extended family and community relationships to expand future possibilities for individuals and relational systems.

Theory of Change

Therapists working from this perspective are interested in opening possibilities for families to understand each other and engage in new experiences. Emotional expression is encouraged as family members are asked to describe their thoughts and feelings in each other's presence. Rigid communication patterns are challenged and often disrupted by spontaneous, playful experiences in the therapeutic encounter. Therapists rely heavily on the use of themselves, their own experiences, stories, intuition, and personal integrity to help families transform. Use of family sculpting, asking family members to use "I" statements, role plays, and psychodrama techniques are also common to this approach.

Whitaker and Satir's Experiential Family Therapy

Carl Whitaker and Virginia Satir are credited as the founders of experiential family therapy. Whitaker is well known for his unique and playful approach to challenging serious family problems. Satir's warmth and genuine interest in the experience of each family member is unparalleled in the field. Both continue to have lasting effects on the ongoing development of experiential approaches today. The underlying assumption that guides experiential therapy is that problems are caused and maintained by families' suppression of emotions. Rather than encouraging emotional expression with age-appropriate regulation, members of many families try to control their own and each other's feelings.

This creates interactional patterns that stunt personal growth, understanding between family members, and family problem solving. Experiential therapists do not focus heavily on theory or structured techniques, relying more on fluid and spontaneous engagement of the family in order to encourage emotional expression and understanding. There are several concepts that are frequently associated with the approach.

1. *Self-actualization.* Experiential therapists maintain a basic belief that all of us have an innate drive toward self-actualization. That is, we naturally move toward understanding ourselves and regulating our emotions over time though our interactions with others. According to experientialists, emotional self-awareness and honest expression of thoughts and emotions are core to this process. When these are blocked because of family and/or societal pressures, problems within and between people arise that prevent actualization of individuals and thwart the relationship potential within systems.

2. *Family myths.* In order to avoid painful feelings and interactions that seem impossible to resolve, families may collectively distort past and present realities. This shapes interaction, governing how and what is talked about, whether or not feelings around certain issues and events can be expressed, and so on. While family myths help families deal with harsh realities, they also contribute to rules and patterns that prevent individual and relational growth.

3. *Inauthentic communication.* Satir held that family members who are avoiding honest emotional and experiential expression tend to distort their interactions through placating, blaming, taking on too much responsibility, and/or focusing on the irrelevant. It is through identifying these patterns and challenging family members to directly and honestly express themselves that therapists are able to help families dislodge themselves from positions that prevent natural growth toward personal and relational fulfillment.

Practice of Experiential Family Therapy   Experiential therapists are primarily interested in personal growth. Symptom removal is secondary to this broader goal. There is also an emphasis on individual experience that often outweighs attention to family interactional patterns. Experiential therapists work with individuals within families to explore the depth of each person's experience and feelings in ways that not only enhance individual self-actualization, but also encourage the potential for family members to connect and support each other toward this ultimate end. A number of here-and-now, in-session techniques are commonly associated with this approach. For example, using a technique called **family sculpting,** therapists may direct members to physically place themselves relative to each other in ways that reflect and express their relationships, thoughts, and feelings. They may interpret or encourage the family to join in interpreting a dream in order to explore the depth of experience of one or more members. The therapist may tell a story about his or her own life that connects in obvious or subtle ways to the family's experience in order to help members gain insight into their own experience. Finally, experiential therapists are known for their spontaneity, use of intuition, playfulness, and personal presence in the therapy encounter.

The work of a family therapist who takes an existential-humanistic perspective is likely to be highly idiosyncratic. In the case of the Olsens, the therapist began a session by telling a story about how she ran away as a teenager. This softened the family's anxiety about being considered problematic. Next, the therapist engaged in playfully asking Rita details about what she decided to pack for her trips and how she coped once her clothes got dirty. As the family began to relax, the therapist asked them to stand and posture themselves in positions that demonstrated their relationships (i.e., sculpt) when Rita and Oscar were both home as well as when either were away. During this process, she carefully elicited the emotional experience of family members by asking them to talk about thoughts and feelings directly with others using "I" statements. As family members became privy to each other's emotional worlds, deep concerns, and perspectives, they were better able to connect and begin solving problems in a more creative manner.

Contemporary Family Therapy: Theory and Practice

Most contemporary family therapy models and approaches build on the knowledge base of traditional family therapy theory. Rather than rejecting the traditional approaches, contemporary approaches integrate concerns about power, culture, and context with the fundamental concepts of family systems theory. We begin this section of the chapter with some of the theoretical sources from which contemporary therapies have been drawn. Then, we look more closely at one model and its practice.

Contributions from Postmodern, Ecological, and Integrative Theories

Postmodern models of family therapy seek to establish a collaborative, co-constructive relationship with the family client system. Drawing on the work of Bronfenbrenner (1979) and Kasambria and Edwards (2000), postmodernist family practitioners look for possibilities within the wider culture and community to help increase the family's capacity for growth. These models adhere to the belief that the power to change inhibiting family behaviors is located in the stories families hold about themselves (e.g., Epston, 2001; Weingarten, 1998). We have many ways to think about and describe our experiences, consciously or unconsciously choosing some experiences and meanings over others. This deeply affects how we make meaning of our lives and how we interact. For someone who grew up in an alcoholic family, for example, the *dominant story* of her life may focus only on the negative and damaging effects of being a parentified child. In therapy, she might make meaning of this experience differently by focusing on an *alternative story* about the strengths and confidence she developed by being in this position. Acting toward others from a self-concept of being "resilient" rather than "damaged" would then create opportunities for different interactions. For therapists who take a narrative approach, helping to deconstruct problem-saturated, dominant stories and restory the content to effect new possibilities and identities are the keys to family treatment. Understanding the meaning family members, and other significant members of the family's wider community, infer from, and imbue to, these stories is the primary goal of treatment. Recognizing that there are multiple interpretations of any story, the work of the family practitioners using this perspective is to empower the family to make adjustments to the primary narrative based on changes inside and outside the family.

Integrative models of family therapy (Anderson & Bagarozzi, 1983; Breunlin et al., 1992; Rigazio-DiGilio, 2000) provide conceptual frameworks for practitioners to design and tailor treatment to the expressed needs of the family. Rather than applying one model in a narrow fashion, the integrative models afford access to a wider repertory of strategies and techniques. Some models (e.g., Jacobson, Christensen, Prince, Cordova, & Eldridge, 2000; Rigazio-DiGilio, 2000; Walsh & McGraw, 2002) also provide specific intervention strategies and planning tools unique to the model itself. These models are also ecological and focus on the full life space of the family-client.

Integrative family theory models provide both overarching metaframeworks to help practitioners select particular therapeutic strategies across the wide field of family therapies and a specific pathway for treatment within the integrative model. Integrative family models require practitioners to become familiar and skillful with a wide range of relational, conceptual, perceptual, and executive skills from discrete theories, therapies, models, and techniques and to know which skills to access to best address the therapeutic, cultural, and contextual needs of their clients. These models help clinicians coordinate assessment and treatment efforts as they work to tailor counseling and therapy to the unique qualities of each family (Rigazio-DiGilio, 1997).

Additional Assumptions of Contemporary Family Therapies

In addition to the basic assumptions that underlie traditional family therapy models, three common guiding assumptions serve as the foundation for most postmodern, ecological, and integrative models.

1. *Individual and family development happens through interaction with the wider environment.* The interaction between the person or the family and the wider sociopolitical environment is viewed as a cultural exchange process. Individuals interact with their wider environment, including their family, and through this interaction certain beliefs, behaviors, and feelings are generated, shared, and reinforced. In a family, the interactions among family members contribute to the evolution of a collective worldview that is spread across all family members.

2. *Individual and family problems are viewed from a developmental, not a pathological, perspective.* Most contemporary family therapy models and approaches are based on a nondeficit perspective. That is, they assume that clients want to adapt successfully within their social and physical environment. When families are constrained or blocked from meeting these needs, patterns of behaving, feeling, and thinking that increase distress become evident. Contemporary models take a positive perspective and help families identify and optimize individual, family, and community resources to deal with their presenting issues and move forward.

From a nondeficit perspective, proponents of traditional diagnoses, as exemplified in the *DSM-IV TR*, tend to pathologize difference, assume that dysfunction resides within the individual, subjugate individuals to the symptoms they exhibit, and perpetuate treatments designed to ameliorate individual dysfunction and its symptoms. While these approaches do address important intrapersonal phenomena, they tend to ignore the relational, social, and cultural systems that may contribute to and construe presumed disorder (Rigazio-DiGilio, Ivey, & Locke, 1997). Issues of racism, sexism, economic deprivation, and others forms of oppression that directly impact family functioning are not considered in the traditional diagnostic process. From most contemporary perspectives, family and individual behavior is viewed as a logical reaction to real or perceived environmental stressors. Rather than simply assigning pathology to the individual or the family, contemporary approaches also consider the toxic external environmental factors that may need to be considered as part of the treatment plan. One tool therapists might use to consider the complexity of individual, relational, community, and cultural influences on the problems presented in treatment is the **community genogram** (Rigazio-DiGilio et al., 2005), which helps trace how individuals and families fit within the broader historical and community environment. The clinical information presented in this graphic assessment tool provides a basis for practitioners to develop hypotheses about presenting issues that may be connected to community and cultural factors. Furthermore, community genograms directly enable clients to assume an active role in determining the focus and course of treatment.

3. *The unique worldviews professionals bring to their work influence how they conceptualize and treat families.* The worldview of a counselor or therapist has two main components: the professional and the personal. The professional worldview, what each of us knows and values about our work and how it should be conducted, is predicated on the professional knowledge, skills, and dispositions we bring to each therapeutic encounter. If a professional is most knowledgeable and comfortable with psychodynamic/historical conceptualizations of treatment, then those methods will tend to dominant her or his work with families. If on the other hand, a professional is competent in a variety of family therapy methods and is skillful at tailoring treatment approaches to the unique qualities of any family-client system, this worldview will lead to integration. Our personal worldview is derived from our own cultural heritage and the experiences and circumstances of our individual lives. Every aspect of the counseling encounter reflects the therapist's culture—such as location, setting, room arrangement, dialogue, treatment goals, and clinical expectations. To the extent possible, counselors should be conscious of the "hidden" cultural aspects of our work patterns and their implications on treatment. For these reasons, it is essential that the practitioner, through reflection and supervision, identify his or her worldview and acknowledge the limitations and strengths of that worldview.

If we are to be effective family therapists, our worldview in working with culturally diverse clients must be premised upon the following.

1. How well we know our own cultural heritage.

2. How well we understand the ways in which sociopolitical factors influence the field of family therapy as well as our own theoretical and therapy approach.

3. How effectively we communicate empathy for members of other cultures.

4. The degree to which we acknowledge that culture may be an essential factor in a treatment plan.

5. The degree to which we eschew homogeneity within groups but instead remain keenly alert to the significant variations of each client and family while noting the broad characteristics that differentiate cultural groups. (Rigazio-DiGilio, in press).

Theory of Change

Therapists working from contemporary perspectives tend to view change as a collaborative process, valuing the uniqueness of each family within its cultural and contextual milieu. How the family co-constructs its history and the meaning of life experiences, including what they define as problematic, takes a front seat as a mechanism for change through conversation and opening space for multiple perspectives. The therapist keeps in mind the interconnectedness of individuals, families, communities, and broader social forces along historic, contemporary, and future timelines as families lead the way toward territories that for them are most relevant and meaningful. At times, possibilities are expanded through the use of reflective teams, the therapist's own thoughts and experiences, and the inclusion of multiple members of extended systems. Therapists working from these perspectives are likely to consider, and when possible intervene in, broader social forces that may be contributing to family problems, including sexism, racism, ableism, and poverty.

Systemic Cognitive Developmental Therapy

Systemic cognitive developmental therapy (SCDT) represents a holistic, nonpathological, and integrative approach to family and wider systems treatment. SCDT is an extension of developmental therapy (DT) (Ivey, Ivey, Myers & Sweeny, 2005), which is a constructivist interpretation of developmental theories. Both models draw on metaphorical reinterpretations of Piagetian constructs to illustrate how human and systemic development occurs over the life span and in therapy.

SCDT links developmental and social constructivist constructs to the therapy process and offers specific assessment and treatment strategies that can be easily learned and applied during the immediacy of the therapeutic encounter. In addition, SCDT provides an *integrative framework* that organizes various family therapy strategies and interventions into a developmental classification matrix that counselors can draw from to tailor treatment to the unique needs of families. Therapists can use the strategies and matrix to identify how families experience, interpret, and operate in their worlds and to construct developmentally tailored and culturally sensitive treatment plans. There are four main components of SCDT theory.

1. *Phases of systemic development.* There are four phases families repeatedly go through in their efforts to adapt to changing developmental and situational demands. During the *systems exploration phase*, members share feelings, perceptions, and reactions about their evolving relationships or particular developmental or situational circumstances. They test the waters to see what type of responses self-disclosure generates. Based on these responses, members determine what information, feelings, and behaviors they will share. Once some common ground is formed, members move toward *system consolidation*. Members find strength in shared beliefs and opinions, but might feel uncertain about ideas or attitudes not mutually

held. The focus is on reinforcing shared ways of experiencing, interpreting, and acting in the world so that thoughts, feelings, and behaviors become somewhat predictable. The foundation achieved in this phase enables families to venture into *system enhancement*. In this phase, members begin to reflect on and modify their unique views of themselves and their life circumstances in ways that do not threaten their sense of mutuality or individuality. Members begin to expand mutual goals, values, and views by elaborating their ideas and beliefs. This is a period of flexibility and creativity when families can evaluate the usefulness of their collective orientation for all members and make modifications as necessary. During *system transformation*, families become aware of various external and internal forces that have influenced collective worldviews and become sensitive to the development and functioning of each member and the family as a whole. As they work to address changing circumstances, families examine outdated or less useful options and develop alternative options that provide continuity for the family while also encouraging new perspectives. Often this returns families to the *system exploration* phase as members seek to discover new ways of making sense of and operating in their world.

SCDT defines adaptive relationships as those that continually recycle through these phases in response to demands for change. Less adaptive families may become arrested in any phase, limiting their ability to appropriately respond to life's demands. For these families, therapy is often indicated.

2. *Collective cognitive-developmental orientations.* The four phases previously described are continually repeated as families grapple with life tasks. The collective orientations that families rely on to experience, interpret, and act on these life tasks are defined using a metaphorical reinterpretation of Piagetian constructs (Piaget, 1965). Piaget proposed that as humans mature, their cognitive abilities develop in four sequential stages: sensorimotory/preoperational (perceiving the world mainly through the senses in infancy); concrete operational (thinking and communicating in childhood in concrete, non-abstract ways); formal operational (still primarily concrete, but gaining some ability to think abstractly in adolescence); and post-formal operational (fully able to think and reason abstractly in adulthood). SCDT reinterpreted Piaget's constructs not as age-related abilities, but as cognitive styles or orientations that all families use, depending on the circumstances.

Within the *sensorimotor-elemental orientation*, families count on sensory experience to understand and relate to their members and their sociocultural environment. Families who rely on this orientation can easily become overwhelmed by slight variations in their environment. Families functioning within the *concrete-situational orientation* view the world as logical and understandable, believe in cause and effect, and can act predictably in the world.

Those who rigidly rely on this orientation use detailed linear descriptions of events with little accompanying affect, analysis, or reflection. Families functioning in the *formal-reflective orientation* rely on pattern recognition and abstract thinking to make sense of their world. Members who analyze their issues but seem unable to act on or change them are overrelying on this orientation. Additionally, they may talk about their feelings rather than really experiencing feelings. Within the *dialectic/systemic orientation*, families understand the interrelated connectedness of the contexts they live in. They rely on systemic thinking to develop complex views of situations they deal with. If they cannot access other orientations, their views may simply be too overwhelming to decipher.

Each orientation is viewed as unique and useful in its own right, depending on the major life issues the family is working through at the moment. One of the goals of SCDT is to assist families to access each of the four orientations in order to effectively adapt to the changing circumstances of their lives. To accomplish this, families need to know how to move *horizontally* and *vertically* through each of the four orientations.

3. *Horizontal and vertical development.* SCDT adapts the Piagetian concepts of horizontal and vertical development (Piaget, 1954) to describe the movement families make within and across the four orientations. *Horizontal development* describes emotional, cognitive, and/or behavioral growth within one orientation. It is particularly useful to establish a deep foundation and master the skills within one orientation. *Vertical development* describes movement from one orientation to another. This movement provides families with the alternative skills, thoughts, and actions associated with different orientations.

4. *Systemic development and adaptation.* Adaptive families can use a well-established horizontal foundation to stretch into other orientations as needed. Because they can access and operate within several orientations, they can call on a wide variety of emotional, cognitive, and behavioral options to handle situational and developmental issues. Nonadaptive families fall within one of two categories. Some may rigidly rely on one or two orientations to handle all of life's issues, and these may be insufficient for the tasks confronting them. Others may haphazardly access underdeveloped resources across orientations that are not in synchrony with demands for adaptation. These families often do not have a strong foundation within any one orientation and are stuck within a useless cycle of trying anything that seems like it should work.

Practice of Systemic Cognitive Developmental Therapy

SCDT suggests that families seeking treatment are experiencing distress because of their inability to master developmental tasks and/or adapt to changing life circumstances. The therapeutic objective is first to assist families to create or reinforce a strong yet flexible foundation within the orientation that is matched to their primary collective orientation. Next, families are assisted to use this foundation as a point of departure to access and develop skills within other orientations more in synchrony with demands for adaptation and change. The ultimate goal is to encourage families to achieve a wide repertory of cognitive, behavioral, and affective options to apply to the developmental and situational demands they encounter during life's journey. This goal is facilitated by helping each family move horizontally and vertically throughout the developmental orientations during the course of treatment.

In the assessment phase, clinicians use *SCDT assessment strategies* and the *SCDT collective cognitive-developmental assessment profile* to access and assess the predominant orientations used by families and the degree to which they have access to other orientations. These linguistically based assessment procedures are used to elicit family dialogue to determine the primary orientations represented by the family as a whole, by subsystems, and by individuals. Responses to the assessment questions also indicate the ability of the family, subsystems, and individuals to access resources in all four orientations.

During the treatment phase, counselors design therapeutic plans that first help families build an adequate foundation within their primary orientation (style matching). This foundation is then used as a steppingstone to assist families in accessing resources available in other orientations (style shifting). *Style matching* occurs when counselors use techniques, interventions, exercises, questions, and language to co-construct environments that are consistent with their clients' predominant collective orientation. *Style shifting* occurs when counselors shift techniques, interventions, exercises, questions, and language in order to assist their clients to explore ancillary orientations. This shift occurs in response to linguistic cues from families that suggest what orientation they appear ready to explore. A return to style matching occurs after a style shift so that families can practice and master their newfound skills.

SCDT defines *four therapeutic environments* that correspond with each of the collective orientations. Each environment reflects a particular style, a set of SCDT questioning strategies, and a set of intervention strategies conducive to work within an associated orientation. The first *environmental structuring environment* offers a context for clients to be in direct contact with the immediacy and depth of their affective sensations and other sensory-based experiences. Interventions assist clients to experience their most basic feelings and can be used to either amplify emotional expression or restrain chaotic affective experience. In the concrete *coaching environment*, the therapist encourages clients to explore their issues within a cause-and-effect perspective and to share family stories and the extended analyses of the antecedents and consequences of specific events. The formal *consulting environment* is co-constructed by clients and the therapist to facilitate a reflective process through which clients identify patterns within their thoughts, feelings, and interactions. Finally, the dialectic/systemic *collaborating environment* is constructed to promote the exploration of ideas and concepts that penetrate the ontological nature of collective worldviews. Clients and clinicians work as colleagues to examine contextual forces (e.g., gender, culture, sociohistorical patterns, economics, politics, intergenerational themes) that might be operating within the sociocultural environment and the therapeutic process.

Using SCDT, the therapist working with the Olsens was able to assess, through carefully listening to how family members described their experiences, that in general, they functioned in concrete-situational and formal-reflective orientations. Ina offered excellent detail about what happened each time Rita ran away, while Oscar drew parallels between how the family handled Rita running away and other issues such as responding to Diana's poor grades or handling problems in the marriage. By thoroughly exploring problems within these preferred orientations (horizontal development), the family was able to open up communication between Ina and Oscar. In time, the therapist found both Rita and Diana more able to express themselves from an elemental orientation and used interventions aimed at vertical development to open space in the family for all to explore emotions more fully. Completing a community genogram with the family helped develop a dialectic/systemic view of the problem as family members became better able to consider their sense of embeddedness with their extended family, cultural histories, community, schools, peers, church, the local economy, and other sociocultural forces. By broadening their access to emotions, recognition of patterns, and understanding of the contextual dimensions of their lives, the family was able to develop strategies within the family and community to deal with problems more effectively.

Now that you have become more familiar with traditional and contemporary family therapy models, look back at your answers to the questions we asked you to consider as you read the case example. Which of your original ideas endure? How have you changed or expanded your thoughts? How might you work with this family using an integrated approach, drawing from ideas across traditional and contemporary models of family therapy?

Evaluation of Family Therapy

There are two major approaches, and a third emerging approach, to researching the process and outcomes of family therapy: nomothetic, idiographic, and idiothetic.

Nomothetic Family Therapy Research: Effectiveness Across Clients

Nomothetic family therapy research represents the accumulated body of knowledge about the relative effectiveness of particular family therapy models or practices across client groups. Research on the traditional family systems models, such as those defined and illustrated in this chapter, on certain integrative models (e.g., Schoenwald, Sheidow, & Letourneau, 2003), and on common factors across family therapy models (e.g., Davis, 2005) reflects the nomothetic approach to research in family therapy.

Findings about the efficacy of family therapy across client groups indicate that it is effective and that it is not harmful (Pinsof & Wynne, 1995). Becvar and Becvar (2003) examined the research findings across client groups and reported the following.

1. When compared to no treatment, nonbehavioral marital and family therapies are twice as likely to reach effective solutions.

2. In cases concerning childhood and adolescent behavioral issues, family therapy methods are successful in about 70% of the cases treated.

3. Conjoint marital therapy is more effective than individual therapy for marital issues.

4. Higher-level "therapist relationship skills" appear necessary for positive outcomes in family therapy. Less than higher-level skills may prevent worsening, merely maintaining the pretherapy status of the family.

5. In terms of efficiency, successful family therapy outcomes occur in relatively few sessions ranging from one to twenty.

6. Co-therapy has not been proven to be superior to family therapy conducted by one therapist.

Nomothetic Family Therapy Research: Effectiveness for Specific Presenting Issues and Populations

Because the originators of the major schools of family therapy were intent on demonstrating the clinical effectiveness of their new theories, the field of family therapy has a long empirical record. Beginning with the conclusion drawn by Gurman, Kirshern, and Pinsof in 1986 that family therapy is effective, and sustained throughout the most influential reviews by leaders in the field (e.g., Liddle & Rowe 2004; Pinsof, Wynne, & Hambright 1996; Sexton & Alexander,

1999; Stanton & Shadish 1997), many positive conclusions about the efficacy of therapy have been validated. For example:

1. Family therapy is as effective as other psychotherapy modalities and is superior to the gains achieved by psychopharmacological interventions (Shadish, Ragsdale, Glaser, & Montgomery, 1995).

2. Family therapy is an effective treatment for conduct disorder problems in children (Serketich & Dumas, 1996).

3. Substance abuse in adolescents and adults is effectively treated with family therapy (Edwards & Steinglass, 1995; Stanton & Shadish, 1997).

4. Couples therapy is more effective than individual therapy for relationship problems, particularly for depressed women (Baucom, Shoham, Mueser, Daiuto, & Stickle, 1998; Green, 2003).

5. Family-based interventions demonstrate greater cost-effectiveness for treatment of delinquency (Henggler, Melton, Smith, Schoenwald, & Hanley, 1993).

6. Family therapy is more efficacious than standard and/or individual treatment for adult schizophrenia, marital distress, eating disorders, and chronic physical illnesses in adults and children (Pinsof & Wynne, 1995).

7. Family therapy is effective for treating issues of childhood, including child abuse and neglect, emotional problems, behavioral problems, enuresis and soiling, and psychosomatic problems (Carr, 2000).

8. Systemic therapy interventions are effective in the treatment of childhood asthma (Lask & Matthew, 1979).

9. Systemic family and couples therapy is effective in the treatment of eating disorders, psychotic illnesses, and mood disorders (Asen, 2002).

10. Couples treatment is effective for sexual dysfunction (Hurlburt, 1993).

The preponderance of evidence suggests that family therapy is effective alone, or in conjunction with pharmacological and other psychological treatments, for a wide range of presenting problems.

Idiographic Family Therapy Research

Idiographic family therapy research reflects trends to capture the uniqueness of each family so that practitioners can tailor interventions on the basis of these unique qualities. Constructivist and social constructionist researchers are increasingly using qualitative, nonnumerical descriptions of family processes that include case studies and multimethod approaches designed to bridge the gap among theory, practice, and research (Guba & Lincoln, 1994; Sells, Smith, & Moon, 1996). Idiographic family therapy research arose in part because of criticisms that nomothetic knowledge tends to characterize families within generic descriptions that subjugate them to the symptoms they exhibit and to decontextualize them from their own cultural heritage and developmental history. These criticisms have been useful in alerting the field to the culture-bound nature of our accumulated research-based knowledge and to the problems that arise when nomothetic findings are elevated to the level of "truth" intended to dictate the work of therapists as applied technicians rather than as backdrops intended to inform clinical inquiry and treatment planning.

The emerging trend in the field is to view clinicians as researchers (Green, 2003; Rigazio-DiGilio, Ivey & Locke, 1997). Borrowing from Kurt Lewin (1951), whose work with groups influenced the creation of family therapy, Lebow (1997) suggests that therapists adopt an action research approach by conducting research on their own caseload. Therapists may employ both quantitative and qualitative methods to best address the questions they have about their practice. By systematically collecting data about treatment processes and family reactions and outcomes, therapist-based research offers a strong alternative to the top-down, theory-driven framework of traditional research approaches. Further, as Lebow suggests, therapists can share their findings with others so that their idiographic research on their own clients can be used nomothetically.

Qualitative family therapy researchers have focused primarily on investigating the processes and outcomes of a single approach to therapy (Gehart, Ratliff, & Randall, 2001). As noted by Burck (2005), the application of qualitative methodologies to researching family therapy processes has provided helpful findings. For example, Coulehan, Friedlander, and Heatherington (1998) developed a conceptual model of a successful process that assists clients in transforming their construction of the presenting problem from an individual, intrapersonal view to an interpersonal, relational, or systemic one using a narrative approach. Helmeke and Sprenkle (2000) found that marital partners do identify specific therapy events as pivotal and that these events tend to be highly individualized accounts, with little overlap between spouses and little overlap between therapist and client identification of pivotal moments. Finally, Kogan and Gale (1997) were able to identify five conversational practices that inform postmodern therapy sessions.

Idiothetic Family Therapy Research

There does seem to be some emerging evidence of a trend toward what Peter Fraenkel (1995) refers to as an integrated, idiothetic approach to family therapy research. Using this approach, family therapy theory and practice can draw from research on general assumptions about families while maintaining respect for the differences that make each family unique. From this framework, research on approaches to family therapy is intended to inform assessment and treatment planning rather than to dictate it. It is how the practitioner uses the information that becomes important. Until recently, practitioners were considered applied technicians of theory and research, which promulgated the idea of theory and research as "truth." As we become increasingly aware of the necessary linkages among theory, practice, and research, the definitions of both knowledge and practice take on a different meaning. From this vantage point, research is not seen as a way to determine how most families are likely to respond within certain ranges of common reactions to particular types of events, but rather as tentative findings about these common reactions for therapists to consider.

Family Therapy and Diverse Populations

Family therapy has been proved effective in mental health prevention and treatment programs, not just in the United States but also all over the world. Kaslow's (2000) history of the international growth of family therapy demonstrates that its core therapeutic concepts have been synthesized and successfully applied within a wide range of cultures. Kaslow details how family therapy is growing in popularity among psychotherapy practitioners, researchers, and academicians in countries on all continents, and how the work in the United States is shaped by the contributions of international experts. "Wherever family therapy was introduced, it met with great resistance but ultimately, based on good interpretation, supportive research findings, and effective treatment outcomes, the resistance has been overcome" (p. 31). Trepper's (2005) review of worldwide activities in family therapy led him to comment, "Some of the most exciting work in the field is now coming from emerging nations in Eastern Europe, from the changing societies in South America, and from areas only recently discovering family therapy, such as Asia" (p. 11).

In the United States, marriage and family therapy methods have been successfully applied with members of diverse cultures. Emerging from a social work and child guidance clinic background, much of the early work in family therapy involved inner-city populations. Families in the cities were living with problems associated with poverty, racism, discrimination, and violence, and these issues were addressed in case formulations and treatment plans. Initially, these issues were viewed as environmental factors and not viewed from a multicultural perspective. That is, poverty was viewed as affecting all members of that group in similar ways regardless of racial, gender, ethnic, and other personal attributes.

By the end of the 1970s, this monolithic perspective of culture and context gave way to a more inclusive and personalized view of how ethnicity, gender, power, privilege, and community factors affect family treatment process and outcomes. Although many professional books, articles, and chapters have been written documenting methods and issues underlying treatment with diverse families, it was only in 2001 that the U.S. Surgeon General issued a report on mental health, culture, race, and ethnicity, stressing the importance of culture in the availability, delivery, and perceived benefits of mental health services. The report concludes that "although effective, well-documented treatments for mental illnesses are available, racial and ethnic minorities are less likely to receive quality care than the general population." A critical consequence of this disparity, according to the report, is that "racial and ethnic minority communities bear a disproportionately high burden of disability from untreated or inadequately treated mental health problems and mental illnesses" (U.S. Department of Health and Human Services, 2001). In order to achieve the aim of the report that "effective treatments for mental illnesses need to benefit every American of every race, ethnicity, and culture" (p. 1), the field needs to ensure that all family practitioners are culturally competent (Ariel, 1999; Hardy & Laszloffy, 1992; Rigazio-DiGilio et al., 1997).

Family therapy has a long history of investigating and documenting how services can be modified to fit within the cultural and social milieu of diverse ethnic groups (Ariel, 1999; Arnold, 2002; Ho, Rasheed, & Rasheed, 2004; McGoldrick, 2002; Okun, 1996). Network therapy used with members of Native American families as reported by Attneave (1969), Speck and Attneave (1973), and Red Horse (1980, 1982) outlines clinical strategies to use when working with members of First Nations Peoples (Yellow Bird, 2001). Family treatment with African Americans has been described by numerous authors, notably Boyd-Franklin (2003), Hines (1989), Cheatham and Stewart (1990), Asante (2003), Karenga (1996), and Pinderhughes (1989). Theories and models of working with Latino families can be found in the works of Garcia-Preto (1996), Flores and Carey (2000), Falicov (1998), Santiago-Rivera, Arredondo, and Gallardo-Cooper (2002), and Morales (1996). Family therapy approaches that have been successful with Asian and Pacific Islander Americans are reported by Hong and Ham (1992), Sluzki (1979), Lee (1997), and Ho and Settles (1984). Beyond the vast resources for providing marriage and family counseling and therapy to members of diverse ethnic groups, approaches to use when working with gay and lesbian families (Morales, 1996; Scrivner & Eldridge, 1995), physical and terminal illness (Campbell & Patterson, 1995; Rolland, 1994; Wood, 1995) and blended families (Visher, 1996) are also well documented. As is evident, family therapy has successfully been used with a wide variety of diverse groups and will be considered the optimal treatment modality for many of the emerging social and cultural issues arising in the United States and abroad.

Family Therapy: Blind Spots, Limitations, and Challenges

Each of the traditional and contemporary family therapies has its blind spots, limitations, and challenges. First, we consider those of the first three models within the traditional group of therapies; then we look at the contemporary models and approaches to family therapy.

Psychodynamic/Historical Approaches

Although psychodynamic/historical treatment methods maintain a focus on the intergenerational family patterns, they do not account for the contextual environment of the family. For instance, issues related to social class, ethnicity or race, and culture are minimized, and therefore, consequences of classism, racism, or sustained discrimination are not acknowledged. Further, developmental patterns are based on a two-parent family structure, which is not always the case in many groups. Psychodynamic/ historical approaches that emphasize self-disclosure and differentiation of the self might be counterproductive when working with families who hold different values about family loyalty and verbal expressiveness, such as members of Asian-American, First Nations Peoples, and Hispanic ethnic groups. The distant and clinical position of the therapist may also be inconsistent with certain minority groups' social framework and environmental perspective. Perceived resistance to therapy may have more to do with a mismatch of therapeutic intervention and a family's values than with avoiding treatment.

Multicultural considerations could guide therapists practicing from psychodynamic/historic approaches to pay attention to intergenerational, cultural, and community history. For example, in relation to the Olsen family, it might be helpful to consider how expectations around connection and parent-child relationships might differ between Oscar and Ina based on nations of origin and gender. Ina's immigration history may be highly relevant to intergenerational family connections. The fact that the fishing industry has become increasingly limited as natural resources dwindle over time and government regulations tighten might be relevant to the level of stress felt throughout the community.

Cognitive-Behavioral/Interactional Approaches

In general, these approaches to family therapy focus on the present and may communicate that the past is not important. This position may not be effective with members of cultural groups who assume a more holistic perspective of time. Because dependency is challenged, some members of Asian-American,

First Nations Peoples, Italian-American, and other cultural groups that ascribe to more communal family structures might reject such direct interventions to align hierarchies and redistribute family roles.

From a multicultural perspective, therapists using cognitive-behavioral/ interactional approaches would also be considering larger system interactions, including the structure of the community. Regarding the Olsen family, the therapist might ask about where Rita goes when she runs away and what the relationships are like between the parents of Rita's friends. The therapist might consider Ina's relationship with Oscar's extended family and her experience as an outsider within a close-knit community. The therapist is likely to find that seasonal changes in family structure are common in fishing communities and help the family access others for support during these transitions.

Existential-Humanistic Approaches

The limitation of existential-humanistic approaches is that they tend to focus on individual expression and the pursuit of freedom. Some clients, especially those whose families have suffered through social oppression and sustained discrimination, may not feel they have much choice because of their environmental circumstances. Many times clients seek therapy for specific direction, and reflecting on freedom of choice and the importance of meaning may create frustration and misunderstanding. The lack of direction in terms of specificity and the concept of individual responsibility may not be consistent with the worldview of many clients from African-American, Asian-American, Italian-American, and Hispanic ethnic groups.

From a multicultural perspective, existential-humanistic therapists would also be paying attention to the level of ease and comfort the Olsen family demonstrates around sharing emotion openly, connecting this to cultural heritage, gender, and community norms. The therapist would need to check her own assumptions about the value of emotional expression so as not to inadvertently interpret the family's reluctance to share emotion as necessarily blocking potential growth. The therapist might find that other cultural and family values conflict with values embedded in an experiential model, such as practicality over spontaneity.

Contemporary Approaches

Contemporary models may be rejected by clients who hold very traditional worldviews and would resist critically analyzing their situation from a variety of perspectives. Issues of power and language may not be salient to many families. Clients who are not comfortable working from a multiperspective orientation may experience frustration as therapists work to open new possibilities within their worldview. Understanding the power of words may not be viewed as important by some clients. As with all the approaches to family therapy described thus far, caution needs to be exercised when using contemporary techniques with particular clients to ensure a cultural and contextual fit that benefits the client. When clients signal that interventions are not working, therapists need to consider alternative strategies that are more consistent with the families' values and environmental circumstances.

Future Development: Family Therapy in a Diverse World

Theoretical research and practice models continue to evolve to meet the changing stressors families are, and will be, dealing with in the first half of the 21st century. Societal trends such as human rights, globalization, the pursuit of self-determination and liberation, and the reduction of domestic, community, and international terrorism and violence will stress family structure and functioning in new ways. It is from the exchange of ideas across disciplines—from philosophy, anthropology, social work, and psychiatry to psychology, mental health counseling, school counseling, and family therapy—that new methods will emerge for working with families and their communities. New models for working together at all levels of the mental health field will accelerate progress toward this goal.

Specifically, some changes that will advance these efforts are to begin determining the quality of effective treatment not merely by the removal of family symptomatic behavior but also by demonstrating consideration of cultural diversity, gender equity, and social justice. We need to continue to explore ways

> to develop knowledge capable of addressing the most serious problems faced by families and larger systems today—poverty, racism, lack of adequate resources, radical changes in the world of work, coping with life in the information society, addictions, serious illness, abuse, trauma, terror, and the critical need for community and families not just to survive, but to thrive. (Imber-Black, 2004, p. 2)

This disposition needs to be based on an international perspective, which validates that we are all members of the human species (Rohner, 2004) regardless of national or ethnic background. Effective tools to assess and intervene at the many levels of family life are needed. This will require an expanded research agenda that examines what works to help individuals and families adjust to their environments, and identifies efficient, cost-effective, and culturally appropriate strategies that address and reduce the aggregate level of stressors in a community. New research and expanded professional goals will change the image of the family therapist to include advocacy for community and policy change, and an emphasis on cultural-political assessment and interventions. As the needs of families change in the postindustrial era, so must the vision and role of the family practitioner. In order for the field to grow over the next 50 years, we need family professionals at all levels who are capable of listening to, and helping to resolve, the issues contemporary families are facing in our ever-diversifying global society.

Summary

1. Beginning in the 1950s, pioneers in family therapy viewed themselves as shifting away from traditional individually oriented treatments toward alternative approaches that relied on systems theory and included all members of the family in the same treatment room working with one clinician. From this systemic perspective, the family is viewed as the primary unit and all members of the family are important contributors to clients' psychological functioning and development.

2. The hallmark of family therapy has been an understanding of the individual in relation to others. Rather than viewing problems as existing within the individual, family therapists have focused their analysis and interventions on relationships within and among individuals, families, and communities.

3. During the early years of family therapy, six foundational models dominated the field. Generally these models embodied European-American male perspectives about normal or healthy family functioning. The basic assumptions and strategies associated with these original models have undergone a series of reevaluations from numerous perspectives, including feminism (which accused the predominant forms of family therapy of minimizing the role of gender, power, and privilege), multiculturalism (which helped the field take a broader look at the social and cultural influences experienced by clients and therapists), social constructionism (which looked at the constructions humans use to view their world and caused family therapists to reexamine their beliefs in the one ideal family structure and to consider multiple images of productive family life), and evidence-based practice (which focused on treatment efficacy and client outcomes and demanded that family therapy be applied in consistent treatment protocols).

4. Family therapy initially developed in the post–World War II context of large-scale social and cultural changes that increased the need for treating families, not just individuals, and in the context of a cultural focus on the nuclear family rather than the extended family. Contemporary family therapy models and approaches developed in the context of instantaneous

worldwide communication, technological advances, and the infusion of racially, culturally, and ethnically diverse individuals, partners, and families.

5. All family therapists view families as systems and understand the unique nuances of client families by exploring family development (for instance, issues related to family bonding), family structure (the variety of family constellations within families), family culture (rituals, beliefs, values, and customs, as well as the ethnic, social, political, religious, educational, and professional communities with which the family identifies), and family functioning (the relative stability and adaptability of families).

6. The traditional approaches to family therapy include the psychodynamic/ historical approach (which emphasizes intrapsychic and intergenerational phenomena), the cognitive-behavioral/interactional approach (which focuses on effective learning processes that expand organizational structures, communication, and interactional processes), and the existential-humanistic approach (which concentrates on current interactional contexts and processes).

7. Rather than rejecting the traditional approaches, contemporary approaches integrate concerns about power, culture, and context with the fundamental concepts of family systems theory. These contemporary approaches advocate recognizing multiple perspectives and realities, not pathologizing clients, and carefully considering all thoughts, behaviors, and interactions within a social context. The approaches include postmodern approaches (which seek to establish collaborative, co-constructive relationships with the family client systems), ecological approaches (in which elements of a client's wider ecology such as immediate and extended family, associates, and historical/ sociocultural/political contexts, are explored), and integrative approaches (which offer frameworks to help clinicians organize theories, therapies, and strategies into broader models of practice).

8. Systemic cognitive developmental therapy (SCDT) is a holistic, nonpatho-logical, and integrative approach to family and wider systems treatment that links developmental and social constructivist constructs to the therapy process and offers both specific assessment and treatment strategies and an integrative framework clinicians can draw on to tailor treatment to specific family needs.

9. Family therapy has provided an effective and alternative treatment setting and modality for working with a wide range of individual, family, and community stressors, diseases, and disorders.

10. Blind spots, limitations, and challenges regarding the traditional family therapy approaches include insufficient focus on multicultural con-cerns (psychodynamic/historical, cognitive-behavioral/interactional, and

existential-humanist), lack of focus on the contextual environment of the family (psychodynamic/historical), potentially culturally inappropriate emphasis on self-disclosure (psychodynamic/historical), potentially culturally inappropriate lack of focus on the past (cognitive-behavioral/interactional), and potentially culturally inappropriate focus on individual expression and the pursuit of freedom (existential-humanist).

11. Contemporary family therapy approaches may experience blind spots, limitations, and challenges insofar as they may be rejected by clients who hold very traditional worldviews and resist critically analyzing their situation from a variety of perspectives.

12. Societal trends such as human rights, globalization, the pursuit of self-determination and liberation, and the reduction of domestic, community, and international terrorism and violence will stress family structure and functioning in new ways.

Key Terms

boundaries (p. 451)
community genogram (p. 469)
differentiation of self (p. 457)
enactments (p. 464)
extended family (p. 447)
family genogram (p. 460)
family map (p. 462)

family sculpting (p. 466)
family structure (p. 445)
feedback loops (p. 451)
nuclear family (p. 447)
reframe (p. 462)
subsystems (p. 462)
triangulation (p. 458)

Resources for Further Study

Professional Organizations

American Association for Marriage and Family Therapy (AAMFT)
112 South Alfred St.
Alexandria, VA 22314-3061
703-838-9808
www.aamft.org

American Psychological Association, Division 43 (Family Psychology)
750 First Street NE
Washington, DC 20002-4242
202-336-5500
www.apa.org/divisions/div43/

American Family Therapy Academy, Inc. (AFTA)
1608 20th Street NW, 4th Floor
Washington, DC 20009
202-483-8001
www.afta.org/

International Family Therapy Association (IFTA, part of AFTA)
c/o Marriage & Family Counseling Service
Safety Building, Room 512
Rock Island, IL 61201
309-786-4491
www.ifta-familytherapy.org/home.html

Professional Journals

Journal of Marital and Family Therapy (primary journal of the AAMFT)
Nova Southeastern University
3301 College Ave.
Ft. Lauderdale, FL 33314
954-262-5398

Journal of Family Psychology (journal of APA Division 43)
(Same mailing address, phone number, and web address as APA)

Journal of Family Psychotherapy (journal of IFTA)
The Haworth Press, Inc.
10 Alice St.
Binghamton, NY 13904
800-429-6784

Suggested Readings

McGoldrick, M. (Ed.). (2002). *Re-visioning family therapy: Race, culture, and gender in clinical practice.* New York: Guilford.

Many contemporary issues in family therapy relative to diversity, power, and privilege.

Ng, K. (Ed.). (2003). *Global perspectives in family therapy: Development, practice, trends.* New York: Brunner-Routledge.

An overview of the development of family therapy in more than a dozen countries, with international authors addressing family issues and practice in diverse cultural contexts.

Rastogi, M., & Weiling, E. (Eds.). (2004). *Voices of color: First person accounts of ethnic minority therapists.* Thousand Oaks, CA: Sage.

Professional and training experiences of therapists of Color are addressed.

Sexton, T., Weeks, G., & Robbins, M. (Eds.). (2003). *Handbook of family therapy.* New York: Brunner-Routledge.

Chapters by leaders in the field; an overview of the history and major family models as well the latest advances in multiculturalism, evidence-based practices, and cutting-edge approaches to therapy and supervision. If you don't want to read the entire handbook, we highly recommend the chapter by Celia Falicov (pp. 37–58), a leader in promoting and understanding family therapy practice from a multicultural perspective.

Other Media Resources

FamilyTherapyResources.net—a service of the AAMFT
(www.familytherapyresources.net/familytherapyresources/index.asp)

Psychotherapy Videos

Psychotherapy Net (http://psychotherapy.net/video/videoframe.html):
John T. Edwards, *Tools and techniques for family therapy.*
Harriet Lerner & Betty Carter, *The legacy of unresolved loss: A family systems approach.*
Monica McGoldrick, *The legacy of unresolved loss.*

IAMFC Family Counseling Videos (www.cmtipress.com/videos.htm):
Harry Aponte, *Structural therapy.*
Kenneth Hardy, *Culture sensitive couples therapy.*
Robert Smith & Patricia Stevens Smith, *Integrative family therapy.*
Marianne Walters, *Marianne Walters' feminist family therapy.*

Chapter 13

Narrative Therapy

KATHIE CROCKET

Problems are produced in the contexts of people's lives—that is, in the stories that shape their lives. The metaphor of story is the primary organizing idea in narrative counseling. Stories are understood to shape and form the world and to shape and form people's lives and identities, as we give meaning to the events of our lives. Our lives are shaped by cultural stories of gender, ethnicity, nationality, and class; by stories told in our families and communities; by stories of our own life experiences.

The central focus of narrative therapy is inquiry into the **dominant stories** that shape and form clients' lives and identities and that shape and produce the problems they encounter. A narrative counselor explores with a client how a problem story has taken on meaning and thus shaped that person's life, that person's identity. As well as exploring the problem story and its effects, narrative counselors listen for **alternative stories,** storylines from clients' lives that go beyond the terms of the problem story and that invite clients to explore other possibilities. The events and values that become alternative stories are already available in the client's own life but tend to lie scarcely noticed and neglected—that is, unstoried—in the face of powerfully shaping problem stories.

A quick example will show how this works in practice. Sue, a young woman, tells me that she has come to counseling to "stop being jealous." As a narrative counselor, I am interested in how this description of herself as jealous has come about in the context of Sue's life. I ask Sue some questions about the history of this description. How has it become meaningful in her life? Together we learn that Steve, Sue's male partner, suggested that Sue is jealous. He first made this claim when Sue objected to his spending "another night out with his friends." A story of Sue as jealous has become familiar to the couple as an explanation for disagreements about how they will each spend time. A story of Sue as jealous leads Sue to counseling to change *herself* for the benefit of the relationship.

I met this story of women as jealous a number of times in my practice at a university counseling service. It was not a story that Steve or Sue, or others I met, made up themselves. Rather, as a narrative counselor, I understand that Steve and Sue, and others, take up ideas circulating in the wider culture and use these ideas to make meaning of events in their own lives. A story of women as jealous is readily available to account for and resolve points of struggle in relationships—in this situation, struggle about how each partner spends her or his time.

A story of women as jealous has effects. For example, it works to require only Sue to change in response to the relationship disagreement. Stories are not neutral in their effects: when a story of young women as jealous is taken for granted, young men are apparently positioned more favorably than young women because the problem is located in the women and they must do the changing.

Through the kind of inquiry that will be described in this chapter, Sue and I investigate the jealousy story. We come to understand how Sue, Steve, and their relationship are affected by the jealousy story. As we explore, it becomes increasingly possible for Sue to evaluate how this story is shaping her life. The effects of a powerfully dominant patriarchal story of women as jealous are exposed as together we learn how the jealousy story is woven into the cultural fabric of gender relations.

On the terms of this larger story of gender, the problem is now located as a point of struggle in a heterosexual relationship. The problem is no longer located in Sue's person, in her gender, in her personality, or in her mental state. Stories other than the jealousy story become more available to make meaning of the objection to Steve's spending "another night out with his friends." Through our conversation, Sue speaks more clearly about her preferences for a relationship with Steve that is based on negotiation and gender equality, not simply on a change in her alone. Previously in the background, these alternative stories of negotiation and equality in relationships are now available to account for and respond to the relationship disagreement.

As well as illustrating how stories work to shape the meanings we make of events, and so to shape our lives, this example shows, in brief overview, how narrative practice works. Narrative practice researches with clients how problems have come to be produced in local and political contexts, how meanings have been made, what the effects of those meanings are, what people make of these effects, and how people might prefer things otherwise.

Narrative counseling is based on the premise that knowledge is contestable. Thus, the process of counseling is a collaborative inquiry into the knowledges carried by the stories that shape people's lives. These knowledges position people within relations of power. Narrative inquiry supports people to take positions to evaluate if the way things are meets their hopes and dreams and intentions for their own lives.

Perhaps there are stories in your own life that come to mind as you read about the shaping effect of stories? Your life will have been shaped by stories others told about you as you grew up, by stories of your family's life, by stories of success or stories of struggle, by stories that come from your cultural identity. Because you are likely to be reading this chapter as part of your education as a counselor, perhaps your life has been shaped by stories of compassion or by a concern for social justice.

There is a link between stories and the words with which stories are told. Narrative counselors carefully select the language forms they use in speaking about both people and problems. This careful selection arises out of the idea that words, like stories, are not neutral. Words do more than mirror reality; they shape and produce reality. If words form and shape the world and form and shape us as people, then speaking and writing become ethical actions (Drewery, 2005). The language we as counselors use and the stories we draw on to understand clients' lives shape the lives of those we speak with. For example, rather than describing a girl as a "troublemaker," a narrative counselor might speak of her as "getting caught up in trouble." The latter description separates the girl from the problem that has beset her and is thus less defining of her identity as a person. Concern for the responsibilities of the shaping effects of stories and language brings the ethics of relationship to the foreground of narrative practice.

This chapter will orient you to three important organizing ideas of narrative therapy and to some of the key practices based on them.

1. *The metaphor of story is central.* Problems are produced in the stories that shape people's lives. Narrative counselors take up a position of genuine inquiry and curiosity about the stories that shape clients' lives.

2. *The stories people call on and the language they use have real effects on their own and others' lives.* One implication of this idea is that we as counselors have a responsibility to consider the effects of the stories we draw on as we meet with clients. Professional stories—that is, our theories about people, problems, and change—are not neutral but shape the lives of the clients we meet.

3. *Counseling has the potential to replicate oppressive practices of the wider culture.* Cognizant of this possibility, counselors must avoid it by being responsible for the effects and the politics of their practices.

Origins and Evolution of Narrative Therapy

Narrative therapy was first articulated in Australia and New Zealand, by Michael White and David Epston. Although the ideas and practices out of which narrative therapy were generated are circulating in many places in the world, this chapter relates a story of this distinctive approach from my perspective in New Zealand.

In New Zealand and Australia in the 1980s, the field of family therapy was energized by the expression of passionate concerns for social justice. At that time these concerns were formulated in terms of gender and culture. Meeting in caucus groups organized by gender or culture was a central strategy employed at professional conferences and in some workplaces to explore and address practices of oppression within family therapy. Central contributors to these processes were workers at the Family Centre in Lower Hutt, New Zealand, whose groundbreaking work for a just approach to family therapy has gained international renown (Tamasese, Waldegrave, Tuhaka, & Campbell, 1998; Waldegrave, 1990). When poverty, or racism, or sexism is the problem, the responses of mainstream psychology are inadequate, the Family Centre team argued. They showed how mainstream psychologies individualized problems and located them inside people, thus giving individuals responsibility for problems not of their making. In 1985, in a landmark address to a national counseling conference, Maori academic and psychiatrist Mason Durie argued that the individualism, reductionism, and dualism foundation of Western therapy models was unhealthy for Maori (the indigenous people of New Zealand). He drew attention to alternative principles central to Maori understandings of well-being (1989), arguing that counseling must be reshaped to the needs of Maori people. At the same time, feminists in Australia and New Zealand (Drewery, 1990; Pilalis, 1987; Pilalis & Anderton, 1984), like feminists elsewhere in the world (e.g., Hare-Mustin, 1978), were critiquing the gendered assumptions of available therapy models and the ways in which therapy reproduced oppressive and sexist practices of the wider culture (Russell & Carey, 2003). Thus, the argument was clearly made, here in New Zealand, that counseling and therapy are indeed political and always potentially oppressive activities.

The limitations of available therapies were also being exposed and explored in other places in the world (see Gergen, 1985; Hare-Mustin, 1978). The potential for counseling and family therapy to reproduce the status quo, and so reproduce inequalities, was being noticed and challenged. New approaches to therapy that responded to some of these challenges began to emerge, especially among family therapists.

Particular to New Zealand was the Family Centre's ongoing development of *just therapy*, an approach that combines therapy with a wider social practice that includes advocacy and social research. Critical to this development was the use of caucuses formed on the basis of cultural identifications (Maori, Pasifika—people from the Pacific Islands—and Pakeha—descendents of New Zealand's original white colonizers). The caucus format opened space to bring forward into therapy cultural knowledges that might not otherwise have been available in a professional context. The result was that based on the concepts of belonging, sacredness, and liberation, the Family Centre developed an approach to therapy that incorporated a much richer expression of Maori and Pasifika worldviews (Waldegrave, 2000) than previously available Western models offered.

Through these years of focus on the politics of therapy, Michael White and David Epston were very active participants in family therapy communities in Australia and New Zealand and internationally. At the same time that the Family Centre was influencing therapy through the development of its unique cultural contribution, Michael and David each also offered his own unique innovative contributions to practice at the cutting edges of the family therapy tradition. Throughout the 1980s, they published and presented widely. Their ideas and practices drew on a broad spectrum of knowledge, including the family therapy tradition, feminism, anthropology, the poststructuralist work of Michel Foucault, critical theory (that body of social theory that aims to critique and transform), and literary theory (for ideas about text and interpretation) (White, 1995). The point to note is the breadth of ideas in which White and Epston were situating their work by the time they presented a substantial body of their own contributions to therapy collected in three books (Epston, 1989; White, 1989; White & Epston, 1989). Their coauthored *Literate Means to Therapeutic Ends* (1989) was republished in the United States in 1990 as *Narrative Means to Therapeutic Ends*. This appears to have been the point at which narrative therapy was named in this way. In response to the body of work published in 1989, Tomm (1989) in North America wrote: "Breaking new ground in any field is a major accomplishment. To do so in different directions at the same time, and in so doing, open up whole new territories, reflects a *tour de force*. In my opinion Michael White and David Epston are engaged in just this kind of trail-blazing for the field of family therapy" (p. 5).

Looking back to this time, it seems to me that the publication of this substantive body of work in 1989 was definitional in the evolution of the approaches that have come to be known collectively as *narrative therapy*. These publications told the story of practices that took seriously the politics of therapy because these practices worked on the basis of an understanding that problems and contexts are intertwined. They showed how alternatives to problems, alternative stories, might be shaped out of people's **local knowledges,** which are ideas that originate from people's own lived experiences in particular settings.

The central organizing metaphor for this practice was the story, and so the idea that stories shape people's lives was taken up for therapeutic purposes. The story, rather than a person's internal state, was the focus for the therapy. The *practice stories* (case studies) in these publications were rich with examples of the exquisite questioning skills that are a hallmark of narrative therapy (as you will see shortly).

Context Then—Context Now

Narrative therapy began within family therapy and in Australia and New Zealand. However, today it is widely used in work with individuals and communities as well as families and in other parts of the world including the United States (Freedman & Combs, 1996; Weingarten, 1998; Zimmerman & Dickerson, 1996), the United Kingdom (Payne, 2006), and South Africa (Kotzé & Kotzé, 2001). Indeed, narrative therapy is now widely enough known to be included in this counseling theory and practice textbook.

In particular, I have found significance in the contribution of feminist theorists and practitioners to the ongoing developments in narrative practice. Here in New Zealand, one of Johnella Bird's (1993, 2000, 2004) continuing contributions has been to show how therapists might practice in ways that expose and explore the working of gender relations. Kaethe Weingarten (1992, 1997, 2003) in the United States exemplifies the feminist praxis of building theory out of one's own life in her writing and practice. Kaethe's work in the areas of motherhood, intimacy, illness narratives, and, most recently, witnessing practices (practices that acknowledge self-in-community in relation with experiences of pain or violence) demonstrates both the politics of everyday actions and the politics of care in everyday actions.

Social justice movements of the 1970s and 1980s offered a clear call to therapists to listen to people whose lives were not described, or lived, in accordance with the terms of mainstream, taken-for-granted professional knowledge. Narrative therapists continue to work with this alternative focus. However, while having a commitment to justice, narrative counselors do not position themselves as liberators who already have certainty about what justice or a better life looks like for others. Rather, a narrative counselor engages in **coresearch** with a client, a collaborative conversational inquiry with the purpose of researching a client's lived experience to generate knowledges previously available to neither party. In this way, a counselor contributes to "an exploration of the possibilities, limitations and possible dangers associated with how things are and with how they are becoming other than what they were" (White, 2000, p. 113) in a particular situation. The emphasis on coresearching local knowledges provides for a "socially and politically sensitive practice" (White, 2000, p. 113) that invites clients to take up authority with respect to their own lives. Narrative counselors work from an *attitude of genuine curiosity* about the lived experiences and knowledges of those who consult them as they *learn with and from clients*. This posture is out of step with the current professional context of managed care and with the standardizing effect of evidence-based practice, for example. Narrative therapists are not alone in being out of step with and critiquing these kinds of universalizing movements, policies, and practices. There is rich scholarly material that exposes the potential and actual oppressions that these kinds of policies and practices enact. Examples of these scholarly ideas are feminist theory and psychology, critical theory in general and critical psychology in particular, and postcolonial theory (critical study of the relations between Eurocentric cultures and colonized societies). Narrative therapists should be familiar with such perspectives so they can work to avoid replication of oppression in their practices. "As narrative therapists, we are ever charged with the exploration of practices that might further contribute to the exposé of the relations of power in our work. It is this scrutiny of our work that makes it possible for us to assume an ethical responsibility for the real effects of this work" (White, 1997, p. 233) in shaping people's lives.

The Author's Journey as a Narrative Therapist

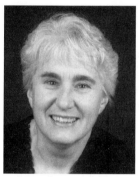

Kathie Crocket

How does one explain where one's journey towards narrative therapy began? Perhaps mine began as my early years were shaped by the care expressed in rural communities on the South Island of New Zealand, where I grew up. I remember these as communities where people pitched in to offer each other practical help—very different from the urban environment of Wellington, New Zealand's capital city, where I completed an undergraduate degree and professional education as a teacher. It was the early 1970s, a time of social change: students marched against the war in Vietnam and protested French nuclear testing in the Pacific; the second wave of feminism arrived; and young Maori, moderate and radical, asserted their Maori identity.

I became a teacher in a small-town community where I found both conservative and activist values around me. I moved between the two. It was here that our children were born, and, like other mothers at home with young children, I expressed care for others in my community by baking cakes, cooking meals, and caring for children. I also attended, organized, and led community education events, and I continued university study. I still experience the shaping effects of these learning experiences. Most significant, I learned a wider repertoire of care behaviors in the form of some counseling skills. This was another marker on my journey.

My formal counselor education was in a university program that taught Carkhuff's (1980) eclectic human resource development model. We were introduced to a wide range of therapies—neurolinguistic programming, transactional analysis, psychodrama, Gestalt therapy, psychodynamic therapy, family therapy, and reality therapy. I graduated with a grab-bag of possible techniques within an

(continued)

overall humanistic orientation. My ongoing professional education continued to add to the eclectic mix.

My professional life was also significantly shaped by the ethos of the vocational guidance service in which I worked for four years as a careers counselor. That service offered staff opportunities to grapple with the challenges of working with Maori in culturally appropriate ways, for those were the clients who came off worst in a time of economic restructuring and high unemployment. While opportunities for bicultural education were ongoing, this was also a time when the appropriateness of Pakeha (my cultural identity) working with Maori was questioned.

It was some years, and many detours, later that perhaps the most significant event in my journey as a narrative therapist took place. It was the early 1990s and I was working as a counselor in a university counseling service. Much of my work was with women from a range of cultural groups but mostly Pakeha, in the areas of eating disorders, sexual abuse, and relationships. The opportunity to learn more about eating disorders practice led me to a workshop with David Epston that was my first serious encounter with narrative therapy. Narrative therapy may still have been in its early stages of development, but the coherence and sophistication of the practice I witnessed was compelling. David demonstrated the exquisite questioning skills and the politics of narrative practice using videos of his work. He drew attention to the fine detail of the progression of the questions he was asking, an approach quite different from that of the traditional therapies with which I was familiar.

In meticulous question after meticulous question, David worked with clients to ease the hold of the eating disorder on their lives. David asked questions such as these: "Can I just ask you why you think it is that anorexia tricks people into going to their death thinking they are fine? Why do you think that is?" (Maisel, Epston, & Borden, 2004, p. 101), and, "Amy, do you think anorexia's real intention is to separate women's minds and spirits from their bodies, and separate you from your mind and spirit?" (p. 209). These questions are examples of a narrative practice called an **externalizing conversation:** the problem, in this case anorexia, is conceptualized and named as *external* to the person and portrayed as a malign force by which a person is tricked, tortured, or imprisoned. David's questions and women's responses each contributed to building an account that exposed the conditions that had made it possible for the eating disorder to take over the women's lives.

Here we see the politics of narrative practice: these questioning approaches are informed by an understanding that eating disorders arise out of the focus of Western cultures on women's appearance and on the promotion of thinness. The purpose of David's questions was to disturb the taken-for-granted cultural stories that link success and approval with thinness and thus render young women vulnerable to eating disorders (Maisel et al., 2004).

At this point, I want to leave the story of my journey to become a narrative therapist and briefly return to the organizing ideas of narrative therapy with which I began the chapter.

1. In the example from Epston's workshop, we see therapeutic use being made of the idea that our lives are shaped by stories. A cultural story that links thinness with success and approval shapes women's lives. David's questions worked to unravel with clients how this story was shaping their lives, and so how anorexia was working in their lives.

2. It is a political action to think about the problem of eating disorders as located in the social world rather than in the pathology of the individual person. This conceptualization offers the person different options for action in the world than an understanding that pathologizes individuals.

3. David takes political action in *naming* the problem as anorexia and in focusing his questions on the investigation of *anorexia as the problem*. The person is not the problem. Clearly, how we use language has real effects on people's lives.

David's workshop had a real effect on my life. To think in terms of links between eating disorders and patriarchal culture was not new for me. But the workshop showed me *practices* that used this idea effectively. The fine detail of narrative questioning practices invites clients to explore and evaluate how culture works in their lives.

The next steps in my own practice were in part supported by the generosity of David's sharing of the archives of an informal anti-anorexia/anti-bulimia league he had organized in New Zealand (Maisel et al., 2004). These archives recorded the **insider knowledges**—that is, the knowledges of those with firsthand experience of problems, in this case the women with whom David worked as they struggled to win back their lives from eating disorders. These archives provided an important link between the workshop, the young women I was working alongside, and my own ongoing learning.

I found the stories of practice and of the changes in people's lives that I read in the three available narrative therapy books (Epston, 1989; White, 1989; White & Epston, 1989) inspiring. Those stories supported me in my practice as I experimented with externalizing conversations that separated people from the problems that beset them. Further workshops with David were opportunities to listen and absorb the practices of narrative questioning and to notice how particular

(*continued*)

questions worked to research local knowledges. As a practitioner trained to offer empathic statements of understanding and not to ask questions, I found this shift in orientation to be substantial. Taping my conversations with clients and reviewing them myself or with my narrative supervisor helped me learn. I came to see more clearly the substance of the transformation narrative practice offered. These were not another set of techniques that might be employed, drawn on to suit a moment or a person, under the umbrella of an eclectic model. Narrative practice depended on quite a different theory than I was familiar with from my study and practice of mainstream counseling approaches. It was grounded in **social constructionism,** the theory that reality is constructed through interactions among and between people and systems of knowledge, as we give meaning to events in the world (Burr, 2003).

By the mid-1990s, my practice had slipped sideways, off its humanistic foundations and into a different landscape of ideas. In this landscape, the focus was on the social world in which meanings are made, in which identity is taken up, and in which problems are produced. As I began using externalizing conversations that coresearched the cultural stories that shaped the lives of those who consulted with me, I saw how clients then used our inquiries to take up authority in living their lives. The effectiveness of the practice was visible in the stories clients told of themselves and their lives.

My move into narrative practice was supported when I became a member of the counselor education team at the University of Waikato in 1993, at the time when the program was also shifting from eclecticism towards a narrative orientation (Monk & Drewery, 1994). Thus, with my colleagues, with counseling program students, and alongside clients in my counseling practice, I worked at further understanding and exploring practice possibilities of the narrative metaphor. For the first time, I was finding ways to satisfactorily theorize my practice and practice my theories.

My present commitment is to a practice that arises out of the narrative metaphor and social constructionist ideas. It is on these terms that other aspects of my professional history are woven into the fabric of my practice. I am not a copy of some other narrative therapist. Rather, I craft my work out of the knowledges available among narrative counselors and social constructionist theorists and out of the experiences and knowledges of my personal and professional life. I make this point to emphasize that there are many styles of narrative practice. Although Michael White and David Epston pioneered this work together, each of them continues to produce a unique practice. I listen carefully to the distinctions others draw in describing their practices; they help me to go about my own work more thoughtfully and purposefully, asking what their ideas might mean for my practice.

Theory of Narrative Therapy

The narrative metaphor suggests that people come to understand themselves and the world through the stories about self and the world that are available to them in their particular cultural context. We inhabit the stories of our culture and make them our own. The narrative metaphor also suggests that we are not passively living out given stories, but actively weaving our lives into the stories currently available to us. Thus, a young woman might actively weave her life into the cultural stories that link slimness and success, and a middle-aged man who has faced several job layoffs might story his life on the terms of a cultural story of failure. As we make stories our own, we contribute to their gaining further authority not only in our own lives but also in the wider culture.

A more theoretical way to talk about cultural stories is to use the term *discourse*. A **discourse** is a metanarrative that tells us how things are in our world and makes particular social processes possible. "Discourse refers to the connection between statements and the prevailing social and power relations in which they are either uttered or silenced" (Law, 1999, p. 117). For example, the terms of gender discourse make it possible to speak of Sue as "jealous" or make it possible for an 85-pound woman to experience her body as fat. As women shape their bodies according to cultural norms, they are said to be engaging in *discursive practices*—that is, in the actions, including speaking, that particular discourses make available. To write a résumé or attend a job interview is to engage in discursive practices of an economic and employment discourse. As a student reading this book, you are engaging in the discursive practices of education, as I am as a teacher writing this chapter.

Social constructionism is the strand of social theory that offers these ideas (Burr, 2003). In a seminal article on social constructionism in psychology, Kenneth Gergen (1985) said that "knowledge is not something people possess, somewhere in their heads, but rather something people *do* together" (p. 270, emphasis added). Narrative therapy makes use of this idea—that people together are shaped by *and* shape the knowledges that circulate in a culture at any particular time. You have seen this idea in the accounts of therapy in this book: times in history, places, and people's personal histories produce particular counseling theories. Narrative therapy is a therapy of postmodern times, shaped by particular people and their interests, and by the concerns and the wider philosophical environment of the time.

Philosophical Foundations

Postmodern ideas are threaded through a range of disciplines; you may have met them in fine arts, theater, literature, architecture, cultural studies, anthropology, gender studies, or sociology, for example. Narrative therapy is situated among diverse but affiliated strands of postmodern social theory. Common to various strands of postmodern theory is the suggestion that claims about knowledge depend upon context. On postmodern terms, knowledge is understood to be subjective, situated, multiple, contested and negotiated, and fragmented; this is in contrast with modernism's emphasis on the search for knowledge as objective, certain, and universally true. Furthermore, the making of knowledge claims is understood not to be neutral, but to have real effects in the world, which include political effects. "Postmodernism suspects all truth claims of masking and serving particular interests in local, cultural and political struggles" (Richardson & St. Pierre, 2005, p. 961).

Among postmodern philosophers, the most significant to narrative therapy has been the French intellectual, Michel Foucault. Michael White (1989; White & Epston, 1989) transported Foucault's analysis of modern systems of power into narrative therapy, showing how—according to Foucault's analysis of the institutions and professional disciplines (e.g., hospitals, prisons, psychological science) of the modern world—people are recruited into "active participation in the fashioning of their own lives, their relationships, and their identities, according to the constructed norms of the culture" (White, 2004, p. 154).

Theoretical Concepts

Clients frequently ask counselors, "Am I normal?" This question rests on the idea that there are universal norms of healthy functioning. Such universal norms are carried in the stories, and the practices those stories produce, that are dominant in one's culture. These metanarratives are known in social constructionist theory as **dominant discourses.** Dominant discourses describe and specify, on the terms of the dominant institutions and disciplines of the culture, universal norms for what is correct and healthy—and normal! Dominant discourses are often so taken for granted that they go without question; people take them up and live their lives on their terms. For example, in many cultures a dominant discourse of family offers the idea that two-parent families produce healthier children than other family forms; this long-established idea continues to hold currency and have real effects on how people live their lives, despite its being contested over recent years (e.g., Baker, 2001). This is not to say that there is anything wrong with the idea that children are well served by two-parent families. However, problems arise when ideas like this exclude and penalize those whose lives do not conform to what becomes a normative prescription.

Michael White has shown the potential for therapists to get caught up, just as clients are, in the truth claims of normative cultural stories, including stories that carry expert psychological knowledges. Practices of **normalizing judgment** would then have counselors and others acting upon people to fit them into norms prescribed on the terms of expert knowledges or on the terms of other dominant discourses. I would have done this with Sue had I not engaged in a kind of **discursive listening** (listening for the discourses at work shaping a person's story) and had I unquestioningly supported the dominant discourses in Sue's initial quest to find ways to be "less jealous." From a narrative perspective, traditional approaches to teaching clients social skills, assertiveness skills, or parenting skills also put counselors at risk for acting in ways that fit people to prescribed norms. The practice section of this chapter shows how a narrative therapist might work to generate approaches to parenting in conversation with a mother. This generative conversation is preferable to imposing a standardized set of parenting skills that come out of a particular worldview that may not fit a particular mother's family, culture, or situation or that may further obscure available knowledges within her own lived experience.

Woven into the fabric of narrative practice are postmodern ideas about power. "We should talk about discourse and power in the same breath," suggested Parker (1991, p. 18). This way of seeing things suggests that power is implicit in all our everyday interactions, in the stories by which we live our lives. Power is understood to be always circulating, in conversations and in stories and so in our lives. Bronwyn Davies (2000) put it this way: "Power is not a thing or essence that can be described, but a complex set of relations amongst people, and in the relations between people and knowledge systems—or patterns of discourse" (p. 18). Narrative therapy makes use of this idea in its investigation of the interrelationships between people's everyday interactions and the knowledge systems of our culture. As people engage with knowledge systems and each other, some storylines are more accessible than others because of history, culture, gender, embodiment, and the other discursive resources on which we have to call.

This point leads us back to the basic idea that the stories that make up our lives are not neutral; some stories get to have more authority in shaping the world and so in shaping lives than others. Within any story, some positions offer speakers more authority than other positions. In a school, for example, the stories told by adults are likely to carry more authority than the stories told by children. For instance, if a child wants to tell a teacher about an injury she received and the teacher greets her with, "Are you going to tell tales?" there is little space available for the child's version of things, the child's story, to be told. In a university, a professor's version of a story is likely to carry more weight than a student's, but, of course, there will be many intersecting stories positioning both people. Perhaps the professor is younger than the student or is struggling with ill health while the student is on the university baseball team; or perhaps the professor is an African-American heterosexual man and the student a White bisexual woman. Stories of normality, gender, sexual orientation, disability, race, cultural identity, and class are all powerfully shaping of lives and relationships. Narrative therapy takes this point seriously: people do not have equal access to any position in any story. Particular stories offer some people more favorable positions than are offered to others. A story of a person caught in the act of committing a crime offers the person less favorable positions than it offers the apprehending police officer, for example. Narrative counseling conversations inquire about and evaluate the effects for a client of the positions a particular story offers, what the client thinks about this situation, and what the client prefers for her or his life.

Practice of Narrative Therapy

In this section I will first introduce some key narrative therapy practices and then illustrate their application in a detailed practice story.

Externalizing Conversations

The idea that people are not problems is played out in practice through the use of externalizing conversations (White, 1989; White & Epston, 1989). In fostering an externalizing conversation, a narrative therapist listens with care to the language that a client is using. However, in responding, the therapist restates what the client has said using **externalizing language,** particular grammatical forms that create a space between the person and the problem. In the following practice story, you will see how externalizing language is used.

The client, Bill, is a 46-year-old African-American man who lost his job as the manager of a supermarket where he had worked for 28 years. After a few months of fruitless job hunting, he suddenly left his wife and four children, ages 10 to 16. Now, a year later, he has a new job, and he wants to come home. His wife has said that she will only accept him back if he agrees to see a counselor who might help him "grow up." This is Bill's second meeting with Adella, a Puerto Rican-American female counselor who has done postgraduate work in narrative therapy.

> *Bill:* I am so disappointed that I was weak and ran away.
>
> *Adella:* What disappoints you, Bill, about the running away?
>
> *Bill:* Well, it looks as though I don't care.

This example demonstrates how a narrative therapist invites a client to take a position in relation with a problem, rather than to assume the problem is located in an internal deficit, in this situation that Bill is weak. The "running away" is the problem, and Bill can take a position in relation with the running away.

Curiosity and Meaning Making

By asking Bill about the disappointment about the running away, Adella brings forward an account of what the disappointment means for Bill rather than assuming that she knows what he means or that they have a shared understanding. Assumptions on her part would exclude from their conversation the possibilities available for the rich storying of the events of Bill's life and the meanings of those events for him. Adella's response is an example of **curious questioning** (McKenzie & Monk, 1997), a narrative therapy technique that consists of asking questions that offer genuine curiosity and are open to learning from clients about the particular knowledges available from clients' lived experience within their particular cultural contexts. The questioning responds very closely to what the person has just said as the therapist and client co-research the influence the problem has on the person and the person has on the problem.

Curious questioning might be informed by what the counselor knows of the wider discursive context. In this situation, Adella knows something about the political context that affects Bill. As devastating as it is for any middle-aged man supporting a family to get laid off, the disadvantage men from minority cultures experience in the labor market implies that it can be even worse for an African-American man in the United States. However, Adella is careful to hold tentatively what she knows and to inquire with curious questions about the specifics of Bill's lived experiences.

Problem Stories and Alternative Stories

At the simplest level, a problem story is told on the problem's terms. As Bill begins his story, for example, running away is evidence that he is weak and that he doesn't care. Or we might imagine a teacher saying to Peta, a school counselor, "That boy Sione is nothing but a troublemaker." A problem story tends to obscure its dependence upon normalizing judgments that pathologize people, their experiences, and their unique ways of living. An alternative story is one that is told on the terms the person prefers as an account of his or her life rather than on terms of the problem story or the dominant discourse (White, 1989). For instance, as Bill's experience is further explored, he might say, "I care very deeply for what has happened to my family, and I wanted to tell them that. However, I left because I didn't want my pain to make things worse for all of them when they were already suffering so much." From a story of Bill as weak, there is the possibility of a story of Bill as a man who cares and who intends to act thoughtfully. An alternative story might also be called a *counterstory*, made up by events that produce a counterplot to that of the problem story.

There will always be the possibility of unearthing other events that counter a problem story. For example, inquiring about the times during the school day when trouble is more or less of a problem to Sione, Peta, the school counselor, might hear that Sione helped another student who was having difficulty with a computer in Technology class. This might be the first event from which a richer counterplot is storied, offering alternative descriptions of Sione and his life that fit better with his hopes for himself and his future.

The Intentions of Inquiry

How does a narrative therapist determine what to inquire about? Here are some guidelines, or steps, based on a map White (2005) offered to outline the scaffolding of inquiry into a problem story.

1. What is the problem that has brought this person to counseling? How might we speak about it in ways that both employ externalizing language and are close to this person's own description of his or her experience?

2. What is the history of this problem? What effects has it had in various areas of this person's life?

3. What does this person make of all this? What is the person's evaluation of how things stand in her or his life?

4. How did the person come to be making this evaluation? What values or commitments stand behind the evaluation?

These questions lead us into richer inquiry about an alternative story, as clients tell us about what they value in their lives. Michael White (2005) suggests a similarly scaffolded approach to inquiry about an alternative story.

1. How does the person prefer to speak about this exception to the problem, or alternative practice, or other way of looking at or going about things?

2. What are the already known effects of this exception or alternative? What other effects might be possible?

3. What does the person make of all this?

4. How does the person come to be making this evaluation?

Counseling is rarely linear in the way a map like this suggests, but rather might interweave these scaffolded steps. The detailed practice story that follows shortly illustrates more of this second phase of the map.

Thin and Thick Descriptions

The concepts of *thin* and *thick descriptions* comes from anthropology (Morgan, 2000; White 1997, p. 15). **Thin descriptions** of people's lives are on the terms of the dominant discourse and exclude the interpretation of the people themselves or of their own community of support. The description of Sue as "jealous" was thin, as was the description of Bill as "weak" and Sione as "a troublemaker." In contrast, **thick descriptions** (or rich descriptions) come from the interpretation of the people whose lives are being described and carry the meanings of their own communities. The type of carefully scaffolded inquiry described earlier is the structure and process of moving from thin to thick descriptions. A richly storied account of one's life and relationships produces more options for ongoing action in the world.

Absent but Implicit

Often people's hopes and intentions and purposes for their lives, or indeed any other possibilities, are obscured by the dominance of a problem story. Narrative counselors employ a kind of radical listening that hears a possible duality in what appears at first to be a singular description (White, 2000, p. 36). They are listening for what is **absent but implicit**—that which is not spoken but is the "other side" of what is spoken. For example, the other side of disappointment is that which is hoped for. Here is an example from the conversation between Bill, the man who left his family, and his counselor, Adella.

> *Bill:* I am so disappointed that I was weak and ran away.

Not named in the problem story but implicit in the disappointment is that which is on the "other side" of disappointment. What unnamed hopes does the disappointment speak to?

> *Adella:* Is there a response you would have preferred, Bill, that seems more fitting, less disappointing for you, than the running away now seems?

This question does not seek to make a plan for the future or to coach Bill in new behaviors. Rather, it asks about and offers room to describe the unrealized hopes that produced disappointment and the values that Bill holds that were contravened by the running away.

> *Bill:* I would have preferred to have just taken a deep breath and told myself I could handle it however painful it was.
>
> *Adella:* Bill, in preferring to have just taken a deep breath and to tell yourself you could handle it, what would you say you are standing for?
>
> *Bill:* I would want my family to know and to see that I care about what is happening for them. And that it is painful for me.

This way of responding, with curiosity, to what is absent but implicit, very quickly opens a space for Bill to speak of what he values. In this way, Bill is already speaking on the terms of an alternative story where a position of moral authority is available to him. In this position, Bill speaks of his hopes in relationship with others while acknowledging the pain of his experience.

Therapeutic Documents

Narrative therapists use therapeutic documents as interventions to record knowledges that are generated in counseling (Epston, 1998; White, 1995; White & Epston, 1989). These knowledges may be the ideas spoken as the problem is coresearched, or they may be ideas that contribute to the alternative story. A typical example of a therapeutic document is a letter the therapist writes to a client between sessions to record the client's account of the effects of a problem and the client's evaluation of those effects. The purpose of a letter might be to support the client, during the counseling, in her or his stand against the influence of a problem. Or the letter might ask further therapeutic questions. For a child, a counselor might prepare a certificate of achievement to show to others who might support a new reputation the child has accomplished (Epston, 1989; Morgan, 2000). David Epston reported that his informal research with clients suggested that a letter was worth "4.5 sessions of good therapy" (White, 2005, p. 200).

Marion was a client who taught me the benefits of re-presenting carefully recorded coresearch in a therapeutic letter (Winslade, Crocket, & Monk, 1997, pp. 70–71). Marion had come to counseling after she has been given a number of psychiatric diagnoses; she wanted me to tell her which was correct. Familiar with experiencing herself as "crazy" as an outcome of telling her story to mental health professionals, Marion was deeply moved by the letter I wrote after our first conversation. That letter recorded her story in ways that showed she had been listened to carefully, and most significant, she experienced it as confirming her sanity. The letter supported Marion in making sense of her life in ways that were acknowledging of her and the struggles she had encountered. How counselors represent clients' lives does matter: words written on a page have an enduring quality (Epston, 1998). The therapeutic letter I sent Marion witnessed the story of her life that we had coresearched. In reading the letter, Marion also got to witness her own life, and on terms other than those previously offered. There was now an alternative story of sanity into which Marion came to stitch her life, as she went on to explore further, in counseling, her hopes for her life and to complete an academic degree.

Therapeutic documents are produced with the agreement of clients, and those for wider circulation (to share with other clients or therapists in training or to use in publications) are produced with clients' consent. In addition to letters, therapeutic documents a counselor might use include declarations, handbooks, notes made in the session, videotapes, lists, and pictures (Morgan, 2000, p. 85).

Audience and Witnessing

Woven into narrative practice is the social constructionist idea that identity is social. The idea that our identities are produced and authenticated as others witness our lives is used to give substance to an alternative story. Narrative counselors might ask questions about present and past relationships with the intention of supporting clients to actively link their lives to the lives of others who share their values and commitments. Michael White calls these exchanges *re-membering conversations* (White, 1997, p. 23), conversations where we invite clients to select, into the membership of their lives, those with whom connection is enriching. For example, I might have asked Sue as she was protesting the effects of her jealousy story, "Who might stand alongside you in your hopes for a negotiated relationship?" The practice story of Maria in the next section illustrates some of the effects of a re-membering conversation, one that clearly links the client's values and hopes for her life with those of another member of her family.

At times, audiences are recruited as witnesses to the preferred developments in people's lives. **Witnessing** is the purposeful positioning of oneself, in relation with community, to hear and respond to another's expression or story.

As Peta, the school counselor, and Sione, her client, work together in support of Sione's achieving a reputation he prefers, together they might write and invite each of Sione's teachers to write a statement in witness to this new reputation. As a university counselor, at times I suggested that a student invite a friend to meet with us to witness the developments in the student's life. Alternatively, we invoked the imagined presence of someone in the student's life who might be a witness. Audiences of other counselors are sometimes recruited to witness; when I visit my counseling students in placement settings, I am available as an outsider witness (White, 2000) to their clients' lives.

The therapist takes responsibility for supporting the shaping of a witnessing response. Witnesses are asked to listen and respond with a purpose: to maximize the effects of knowing clients in relation to the stories they tell about themselves and others tell about them. The effect of this kind of witnessing is to further enrich preferred developments and thus alternative storylines for the client who is at the center of the consultation. At the same time, there is potential for all of the people who participate to become other than who they were, through witnessing practices as well as through engagement in therapeutic conversations (White, 2000).

Michael White uses the word **transport** to describe this movement, this becoming other than who we were (2004, p. 224). I think this word is beautifully evocative of the kinds of change that a storying approach produces: we are carried—by the stories we tell together, hear together, and witness together—into new possibilities for understanding self and the world, and thus for living.

A Counseling Conversation: Theory of Change in Action

The example that follows shows the development of an alternative story. You will notice how, as counselor, I pay careful attention to words, phrases, and sentences that might otherwise slip by. I am interested in them because they may be fragile threads of apparently neglected storylines in the life of the client, Maria. My responses are intended to explore the possibilities for us together to weave those threads into the fabric of a story of more substance that will be available to Maria in living her life.

The Context of the Counseling

Maria has come for counseling referred by Hera, a social worker with the New Zealand government agency that has statutory (legal) responsibility for the care and protection of children. The referral has come about because of concerns that the care and protection of Maria's two young children, Sam and Kara, is not adequate. Maria and Hera are both Maori. I am Pakeha. Hera has told me there are no Maori counselors available at this time. Maria says she just wants to get on with the counseling because she does not want to lose her kids.

On the statutory agency's terms, my purpose is to work with Maria to coach her in parenting skills and to report back to the agency on her progress. This report will form part of the agency's assessment of whether further intervention is needed to provide care for Maria's children. Also in this practice story is Maria's Pakeha partner, Joe. He comes and goes from Maria's home. Joe is not the children's father.

Starting Points in This Therapy Conversation: Ethics and Politics

Maria enters our second session complaining that Hera has been "giving me the hassle," and "getting on my case." Maria's objection to "the hassle" is palpable. As I listen, I think about the discursive context of our conversation, the discourses that shape our conversation. For example, I know that antagonism between mothers and statutory agency social workers is not unusual. The degrading effects of state scrutiny frequently produce either resistance or resignation in mothers. I thus identify the difficulty between Hera and Maria as produced by the wider discursive context. In doing so, I am enacting the belief that people are not problems: I see neither Hera nor Maria as the problem here.

At the same time, I take seriously the responsibility of adults to protect and care for children. I want to have a coresearching conversation with Maria about safe care for her children. As a narrative practitioner, my purpose is not to prescribe particular versions of motherhood or to teach particular parenting skills. Responding to what Maria says, I will ask questions to bring forward ideas and beliefs about, and practices of, mothering that will assist her and support her in providing safe care for Kara and Sam.

As we begin, I listen closely to what Maria is saying about her experiences of "the hassle" from Hera. Speaking at length, she concludes, "When it's not even me whose case she should be on. At least I'm not like Joe."

Selecting a Response: Listening for Storylines

I ask Maria, "When you say at least you're not like Joe, can you say some more about that?" I ask this question, not to focus blame on Joe, but because within Maria's statement, distinguishing between her and Joe, I hear echoes of the possibility of an alternative story about Maria and mothering.

"Well, like last night," Maria begins, "our basketball team was playing at dinner time, and I asked Joe to look after the kids while I played. I thought that would be okay. I wasn't away long. I gave him money to get the kids pizza. Anyway, I get home and he's used the money to buy them ice cream and candy and to buy himself beer and get one of his sleazy videos. He's drinking beer and watching his videos, and the kids are outside and it was freezing cold," she says with considerable emphasis. Then, almost under her breath, she adds, "Kids shouldn't have to put up with that."

Maria speaks first about what happened the previous night, about actions. Then she offers an evaluation of those actions: "Kids shouldn't have to put up with that." I am immediately curious about the ideas that stand behind her evaluation: What is Maria saying here about her knowledge, as a mother, about caring for kids?

I ask, "Maria, when you say that kids shouldn't have to put up with that, what is it that you say kids shouldn't have to put up with?"

"Ice creams aren't dinner. You don't buy beer with money for food," Maria responds. Again, her objection is palpable.

My question has opened a space for Maria to speak further about what she stands for as a mother. We have here the beginnings of an alternative story. My task is to continue coresearching with Maria her ideas about what kids need. The richer telling of that story might offer Maria and her children the options for care that Hera and Maria both seek.

Narrative therapists take careful notes when these kinds of developments take place in a session. Sometimes I gather these notes on a whiteboard where both my client and I can read them or write them (Winslade et al., 1997, p. 71).

Asking Permission: Attending to Power Relations

I ask Maria for permission to gather these thoughts together on the whiteboard on the wall beside our chairs. I ask for her permission, aware that in the background of our conversation is an agency with the statutory power to remove Maria's children. I bring a concern for the relations of power that get produced as we work: I will be of little use to Maria if I get myself positioned as another worker who is "on her case" or who "gives her the hassle." So I check with Maria, wanting to build a partnership that offers respect for the perspective Maria has to offer. Narrative therapy is a practice of collaboration. The questions I ask are critical to the story that gets told. The skills of narrative therapists lie in how they listen and the questions they go on to ask. But it is the client's responses that become the substance of the knowledge we produce together.

With Maria's permission, I write a heading, using Maria's words, "Kids shouldn't have to put up with." Underneath, I write Maria's words, "Food money being spent on beer." The writing offers a visible record, pulling these aspects of our conversation down into a possible storyline of Maria's ideas about parenting. As I write, Maria adds, "And not ice creams for dinner. Kids should be properly fed."

Hearing and Using a Distinction

This second part of Maria's response goes beyond what she stands *against* as a parent. She now speaks about what she stands *for*. There is a subtle shift as Maria offers the idea that kids should be properly fed. Wanting to make the most of this distinction, I say, "Maria, I wrote up here, 'what kids shouldn't have to put up with' because you told me that there were things that went on last night that kids shouldn't have to put up with. And now I'm wondering if maybe you think we might have another heading, too?"

Maria looks at me, and I repeat what she told me. "You said, 'Kids should be properly fed.'"

"Yeah, well, they should," Maria replies.

"May I put that over on this side?" I ask, writing on the left of the board: "Kids should be properly fed." Having written, I check again, "Is this okay to write this part here?" When Maria agrees, I ask her a further checking question: Would she like a heading for this second side, for what kids should get, or will we leave it for now and come back to it once we have heard some more about her ideas about what kids shouldn't have to put up with? At the same time that I am asking Maria's guidance about the next step in our conversation, implicit in my question is that there will be more ideas to add to this storyline if we continue our inquiry.

I offer options to Maria about our conversation. I guide and take responsibility for the construction of the conversational process, but I also ask for guidance from Maria about what she is making of our conversation. My belief is that Maria will be best positioned as a mother in her everyday life if she is positioned to speak with authority in our conversation.

My purpose is to open a space for Maria to make claims about what she believes about parenting on the basis that these claims shape her life as a mother. Because these claims shape her life, it is my responsibility to take them seriously. Michael White (2000) wrote of *honoring* such claims. He contrasted this practice with the culture of doubt and cynicism that frequently meets and dismisses identity claims like these with words such as, "She's just saying what she thinks you want to hear" (pp. 111–112). My purpose is to attend to these fragments of an identity claim Maria offers and to work carefully with her to open space for other aspects of a story of which they are part. I hear Maria's experiences of indignation as supporting her to give expression to some subtle but potentially significant claims about parenting. These claims will become more meaningful as they are connected to other events and values in Maria's life.

Coresearching within Maria's Experience

Maria elects to continue talking about what kids shouldn't have to put up with. "Joe shouldn't have left them outside by themselves. The big one is too little to look after the little one; he's just a baby himself, really," she says.

I am curious about what it is that Maria is standing *for* in the care of children as she objects to Joe's actions. Absent from but implicit in what she has said is some idea about what I might call age-appropriate care. What might come of this idea being brought into the foreground of our conversation? I ask Maria about how she decides what Sam, her older child, is old enough to do, and what he isn't. She tells me that she expects him to dress himself in the mornings but that she helps Kara get dressed. With this example, Maria's ideas about parenting are grounded in actions she has already taken. Ideas grounded in her own actions and knowledge are likely to have credibility for her.

Storying What Is Implicit

As our conversation continues and the record on the whiteboard grows, I often ask Maria about the ideas that stand behind what she says. I don't take for granted that I already understand what is implicit in what she says. My purpose is to coresearch the potential meanings of the story fragments she offers to bring forward a richer account of the values Maria holds with respect to care of her children.

> *Kathie:* Maria, you are saying that you don't like Joe watching sleazy videos when Sam and Kara are around. I don't want to assume your reasons for that would be the same as mine might be, so can I ask about what you are thinking here?
>
> *Maria:* Well, they are only kids, they're just babies.
>
> *Kathie:* What does it mean that they are only kids, they're only babies?
>
> *Maria:* You know, I don't even like his videos much myself, and I'm an adult.

Discursive Listening

Let me take you back to the concept of discourse, the idea that cultural stories shape our lives. I have listened to the fine details of Maria's words and to her particular story and have been responding to them. At the same time, I hear echoes of cultural stories by which Maria's particular story is shaped.

I think about gender discourse and the effects for women and children of the patriarchal heritages and practices of our society. I know that stories and practices that take for granted male privilege may have the effect that a woman lets go of preferences for care for herself or her children in order to preserve a relationship with a male partner. This being the case, how I respond to a comment such as Maria's statement that she doesn't like Joe's videos much herself will have real effects for what it becomes possible to speak about in counseling (Hare-Mustin, 1994) and potential effects in the lives of Maria and her children. I believe that it is my responsibility to inquire further about the experiences and ideas that stand behind Maria's statement.

At this moment in the counseling, as I listen to Maria, I think of the stories women have told me about not having much say about something as everyday as what is shown on the television screens in their living rooms. Young women students whom I worked with in the area of eating disorders and body image first taught me about the harmful effects for them of being subjected to television programs not of their choosing when they entered the shared living spaces of their student accommodations. I learned that television and video remote controls represent a significant way in which gender relations are played out daily in family homes, student suites, and public spaces. I learned that men are more likely to get to select what is shown on television screens because the remote controls usually seem to be found in their hands. Echoing Maria's words, I hear this cultural story that positions men with more access to determine what is viewed on television screens and that tends to position women poorly in this regard.

While thinking about this big picture of the discursive context, right now in this conversation I want to stay close to Maria's experience in order to continue to research it with her. Responding using her own words, I ask Maria to tell a little more of her objection to Joe's videos and the values and ideas that support it. My purpose is to give her authority in this matter more substance.

> *Kathie:* You don't like the videos much yourself, Maria. What is it you don't like?
>
> *Maria:* Some of it is pretty gross. Unless I'm drinking, I never sit down and watch them with him.

I choose not to take up Maria's reference to drinking because my focus is on making space for Maria to tell of the values implicit in her objection to the videos.

> *Kathie:* Maria, the not watching, what's that about?

Do you hear the externalizing language? "Not watching" is an action Maria takes rather than something inside her. My question gives her action significance. I intend my question to invite her to say more about the meanings of this action.

> *Maria:* They're disgusting really. Why would I want to watch that stuff?

Possible Links with a Community of Others

In response, I tentatively offer Maria a connection with the objections of other women in similar situations.

> *Kathie:* Maria, over the years I have met other women who have objected to what was being shown on the television screens in their living rooms because they did not like the ways women were being treated. They did

not want degrading images of women on their screens—for themselves, for their children, and for the men in their lives. Does their objection have any connection with what you said: that you find that the videos Joe watches are "disgusting"? Or does it not connect? Is it something else about them that you find "disgusting"?

The naming of the images as "degrading of women" is purposive political action on my part. At the same time, the tentativeness of the latter part of my question leaves space for Maria to take up, or not, the way I named the problem with the videos. However, if there is resonance for Maria in the protests of other women, their voices can help to support her as she speaks to the values on which she might call in acting to care for and protect her young children.

Do you notice, too, that I suggest that such degrading images have effects not only for women and children, but also for men? It is the taken-for-granted practices that are objectionable, and I am careful to speak in ways that focus Maria's evaluation on practices, not on people, either as individuals or as a group. The problem is the problem; the person is not the problem.

Building the Plot of the Alternative Story: Coresearching History

Our conversation continues and the account of what kids shouldn't have to put up with grows. Maria suggests a heading for the account we have built towards on the left side of the board: "What I want Sam and Kara to have." My questions offered the potential to generate the knowledges we have gathered; Maria's responses to the questions have provided the substance. This is coresearching in action.

The ideas we have gathered begin to form an alternative story. It is alternative in that the story it tells is not one of Maria as a mother who has failed to care for and protect her children, but rather one of Maria as a woman with knowledge about and experience in caring for her children. I decide now to investigate something of the history of this alternative story. Tracing its history, we may give it further richness, and also further credibility, by connecting the story so far with other people and events in Maria's life.

> *Kathie:* Maria, I am thinking about all these ideas you have told me about caring for Kara and Sam that we have gathered here on the board. I am wondering about who, or where, these ideas connect you with. Are these ideas and things to do that you have learned from somewhere in particular? Did you learn them maybe from your family, or from friends, or from watching someone, or are they something you have been thinking about for yourself more recently?
>
> *Maria:* I'm not sure. I didn't know I thought all those things, really.

Kathie: You didn't know you thought these things about caring for kids?

Maria: Not really. Well, I guess I did in some ways. I did say to you that my kids shouldn't have to put up with stuff like adults who aren't reliable. I did say kids should be safe—and I really believe that even though Hera doesn't trust me. But I hadn't put it all together like that. It looks different all there together on the board.

I do not take for granted what Maria means when she tells me that it looks different on the board. Have I inadvertently imposed upon Maria an agenda of a story of parenting that interests me more than her? What does looking different mean to her? I invite Maria to evaluate what we have done.

Inviting Evaluation and Justification

Kathie: What do you think about it all there together like that [on the whiteboard]? Is that okay? Is there something else you would rather we did?

Maria: No, I like them together like that. It's good. When I see that, I look at it, and I think, "Gee, I am a good mum. I can be a good mum." When I see that, I think that there's no way I'm going to let Hera take Sam and Kara away from me.

The invitation to Maria to evaluate what we have done has the effect of Maria's taking a position in relation to the local knowledges that we have generated in our coresearch. Maria likes these knowledges. They suit her. But more than that, the evaluation of these knowledges has opened space for her to make a further significant identity claim about her abilities as a mother: "I am a good mum." I am very interested in this identity claim.

My interest is not because I agree with the idea that mothers can be divided into good and bad mothers. A good mother/bad mother story is one that circulates in our culture, and it contributes to the problem story in which Maria has found herself. I am interested in what this claim about herself as a mother might stand for and mean. I am interested in how it will contribute to this increasingly rich story of Maria's relationships with and responsibilities to her children. I take her identity claim as an event along the way that contributes to the account we are weaving. Similarly, when later Maria speaks of putting kids first, I see this idea as an event along the way of the conversation rather than a practice that I am advocating for Maria.

I let go, for now, of the focus on the history of these ideas in Maria's life. My next question offers Maria the opportunity to further substantiate her claim. I ask it not because of doubt or cynicism on my part, but to story the claim more richly by tracing carefully the steps of our coresearch. An invitation to Maria to speak the evidence herself is likely to enhance the credibility of the account to her.

> *Kathie:* Maria, what do you see on that list which says to you that you are a good mum?
>
> *Maria:* Well, it does say that I believe in looking after kids properly, like putting the kids first, like talking to them when I put them to bed, like cuddling them when they get hurt, like thinking about being reliable. [Pauses.] It's only because of Joe that things have gone wrong.

Maria's eyes fill with tears. I do not know what this event means, but I am interested in its meanings being spoken. Maria has just taken, again, a position of evaluation. Her evaluation of her ideas about caring for Sam and Kara, gathered on the board, has evoked a turning back to the context of her life and family that has brought us together. She moves to an evaluation of things there. Something has moved her, and I am interested in the transport—that is, I am interested in the possibilities for her life to which this evaluation has carried her. I hope the words I use in the following dialogue convey the gentleness and reverence I intended.

> *Kathie:* What are your tears for, Maria?
>
> *Maria:* I haven't been doing that, have I?
>
> *Kathie:* Maria, what is it you haven't been doing?
>
> *Maria:* I haven't been putting the kids first.
>
> *Kathie:* Your tears are for not putting the kids first? [Maria nods "yes."]

Maria is living out the identity of a "good mum" that she had just a short time ago claimed. As a "good mum," she is evaluating for herself recent events in her family and her part in them. My questions invite meaning making and gently support her to name her evaluation. I have used the word *evaluation* purposefully: Maria's speaking position is as moral agent in her life. She is positioned, in our coresearch, to evaluate how things have been and whether or not they suit the preferences for parenting that she has articulated earlier in our conversation. Maria is *witnessing* to how some things have been in recent times, to her hopes for and values in her parenting, to the gap between those hopes and values and how things have been.

Hearing Maria witnessing to these gaps, I return to my question about the possible histories of the values and practices represented on the whiteboard. I do not want her to be immobilized by pain or shame about having been separated from these hopes and from what she knows about caring for children. I am interested in what we might bring forward here to give more substance to the story of practices of care for children by making more links across time in this alternative story of care.

Coresearching History to Strengthen Connection

> *Kathie:* Maria, I asked a few minutes ago where you might have learned these ideas about being a mother that we have up here [on the board], these ideas about "putting kids first." Is it okay if I ask you about that again now? Who might have taught you these ideas, in your own growing up or in your adult life?

> *Maria:* Well, it sure wasn't my mother. She just left us kids whenever she felt like it. When a new man came along, we sure weren't her first thought. It was Koro who was there for us, he brought us up, really. [*Koro* is the Maori word for grandfather.]

> *Kathie:* Koro, he brought you up, really? He was there for you?

> *Maria:* Yes, he just was always there. He put us first.

> *Kathie:* Koro put kids first. He put you first.

> *Maria:* He did. He always put us first. If it wasn't for him . . .

Here, I work slowly and carefully, reflecting back to Maria these fragments of a storyline of a caregiver in her life putting kids first. Stepping back from questioning, I retell, in Maria's own words, this very moving turn in the story. I experience reverence in this moment as I witness Maria's remembering the care her Koro offered her. As Maria's voice fades, my choice of response is guided by the possibilities of supporting a story of care.

> *Kathie:* Maria, you said that Koro put you first. And on the board here, we have the ideas you have talked about today that have to do with putting children first. Do you think there's a connection between the ideas you have talked about today and the ideas Koro might have had when he cared for you?

Maria pauses. As I wait, I wonder if the pausing is produced by Maria experiencing a resonance between these two accounts of care. Is it possible that our conversation has generated reverberations that have reached down into Maria's own history and made the telling of this particular story of care possible? (For a discussion of the idea of reverberations with our histories, see White [2005].) What might Koro's legacy of care contribute to Maria's claim about being a "good mum," I ask myself. How might Koro act as an audience to Maria's identity claims and thus authenticate them? As I wait alongside Maria's pausing, I listen to my silent questions. I do not rush to continue, for I do not know where Maria's thinking is taking her. After a time, I offer another question about the link between these two accounts.

> *Kathie:* What would Koro say about what's on the board here, Maria?
>
> *Maria:* I didn't know it before, but I think Koro taught me those things. And I think I forgot them a bit. But those things are what Koro would say. I just hadn't thought about Koro when we were putting them up there.

I notice that we now have Koro's voice alive to us in the room—"those things are what Koro would say"—and that his ways of caring for children are strongly connected with the practices that Maria has spoken of today.

I also notice Maria's evaluation of her situation: "I think I forgot them a bit." If any small voice of professional cynicism had led me to harbor any doubt about the alternative story Maria has been telling, here was yet another counter to that voice. I note Maria's words as they may be useful to return to later.

For now I want to thicken the connections between these two "episodes" in the story of care. I invite Maria to weigh up the effects for her of the connections we are building between her and Koro in this story.

> *Kathie:* What's it like to be thinking about these ideas on the board—that there are ways of caring for children that Koro taught you, that you learned from Koro, that what is here is what Koro would say?
>
> *Maria:* It's good. It's really good.
>
> *Kathie:* Koro, who cared for you, taught you those things about caring for children, Maria. Do you think Koro knew how much you learned from him?
>
> *Maria:* He would have wanted me to learn. But look what's happening to my kids.

I believe that it is not by chance that again Maria is taking up a position of commentary on her own situation, noticing shortfalls in the provision of care for her children. The therapeutic space is such that there has been no loss of dignity for Maria, no shaming or blaming when she has spoken of a distance between her preferences and the ways things have been recently for her children. There is no sense that she has been evaluated as a person. Rather, through co-researching, the conversation has positioned Maria as a person who has ideas about care for children, even though some of her actions may have temporarily separated her from her preferences for living her life and parenting her children.

Again, as Maria notices this separation from her preferences, I do not want her to be immobilized by the pain of recognition or to experience blame. Noticing Maria's evaluation, I want to inquire about her link with Koro for its potential to support her to further take up the care for her children in the ways she has told it today.

> *Kathie:* Maria, you said that Koro would have wanted you to learn from him. Is Koro still alive?
>
> *Maria:* He passed on when I was 18.
>
> *Kathie:* I am sorry. Maria, what do you think Koro would say about these things here [on the board] that we are talking about today?
>
> *Maria:* He'd say, "Good on you, girl. Good on you." But he'd also tell me that I am just like my mum, taking on no-good men.

While I notice the expression of encouragement that Maria has spoken in Koro's voice, my attention is also on the evaluation of her situation Maria has offered in Koro's voice. There is a resonance with the evaluation Maria offered much earlier in our conversation, of the part Joe has played in producing the current situation where Maria's parenting is under scrutiny. Maria is not the first woman I have met whose partner's behaviors threaten the well-being of her children, and I have kept this aspect of the situation in mind as we have been in conversation.

At this point in the conversation, Maria and I are better positioned in our working together to consider an evaluation of this aspect of her situation. Rather than reproducing Maria's words, I speak in terms of the implicit expression of Koro's care and hopes for Maria with respect to her relationships with men. I respond this way to lessen opportunities for blame to enter our conversation: women who are subject to abuse or poor treatment by men with whom they are in relationship are frequently the target of blame for their situation. In this context, blame of women is produced by another of the cultural stories that shapes lives in a patriarchal society.

> *Kathie:* For you and for your mum, Maria, Koro would have wanted relationships with men to be with good men?
>
> *Maria:* He'd sure give me a growling about Joe, if he knew.
>
> *Kathie:* What would he be intending if he gave you a growling about Joe, Maria?

My question, again, reduces the space for blame to enter our conversation. The inquiry focuses on Koro's hopes for Maria's life, expressed through "giving her a growling." My question seeks to name what is absent from but implicit in the "growling."

> *Maria:* He'd say, "Look after your tamariki [children], girl, look after my mokopuna [grandchildren]."

Maria's response further thickens the account of her connections with Koro. Sam and Kara are not only her tamariki, her children, but they are also Koro's mokopuna, his grandchildren. Maria and her children are now woven a little further into a storyline of whanau [family] connection and care. I repeat Maria's words so that she hears them retold, but I am also aware that we are at the end of our time together. We have both been intensely involved in conversation. I think both of savoring with Maria this moment and its meanings and of closing our meeting.

> *Kathie:* Koro would say, "Look after your tamariki, girl; look after my mokopuna." [Pause.] Do you have any ideas about how Koro would want you to do that, Maria?
>
> *Maria:* Just what's up there [on the board]. That's not just me, that's Koro, too, saying that.
>
> *Kathie:* Maria, it's time for us to be finishing here for today, but can I just put those words up here, too?

"Look after your tamariki; look after my mokopuna," I say as I write. Then I ask Maria directly what this conversation has been like for her today. Again, this question calls Maria into a position of evaluating, rather than being evaluated. I ask her if I may send her a letter with the ideas recorded on the board from our conversation today and the story of Koro teaching her about caring for children.

As we part, having agreed to meet again, among my thoughts are warm rememberings of my own grandfathers and their care for me. My conversation with Maria has gifted this connection to me; there may be a time when I can acknowledge this to her.

The Effects of Coresearch

Maria's life has been directly shaped by the responses I have offered her. The language I used and the stories to which I paid attention were profoundly shaping of the direction of our conversation. Maria began the conversation with the subject of intervention by governmental authorities, experiencing herself as acted upon and identified as failing at parenting. The narrative therapy skills of inquiry into what might otherwise have been neglected storylines in Maria's life leave her quite differently positioned by the end of our conversation.

A collaborative practice of coresearching inquiry has supported Maria to stitch herself and Sam and Kara into an alternative storyline. This alternative storyline positions her more strongly as a mother in her care for her children. The resources for this story were already available in the experiences of Maria's life. Local knowledges from within Maria's own experience have given substance to the alternative story that now shapes her life.

Role of the Client-Counselor Relationship

Narrative counselors pay micro attention to relationship practices; this stance is central to the epistemology and practice of narrative counseling. The following are some aspects of a counseling relationship that were demonstrated by the illustration of practice you have just read.

- *Active attention is given to the relation of power and the position of privilege of a counselor.* For instance, the counselor consults the client about the direction the conversation has taken, or might take, and invites the client's evaluation. Clients are thus positioned as active in the construction of the therapeutic relationship.

- *Narrative counselors operate on the basis that there is no neutral position for them to occupy.* They therefore work to avoid replicating the normalizing judgments and other oppressive practices offered on the terms of dominant discourses.

- *Counselors and clients work together to coresearch clients' lived experiences.* These coresearching practices position clients as knowledgeable about and active in their own lives and in the work of counseling.

- *The therapeutic relationship offers counselors positions from which they witness to the lives of those who consult them, to the stories clients tell about their lives, and to the alternative stories produced in the counseling room.* Because witnesses act to authenticate identity claims, our responding actively shapes the identities of those we meet with.

- *Counselors' experiences in a witnessing position also shape their own lives so that they may become other than who they were.*

- *This enrichment of our own lives, through the privilege of the conversations we have with clients, might be acknowledged to our clients.* This acknowledgment is a way of offering ourselves as accountable to those who consult us (White, 2000); it disturbs the more familiar one-way accountability of client to therapist and the familiar assumption that only the client is changed by therapy.

> • *A counselor might, with appropriate permissions, pass the fruits of coresearch between one client and another* (Epston, 1998). In this way the counselor is, at times, a conduit passing on local knowledges between clients, with the effect that clients join one another as cotherapists.

Practices of inquiring about clients' local knowledges and connecting clients with others in their lives contribute to what Michael White (1997) describes as a *de-centered* but influential position for the therapist. Aileen Cheshire (personal communication, February 1997) has characterized this relationship by suggesting that a counselor is a "guest" in someone's life. Thus, counselors are present only at the client's invitation, and we must understand and negotiate the invitation each client offers. At the same time, we have a responsibility for the way we host the therapeutic meeting and conversation. White (1993) suggested that therapists meet clients from a position of solidarity, ". . . a solidarity that is constructed by therapists who refuse to draw a sharp distinction between their lives and the lives of others, who refuse to marginalize those persons who seek help" (p. 132). It is also a position of solidarity in which therapists realize that if they were faced with the same life circumstances, they might not do as well as their clients are doing. Our hope is that this kind of solidarity would invite a client such as Maria to notice herself acting as "a significant agent in the production of the counselling process from which she is benefiting" (Winslade et al., 1997, p. 53).

Long-Term Versus Short-Term Applications

My own experience is that narrative practices have been useful across a range of concerns that people have brought to counseling, from a single conversation about making a decision between two job offers to managing an obsessive-compulsive disorder over time. The narrative therapy literature shows a similar range, from briefer to longer-term work, including both time-limited and ongoing groups and community work of many kinds. For example, Brigitte, Sue, Mem, and Veronika (1997) recorded their experiences of "rekindling our love for life" (p. 26) in an ongoing narrative group for people who had been troubled by voices (in *DSM* terms, schizophrenic hallucinations); Yvonne Sliep (2005) described her use, over a more defined time, of narrative theater practice in "strengthening the social fabric" (p. 52) in communities affected by trauma, conflict, and war in Malawi, Uganda, Burundi, and East Congo; and Lorraine Hedtke (2000), writing of her work in hospice settings in the United States, offered a moving account of her conversations with Ellen, all of which took place on the day that Ellen's husband died. These are examples of accounts of innovative practices, both long term and short term, generated to respond to particular situations. The narrative therapy emphasis is on (1) generating responsive practice rather than replicating standardized practices and (2) evaluating with our clients how useful the practice is for them and on that basis, making decisions about the time frames within which we work.

Evaluation of Narrative Therapy

By this stage of the chapter, it will perhaps not be surprising to you that a discussion of evaluation of narrative therapy from a narrative counseling perspective might begin with some *questions* about evaluation. Whose voices are both explicitly and implicitly present in evaluation studies? On whose terms was the evaluation conducted? What criteria are used in the evaluation? Who chose these criteria? Why did they choose these terms? What are the effects of these terms? What political purposes are at work in this approach to evaluation? What do the results really tell us about the effects of the approach in the lives of the people who have consulted us?

The purpose of such questions is not to sidestep accountability, but rather to emphasize that evaluation is not a neutral process. Narrative therapist Jane Speedy (2004) wrote of experiencing "dis-ease with the ways that most participants are re-presented in traditional research studies" (p. 45). In the modernist project with its emphasis on universality and the management of populations, generalizability is a central value, both for research and for approaches to practice; thus, nomothetic research makes sense. Postmodern research and therapeutic practice aim to make much more modest claims; their emphasis is on local, interpretive accounts that are idiographic in nature. However, such modesty does not readily find a place in a dominant positivist evaluation culture where ideas about empirically supported practice demand nomothetic studies. In their discussion of the current empirically supported culture of professional practice, Stephen Goss and Suzanna Rose (2002) wrote, "It can be argued that some forms of research are inherently biased in favour of those therapeutic models that are most amenable to the types of data they produce" (p. 69). Narrative therapy is philosophically at odds with the principles that produce nomothetic studies. Despite Peter Fraenkel's (1995, p. 121) particular demonstrations that idiographic or nomothetic claims may each carry traces of the other, I know of no studies evaluating narrative therapy that have successfully taken up the kind of "ideothetic" approach, employing both nomothetic and idiographic strategies, that Fraenkel envisioned.

Accountability in Narrative Practice

Social constructionist therapies are associated with a "mistrust" of nomothetic knowledge (Fraenkel, 1995, p. 115). What does this mean, then, for accountability in narrative therapy? What do narrative counselors have to offer those who want access to information about the effects of narrative practice on clients' lives?

Narrative counselors most often look to research practices that offer some resonance with the ethics of their therapeutic practice (e.g., Crocket, 2004; Crocket, Drewery, McKenzie, Smith, & Winslade, 2004; Gaddis, 2004; Ingram & Perlesz, 2004; Kotzé & Kotzé, 2001; O'Neill, 2004; Redstone, 2004; Speedy, 2004; Tootell, 2004). To this end, Jane Speedy (2004) argued for documenting the outcomes of narrative practice through "an extensive (cumulative rather than conclusive) narrative practice outcomes archive" that would offer "diverse and thick descriptions of the outcomes, aftermaths and reverberations of these [therapy] experiences in the lives of different people at different times across different continents" (p. 51). Such an archive, she suggested, would be produced by practitioners and the people who consult them and would include in its potential audience policy makers and those who make decisions about service provision.

There already exists in the narrative therapy literature a symphony of compelling accounts of practice with particular individuals, groups, and communities. In this literature, there is often at least a dual focus on the process and the effects of the practice. In these accounts, the effects ("outcome") story comes directly out of the story of the therapy itself (the process). An evaluation of such accounts is possible. These are some of the questions I might ask: Was the practice story credible? Was its ethical purpose and theoretical rationale clear and transparent? Was there evidence of benefit to the person seeking help, and on the terms of the person seeking help? How was the person seeking help represented in the account? Did this account move (transport) me?

Consulting your consultants (i.e., your clients) is a further narrative practice that serves as a form of evaluation (Epston & White, 1992). This practice involves documenting with clients the knowledges and strategies that they believe are important, both in managing what had been problematic to them and in asserting their own preferences for their lives. The documenting is useful as a retelling for clients in that it provides a potential, or actual, audience for them. It is also useful as a document that might be circulated to others meeting the same difficulties, who will thus be joined in what they face and who are in a position to evaluate these insider knowledges for what they might offer them. These documents also educate counselors.

An ethic of collaboration means that narrative practitioners see evaluation as an ongoing project throughout the therapy. At any point in a counseling conversation, it might be relevant for a counselor to pause and inquire, genuinely, how the conversation is going for the client: Is the conversation meeting what the person came for, and does the person have any suggestions for other directions (see White, 1995, 1997)? As well, a similar kind of accountability back to clients is practiced when we situate our questions—that is, when we tell clients why we are asking what we are asking.

In a further accountability strategy, practitioners acknowledge the ways in which the lives of clients shape and contribute to their own lives. This practice is part of what Michael White calls a *two-way account of therapy* (1997, pp. 130–131). The shaping of our own lives is another of those experiences that might go unnoticed and therefore unstoried. The ethic here is of a direct accountability to the clients we meet with in our work, whether accounting for our contributions to the conversation, accounting for the meaningfulness of the conversation for us, or genuinely consulting about how the conversation is suiting our clients and what they might prefer.

These kinds of approaches to evaluation yield more modest measures of the usefulness of narrative practices than traditional nomothetic approaches. Yet they provide an alternative story of evaluation of practice. As Busch, Strong, and Lock (2004) note, "The positivist domination and saturation of evaluation is just the way things have turned out so far in psychological and psychotherapeutic research" (p. 10). Implicit in this observation is the possibility that things might turn out otherwise as we pursue different options for evaluation of counseling.

Narrative Therapy: Blind Spots, Limitations, and Challenges

In introducing narrative practices, this chapter contains simplifications and leaves much out. Perhaps some of these simplifications, incomplete descriptions, and omissions have had you asking as you read, "But what does a narrative therapy approach say about. . . ?" or, "How does narrative practice deal with. . . ?" I hope you might have been thinking not only about the gaps in my account, but also the questions about narrative practice that your own life experiences raised for you as you read. The questions you bring to your reading are as important in identifying potential limitations of narrative practice as any identified by narrative therapists or other writers.

An important starting point in thinking about limitations is to acknowledge that a therapy that takes knowledge to be subjective, situated, fragmented, multiple, and contested does not expect that everything can be seen and known, in advance or at all. Narrative therapists expect that there is much that we do not know and that we have yet to learn (White, 1995). My colleague, Elmarie Kotzé, often refers to Maturana and Varela's (1997) question: "What might we not see that we do not see?" (p. 19). This kind of inquiry is an expression of the ethics of narrative practice, one to which I aspire.

Blind Spots

Counselors centered in both traditional family therapy and individual counseling find much that is unfamiliar, discomforting, and disconcerting in narrative therapy. This is not surprising because narrative therapy does not rely on the structuralist assumptions about persons and family systems that have produced familiar mainstream therapies. Rather, narrative therapy tells a story of both continuity with (Freedman & Combs, 1996) and discontinuity from (White, 1997) traditional therapies. An emphasis on discontinuity has led to some criticisms. For example, in a written dialogue about relationships between narrative therapy and systemic family therapy, Brian Stagoll claimed that White (1997) offered "strident insistence on severing narrative therapy from the culture of psychotherapy from which it arose" (Stagoll, 2000, p. 126). Another who expressed regret about a break from previous modalities was Salvador Minuchin (1998), the central figure in structural family therapy. He criticized narrative therapy for what he saw as a return to an emphasis on the individual, in its move away from systemic principles that emphasize "social relatedness."

Because of narrative therapy's strong concern for social justice, narrative therapists run the risk of imposing a social justice agenda in the consulting they do (Smith, 1997; see Monk & Gerhart, 2003). Steve de Shazer (1993) drew attention to the effects of narrative therapy's taking an "anti-problem approach" (e.g., an anti-anorexia approach). From his solution-focused perspective, he suggested that an anti-problem orientation continues to organize solutions around problems; his preference is for a more "radical distinction between 'problem' and 'solution'" (p. 119).

These criticisms echo Lynn Hoffman's (1990) suggestion that "an art of lenses" (p. 1) is involved in the selection of approaches to practice: the conceptual lens we use cannot make everything visible all at once. Any critique is made through some particular lens. Whether the critique and any response that might be made is satisfying both to the person offering the critique and to a narrative therapist depends on the degree to which they can create shared meaning despite their differences in philosophical positions and conceptual lenses. This point brings us to some of the limitations of narrative therapy.

Limitations

Because of its postmodern epistemological base, narrative therapy does not blend readily into an integrated approach. Some would see this as a limitation. For example, I described earlier my own experience of coming to understand that externalizing conversations depend upon an understanding of personhood that is at odds with humanistic approaches. I also noted that the counselor education program in which I teach has a single focus on narrative therapy, thus offering students the opportunity to develop a sound basis of skills in narrative practice rather than to learn a little about multiple approaches to practice. While preferring this soundness, I sometimes regret that our program's curricular focus does not offer our students richer engagement with the wider histories of our field.

In most agencies, schools, and social service settings, practice approaches with longer histories dominate and thus set the agenda invisibly. In such contexts, narrative counselors might be seen to be pedantic in questioning seemingly ordinary practices, such as the language of everyday professional talk that is taken for granted by those whose theories may not pay these matters explicit attention in the way that narrative therapists do. Because narrative practitioners hold that language produces reality—that is, words speak people into being—we do not reproduce uncritically what may have become everyday professional talk or practice. For example, we might speak with a receptionist about alternatives to a familiar statement such as, "Your two o'clock is here" (Winslade et al., 1997, p. 57), in order to offer a less objectifying way of speaking about a client. The unusualness of this kind of attention to the nuance of language might set us apart from colleagues and leave us at risk of some of the kinds of critique noted earlier. It is not always comfortable for our colleagues, or for us, to have attention drawn to taken-for-granted practices that have unintended objectifying effects. While narrative therapists in some circumstances might prefer to work at the margins of agencies, we would also have to ask ourselves whether this is a position from which we can best work with and advocate for clients who are experiencing serious social, political, or economic marginalization.

In the wider professional world in New Zealand and internationally, narrative practitioners not infrequently find themselves at the edge of professional communities, not readily understood by those whose knowledge bases do not encompass postmodern therapies. I believe that it is to my professional peril, and to my clients', if I do not understand the dominant terms of mainstream therapies—that is, I must be multilingual in the languages of traditional therapies. However, there is not the same risk for those professionals who speak only on the terms of their own preferred traditional approach, which means that the responsibility to translate is shared unevenly.

Questions might also be asked about the limitations of narrative therapy at the level of daily practice. For example, questions are often asked about narrative therapy and individual responsibility. "Doesn't externalizing remove personal responsibility?" people ask. Such a question depends upon dominant Western ideas about the self and about individual responsibility. Narrative therapy construes responsibility differently. This difference is seen clearly in Alan Jenkins's (1990) groundbreaking work on violence in which he suggested an approach that involves "invitations to responsibility." Such invitations offer people possibility rather than blame while holding them accountable for violent actions. The difference is also visible in narrative therapy's emphasis on the social construction of alcoholism (Winslade & Smith, 1997) rather than an emphasis on a personal deficit of the individual. In these examples, we see an interrelationship between story and lived experiences. Narrative therapists believe that how we story people's lived experience does have effects in the world: it is the space between experience and our making meaning of experience that narrative therapists negotiate.

Challenges

Because a search for certainties remains a dominant organizing feature of everyday life in the modern world, narrative practitioners are not impervious to becoming caught up in certainty about our own theories. This chapter began with the idea of narrative as a metaphor, the idea of lives as storied as a possible account of personhood. Narrative therapists may lose sight of this point and act as though their theoretical and philosophical position is an exact match with some fixed reality. The implications of Hoffman's (1990) review of the changing lenses through which she has viewed therapy are that the lenses available to us now are limited and will be replaced. Johnella Bird (2000) warned against both complacency—a self-satisfaction that might have us cease to question our practices—and an intolerance that might arise out of taking positions of certainty and applying normalizing judgments to others. "Complacency and intolerance of difference are the forerunners of a therapy or counseling practice that alienates and subjugates others" (Bird, 2000, p. 129). With Johnella's words in mind, I think an important challenge we face is to work for modesty about the claims we make for narrative practice.

Future Development: Narrative Therapy in a Diverse World

Narrative therapy came out of concern about alienation and subjugation in a number of arenas, including within the practice of therapy itself. Narrative therapy's situation originally was family therapy; David Epston suggests it is now community (2001, p. 182). In terms of future developments in narrative practices, I imagine practitioners looking to local communities, and to clients, for guidance about the kinds of practices that are most useful to them and about the situations in which we might practice. Here in New Zealand, for example, immigrants now come from many more ethnic, cultural, and national backgrounds than at any time in the past. What effects will learning with and from them have for our practices? The New Zealand government is one of the few who sponsor refugee immigrants, many of whom have suffered the most serious injustices and violations. How might we serve their hopes for new lives? In our country, the distribution of wealth is increasingly uneven; domestic violence and sexual abuse continue; and the access Maori, and in particular Maori women and children, have to the economic and social resources of the community is inequitable. Although in New Zealand women currently hold the positions of prime minister, governor general, chief justice, and speaker of the House of Representatives, there are many women who continue to be poorly positioned to care for themselves and their families. What responsibilities do counselors and the counseling profession have to these issues? And what about counseling in your country? What concerns do you see to which counselors might have responsibility to respond? I believe that how we meet with women and men in therapy does make a difference in shaping their lives.

Perhaps our ways forward might come from remaining curious about what communities want from us. We may benefit from the modesty of acknowledging the limits of our own location and history, and so the limits of the thinking and understanding available to us. Continuing curiosity about alternative histories, locations, understandings, and ways of practicing holds the possibilities of new options for counseling practice. The challenge is to find ways to be open to such possibilities.

Summary

1. The metaphor of story is the primary organizing idea in narrative counseling. Stories are understood to shape and form the world and to shape and form people's lives and identities, as we give meaning to the events of our lives. Our lives are shaped by cultural stories of gender, ethnicity, nationality, and class; by stories told in our families and communities; by stories of our own life experiences.

2. Narrative counseling is based on the premise that knowledge is contestable. Thus, the process of counseling is a collaborative inquiry into the knowledges carried by the stories that shape clients' lives. Narrative inquiry supports people to take positions to evaluate whether the way things are meets their hopes, dreams, and intentions for their own lives.

3. There is a link between stories and the words with which stories are told. Narrative counselors carefully select the language forms they use in speaking about both people and problems. This careful selection arises out of the idea that words, like stories, are not neutral. Words do more than mirror reality; they shape and produce reality.

4. The key practices of narrative therapy are that (1) the metaphor of story is central, (2) the stories people call on and the language they use have real

effects on their own and others' lives, and (3) counseling has the potential to replicate oppressive practices of the wider culture.

5. Narrative therapy was first articulated from Australia and New Zealand by Michael White and David Epston and developed out of an exploration (at the Family Centre in Lower Hutt, New Zealand) of the limitations of mainstream psychology with regard to poverty, racism, and sexism. Although it began within family therapy, narrative therapy is now widely used in work with individuals and communities.

6. The narrative metaphor suggests that people come to understand themselves and the world through the stories about self and the world that are available to them in their particular cultural context. Cultural norms are referred to as discourses, and they tell us how things are in our world and make particular social processes possible. People responding to these discourses are said to be engaging in discursive practices, or actions, including speaking, that particular discourses make available.

7. Dominant discourses carry within them taken-for-granted ideas about how things should be. They thus shape our actions, our lives, and so the stories we have about our lives, even when we might not seem to be performing in our lives particularly well on the terms of those discourses. Discourses make available normalizing judgments by which we measure and scrutinize our own and others' lives.

8. Several methods are employed in the practice of narrative therapy, including externalizing conversations (in which the therapist reproduces the client's language in a way that externalizes the problem rather than maintains the client's internalized focus on the problem), using curious questioning (an assumption-free stance that helps the therapist understand the client's story more fully), listening for problem stories versus alternative stories (the overpowering story the client perceives as causing his or her problem versus the storylines that go beyond the terms of the problem story), listening for thin versus thick descriptions (a client's descriptions based on the terms of the dominant discourse versus a richly storied account of the client's life and relationships), listening for absent but implicit descriptions (hopes, intentions, and purposes in clients' lives that are obscured by the dominance of a problem story), using therapeutic documents with the client (recording, for therapeutic effect, knowledges that are generated in counseling), and using audiences and witnessing (which speaks to the narrative therapy concept that identity is socially constructed).

9. In narrative therapy, change is brought about by "opening space" in places where previously none was visible because of the stranglehold a problem may have had. In other words, clients are assisted in moving past the problem story and developing the alternative story, the unstoried experiences and

ideas that might contribute to clients living their lives on terms that are more attuned to their own hopes, intentions, and purposes for their lives.

10. Narrative therapy is useful across a wide range of concerns people have brought to counseling, in short and long-term work, and in a wide range of settings, including work with individuals, groups, and communities.

11. Evaluation of narrative typically doesn't involve nomothetic knowledge. Rather, evaluation involves consulting the consultants (documenting knowledges and strategies with clients during the therapeutic process), using inquiry (pausing during the therapy to directly ask clients about their thoughts and suggestions regarding the process), and employing a two-way account of therapy (exploring the ways in which clients' lives contribute to therapists' lives).

12. Narrative therapy is limited in that it views knowledge to be subjective, situated, fragmented, multiple, and contested, and therefore it does not expect that everything can be seen and known. In addition, it does not blend well with an integrated therapy approach, its focus on language might be regarded as pedantic, it is sometimes perceived as an outsider therapy, and some might view its externalizing focus as removing clients' personal responsibility. A challenge to narrative therapists is to keep in mind that the therapy is a philosophy, not a certainty.

13. Narrative therapy developed out of a concern about alienation and subjugation in a number of arenas, including counseling. In the future, narrative therapy is likely to be situated in communities, and narrative therapists will be looking to local communities for guidance regarding their needs for consultation.

Key Terms

absent but implicit (p. 505)
alternative stories (p. 489)
consulting your consultants (p. 524)
coresearch (p. 494)
curious questioning (p. 503)
discourse (p. 499)
discursive listening (p. 501)
dominant discourses (p. 500)
dominant stories (p. 489)
externalizing conversation (p. 496)

externalizing language (p. 502)
insider knowledges (p. 497)
local knowledges (p. 493)
normalizing judgment (p. 500)
social constructionism (p. 498)
thick descriptions (p. 505)
thin descriptions (p. 505)
transport (p. 508)
witnessing (p. 507)

Resources for Further Study

Professional Organizations

Professional education in narrative therapy:

Dulwich Centre
Adelaide, Australia
www.dulwichcentre.com.au/

Evanston Family Therapy Center
Chicago, IL
www.eftc.info/ (with useful links to other narrative therapy sites)

Family Institute of Cambridge, MA
www.familyinstitutecamb.org/about/

University of Waikato
Hamilton, New Zealand
http://soe.waikato.ac.nz/counselling/

Professional Journals

International Journal of Narrative Therapy and Community Work
Dulwich Centre
Adelaide, Australia
www.dulwichcentre.com.au/

Suggested Readings

Introductions to narrative practice:

Dulwich Centre. For many published articles on narrative therapies, go to its website at www.dulwich.centre.com.au/.

Morgan, A. (2000). *What is narrative therapy? An easy-to-read introduction.* Adelaide, Australia: Dulwich Centre Publications.

A clear, accessible, step-by-step introduction and guide to narrative practice.

Winslade, J., & Monk, G. (1999). *Narrative counseling in schools: Powerful and brief.* Thousand Oaks, CA: Corwin Press.

Another clearly written, carefully sequenced overview of and guide for narrative practice. Many practice illustrations from school counseling.

Overview accounts:

Freedman J., & Combs, G. (1996). *Narrative therapy: The social construction of preferred realities.* New York: Norton.

Telling a United States story, a rich introductory chapter traces the authors' own routes towards narrative practice and social constructionist ideas. Accessible and practical.

Monk, G., Winslade, J., Crocket, K., & Epston, D. (Eds.). (1997). *Narrative therapy in practice: The archaeology of hope*. San Francisco: Jossey-Bass.

A group of New Zealand practitioners describe practice in a range of contexts: schools, alcohol counseling, health education, psychiatry, male sexual abuse, group work, mediation.

Zimmerman, J., & Dickerson, V. (1996). *If problems talked: Narrative therapy in action*. New York: Guilford.

Rich in practice examples from the United States.

Theory, philosophy, and professional context:

Burr, V. (2003). *An introduction to social constructionism* (2nd ed.). London: Routledge.

We use this book as a text in the University of Waikato M.Couns. degree program because it offers a thorough overview of and introduction to social constructionist ideas.

Denborough, D. (Ed.). (2001). *Family therapy: Exploring the field's past, present and possible futures*. Adelaide, Australia: Dulwich Centre Publications.

A delightful collection of conversational interviews with influential family therapists. Narrates a context for narrative practice.

Gergen, K. (1991). *The saturated self: Dilemmas of identity in contemporary life*. New York: Basic Books.

An accessible introduction to ideas about how the self is produced by the traditions and practices of romantic, modern, and postmodern life.

Thomas, L. (2002). Poststructuralism and therapy: What's it all about? *The International Journal of Narrative Therapy and Community Work, 2,* 85–89.

A brief and accessible response to questions commonly asked about poststructuralist ideas and therapy.

Other Media Resources

Videotape

White, M. (1992). *Recent developments in the narrative approach* [AAMFT Learning Edge Series]. Alexandria, VA: American Association for Marriage and Family Therapy.

No longer recent, but a clear introduction to externalizing conversations.

Websites

www.narrativeapproaches.com/
www.heartsnarrative.cc/
http://masterswork.com/shopsite_sc/store/html/nartherapy.html#White

Glossary

The chapter in which each term appears as a key term is indicated as follows: Chapter 3, Psychoanalytic Therapy (3-PS); Chapter 4, Adlerian Therapy (4-AD); Chapter 5, Existential Therapy (5-EX); Chapter 6, Person-Centered Therapy (6-PC); Chapter 7, Gestalt Therapy (7-GE); Chapter 8, Behavior Therapy I: Traditional Behavior Therapy (8-BE); Chapter 9, Behavior Therapy II: Cognitive-Behavioral Therapy (9-CB); Chapter 10, Reality Therapy (10-RE); Chapter 11, Feminist Therapy (11-FE); Chapter 12, Family Therapy (12-FA); and Chapter 13, Narrative Therapy (13-NA).

ABC model   (8-BE) A term that delineates the temporal sequence of antecedents, behavior, and consequences.

absent but implicit   (13-NA) That which is not spoken but is the "other side" of what is spoken. For example, the other side of disappointment is that which was hoped for.

activity schedule   (9-CB) A written, hour-by-hour plan of what a client will do on a given day that gives the client structure to guide and encourage adaptive behaviors.

actualizing tendency   (6-PC) An inherent tendency within the individual to strive toward fulfillment, autonomy, and independence, and generally toward optimal development of the total organism.

alternative stories   (13-NA) Stories that are outside or beyond the terms of the dominant or problem story.

androcentric   (11-FE) Describing a situation in which men and boys are used as the standard for normal and valued behavior and characteristics. Using a male-centered perspective.

androgyny   (11-FE) Having a balance of male and female stereotypic traits.

animism   (5-EX) The belief that everything in the universe is connected by a common spirit.

antecedents   (8-BE) Prerequisites (knowledge, skills, and resources) and environmental cues that are present or occur before a behavior is performed and that set the stage for and initiate behaviors.

anxiety hierarchy   (8-BE) A list of events that elicit anxiety, ranked by the client in order of increasing anxiety.

archetypes   (3-PS) In Jungian theory, shared symbols in the collective unconscious.

assertion training   (8-BE) A skills training treatment package to teach people both how and when to behave assertively.

assimilation   (7-GE) The subjective experience that one is different or has changed in some way as a result of contact with the environment.

authenticity   (5-EX) The state of being real or genuine.

automatic thoughts   (9-CB) Cognitive therapy term for irrational, maladaptive cognitions.

awareness   (7-GE) The process of directing one's attention to the most salient aspect of the individual/environmental field at the present moment.

backup reinforcers   (8-BE) In a token economy, reinforcers for which clients can exchange tokens that they earned for desirable behaviors.

basic mistakes   (4-AD) Adler's term for self-defeating cognitions, such as making overgeneralizations and setting impossible-to-reach goals.

becoming   (5-EX) A term used to indicate that each individual continuously creates the self.

behavior rehearsal   (8-BE) Therapy procedure in which a client practices performing an adaptive behavior.

birth order   (4-AD) Notion that the order in which siblings are born and the way in which each sibling's psychological position in the family is interpreted strongly predict their life-styles.

boundaries   (12-FA) Conceptual demarcations between individuals and parts of systems that describe who participates and how.

brief/graduated exposure therapies   (8-BE) Procedures that expose clients to threatening events for a short period and incrementally, beginning with low anxiety-inducing events and progressing to high anxiety-inducing events.

choice theory   (10-RE) The theoretical underpinning of reality therapy, which posits that behavior originates from within and that most behaviors are chosen.

closure   (7-GE) The end point of a figure formation and destruction process.

cognitive modeling   (9-CB) A model's talking aloud about what he or she is thinking.

cognitive restructuring   (9-CB) Replacing maladaptive cognitions with adaptive cognitions.

cognitive therapy   (9-CB) Cognitive restructuring therapy in which clients are taught to view their irrational beliefs as tentative hypotheses that they can test by gathering evidence that refutes the beliefs.

cognitive-behavioral therapy   (9-CB) Interventions that directly or indirectly change clients' cognitions that are maintaining their problem behaviors.

collaborative empiricism   (9-CB) Cognitive therapy procedure in which the therapist and client work together to frame the client's irrational beliefs as hypotheses and design homework "experiments" that the client uses to test these hypotheses.

collective unconscious   (3-PS) In Jungian theory, a realm of the unconscious in which there are symbols that are shared by all humanity.

community genogram   (12-FA) A graphic tool that emphasizes strengths and resources that can be accessed in the contexts of family, community, and culture.

condensation   (3-PS) Two ideas being expressed with a single image.

conditions of worth   (6-PC) An individual's attempt to behave in certain ways to create the conditions in which he or she is most likely to be positively regarded and accepted.

confluence   (7-GE) Denial of any difference between the self and the environment; a subjective sense that there is no contact boundary.

congruence (6-PC) An optimal state of functioning or mental health in which an individual's thoughts, behaviors, and emotions are aligned with the person's self-concept.

conscious (3-PS) The part of the mind containing all that we are aware of.

consciousness raising (11-FE) Increasing awareness about the existence of societal oppression and privilege.

consequences (8-BE) Events that occur after and as a result of performing a behavior and that determine whether the person will engage in the specific behavior or similar behaviors again.

consulting your consultants (13-NA) Therapists' consulting with clients—those who have consulted with them—about the knowledges the clients have generated that may be of use to others and about the therapy itself in order to further develop therapists' practices.

contact (7-GE) A behavior that establishes a relationship with the figure of interest.

contact boundary (7-GE) The meeting point between self and other.

coping model (8-BE) A model who is initially fearful about and somewhat incompetent in performing a behavior but who then becomes more comfortable and skilled in performing it.

coresearch (13-NA) The narrative practice of collaborative conversational inquiry with the purpose of researching a person's lived experience to generate knowledges previously unavailable to either party.

countertransference (3-PS) In classical psychoanalysis, the process by which the therapist displaces unconscious feelings and impulses from the therapist's past onto the client. In contemporary psychoanalysis, the totality of the therapist's perception of and responses to the client.

courage (5-EX) The heart or spirit to confront life and its demands.

covert self-modeling (8-BE) A procedure in which clients imagine themselves performing the target behavior.

creative adjustment (7-GE) An accommodation made by an individual who is striking a balance between getting a need met and fitting into the dominant field conditions that have power and control over his or her well-being.

curious questioning (13-NA) Therapists' asking questions that offer genuine curiosity and are open to learning from clients about the particular knowledges available from clients' lived experience within their particular cultural contexts.

cycle of awareness and contact (7-GE) A model that describes the figure formation and destruction process in detail, designating stages in that process and points of potential interpretation.

Dasein (5-EX) The human being that exists; a German term coined by Ludwig Binswanger, which literally translated means "there being."

death drive (3-PS) Freud's term for the source of aggression and destructiveness.

defense mechanisms (3-PS) Processes by which people ward off anxiety-provoking impulses, thoughts, and feelings.

deflection (7-GE) Engagement of the environment in an indirect way that diffuses or dilutes the intensity of full-on contact.

denial   (3-PS) A defense mechanism in which people negate the presence of a thought, feeling, or impulse in themselves or an aspect of external reality.

dereflection   (5-EX) A therapeutic technique used by Victor Frankl in which the client is encouraged to "think away" from whatever causes presenting anxiety.

dialogue   (7-GE) A term that describes a relationship between two individuals that alternates between moments of I-It and I-Thou relating.

differential reinforcement   (8-BE) Indirectly decelerating an undesirable behavior by reinforcing an alternative, more desirable behavior.

differential relaxation   (8-BE) Relaxing all muscles not needed to perform required behaviors (used in in vivo exposure therapy).

differentiation of self   (12-FA) The separation of emotions and intellect as reflected by the ability to maintain a sense of self in relation to others.

discouragement   (4-AD) Lacking courage; feeling that one does not belong to society in a useful, constructive manner.

discourse   (13-NA) A metanarrative that tells us how things are in our world and that makes particular social processes possible.

discursive listening   (13-NA) Listening for the discourses that shape the personal stories being told by clients.

displacement   (3-PS) A defense mechanism in which a conflict is experienced in a context remote from the one in which it originated and in which it is most emotionally charged.

dissociation   (3-PS) A defense mechanism in which certain experiences are allowed into consciousness only in certain states of mind.

dominant discourses   (13-NA) Those discourses or metanarratives that produce the taken-for-granted norms and politics of social life.

dominant stories   (13-NA) Cultural, community, and family stories whose terms are taken for granted and accepted by individuals as norms.

early recollection   (4-AD) A single incident in early childhood (under age 8) that an individual can vividly recall and describe.

ego   (3-PS) The part of the mind that mediates among the id, the superego, and the external world.

ego psychology   (3-PS) A form of psychoanalysis focusing on the activities of the ego and aiming, in therapy, to strengthen that part of the mind.

Eigenwelt   (5-EX) The personal environment; a German term coined by Ludwig Binswanger as part of his three-world model (Eigenwelt, Mitwelt, and Umwelt).

Electra complex   (3-PS) A syndrome in which a girl around the age of 5 has impulses to have sex with her father and to kill her mother.

empathy   (6-PC) A process in therapy in which the counselor communicates that he or she accurately perceives the client's internal experience and the meaning of that experience.

empowerment   (11-FE) Exerting influence over the personal, interpersonal, and institutional factors that impact health and well-being.

empty chair   (7-GE) A technique that allows the client to imagine talking to another who is not present.

enactments (12-FA) Therapist-directed in-session interventions in which clients are asked to engage in new behaviors, including speaking directly to each other.

encouragement (4-AD) Technique of building the therapy relationship and fostering client change by helping clients to feel that they have worth as they are.

energic model (3-PS) Freud's model of the mind that depicts mental functioning as deriving from the interplay of various forces or forms of energy.

environment (7-GE) The context and culture in which the client lives.

eros (3-PS) The life force that gives rise to libido.

essence (5-EX) The essential being of a person, which is created solely by the person.

ethnocentric (11-FE) Describing a situation in which the dominant ethnic group's values and perceptions serve as the norm against which subordinate ethnic groups are evaluated.

existence (5-EX) The state of existing.

existential anxiety The human being's inherent fear of nonbeing or death.

existentialism (5-EX) A philosophical and literary movement based on the doctrine that existence precedes essence; it holds that humans are totally free and responsible for their acts and that this responsibility is the source of their dread and anguish.

experiment (7-GE) A method that shifts the focus of counseling from talking about a topic to an activity that will heighten the client's awareness and understanding through experience.

exposure therapies (8-BE) Treatment procedures that expose clients to anxiety-inducing events in order to reduce the anxiety.

extended family (12-FA) Groups of people beyond the nuclear family who are related by blood and/or consider themselves part of enduring, close relationships with each other.

externalizing conversation (13-NA) A practice in which the problem is conceptualized and named as distinct from the person and seen as a malign force by which a person is tricked, tortured, or imprisoned.

externalizing language (13-NA) Linguistic and political practice that locates the problem outside the person, thereby producing a gap between person and problem that can be explored by externalizing conversations.

extinction (8-BE) Treatment that eliminates reinforcers for a behavior in order to decelerate the behavior.

family constellation (4-AD) Siblings, parents, and other key people who have early developmental influences upon an individual.

family genogram (12-FA) A diagram of intergenerational and extended family systems using symbols to represent family members and events.

family map (12-FA) A diagram that reflects family structural arrangements using symbols to represent family members and their relationships to each other.

family sculpting (12-FA) An experiential method in which family members physically place themselves relative to each other in ways that reflect and express their relationships, thoughts, and feelings.

family structure (12-FA) Family organization and definition of relationships reflected by recurring patterns of interaction.

faulty logic   (4-AD) Adler's term for convictions that run counter to social interest, are unique to the individual, and do not facilitate useful, constructive belonging.

feedback loops   (12-FA) Circular mechanisms through which information is taken out and brought into a system, creating change and/or stability.

field   (7-GE) A dynamic interrelated system of relationships, each part of which influences every other part.

figure   (7-GE) The aspect of the environment that stands out to the perceiver.

figure formation and destruction   (7-GE) An ongoing process in which individuals become aware of a need or interest and make contact with some aspect of the environment in a way that satisfies or "destroys" that figure, allowing it to recede to the background.

flooding   (8-BE) Common behavior therapy term for prolonged/intense exposure therapies.

free association   (3-PS) Client's reporting every thought or feeling that comes to mind, no matter how seemingly trivial or embarrassing.

freedom   (5-EX) The state of psychological independence that is inescapable and comes from being in the world.

gestalt   (7-GE) A German word meaning a "form," "whole," or "configuration."

graded task assignments   (9-CB) Cognitive therapy technique in which clients are prompted and shaped to engage in small, sequential steps that lead to a therapeutic goal.

ground   (7-GE) The backdrop from which figures emerge.

holism   (4-AD) An understanding of each person as an integrated being in which the whole is greater than the sum of its parts.

holistic   (7-GE) All aspects of an individual's experience are regarded as equally important and connect to form an organismic whole.

homework assignments   (8-BE) Between-session therapy tasks clients engage in.

id   (3-PS) The part of the mind containing instincts and biological urges.

ideal self   (6-PC) An individual's desired sense of self or the self the person would like to be.

identification   (3-PS) A defense mechanism involving taking on other people's characteristics.

identity development models   (11-FE) Theories that describe the processes by which individuals' social identities are impacted by the advantaged or disadvantaged social positions of their social locations.

in vivo   (8-BE) Describes procedures implemented in actual situations (as opposed to imagining them).

in vivo exposure therapy   (8-BE) Essentially systematic desensitization in which the client is exposed to the actual anxiety-evoking events (rather than imagining them).

incongruence   (6-PC) A state in which individuals experience a sense of discord between their self-concept and their present thoughts, behaviors, and emotions.

inferiority complex   (4-AD) A behavioral manifestation of a strong and exaggerated subjective belief that one is not as good as other people.

inner world (or internal world)   (3-PS) Fantasies containing stable representations of self and others.

insider knowledges (13-NA) Knowledges produced by those with firsthand experience of problems or difficulties.

interactionist (11-FE) Counseling theories that view client problems as arising from a combination of internal and external factors.

internal frame of reference (6-PC) The realm of experience available to the awareness of the individual at any moment.

internal object (3-PS) In object relations theory, a stable representation of other people.

interpretation (3-PS) In classical psychoanalysis, the activity of the therapist in conveying to the client the unconscious meaning of his or her dreams and free associations. In contemporary psychoanalysis, the process of the therapist's addressing the meanings emerging from the analytic interaction.

intrapsychic (11-FE) Counseling theories that view the source of clients' problems as internal to the client.

introjection (7-GE) The "swallowing whole" of some aspect of the environment without discrimination.

I-thou (5-EX) A way of relating to another person as a subject with care and authenticity as opposed to "I-It," which is relating to the other as an object or a thing.

libido (3-PS) Freud's term for sexual energy.

life goals (4-AD) An individual's goals that are beneficial to others or, at least, do not interfere with those of others.

life tasks (4-AD) The main challenges people experience in life, which must be addressed in order to function effectively.

life-style (4-AD) Adler's term for the attitudes and convictions people have about how to find their place in the world; the instructions for how to belong.

local knowledges (13-NA) Ideas that originate out of people's own lived experiences in particular settings.

locus of evaluation (6-PC) The source of a person's valuing process, existing either internally, with evidence being provided by the person's own senses, or externally, with the person looking to others to assess the value of an experience.

logotherapy (5-EX) Based on existential principles, a psychotherapeutic model developed by Victor Frankl.

maieutic method (5-EX) Therapeutic process, adapted from Socrates' teaching method, in which the counselor solicits ideas from the client by posing a series of questions to the client.

maintaining conditions (8-BE) Antecedents and consequences of a behavior that result in a behavior being performed.

mastery and pleasure ratings (9-CB) Cognitive therapy technique in which clients use a rating scale to assess their daily activities for mastery (sense of accomplishment) and for pleasure (feelings of enjoyment).

meaning (5-EX) An individual's sense of significance and purpose. To be devoid of meaning in life is to be devoid of hope or reason for being.

mistaken goals (4-AD) Adler's term for an individual's goals that are detrimental to other people and run counter to social interest.

Mitwelt (5-EX) The social environment; a German term, which literally translated means "with-world," coined by Ludwig Binswanger as part of his three-world model (Eigenwelt, Mitwelt, and Umwelt).

modeling therapies (8-BE) Procedures that expose a client (an observer) to a person (a model) whose behavior the client could benefit from by imitating.

needs (10-RE) The basic innate motivators of behaviors: survival or self-preservation; love or belonging; power, achievement, or inner control; freedom or independence; fun or enjoyment.

neuroses (3-PS) Patterns of self-defeating behavior and symptomatology.

normalizing judgment (13-NA) A perspective on what is normal that leads to the shaping of lives in reference to established norms.

nuclear family (12-FA) Members of intimate, enduring relational systems that offer contact and support to each other in daily living.

object (5-EX) The person in an interaction who is seen or acted upon (as opposed to the subject who sees or acts).

object relations theories (3-PS) Psychoanalytic theories that emphasize the influence of preconceptions, schemata, and templates through which self and others are perceived and experienced.

Oedipus complex (3-PS) A syndrome in which a boy around the age of 5 has impulses to have sex with his mother and to kill his father.

openness to experience (6-PC) An individual's ability to readily accept information from the environment without distortion or defensiveness.

oppression (11-FE) Forces that cause certain social groups to be disadvantaged and subordinated by being denied access to societal resources and power.

organismic self-regulation (7-GE) Maintaining one's health and well-being by attending to the most salient or figural need or interest at a particular moment and initiating some action with the environment to satisfy that interest or need.

organismic valuing process (6-PC) An individual's ability to make judgments or assessments of the desirability of an action or behavior on the basis of sensory evidence and life experience.

overcorrection (8-BE) Deceleration therapy in which clients correct the effects of their maladaptive or harmful actions (restitution) and then intensively practice an appropriate alternative behavior (positive practice).

paradoxical intention (5-EX) A therapeutic technique used by Victor Frankl, in which he encouraged the client to think about or focus on the thing or person that causes anxiety.

paradoxical intervention (12-FA) A request designed to be inherently incongruent to encourage family members to reject the directive in favor of giving up a symptom.

paradoxical theory of change (7-GE) Change occurs by more fully experiencing "what is," not by trying to get to "what is not."

participant modeling (8-BE) A treatment package in which the therapist models an anxiety-evoking behavior and then encourages and guides the client's practicing the behavior.

patriarchal (11-FE) Referring to a society in which dominant and valued social roles are assigned to males and subordinate ones to females.

penis envy (3-PS) Freud's idea that women universally wish to have a penis and envy men their possession of a penis.

phenomenological inquiry (7-GE) A way of understanding and assisting clients by encouraging them to describe their experiences and the meanings they ascribe to those experiences.

phenomenology (7-GE) The description of data available to the senses; what is given and evident in any immediate experience.

physically aversive consequences (8-BE) Decelerating a maladaptive behavior by making its consequences physically unpleasant.

positive regard (6-PC) An attitude and feeling communicated by the therapist that the client is genuinely accepted and prized for who he or she is in the present moment.

power (11-FE) The ability to access personal and environmental resources to effect personal and/or external change.

preconscious (3-PS) The part of the mind containing content that has not become conscious but is potentially accessible to consciousness.

private logic (4-AD) Adler's term for ideas conceived in childhood that comprise one's deeply established personal beliefs or constructs.

privilege (11-FE) The experience of social groups that are advantaged and have access to societal resources and power.

problem-solving therapy (9-CB) Coping skills therapy in which clients sequentially follow a series of seven interrelated steps or stages to treat a psychological problem for which they specifically have sought treatment.

process (7-GE) The way in which an individual experiences and interacts with the environment and the present moment.

progressive relaxation (8-BE) Muscle relaxation technique that involves alternately tensing and relaxing various muscle groups to train clients to differentiate between tension and relaxation, which allows them to create bodily relaxation.

projection 1. (3-PS) A defense mechanism that involves attributing disavowed aspects of self to another person. 2. (7-GE) Attribution of a part of the self to the environment such that it is experienced in another, not in the self.

projective identification (3-PS) In object relations theory, the process of attributing disavowed aspects of self to another person and then maintaining an unconscious identification with that aspect of self in the other person.

prolonged/intense exposure therapies (8-BE) Treatments in which clients experience highly anxiety-evoking events for lengthy periods in order to reduce anxiety.

prompts (8-BE) Cues that remind or instruct a client to perform a behavior.

psychological adjustment (6-PC) An individual is seen as psychologically adjusted when there is consistency between sensory and visceral experience and the concept of self.

psychological maladjustment (6-PC) This state occurs when there is inconsistency between experience and self-concept and when the individual denies or distorts awareness of experience which creates incongruence.

psychotherapeutic eros (5-EX) A close, intimate, but nonsexual feeling that the therapist has for the client.

punishment (8-BE) A process by which the consequence of a behavior decreases the likelihood that the behavior will be repeated.

quality world (10-RE) A collection of specific wants or pictures of wants unique to each individual that develops from choices designed to satisfy needs.

rational emotive behavior therapy (REBT) (9-CB) Cognitive restructuring therapy in which clients' irrational thoughts are directly challenged and replaced with rational thoughts.

rationalization (3-PS) A defense mechanism in which an irrational emotional response is framed as having a rational basis.

reaction formation (3-PS) Defense mechanism in which an idea is represented by its opposite.

reframe (12-FA) To relabel the conceptual understanding of problems so as to expand possibilities for change.

regression (3-PS) A defense mechanism in which an individual returns to a mode of functioning characterizing an earlier development phase.

reinforcement (8-BE) A process by which the consequence of a behavior increases the likelihood that the behavior will be repeated.

reinforcer (8-BE) Consequence of a behavior that increased the likelihood that the behavior will be repeated.

relational model (3-PS) A form of contemporary psychoanalysis in which mental life is believed to be organized by one's past and present interpersonal context.

repression (3-PS) A defense mechanism in which psychic material is rendered unconscious.

resistance (3-PS) The process by which the client wards off the therapist's efforts to bring unconscious psychic content to awareness.

response cost (8-BE) Deceleration therapy in which a client is temporarily deprived of a valued item or a privilege as a consequence of performing a deceleration target behavior.

response prevention (8-BE) Procedure in which clients are prevented from engaging in their typical anxiety-reducing responses; used as part of in vivo flooding.

retroflection (7-GE) A term used in two ways in Gestalt theory: (1) energy, emotions, and words necessary to make contact with another are cut off and redirected back (retro) toward the self; and (2) doing something for yourself rather than asking someone to do it for you.

schema (9-CB) A broad, pervasive, and rigid cognitive theme about oneself, others, or the world that a person uses to interpret particular events.

schema-based cognitive therapy (9-CB) Technique that identifies and modifies clients' schemas that are maintaining their problem behaviors.

self (6-PC) An individual's organized and consistent set of perceptions of the characteristics of the *I* or *me* coupled with the values attached to these perceptions.

self-actualization (6-PC) A basic human drive toward growth or completeness that is realized when a person experiences the self as the ideal self.

self-concept (4-AD) The sum total of all of the convictions and attitudes one has about oneself.

self-ideal (4-AD) A person's idea of what he or she ought to be in relation to the world and people.

self-instructional training (9-CB) Coping skills therapy that teaches clients to instruct themselves to cope effectively with difficult situations.

self-knowledge (5-EX) Individuals' awareness of their personality traits, abilities, limitations, preferences, and other key aspects of themselves.

self-modeling (8-BE) Therapy in which clients serve as their own models of adaptive functioning.

self-talk (9-CB) What people say to themselves when they are thinking.

setting events (8-BE) Broad environmental conditions that influence the likelihood that a person will engage in a particular behavior.

sexism (11-FE) Institutional and personal bias based on gender; most commonly a form of oppression that subordinates girls and women.

shaping (8-BE) A process of reinforcing successively closer approximations or components of a behavior so that eventually the individual performs the complete behavior.

skills training (8-BE) Treatment packages—consisting of modeling, direct instruction, prompting, shaping, role playing, and behavior rehearsal—that teach clients skills.

social constructionism (13-NA) The theory that reality is constructed through interactions among and between people and systems of knowledge, as we give meaning to events in the world.

social identities (11-FE) How individuals perceive their social locations.

social interest (4-AD) Concern for the interest of others; behaviors and attitudes that display a sense of responsibility for and community with others.

social locations (11-FE) Culturally constructed categories that place people into social groups; the social positions that people hold in a given culture.

social skills training (8-BE) Skills training specifically for developing interpersonal skills.

Socratic dialogue (5-EX) A method of teaching first used by Socrates in which the master imparts no information but asks a sequence of questions. By answering the questions, the pupil eventually comes to acquire the desired knowledge.

stimulus control (8-BE) Treatments that modify the antecedent stimuli that are maintaining a target behavior.

stress inoculation training (9-CB) Coping skills therapy to prevent stress; clients learn coping skills and then practice using the skills while being exposed to stress-evoking events.

structural model (3-PS) Freud's model that divides the mind according to psychic functions—specifically, id, ego, and superego.

subject (5-EX) The person in an interaction who sees and acts (as opposed to the object who is seen or acted upon).

sublimation (3-PS) The most mature defense mechanism in which the energy of an instinctual impulse is turned toward a socially productive end.

subsystems (12-FA) Units within larger systems that are defined by numerous functions including roles, interests, goals, gender, and generational status. Each member of a family system simultaneously belongs to numerous subsystems.

superego (3-PS) Freud's term for the part of the mind that contains societally derived ideals and values.

systematic desensitization   (8-BE) Exposure therapy in which the client imagines successively more anxiety-arousing situations while engaging in a behavior that competes with anxiety.

target behavior   (8-BE) A discrete, measurable aspect of a client's problem that is changed to alleviate the problem.

technique   (7-GE) A standard operating procedure used in many psychotherapy orientations by a counselor to achieve a particular outcome when certain conditions are present.

thick description   (13-NA) Description of a person that comes from the interpretation of the person being described and carries the meanings of the person's community of support.

thin description   (13-NA) Description of a person that comes from the dominant discourse and excludes the interpretation of the person being described and the interpretations of the person's community of support.

thought stopping   (9-CB) Technique to decrease persistent, disturbing thoughts by first interrupting the disturbing thought and then substituting a nondisturbing, competing thought.

time out from positive reinforcement   (8-BE) Temporarily withdrawing a client's access to generalized reinforcers when a client performs a deceleration target behavior.

token economy   (8-BE) Treatment system for motivating clients to perform desirable behaviors and to refrain from performing undesirable behaviors by earning and losing token reinforcers (such as points).

tonic behaviors   (10-RE) Healthy counselor behaviors that enable the client to feel safe, secure, and motivated.

top dog–underdog dialogue   (7-GE) A technique in which a therapist coaches a client to enact a conversation between two parts of the self that are unintegrated or in conflict.

topographic model   (3-PS) Freud's model of the mind that postulates varying levels of consciousness: conscious, preconscious, and unconscious.

total behavior   (10-RE) The composite of four components of behavior: actions, cognition or thinking, emotions or feelings, and physiology.

toxic behaviors   (10-RE) Unhealthy counselor behaviors that cast a negative pall on the counseling process and result in client resistance rather than change.

transference   (3-PS) In classical psychoanalysis, the process by which clients displace unconscious feelings and impulses from the past onto the therapist. In contemporary psychoanalysis, the totality of the client's perceptions of, and responses to, the therapist.

transport   (13-NA) Being "carried across" by the stories we have told or witnessed and thus becoming other than who we were.

treatment package   (8-BE) Combination of two or more therapies to increase the effectiveness of the treatment.

triangulation   (12-FA) Process in which members of an unstable dyad detour conflict onto a third person or issue in order to stabilize their relationship.

Uberwelt   (5-EX) The spiritual world (literally the "overworld"); German term introduced by Van Deurzen-Smith to supplement Binswanger's three-world model (Eigenwelt, Mitwelt, and Umwelt).

Umwelt   (5-EX) The natural environment, a German term coined by Ludwig Binswanger as part of his three-world model (Eigenwelt, Mitwelt, and Umwelt).

unconditional positive regard   (6-PC) An attitude and feeling communicated by the therapist that the regard and acceptance being shown to a client is absolute.

unconscious   (3-PS) The part of the mind that is the repository of content that is repressed and out of awareness.

vicarious extinction   (8-BE) Modeling therapy to reduce fear or anxiety by exposing a client to a model who performs the anxiety-evoking behavior without any negative consequences occurring.

video self-modeling therapy   (8-BE) Technique in which clients watch videos of themselves performing adaptive behaviors.

wants   (10-RE) The specific things in our lives that we believe will satisfy our basic needs.

WDEP system   (10-RE) Teaching and learning tool comprising the most significant reality therapy interventions: helping clients define their wants and needs (W), examining their doing (behavior) and direction in which the behavior takes clients (D), conducting self-evaluation focused on the attainability of their wants and the effectiveness of their behaviors (E), and formulating plans of action (P).

witnessing   (13-NA) The purposeful positioning of oneself, in relation with community, to hear and respond to another's expression or story.

References

Abrahms, J. L. (1983). Cognitive-behavioral strategies to induce and enhance a collaborative set in distressed couples. In A. Freeman (Ed.), *Cognitive therapy with couples and groups* (pp. 125–155). New York: Plenum.

Abramowitz, J. S. (2001). Treatment of scrupulous obsessions and compulsions using exposure and response prevention: A case report. *Cognitive and Behavioral Practice, 8,* 79–85.

Abrams, M., & Ellis, A. (1994). Rational emotive behaviour therapy in the treatment of stress. *British Journal of Guidance and Counselling, 22,* 39–50.

Ackerman, N. W. (1958). *The psychodynamics of family life.* New York: Basic Books.

Adler, A. (1931/1992). *What life could mean to you* (C. Brett, Trans.). Oxford, UK: Oneworld.

Adler, A. (1956). *The Individual Psychology of Alfred Adler: A systematic presentation in selections from his writings* (H. L. Ansbacher & R. R. Ansbacher, Eds.). New York: Basic Books.

Alford, B. A., & Beck, A. T. (1994). Cognitive therapy of delusional beliefs. *Behaviour Research and Therapy, 32,* 369–380.

Alford, B. A., & Correia, C. J. (1994). Cognitive therapy of schizophrenia: Theory and empirical status. *Behavior Therapy, 25,* 17–33.

Allen, K. D., Danforth, J. S., & Drabman, R. S. (1989). Videotaped modeling and film distraction for fear reduction in adults undergoing hyperbaric oxygen therapy. *Journal of Consulting and Clinical Psychology, 57,* 554–558.

Alliance of Psychoanalytic Organizations. (2006). *Psychodynamic diagnostic manual.* Silver Spring, MD: Author.

Altman, N. (1995). *The analyst in the inner city: Race, class, and culture through a psychoanalytic lens.* Hillsdale, NJ: The Analytic Press.

Altman, N. (2004). History repeats itself in transference and countertransference. *Psychoanalytic Dialogues, 14,* 807–816.

Alvarez, M. F. (1997). Using REBT and supportive psychotherapy with post-stroke patients. *Journal of Rational-Emotive & Cognitive-Behavior Therapy, 15,* 231–245.

American Counseling Association. (1999). *Ethical standards for Internet online counseling of the American Counseling Association.* Alexandria, VA: Author.

American Counseling Association. (2002). *Multicultural counseling competencies.* Alexandria, VA: Author.

American Counseling Association. (2005). *Code of Ethics.* Retrieved February 11, 2006, from http://www.counseling.org

American Psychiatric Association. (2000). *Diagnostic and statistical manual of mental disorders–Text revision* (4th ed.). Washington, DC: Author.

American Psychological Association. (1975). Report of the task force on sex bias and sex-role stereotyping in psychotherapeutic practice. *American Psychologist, 30,* 1169–1175.

American Psychological Association. (1992). Ethical principles of psychologists and code of conduct. *American Psychologist, 47,* 1597–1611.

American Psychological Association. (1993). Guidelines for providers of psychological services to ethnic, linguistic, and culturally diverse populations. *American Psychologist, 48,* 45–48.

American Psychological Association. (1995). Training in and dissemination of empirically-validated psychological treatments: Report and recommendations. *The Clinical Psychologist, 48,* 3–24.

American Psychological Association. (2002a). Ethical principles of psychologists and code of conduct. *American Psychologist, 57,* 1060–1073. Available from APA website, http://www.apa.org/ethics

American Psychological Association. (2002b). *Guidelines on multicultural education, training, research, practice, and organizational change for psychologists.* Retrieved June 2005 from www.apa.org

American Psychological Association. (2003a). Guidelines on multicultural education, training, research, practice, and organizational change for psychologists. *American Psychologist, 58,* 377–402.

American Psychological Association. (2003b). Guidelines for psychological practice with older adults. Retrieved from http://www.apa.org/practice/Guidelines_for_Psychological_Practice_with_Older_Adults.pdf

American Psychological Association, Division 44/Committee on Lesbian, Gay, and Bisexual Concerns Joint Task Force on Guidelines for Psychotherapy with Lesbian, Gay, and Bisexual Clients. (2000). Guidelines for psychotherapy with lesbian, gay, and bisexual clients. *American Psychologist, 55,* 1440–1451.

Anderson, C. (1995). *Flying solo.* New York: Norton.

Anderson, H., & Goolishian, H. (1988). Human systems as linguistic systems: Preliminary and evolving ideas about the implications for clinical theory. *Family Process, 27,* 371–93.

Anderson, H., Goolishian, H. A., & Winderman, L. (1986). Problem determined systems: Toward transformation in family therapy. *Journal of Strategic and Systemic Therapies, 5,* 1–14.

Anderson, S. A., & Bagarozzi, D. (1983). The use of family myths as an aid to strategic therapy. *Journal of Family Therapy, 5,* 145–164.

Anderson, S. A., & Sabatelli, R. M. (1999). *Family interaction: A multigenerational developmental perspective* (2nd ed.). Boston: Allyn & Bacon.

Andersson, G., Melin, L., Scott, B., & Lindberg, P. (1995). An evaluation of a behavioural treatment approach to hearing impairment. *Behaviour Research and Therapy, 33,* 283–292.

Ansbacher, H. L. & Ansbacher, R. R. (Eds.). (1956). *The Individual Psychology of Alfred Adler: A systematic presentation in selections from his writings.* New York: Harper Torchbooks.

Ansbacher, H. L., & Ansbacher, R. (Eds.). (1970). *Superiority and social interest by Alfred Adler.* Evanston, IL: Northwestern University Press.

Anton, W. D. (1976). An evaluation of outcome variables in the systematic desensitization of test anxiety. *Behaviour Research and Therapy, 14,* 217–224.

Antoni, M. H., Kumar, M., Ironson, G., Cruess, D. G., Lutgendorf, S., Klimas, N., et al. (2000). Cognitive-behavioral stress management intervention effects on anxiety, 24Hr urinary norepinephrine output, and T-Cytotoxic/suppressor cells over time among symptomatic HIV-infected gay men. *Journal of Consulting and Clinical Psychology, 68,* 31–45.

Antoni, M. H., Lehman, J. M., Kilbourn, K. M., Boyers, A. E., Culver, J. L., Alferi, S. M., et al. (2001). Cognitive-behavioral stress management intervention decreases the prevalence of depression and enhances benefit finding among woman under treatment for early-stage breast cancer. *Health Psychology, 20,* 20–32.

Antoninus, M. A. (1944). *The meditations of Marcus Antonius* (A. Farquharson, Ed.). London: Oxford University Press.

Aponte, H. J. (1987). The treatment of society's poor: An ecological perspective on the underorganized family. *Family Therapy Today, 2*(1), 1–7.

Arciniega, G. M., & Newlon, B. J. (1999). Counseling and psychotherapy: Multicultural considerations. In D. Capuzzi & D. F. Gross (Eds.), *Counseling & psychotherapy: Theories and interventions* (2nd ed., pp. 435–458). Upper Saddle River, NJ: Merrill/ Prentice-Hall.

Arean, P. A., Perri, M. G., Nezu, A. M., Schein, R. L., Christopher, F., & Joseph, T. X. (1993). Comparative effectiveness of social problem-solving therapy and reminiscence therapy as treatments for depression in older adults. *Journal of Consulting and Clinical Psychology, 61,* 1003–1010.

Ariel, S. (1999). *Culturally competent family therapy.* Westport, CT: Greenwood.

Arkowitz, H. (1992a). Integrative theories of therapy. In D. K. Freedheim (Ed.), *History of psychotherapy: A century of change* (pp. 261–303). Washington, DC: American Psychological Association.

Arkowitz, H. (1992b, Summer). Psychotherapy integration: Bringing psychotherapy back to psychology. *The General Psychologist,* 11–20.

Armstrong, K. J., & Drabman, R. S. (1998). Treatment of a nine-year-old girl's masturbatory behavior. *Child and Family Behavior Therapy, 20,* 55–62.

Arnold, M. S. (2002). Culture-sensitive family therapy. In J. Carlson & D. Kjos (Eds.), *Theories and strategies of family therapy* (pp. 19–40). Boston: Allyn & Bacon.

Asante, M. K. (2003). *Afrocentricity: The theory of social change* (2nd ed.). Chicago: African American Images.

Asarnow, J. R., & Callan, J. W. (1985). Boys with peer adjustment problems: Social cognitive processes. *Journal of Consulting and Clinical Psychology, 53,* 80–87.

Asay, T. P., & Lambert, M. J., (1999). The empirical case for the common factors in therapy. In M. A. Hubble, B. L. Duncan, & S. D. Miller (Eds.), *The heart and soul of change* (pp. 23–55). Washington, DC: American Psychological Association.

Asen, E. (2002). Outcome research in family therapy. *Advances in Psychiatric Treatment, 8,* 230–238.

Attneave, C. (1969). Therapy in tribal settings and urban network interventions. *Family Process, 8,* 192–210.

Aubrey, R. F. (1977). Historical development of guidance and counseling and implications for the future. *Personnel and Guidance Journal, 55,* 288–295.

Auerswald, E. (1968). Interdisciplinary versus ecologicial approach. *Family Process, 2,* 202–216.

Aydin, G., & Yerin, O. (1994). The effect of a story-based cognitive behavior modification procedure on reducing children's test anxiety before and after cancellation of an important examination. *International Journal for the Advancement of Counselling, 17,* 149–161.

Ayllon, T., & Azrin, N. H. (1968). *The token economy: A motivational system for therapy and rehabilitation.* New York: Appleton-Century-Crofts.

Baker, M. (2001). *Families, labour and love: Family diversity in a changing world.* Crows Nest, NSW Australia: Allen & Unwin.

Baldwin, M. (1987). Interview with Carl Rogers on the use of self in therapy. In M. Baldwin & V. Satir (Eds.), *The use of self in therapy* (pp. 45–52). New York: Haworth Press.

Ballard, K. D., & Crooks, T. J. (1984). Videotape modeling for preschool children with low levels of social interaction and low peer involvement in play. *Journal of Abnormal Child Psychology, 12,* 95–110.

Balter, R. & Unger, P. (1997). REBT stress management with patients with chronic fatigue syndrome. *Journal of Rational-Emotive & Cognitive-Behavior Therapy, 15,* 223–230.

Bandura, A. (1977). *Social learning theory.* Englewood Cliffs, NJ: Prentice-Hall.

Bandura, A. (1986). *Social foundations of thought and action: A social cognitive theory.* Englewood Cliffs, NJ: Prentice-Hall.

Bandura, A. (1997). *Self-efficacy: The exercise of control.* San Francisco: Freeman.

Bandura, A., & Menlove, F. L. (1968). Factors determining vicarious extinction of avoidance behavior through symbolic modeling. *Journal of Personality and Social Psychology, 8,* 274–281.

Bandura, A., & Walters, R. H. (1963). *Social learning and personality development.* New York: Holt, Rinehart & Winston.

Bankart, C. P. (1997). *Talking cures: A history of Western and Eastern psychotherapies.* Pacific Grove, CA: Brooks/Cole.

Baptiste, D. A. (1987). Family therapy with Spanish-heritage immigrant families in cultural transition. *Contemporary Family Therapy, 9*(4), 229–251.

Barnhill, L. H., & Longo, D. (1978). Fixation and regression in the family life cycle. *Family Process, 17,* 469–478.

Baruth, L. G., & Manning, M. L. (1987). God, religion, and the life tasks. *Individual Psychology, 43,* 429–436.

Bateson, G. (1951). Information and codification: A philosophical approach. In J. Ruesch & G. Bateson (Eds.), *Communication: The social matrix of psychiatry* (pp. 168–211). New York: Norton.

Bateson, G., Jackson, D., Haley, J., & Weakland, J. (1956). Towards a theory of schizophrenia. *Behavioral Science, 1,* 251–64.

Baucom, D. H., & Epstein, N. (1990). *Cognitive-behavioral marital therapy.* New York: Brunner/Mazel.

Baucom, D., Shoham, V., Mueser, K. T., Daiuto, A. D., & Stickle, T. R. (1998). Empirically supported couple and family interventions for marital distress and adult mental health problems. *Journal of Consulting and Clinical Psychology, 66,* 53–88.

Beauvoir, S. de. (1953). *The second sex* (H. M. Parshley, Ed. & Trans.). London: Jonathan Cape.

Beck, A. T. (1963). Thinking and depression. *Archives of General Psychiatry, 9,* 324–333.

Beck, A. T. (1967). *Depression: Clinical, experimental, and theoretical aspects.* New York: Harper & Row.

Beck, A. T. (1976). *Cognitive therapy and the emotional disorders.* New York: International Universities Press.

Beck, A. T. (1988). Cognitive approaches to panic disorder: Theory and therapy. In S. Rachman & J. D. Maser (Eds.), *Panic: Psychological perspectives* (pp. 91–109). Hillsdale, NJ: Erlbaum.

Beck, A. T., & Freeman, A. (1989). *Cognitive therapy of personality disorders.* New York: Guilford.

Beck, A. T., Rush, A. J., Shaw, B. F., & Emery, G. (1979). *Cognitive therapy of depression.* New York: Guilford.

Beck, A. T., & Weishaar, M. (1989). Cognitive therapy. In A. Freeman, K. M. Simon, L. E. Beutler, & H. Arkowitz (Eds.), *Comprehensive handbook of cognitive therapy* (pp. 21–36). New York: Plenum.

Beck, A. T., Wright, F. D., Newman, C. F., & Liese, B. S. (1993). *Cognitive therapy of substance abuse.* New York: Guilford.

Becker, W. (1971). *Parents are teachers: A child management program.* Champaign, IL: Research Press.

Becvar, D., & Becvar, R. (2003). *Family therapy: A systemic integration* (5th ed.). Needham Heights, MA: Allyn & Bacon.

Becvar, R. J., & Becvar, D. S. (1994). The ecosystemic story: A story about stories. *Journal of Mental Health Counseling, 16,* 22–32.

Bedford, M. (1972). *Existentialism and creativity.* New York: Philosophical Library.

Beels, C. C. (2002). Notes for a cultural history of family therapy. *Family Process, 41,* 67–82.

Beisser, A. R. (1970). The paradoxical theory of change. In J. Fagan & I. L. Shepherd (Eds.), *Gestalt therapy now* (pp. 77–80). New York: Harper & Row.

Bell-Dolan, D. J. (1995). Social cue interpretation of anxious children. *Journal of Clinical Child Psychology, 24,* 1–10.

Bergin, A. E., & Garfield, S. L. (Eds.). (1994). *Handbook of psychotherapy and behavior change* (4th ed.). New York: Wiley.

Bernard, M. E., & DiGiuseppe, R. [A.]. (1989). Rational-emotive therapy today. In M. E. Bernard & R. [A.] DiGiuseppe (Eds.), *Inside rational-emotive therapy: A critical appraisal of the theory and therapy of Albert Ellis* (pp. 1–7). San Diego: Academic Press.

Beutler, L. E. (1998). Identifying empirically supported treatments: What if we didn't? *Journal of Consulting and Clinical Psychology, 66,* 113–120.

Bhabha, H. (1990). *Nation and narration.* New York: Routledge.

Bigelow, K. M., Huynen, K. B., & Lutzker, J. R. (1993). Using a changing criterion design to teach fire escape to a child with developmental disabilities. *Journal of Developmental and Physical Disabilities, 5,* 121–128.

Biggam, F. H., & Power, K. G. (1999). Social problem-solving skills and psychological distress among incarcerated young offenders: The issue of bullying and victimization. *Cognitive Therapy and Research, 23,* 307–326.

Binswanger, L. (1975). *Being-in-the-world: Selected papers of Ludwig Binswanger* (J. Needleman, Trans.). London: Souvenir Press.

Binswanger, L. (1991). Existential analysis and psychotherapy. In J. Ehrenwald (Ed.), *The history of psychotherapy* (pp. 374–379). Northvale, NJ: Aronson.

Bird, J. (1993). Coming out of the closet: Illuminating the therapeutic relationship. *Journal of Feminist Family Therapy, 5*(2), 47–64.

Bird, J. (2000). *The heart's narrative: Therapy and navigating life's contradictions.* Auckland, New Zealand: Edge Press.

Bird, J. (2004). *Talk that sings: Therapy in a new linguistic key.* Auckland, New Zealand: Edge Press.

Bird, M., Alexopoulos, P., & Adamowicz, J. (1995) Success and failure in five case studies: Use of cued recall to ameliorate behaviour problems in senile dementia. *International Journal of Geriatric Psychiatry, 10,* 305–311.

Black, D. (1987). A minimal intervention program and a problem-solving program for weight control. *Cognitive Therapy and Research, 11,* 107–120.

Blampied, N. M., & Kahan, E. (1992). Acceptability of alternative punishments: A community survey. *Behavior Modification, 16,* 400–413.

Bloom, J. W., & Walz, G. R. (Eds.). (2000). *Cybercounseling and cyberlearning: Strategies and resources for the millennium.* Alexandria, VA: American Counseling Association.

Bloom, J. W., & Walz, G. R. (Eds.). (2004). *Cybercounseling and cyberlearning—An encore.* Alexandria, VA: American Counseling Association.

Bohart, A. C., & Greenberg, L. S. (1997). *Empathy reconsidered: New directions in psychotherapy.* Washington, DC: American Psychological Association.

Bohart, A., & Tallman, K. (1999). *How clients make therapy work: The process of active self-healing.* Washington, DC: American Psychological Association.

Bollas, C. (1987). *The shadow of the object.* New York: Columbia University Press.

Bootzin, R. R. (1972). Stimulus control treatment for insomnia. *Proceedings of the 80th annual convention of the American Psychological Association, 7,* 395–396.

Bootzin, R. R., Epstein, D., & Wood, J. M. (1991). Stimulus control instructions. In P. Hauri (Ed.), *Case studies in insomnia* (pp. 19–28). New York: Plenum.

Boss, M. (1963). *Psychoanalysis and daseinsanalysis* (L. B. Lefebre, Trans.). New York: Basic Books.

Boszormenyi-Nagy, I. (1987). *Foundations of contextual therapy.* New York: Brunner/Mazel.

Boudin, H. M. (1972). Contingency contracting as a therapeutic tool in deceleration of amphetamine use. *Behavior Therapy, 3,* 602–608.

Bowen, M. (1960). A family concept of schizophrenia. In D. D. Jackson (Ed.), *The etiology of schizophrenia* (pp. 346–372). New York: Basic Books.

Bowen, M. (1972). On the differentiation of self. In J. Framo (Ed.), *Family interaction: A dialogue between family researchers and family therapists* (pp. 111–173). New York: Springer.

Bowen, M. (1974). Toward the differentiation of self in one's family of origin. In E. Andres & J. Lorio (Eds.), *Georgetown Family Symposium* (Vol. 1, pp. 171–191). Washington, DC: Georgetown Medical Center.

Bowen, M. (1975). Bowen on triangles, Part II. *Family, 2*(1), 35–38.

Bowen, M. (1978). *Family therapy in clinical practice.* New York: Aronson.

Bowers, W. A. (1989). Cognitive therapy with inpatients. In A. Freeman, K. M. Simon, L. E. Beutler, & H. Arkowitz (Eds.), *Comprehensive handbook of cognitive therapy* (pp. 583–596). New York: Plenum.

Boyd-Franklin, N. (1989a). *Black families in therapy*. New York: Guilford.

Boyd-Franklin, N. (1989b). Five key factors in the treatment of Black families. *Journal of Family Therapy and the Family, 6*, 53–69.

Boyd-Franklin, N. (2003). *Black families in therapy* (2nd ed.). New York: Guilford.

Bozarth, J. D., Zimring, F. M., & Tausch, R. (2002). Research in client-centered therapy: The evolution of a revolution. In D. Cain & J. Seeman (Eds.), *Humanistic psychotherapies: Handbook of research and practice* (pp. 147–188). Washington, DC: American Psychological Association.

Brabeck, M. M. (Ed.). (2000). *Practicing feminist ethics in psychology*. Washington, DC: American Psychological Association.

Brabeck, M. M., & Brown, L. (with Christian, L., Espin, O., Hare-Mustin, R., Kaplan, A., et al.). (1997). Feminist theory and psychological practice. In J. Worrell & N. G. Johnson (Eds.), *Shaping the future of feminist psychology: Education, research, and practice* (pp. 15–35). Washington, DC: American Psychological Association.

Brabeck, M. M., & Ting, K. (2000). Feminist ethics: Lenses for examining ethical psychological practice. In M. M. Brabeck (Ed.), *Practicing feminist ethics in psychology* (pp. 17–35). Washington, DC: American Psychological Association.

Braswell, L., & Kendall, P. C. (2001). Cognitive-behavioral therapy with youth. In K. S. Dobson (Ed.), *Handbook of cognitive-behavioral therapies* (2nd ed., pp. 246–294). New York: Guilford.

Breuer, J., & Freud, S. (1895). Studies on hysteria. *Standard edition of the complete psychological works of Sigmund Freud* (Vol. 2). London: Hogarth Press.

Breunlin, D., Schwartz, R., & MacKune-Karrer, B. (1992). *Metaframeworks: Transcending the models of family therapy*. San Francisco: Jossey-Bass.

Brickman, J. (1984). Feminist, non-sexist, and traditional models of therapy: Implications for working with incest. *Women and Therapy, 3*, 49–67.

Brigitte, Sue, Mem, & Veronika. (1997). Power to our journeys. *Dulwich Centre Newsletter, (1)*, 25–33.

Broder, M. S. (2000). Making optimal use of homework to enhance your therapeutic effectiveness. *Journal of Rational-Emotive & Cognitive-Behavior Therapy, 18*, 3–18.

Brodsky, A. M., & Hare-Mustin, R. T. (1980). *Women and psychotherapy: An assessment of research and practice*. New York: Guilford.

Bronfenbrenner, U. (1979). *The ecology of human development*. Cambridge, MA: Harvard University Press.

Broverman, I. K., Broverman, D. M., Clarkson, F. E., Rosenkrantz, P. S., & Vogel, S. R. (1970). Sex-role stereotypes and clinical judgments of mental health. *Journal of Counseling and Clinical Psychology, 34*, 1–7.

Brown, G. K., Ten Have, T., Henriques, G. R., Xie, S. X., Hollander, J. E., & Beck, A. T. (2005). Cognitive therapy for the prevention of suicide attempts: A randomized controlled trial. *Journal of the American Medical Association, 294*, 563–570.

Brown, L. (2003). *When mainstream and feminist ethics collide* presented at the annual convention of the American Psychological Association, Toronto, Ontario, Canada.

Buber, M. (1967). *A believing humanism: Gleanings*. New York: Simon & Schuster.

Buber, M. (1958/1970). *I and Thou* (W. Kaufmann, Trans.). New York: Scribner's.

Bugental, J. F. T. (Ed.). (1967). *Challenges of humanistic psychology.* New York: McGraw-Hill.

Bujold, A., Ladouceur, R., Sylvain, C., & Boisvert, J. (1994). Treatment of pathological gamblers: An experimental study. *Journal of Behavior Therapy and Experimental Psychiatry, 25,* 275–282.

Burck, C. (2005). Comparing qualitative research methodologies for systemic research: The use of grounded theory, discourse analysis and narrative analysis. *Journal of Family Therapy, 27,* 237–262.

Burns, D. D., & Nolen-Hoeksema, S. (1992). Therapeutic empathy and recovery from depression in cognitive-behavioral therapy: A structural equation model. *Journal of Consulting and Clinical Psychology, 60,* 441–449.

Burr, V. (2003). *An introduction to social constructionism* (2nd ed.). London: Routledge.

Burton, A. (1972). *Twelve therapists.* San Francisco: Jossey-Bass.

Busch, R., Strong, T., & Lock, A. (2004, August). *Evaluation and the challenges of evaluating narrative therapy.* Paper presented at the annual conference of the New Zealand Psychological Society, Wellington, New Zealand.

Cain, D. J. (1989). The paradox of nondirectiveness in the person-centered approach. *Person-Centered Review, 4*(2), 123–131.

Cain, D. J. (1990). Further thoughts about nondirectiveness and client-centered therapy. *Person-Centered Review, 5*(1), 89–99.

Calamari, J. E., Faber, S. D., Hitsman, B. L., & Poppe, C. J. (1994). Treatment of obsessive compulsive disorder in the elderly: A review and case example. *Journal of Behavior Therapy and Experimental Psychiatry, 25,* 95–104.

Campbell, T. J., & Patterson, J. M. (1995). The effectiveness of family interventions in the treatment of physical illness. *Journal of Marital and Family Therapy, 21,* 545–584.

Camus, A. (1947). *La peste.* [The plague]. Paris: Gallimard.

Camus, A. (1972). *The plague* (S. Gilbert, Trans.). New York: Vintage.

Capuzzi, D., & Gross, D. R. (1995). *Counseling and psychotherapy: Theories and interventions.* Englewood Cliffs, NJ: Merrill/Prentice Hall.

Carey, M. P., Braaten, L. S., Maisto, S. A., Gleason, J. R., Forsyth, A. D., Durant, L. E., et al. (2000). Using information, motivation enhancement, and skills training to reduce the risk of HIV infection for low-income urban women: A second randomized clinical trial. *Health Psychology, 19,* 3–11.

Carey, R. G., & Bucher, B. B. (1986). Positive practice overcorrection: Effects of reinforcing correct performance. *Behavior Modification, 10,* 73–92.

Cariaga, J., Burgio, L. F., Flynn, W., & Martin, D. (1991). A controlled study of disruptive vocalizations among geriatric residents in nursing homes. *Journal of the American Geriatric Society, 39,* 501–507.

Carkhuff, R. (1980). *The art of helping* (4th ed.). Amherst, MA: HRD Press.

Carlson, J. D. (1989). On beyond Adler. *Journal of Individual Psychology, 45,* 411–413.

Carlson, J. D. (2000). Individual psychology in the year 2000 and beyond: Astronaut or dinosaur? Headline or footnote? *Journal of Individual Psychology, 56,* 3–13.

Carlson, J. [D.], & Dinkmeyer, D. (2003). *Time for a better marriage.* Atascadero, CA: Impact.

Carlson, J. D., & Slavik, S. (1997). *Techniques in Adlerian psychology.* Philadelphia: Taylor & Francis.

Carlson, J. [D.], & Sperry, L. (1998). Adlerian psychotherapy as a constructivist psychotherapy. In M. F. Hoyt (Ed.), *The handbook of constructive therapies: Innovative approaches from leading practitioners* (pp. 68–82). San Francisco: Jossey-Bass.

Carlson, J. D., Watts, R. E., & Maniacci, M. (2006). *Adlerian therapy: Theory and practice.* Washington, DC: American Psychological Association.

Carlson, J. M., & Carlson, J. D. (2000). The application of Adlerian psychotherapy with Asian Americans. *Journal of Individual Psychology, 56,* 214–225.

Carmin, C. N., Wiegartz, P. S., Yunus, U., & Gillock, K. L. (2002). Treatment of late-onset OCD following basal ganglia infarct. *Depression and Anxiety, 15,* 87–90.

Carr, A. (2000). Evidence-based practice in family therapy and systemic consultation 1. Child-focused problems. *Journal of Family Therapy, 22,* 29–60.

Carstensen, L. L., & Fisher, J. E. (1991). Treatment applications for psychological and behavioral problems of the elderly in nursing homes. In P. A. Wisocki (Ed.), *Handbook of clinical behavior therapy with the elderly client* (pp. 337–362). New York: Plenum.

Carter, B., & McGoldrick, M. (1988). *The changing family life-cycle.* Boston: Allyn & Bacon.

Cass, V. (1979). Homosexual identity formation: A theoretical model. *Journal of Homosexuality, 4,* 219–235.

Chambless, D. L., & Hollon, S. D. (1998). Defining empirically supported therapies. *Journal of Consulting and Clinical Psychology, 66,* 7–18.

Chambless, D. L., & Ollendick, T. H. (1996). An update on empirically validated therapies. *The Clinical Psychologist, 49,* 5–18.

Chambless, D. L., & Ollendick, T. H. (2001). Empirically supported psychological intervention: Controversies and evidence. *Annual Review of Psychology, 52,* 685–716.

Chambless, D. L., Sanderson, W. C., Shoham, V., Johnson, S. B., Pope, K. S., Crits-Christoph, P., et al. (2001). Empirically supported psychological intervention: Controversies and evidence. *Annual Review of Psychology, 52,* 685–716.

Chambless, D. L., & Williams, K. E. (1995). A preliminary study of African Americans with agoraphobia: Symptoms severity and outcome of treatment with in vivo exposure. *Behavior Therapy, 26,* 501–515.

Chandler, C. K. (1995). Contemporary Adlerian reflections on homosexuality and bisexuality. *Journal of Individual Psychology, 51,* 82–89.

Chandler, R., Worell, J., Johnson, D., Blount, A., & Lusk, M. (1999, August). Measuring long-term outcomes of feminist counseling and psychotherapy. In J. Worell (Chair), *Measuring process and outcomes of feminist counseling and therapy.* Paper presented at the annual meeting of the American Psychological Association, Boston, MA.

Charlop, M. H., & Milstein, J. P. (1989). Teaching autistic children conversational speech using video modeling. *Journal of Applied Behavior Analysis, 22,* 275–285.

Charlop, M. H., Schreibman, L., & Tryon, A. S. (1983). Learning through observation: The effects of peer modeling on acquisition and generalization in autistic children. *Journal of Abnormal Child Psychology, 11,* 355–366.

Cheatham, H., & Stewart, J. (1990). *Black families: Interdisciplinary perspectives.* New Brunswick, NJ: Transactional Publishers.

Chemtob, C. M., Novaco, R. W., Hamada, R. S., & Gross, D. M. (1997). Cognitive-behavioral treatment for severe anger in posttraumatic stress disorder. *Journal of Consulting and Clinical Psychology, 65,* 184–189.

Chessick, R. D. (1987). *Great ideas in psychotherapy.* Northvale, NJ: Aronson.

Cheston, S. E. (2000). The spirituality of encouragement. *Journal of Individual Psychology, 56,* 296–303.

Chorpita, B. F. (1995). Eventual responders: What do we do when treatments do not work? *the Behavior Therapist, 18,* 140–141.

Christian, J. L. (1977). *Philosophy: An introduction to the art of wondering* (2nd ed.). New York: Holt, Rinehart & Winston.

Christophersen, E. R. (1977). *Little people: Guidelines for common sense child rearing.* Lawrence, KS: H & H Enterprises.

Chung, R. C., & Bemak, F. (1998). Life-style of Vietnamese refugee women. *Journal of Individual Psychology, 54,* 373–384.

Church, M. (1983). Psychological therapy with elderly people. *Bulletin of the British Psychological Society, 36,* 110–112.

Cloitre, M. (1995). An interview with Edna Foa. *The Behavior Therapist, 18,* 177–181.

Cohen, D. B. (1994). *Out of the blue: Depression and human nature.* New York: Norton.

Colvin, C., & Boddington, S. J. A. (1997). Behaviour therapy for obsessive compulsive disorder in a 78-year-old woman. *International Journal of Geriatric Psychiatry, 12,* 488–491.

Congress, E. P. (1994). The use of culturagrams to assess and empower culturally diverse families. *Families in Society, 75,* 531–539.

Constantine, M. G., & Sue, D. W. (2005). The American Psychological Association's guidelines on multicultural education, training, research, practice, and organizational psychology: Initial development and summary. In M. G. Constantine & D. W. Sue (Eds.), *Strategies for building multicultural competence in mental health and educational settings* (pp. 3–18). Hoboken, NJ: Wiley.

Cook, D. A. (1999). Gestalt treatment of adolescent females with depressive symptoms: A treatment outcome study. *Dissertation Abstracts International, 60* (8b), 4210.

Cooper, M. (2004). Existential approaches to therapy. In P. Sanders (Ed.), *The tribes of the person-centered nation: An introduction to the schools of therapy related to the person-centered approach* (pp. 95–124). Ross-on-Wye, UK: PCCS Books.

Corey, G. (2001). *Theory and practice of counseling and psychotherapy* (6th ed.). Belmont, CA: Brooks-Cole.

Cornelius-White, J., & Cornelius-White, C. (2005). Reminiscing and predicting: Rogers's beyond words speech and commentary. *Journal of Humanistic Psychology, 45*(3), 383–396.

Corsini, R. J., & Auerbach, A. J. (Eds.). (1998). *Concise encyclopedia of psychology.* New York: Wiley.

Cotharin, R. L., & Mikulas, W. L. (1975). Systematic desensitization of racial emotional responses. *Journal of Behavior Therapy and Experimental Psychiatry, 6,* 347–348.

Coulehan, R., Friedlander, M. L., & Heatherington, L. (1998). Transforming narratives: A change event in constructivist family therapy. *Family Process, 37,* 17–33.

Creswell, J. W. (1998). *Qualitative inquiry and research design.* Thousand Oaks, CA: Sage.

Crits-Christoph, P., Wilson, T. G., & Hollon, S. D. (2005). Empirically supported psychotherapies: Comment on Westen, Novotny, and Thompson-Brenner (2004). *Psychological Bulletin, 131,* 412–417.

Croce, B. (1910). *Ce qui est vivant et ce qui est mort de la philosophie de Hegel* [The legacy of Hegel's philosophy] (H. Duriot, Trans.). Paris: V. Giard & E. Brière.

Crocket, K. (2004). From narrative practice in counselling to narrative practice in research: A professional identity story. *International Journal of Narrative Therapy and Community Work,* (2), 63–67.

Crocket, K., Drewery, W., McKenzie, W., Smith, L., & Winslade, J. (2004). Working for ethical research in practice. *International Journal of Narrative Therapy and Community Work,* (3), 61–66.

Cross, W. E. (1980). Models of psychological nigrescence. In R. L. Jones (Ed.), *Black psychology* (pp. 81–98). New York: Harper & Row.

Cunningham, P. (2000). A sociology of adult education. In A. Wison & E. Hayes (Eds.), *Handbook of adult and continuing education* (pp. 573–591). San Francisco: Jossey-Bass.

D'Andrea, M., & Daniels, J. (2003). *Multicultural counseling: Empowerment strategies for a diverse society.* Pacific Grove, CA: Brooks/Cole.

Dagley, J. C. (2000). Adlerian family therapy. In A. M. Horne (Ed.), *Family counseling and therapy* (3rd ed., pp. 366–419). Itasca, IL: Peacock.

Danto, E. A. (2005). *Freud's free clinics.* New York: Columbia University Press.

Dapcich-Miura, E., & Hovell, M. F. (1979). Contingency management of adherence to a complex medical regimen in an elderly heart patient. *Behavior Therapy, 10,* 193–201.

Dattilio, F. M., & Padesky, C. A. (1990). *Cognitive therapy with couples.* Sarasota, FL: Professional Resource Exchange.

Davies, B. (2000). *A body of writing, 1990–1999.* Walnut Creek, CA: AltaMira Press.

Davis, S. (2005). Common and model-specific factors: What marital therapy model developers, their former students, and their clients say about change. Unpublished doctoral dissertation: Virginia Polytechnic Institute and State University, Blacksburg.

Davison, G. C. (1995). A failure of early behavior therapy (circa 1960): Or why I learned to stop worrying and to embrace psychotherapy integration. *Journal of Psychotherapy Integration, 5,* 107–112.

Dawson, B., de Armas, A., McGrath, M. L., & Kelly, J. A. (1986). Cognitive problem-solving training to improve child-care judgement of child neglectful parents. *Journal of Family Violence, 1,* 209–221.

de Shazer, S. (1993). Commentary: de Shazer & White: Viva la difference. In S. Gilligan & R. Price (Eds.), *Therapeutic conversations* (pp. 112–120). New York: Norton.

DeBarry, S. (1982a). The effects of meditation-relaxation on anxiety and depression in a geriatric population. *Psychotherapy: Theory, Research, & Practice, 19,* 512–521.

DeBarry, S. (1982b). An evaluation of progressive muscle relaxation on stress related symptoms in a geriatric population. *International Journal of Aging and Human Development, 14,* 255–269.

DeBarry, S., Davis, S., & Reinhard, K. E. (1989). A comparison of meditation-relaxation and cognitive-behavioral techniques for reducing anxiety and depression in a geriatric population. *Journal of Geriatric Psychiatry, 22,* 231–247.

Deegear, J., & Lawson, D. M. (2003). The utility of empirically supported treatments. *Professional Psychology: Research and Practice, 34*, 271–277.

DeMaria, R., Weeks, G., & Hof, L. (1999). *Intergenerational assessment of individuals, couples, and families: Focused genograms.* Castleton, NY: Hamilton Printing.

Deming, W. E. (1986). *Out of the crisis.* Cambridge, MA: MIT Press.

Derrida, J. (1978). *Writing and difference.* Chicago: University of Chicago Press.

D'Haene, M. T. (1995). Evaluation of feminist-based adolescent group therapy. *Smith College Studies in Social Work, 65*(2), 153–165.

Dick-Siskin, L. P. (2002). Cognitive-behavioral therapy with older adults. *The Behavior Therapist, 25*, pp. 3–4, 6.

Diller, A., Houston, B., Morgan, K. P., & Ayim, M. (1996). *The gender question in education: Theory, pedagogy, and politics.* Boulder, CO: Westview Press.

DiNicola, V. F. (1986). Beyond babel: Family therapy as cultural translation. *International Journal of Family Psychiatry, 7*(2), 179–191.

Dinkmeyer, D. C., Dinkmeyer, D. C., Jr., & Sperry, L. (1987). *Adlerian counseling and psychotherapy* (2nd ed.). Columbus, OH: Merrill.

Dinkmeyer, D. C., & Losconcy, L. E. (1980). *The encouragement book.* Englewood Cliffs, NJ: Prentice-Hall.

Dinkmeyer, D. C., McKay, G. D., & Dinkmeyer, D. C., Jr. (1997). *The parent's handbook: Systematic training for effective parenting.* Circle Pines, MN: American Guidance Service.

Dinkmeyer, D. C., Jr., & Sperry, L. (2000). *Counseling and psychotherapy: An integrated, Individual Psychology approach* (3rd ed.). Upper Saddle River, NJ: Merrill/Prentice-Hall.

Doherty, W., & Carroll, J. (2003). The citizen therapist and family centered community building. Introduction to a new section of the journal. *Family Process, 41*(4), 561–568.

Donohue, B., Thevenin, D. H., & Runyon, M. K. (1997). Behavioral treatment of conversion disorder in adolescence: A case example of *globus hystericus. Behavior Modification, 21*, 231–251.

Downing, N. W., & Roush, K. L. (1985). From passive acceptance to active commitment: A model of feminist identity development for women. *The Counseling Psychologist, 13*, 696–709.

Dowrick, P. W. (1991). *Practical guide to using video in the behavioral sciences.* New York: Wiley.

Dowrick, P. W. (1994). Video psychology. In R. J. Corsini (Ed.), *Encyclopedia of psychology* (2nd ed., pp. 566–567). New York: Wiley.

Dreikurs, R. (1967). *Psychodynamics, psychotherapy, and counseling: Collected papers.* Chicago: Alfred Adler Institute.

Dreikurs, R., & Cassell, P. (1972). *Discipline without tears.* New York: Penguin.

Dreikurs, R., & Mosak, H. H. (1967). The tasks of life. II. The fourth life task. *Individual Psychology, 4*, 51–55.

Dreikurs, R., & Soltz, V. (1964). *Children: The challenge.* New York: Hawthorn.

Drewery, W. (1990). Listening, hearing and power relations: The problem of unconditional positive regard. *New Zealand Association of Counsellors Journal, 12*(1), 27–38.

Drewery, W. (2005). Why we should watch what we say: Position calls, everyday speech and the production of relational subjectivity. *Theory and Psychology, 15*, 305–324.

Droit, R.-P. (2004, August 19). Socrate et ses galaxies [Socrates and his colleagues]. *Le point, 1665,* 62–63.

Dryden, W., & Ellis, A. (2001). Rational emotive behavior therapy. In K. S. Dobson (Ed.), *Handbook of cognitive-behavioral therapies* (2nd. ed., pp. 295–348). New York: Guilford.

Dryden, W., & Hill, L. K. (Eds.). (1993). *Innovations in rational-emotive therapy.* Newbury Park, CA: Sage.

Duhl, B. S., & Duhl, E. J. (1981). Integrative family therapy. In A. S. Gurman & D. P. Knishern (Eds.), *Handbook of family therapy.* New York: Brunner/Mazel.

Dupree, L. W. (1993). Treatment of paranoid ideation and hostile verbalizations in an elderly woman using thought-stopping, assertiveness training, and marital discharge contracting: A case study. *Clinical Gerontologist, 13,* 29–43.

Durant, W. (1954). *Our oriental heritage.* New York: Simon & Schuster.

Durie, M. (1989). A move that's well overdue: Shaping counselling to meet the needs of Maori people. *New Zealand Counselling and Guidance Association Journal, 11*(1), 13–23.

Duvall, E. M. (1977). *Marriage and family development* (5th ed.). New York: Lippincott.

D'Zurilla, T. J., & Chang, E. C. (1995). The relations between social problem solving and coping. *Cognitive Therapy and Research, 19,* 547–562.

D'Zurilla, T. J., Chang, E. C., Nottingham, E. J., & Faccini, L. (1998). Social problem-solving deficits and hopelessness, depression, and suicide risk in college students and psychiatric inpatients. *Journal of Clinical Psychology, 54,* 1–17.

D'Zurilla, T. J., & Goldfried, M. R. (1971). Problem solving and behavior modification. *Journal of Abnormal Psychology, 78,* 107–126.

D'Zurilla, T. J., & Nezu, A. M. (2001). Problem solving therapies. In K. S. Dobson (Ed.), *Handbook of cognitive behavioral-therapies* (2nd ed., pp. 211–245). New York: Guilford.

Ecrement, E. R., & Zarski, J. J. (1987). The pastor-as-counselor: Adlerian contributions to the process. *Individual Psychology, 43,* 461–467.

Edelman, R. E., & Chambless, D. L. (1993). Compliance during sessions and homework in exposure-based treatment of agoraphobia. *Behaviour Research and Therapy, 31,* 767–773.

Edwards, D. J., Dattilio, F. M., & Bromley, D. B. (2004). Evidence-based practice: The role of case-based research. *Professional Psychology: Research and Practice, 35,* 589–597.

Edwards, M. E., & Steinglass, P. (1995). Family therapy treatment outcomes for alcoholism. *Journal of Marital and Family Therapy, 21,* 475–510.

Efran, J., Lukens, M., & Lukens, R. (1990). *Language, structure and change.* New York: Norton.

Egel, A. L., Richman, G. S., & Koegel, R. L. (1983). Cognitive-behavioral strategies to induce and enhance a collaborative set in distressed couples. In A. Freeman (Ed.), *Cognitive therapy with couples and groups* (pp. 125–155). New York: Plenum.

Eissler, K. (1958). Remarks on some variations in psychoanalytic technique. *International Journal of Psychoanalysis, 39,* 222–229.

Elkin, I., Shea, M. T., Watkins, J. T., Imber, S. D., Sotsky, S. M., Collins, J. F., et al. (1989). National Institute of Mental Health Treatment of Depression Collaborative Research Program: General effectiveness of treatments. *Archives of General Psychiatry, 46,* 971–982.

Elliott, R., Watson, J. C., Goldman, R. N., & Greenberg, L. S. (2004). *Learning emotion focused therapy.* Washington, DC: American Psychological Association.

Ellis, A. (1962). *Reason and emotion in psychotherapy.* New York: Lyle Stuart.

Ellis, A. (1970). Tribute to Alfred Adler. *Journal of Individual Psychology, 26,* 11–12.

Ellis, A. (1989a). Comments on my critics. In M. E. Bernard & R. [A.] DiGiuseppe (Eds.), *Inside rational-emotive therapy: A critical appraisal of the theory and therapy of Albert Ellis* (pp. 199–233). San Diego: Academic Press.

Ellis, A. (1989b). The history of cognition in psychotherapy. In A. Freeman, K. M. Simon, L. E. Beutler, & H. Arkowitz (Eds.), *Comprehensive handbook of cognitive therapy* (pp. 5–20). New York: Plenum.

Ellis, A. (1993). Changing rational-emotive therapy (RET) to rational emotive behavior therapy (REBT). *The Behavior Therapist, 16,* 257–258.

Ellis, A. (1994a). Ellis, Albert. *Current Biography, 65,* 6–10.

Ellis, A. (1994b). General semantics and rational emotive behavior therapy. In P. D. Johnston, D. D. Bourland, & J. Klein (Eds.), *More E-prime: To be or not II* (pp. 213–240). Concord, CA: International Society for General Semantics.

Ellis, A. (1994c). Post-traumatic stress disorder (PTSD): A rational emotive behavioral theory. *Journal of Rational-Emotive & Cognitive-Behavior Therapy, 12,* 3–25.

Ellis, A. (1994d). Radical behavioral treatment of private events: A response to Michael Dougher. *The Behavior Therapist, 17,* 219–221.

Ellis, A. (1995). Changing rational-emotive therapy (RET) to rational-emotive behavior therapy (REBT). *Journal of Rational-Emotive & Cognitive-Behavior Therapy, 13,* 85–89.

Ellis, A. (1999). Rational emotive behavior therapy and cognitive behavior therapy for elderly people. *Journal of Rational-Emotive & Cognitive-Behavior Therapy, 17,* 5–18.

Ellis, A. (2000). Spiritual goals and spirited values in psychotherapy. *Journal of Individual Psychology, 56,* 277–284.

Ellis, A., & Bernard, M. E. (1985). What is rational-emotive therapy (RET)? In A. Ellis & R. M. Grieger (Eds.), *Handbook of rational-emotive therapy* (pp. 1–30). New York: Springer.

Ellis, A., & Dryden, W. (1987). *The practice of rational-emotive therapy.* New York: Springer.

Ellis, C. R., Singh, N. N., Crews, W. D., Bonaventura, S. H., Gehin, J. M., & Ricketts, R. W. (1997). In N. N. Singh (Ed.), *Prevention and treatment of severe behavior problems: Models and methods in developmental disabilities* (pp. 253–269). Pacific Grove, CA: Brooks/Cole.

Engle-Friedman, M., & Bootzin, R. R. (1991). Insomnia as a problem for the elderly. In P. A. Wisocki (Ed.), *Handbook of clinical behavior therapy with the elderly client* (pp. 273–298). New York: Plenum Press.

Enns, C. Z. (1997). *Feminist theories and feminist psychotherapies: Origins, themes, and variations.* Binghamton, NY: Harrington Park Press.

Epstein, N. (1983). Cognitive therapy with couples. In A. Freeman (Ed.), *Cognitive therapy with couples and groups* (pp. 107–123). New York: Plenum.

Epston, D. (1989). *Collected papers.* Adelaide, Australia: Dulwich Centre Publications.

Epston, D. (1998). *'Catching up' with David Epston: A collection of narrative practice-based papers published between 1991 and 1996.* Adelaide, Australia: Dulwich Centre Publications.

Epston, D. (2001). Anthropology, archives, co-research and narrative therapy. In D. Denborough (Ed.), *Family therapy: Exploring the field's past, present and possible futures* (pp. 177–182). Adelaide, Australia: Dulwich Centre Publications.

Epston, D., & White, M. (1992). *Experience, contradiction, narrative and imagination.* Adelaide, Australia: Dulwich Centre Publications.

Erikson, E. H. (1982). *The life cycle completed: A review.* New York: Norton.

Eysenck, H. J. (1952). The effects of psychotherapy: An evaluation. *Journal of Consulting Psychology, 16,* 319–324.

Fairbairn, W. R. D. (1952). *Psychoanalytic studies of the personality.* London: Routledge & Kegan Paul.

Fairbairn, W. R. D. (1958). On the nature and aims of psychoanalytic treatment. *International Journal of Psychoanalysis, 39,* 374–385.

Falicov, C. (1988). *Cultural perspectives in family therapy.* Rockville, MD: Aspen.

Falicov, C. (1998). From rigid borderlines to fertile borderlands: Reconfiguring family therapy. *Journal of Marital and Family Therapy, 24,* 157–163.

Fall, K. A., Holden, J. M., & Marquis, A. (2004). *Theoretical models of counseling and psychotherapy.* New York: Brunner-Routledge.

Fang, S., & Wark, L. (1998). Developing cross-cultural competence with traditional Chinese Americans in family therapy: Background information and the initial therapeutic contact. *Contemporary Family Therapy, 20*(1), 59–77.

Fanon, F. (1963). *The wretched of the earth.* New York: Grove Press.

Farrell, S. P., Hains, A. A., & Davies, W. H. (1998). Cognitive behavioral interventions for sexually abused children exhibiting PTSD symptomology. *Behavior Therapy, 29,* 241–255.

Fassinger, R. E. (2001). Women in non-traditional occupational fields. In J. Worell (Ed.), *Encyclopedia of women and gender: Sex similarities and differences and the impact of society on gender* (Vol. 2, pp. 1269–1280). San Diego, CA: Academic Press.

Feminist Therapy Institute. (1990). Feminist Therapy Institute code of ethics. In H. Lerman & N. Porter (Eds.), *Feminist ethics in psychotherapy* (pp. 38–40). New York: Springer.

Fenichel, O. (1945). *The psychoanalytic theory of neurosis.* New York: Norton.

Ferguson, E. D. (2001). Adler and Dreikurs: Cognitive-social dynamic innovators. *Journal of Individual Psychology, 57,* 324–341.

Feske, U. (2001). Treating low-income and African-American women with posttraumatic stress disorder: A case series. *Behavior Therapy, 32,* 585–601.

Fink, C. M., Turner, S. M., & Beidel, D. C. (1996). Culturally relevant factors in the behavioral treatment of social phobia: A case study. *Journal of Anxiety Disorders, 10,* 201–209.

Fitzgerald, L. F., & Nutt, R. (1986). The Division 17 principles concerning the counseling/psychotherapy of women: Rationale and implementation. *The Counseling Psychologist, 14,* 180–216.

Fleece, L. (1995). [Review of the book *The therapeutic relationship in behavioural psychotherapy*]. *The Behavior Therapist, 18,* 142.

Flew, A. (1979). *A dictionary of philosophy* (Rev. 2nd ed.). New York: Gramercy.

Flores, M. T., & Carey, G. (2000). *Family therapy with Hispanics.* Boston: Allyn & Bacon.

Foa, E. B., & Rothbaum, B. O. (1998). *Treating the trauma of rape: Cognitive-behavioral therapy for PTSD*. New York: Guilford.

Fonagy, P. (2001). The talking cure in the cross fire of empiricism—The struggle for the hearts and minds of psychoanalytic clinicians. *Psychoanalytic Dialogues, 11*(4), 621–632.

Forsyth, J. P. (1997). It was the age of wisdom, it is the age of hope: Commentary on "It was the best of times, it was the worst of times." *Behavior Therapy, 28*, 397–401.

Foucault, M. (1980). *The history of sexuality*, (Vol. 1). New York: Vintage.

Foxx, R. M., & Azrin, N. H. (1972). Restitution: A method of eliminating aggressive-disruptive behavior of retarded and brain damaged patients. *Behaviour Research and Therapy, 10*, 15–27.

Fraenkel, P. (1995). The nomothetic-idiographic debate in family therapy. *Family Process, 34*, 113–121.

Frame, C. L., & Matson, J. L. (1987). *Handbook of assessment in childhood psychopathology: Applied issues in differential diagnosis and treatment evaluation*. New York: Plenum.

Frame, M. (2000). The spiritual genogram in family therapy. *Journal of Marital and Family Therapy, 26*, 211–216.

Frank, J. D., & Frank, J. B. (1991). *Persuasion and healing: A comparative study of psychotherapy* (3rd ed.). Baltimore: Johns Hopkins University Press.

Frank, K. A. (1999). *Psychoanalytic participation: Action, interaction, and integration*.

Frankl, V. E. (1963/1984). *Man's search for meaning*. New York: Washington Square Press.

Frankl, V. E. (1967). *Psychotherapy and existentialism: Selected papers on logotherapy*. New York: Simon & Schuster.

Frankl, V. E. (1975). *The unconscious God*. New York: Simon & Schuster.

Freedman J., & Combs, G. (1996). *Narrative therapy: The social construction of preferred realities*. New York: Norton.

Freidman, M. (1985). *The healing dialogue in psychotherapy*. New York: Aronson.

Freire, P. (1970). *Pedagogy of the oppressed*. New York: Pantheon Books.

Freud, A. (1966). *The ego and the mechanisms of defense* (Rev. ed.). Madison, CT: International Universities Press.

Freud, S. (1919). Lines of advance in psychoanalytic therapy. *Standard edition of the complete psychological works of Sigmund Freud* (Vol. 17, pp. 157–168). London: Hogarth Press.

Frevert, V. S., & Miranda, A. O. (1998). A conceptual formulation of the Latin culture and the treatment of Latinos from an Adlerian psychology perspective. *Journal of Individual Psychology, 54*, 291–309.

Frew, J. E. (2003). Gestalt in a CBT world. *British Gestalt Journal, 12*, 115–116.

Friedman, M. (1985). *The healing dialogue in psychotherapy*. New York: Aronson.

Friedman, M. (1986). Carl Rogers and Martin Buber. *Person-Centered Review, 1*(4), 409–435.

Friedman, S., Smith, L. C., Halpern, B., Levine, C., Paradis, C., Viswanathan, R., et al. (2003). Obsessive-compulsive disorder in a multi-ethnic urban outpatient clinic: Initial presentation and treatment outcome with exposure and ritual prevention. *Behavior Therapy, 34*, 397–410.

Frye, A. A., & Goodman, S. H. (2000). Which social problem-solving components buffer depression in adolescent girls? *Cognitive Therapy and Research, 24*, 637–650.

Fudge, R. C. (1996). The use of behavior therapy in the development of ethnic consciousness: A treatment model. *Cognitive and Behavioral Practice, 3,* 317–335.

Gaddis, S. (2004). Repositioning traditional research: Centering clients' accounts in deconstruction of professional therapy knowledges. *International Journal of Narrative Therapy and Community Work, 2,* 37–48.

Gallagher, K. T. (1975). *The philosophy of Gabriel Marcel.* New York: Fordham University Press.

Gambrill, E. (1995). Assertion skills training. In W. O'Donohue & L. Krasner (Eds.), *Handbook of psychological skills training: Clinical techniques and applications* (pp. 81–118). Boston: Allyn & Bacon.

Garcia-Preto, N. (1996). Latino families: Another view. In M. McGoldrick, J. Giordano, & J. K. Pearce (Eds.), *Ethnicity and family therapy* (pp. 141–154). New York: Guilford.

Garfield, S. L. (1998). Some comments on empirically supported treatments. *Journal of Consulting and Clinical Psychology, 66,* 121–125.

Gaston, L., Goldfried, M. R., Greenberg, L. S., Horvath, A. O., Raue, P. J., & Watson, J. (1995). The therapeutic alliance in psychodynamic, cognitive-behavioral, and experimental therapies. *Journal of Psychotherapy Integration, 5,* 1–26.

Gehart, D., Ratliff, D., & Randall. L. (2001). Qualitative research in family therapy: A substantive and methodological review. *Journal of Marital and Family Therapy, 27,* 261–274.

Gendlin, E. T. (1986, March). Talk on experiential focusing and Rogers's contributions. Videotape presented at "Beyond Words" symposium at the Chicago Counseling and Psychotherapy Center.

Gendlin, E. T. (1996). *Focusing-oriented psychotherapy.* New York: Guilford.

Gergen, K. (1985). The social constructionist movement in modern psychology. *American Psychologist, 40,* 266–275.

Gil, K. M., Wilson, J. J., Edens, J. L., Workman, E., Ready, J., Sedway, J., et al. (1997). Cognitive coping skills training with sickle cell disease pain. *International Journal of Behavioral Medicine, 4,* 364–377.

Gilbert, L. A. (1980). Feminist therapy. In A. M. Brodsky & R. T. Hare-Mustin (Eds.), *Women and psychotherapy: An assessment of research and practice* (pp. 245–265). New York: Guilford.

Gill, M. (1982). *Analysis of transference* (Vol. 1). New York: International Universities Press.

Gilligan, C. (1982). *In a different voice: Psychological theory and women's development.* Cambridge, MA: Harvard University Press.

Gilman, S. (1993). *Freud, race, and gender.* Princeton, NJ: Princeton University Press.

Glass, D. C., & Singer, J. E. (1971). Behavioral consequences of adaptation to controllable and uncontrollable noise. *Journal of Experimental Social Psychology, 7,* 244–257.

Glasser, W. (1965). *Reality therapy: A new approach to psychiatry.* New York: Harper Row.

Glasser, W. (1968). *Schools without failure.* New York: HarperCollins.

Glasser, W. (1972). *The identity society.* New York: HarperCollins.

Glasser, W. (1985). *Control theory.* New York: HarperCollins.

Glasser, W. (1998). *Choice theory.* New York: HarperCollins.

Glasser, W. (2003). *Warning: Psychiatry can be hazardous to your mental health.* New York: HarperCollins.

Glasser, W. (2004). A new vision for counseling. *Family Journal, 12*, 339–341.

Glasser, W., & Wubbolding, R. E. (1995). Reality therapy. In R. J. Corsini & D. Wedding (Eds.), *Current psychotherapies* (5th ed., pp. 293–321). Itasca, IL: Peacock.

Glasser, W., & Zunin, L. (1973). Reality therapy. In R. Corsini (Ed.), *Current psychotherapies* (2nd ed., pp. 283–297). Itasca, IL: Peacock.

Gold, J. (1996). *Key concepts in psychotherapy integration.* New York: Plenum.

Goldenberg, H., & Goldenberg, I. (2002). *Counseling today's families.* Pacific Grove, CA: Brooks/Cole.

Goldfried, M. R. (1988). Application of rational restructuring to anxiety disorders. *The Counseling Psychologist, 16*, 50–68.

Goldfried, M. R. (1995). *From cognitive-behavior therapy to psychotherapy integration: An evolving view.* New York: Springer.

Goldstein, H., & Mousetis, L. (1989). Generalized language learning by children with severe mental retardation: Effects of peers' expressive modeling. *Journal of Applied Behavior Analysis, 22*, 245–259.

Gonzales, R. (2001). ABC relaxation training as a treatment for depression for Puerto Rican elderly. In J. C. Smith (Ed.), *Advances in ABC relaxation: Applications and inventories* (pp. 209–211). New York: Springer.

Goodman, D. J. (2001). *Promoting diversity and social justice: Educating people from privileged groups.* Thousand Oaks, CA: Sage.

Goodman, L. A., Liang, B., Helms, J. E., Latta, R. E., Sparks, E., & Weintraub, S. R. (2004). Training counseling psychologists as social justice agents: Feminist and multicultural principles in action. *The Counseling Psychologist, 32*, 793–837.

Gorenstein, E. E., Papp, L. A., & Kleber, M. S. (1999). Cognitive behavioral treatment of anxiety in later life. *Cognitive and Behavioral Practice, 6*, 305–320.

Goss, S., & Rose, S. (2002). Evidence based practice: A guide for counsellors and psychotherapists. *New Zealand Journal of Counselling, 23*(2), 67–76.

Grant, B. (2004). The imperative of ethical justification in psychotherapy: The special case of client-centered therapy. *Person-Centered and Experiential Psychotherapies, 3*(3), 152–165.

Greaves, D. (1997). The effects on rational-emotive parent education on the stress of mothers with young children with Down Syndrome. *Journal of Rational-Emotive & Cognitive-Behavior Therapy, 15*, 249–267.

Green, J. B. (2003). *Introduction to family theory and therapy.* Pacific Grove, CA: Brooks/Cole.

Greenberg, J. R. (1986). Theoretical models and the analyst's neutrality. *Contemporary Psychoanalysis, 22*, 87–106.

Greenberg, J. R., & Mitchell, S. A. (1983). *Object relations in psychoanalytic theory.* Cambridge, MA: Harvard University Press.

Greenberg, L. S., & Foerster, F. S. (1996). Task analysis exemplified: The process of resolving unfinished business. *Journal of Counseling and Clinical Psychology, 64*, 439–446.

Greenberg, L. S., Korman, L. M., & Pavio, S. C. (2002). Emotion in humanistic psychotherapy. In D. J. Cain & J. Seeman, *Humanistic psychotherapies: Handbook of research and practice* (pp. 499–530). Washington, DC: American Psychological Association.

Greenberg, L. S., & Paivio, S. C. (1997). *Working with emotions in psychotherapy.* New York: Guilford.

Greenberg, L. S., & Rice, L. N. (1981). The specific effects of a Gestalt intervention. *Psychotherapy: Theory, Research, and Practice, 18,* 31–37.

Greenberg, L. S., & Van Balen, R. (1999). The theory of experience-centered therapies. In L. S. Greenberg, J. C. Watson, & G. Lietaer (Eds.), *Handbook of experiential psychotherapy* (pp. 28–57). New York: Guilford.

Greenberg, L. S., & Watson, J. (1998). Experiential therapy of depression: Differential effects of client-centered relationship conditions and process experiential interventions. *Psychotherapy Research, 8,* 210–224.

Greene, B. (1994). Lesbian women of color: Triple jeopardy. In L. Comas-Diaz & B. Greene (Eds.), *Women of color: Integrating ethnic and gender issues in psychotherapy* (pp. 389–427). New York: Guilford.

Greenspan, M. (1983). *A new approach to women and therapy.* New York: McGraw-Hill.

Greyson, J. B., Foa, E. A., & Steketee, G. (1985). Obsessive-compulsive disorder. In M. Hersen & A. S. Bellack (Eds.), *Handbook of clinical behavior therapy with adults* (pp. 133–165). New York: Plenum.

Griffith, E. H., Ezra, E., & Baker, F. M. (1993). Psychiatric care of African Americans. In A. C. Gaw (Ed.), *Culture, ethnicity & mental illness* (pp. 147–173). Washington, DC: American Psychiatric Press.

Griffith, J. (2006). Adler's organ jargon. In S. Slavik & J. Carlson (Eds.), *Readings in the theory of Individual Psychology* (pp. 83–90). New York: Taylor and Francis.

Grunebaum, H., & Chasin, R. (1978). Relabeling and reframing reconsidered: The beneficial effects of a pathological label. *Family Process, 17,* 449–456.

Grunebaum, H., & Chasin, R. (1982). Thinking like a family therapist: A model for integrating the theories and methods of family therapy. *Journal of Marital and Family Therapy, 8,* 403–416.

Guba, E. G., & Lincoln, Y. S. (1994). Competing paradigms in qualitative research. In N. K. Denzin & Y. S. Lincoln (Eds.), *Handbook of qualitative research* (pp. 105–117). Thousand Oaks, CA: Sage.

Guevremont, D. C., Tishelman, A. C., & Hull, D. B. (1985). Teaching generalized self-control to attention-deficit boys with mothers as adjunct therapists. *Child and Family Behavior Therapy, 7,* 23–36.

Gumpel, T. P., & Frank, R. (1999). An expansion of the peer-tutoring paradigm: Cross-age peer tutoring of social skills among social rejected boys. *Journal of Applied Behavior Analysis, 32,* 115–118.

Gurman, A., & Fraenkel, P. (2002). The history of couple therapy: A millennial review. *Family Process, 41*(2), 199–224.

Gurman, A., Kirshern, D. P., & Pinsof, W. M. (1986). Research on the process and outcome of marital and family therapy. *Psychotherapy, 29,* 65–71.

Haaga, D. A. F., & Davison, G. C. (1989). Outcome studies of rational-emotive therapy. In M. E. Bernard & R. [A.] DiGiuseppe (Eds.), *Inside rational-emotive therapy: A critical appraisal of the theory and therapy of Albert Ellis* (pp. 155–197). San Diego: Academic Press.

Haley, J. (1963). *Strategies of psychotherapy.* New York: Grune & Stratton.

Haley, J. (1973). *Uncommon therapy: The psychiatric techniques of Milton H. Erikson.* New York: Norton.

Hall, C. (1997). Cultural malpractice: The growing obsolescence of psychology with the changing U.S. population. *American Psychologist, 52,* 642–651.

Hammond, W., & Romney, D. (1995). Cognitive factors contributing to adolescent depression. *Journal of Youth and Adolescence, 24,* 667–682.

Handlbauer, B. (1998). *The Freud-Adler controversy.* Oxford, UK: Oneworld Publications.

Hanly, C. (1979). *Existentialism and psychoanalysis.* New York: International Universities Press.

Hanna, F. J. (1998). A transcultural view of prejudice, racism, and community feeling: The desire and striving for status. *Journal of Individual Psychology, 54,* 336–345.

Hanna, S. M., & Brown, J. H. (2004). *The practice of family therapy* (3rd ed.). Pacific Grove, CA: Brooks/Cole.

Hansen, J., & L'Abate, L. (1982). *Approaches to family therapy.* New York: Macmillan.

Hardy, K. V., & Laszloffy, T. A. (1992). Training racially sensitive family therapists: Context, content, and contact. *Families in Society, 73,* 363–370.

Hardy, K. V., & Laszloffy, T. A. (1995). The cultural genogram: Key to training culturally competent family therapists. *Journal of Marital and Family Therapy, 21,* 227–237.

Hare-Mustin, R. (1994). Discourses in the mirrored room: A postmodern analysis of therapy. *Family Process, 33,* 19–35.

Hare-Mustin, R. T. (1978). A feminist approach to family therapy. *Family Process, 17,* 181–194.

Harris, S. L., & Romanczyk, R. G. (1976). Treating self-injurious behavior of a retarded child by overcorrection. *Behavior Therapy, 7,* 235–239.

Hartmann, D. P. (1988). Measurement and analysis. M. H. Bornstein & M. E. Lamb (Eds.), *Developmental psychology: An advanced textbook* (2nd ed., pp. 85–147). Hillsdale, NJ: Erlbaum.

Harway, M. (1979). Training counselors. *The Counseling Psychologist, 8,* 8–10.

Hatch, M. L., Friedman, S., & Paradis, C. M. (1996). Behavioral treatment of obsessive-compulsive disorder in African Americans. *Cognitive and Behavioral Practice, 3,* 303–315.

Hayes, S. C., Strosahl, K. D., & Wilson, K. G. (1999). *Acceptance and commitment therapy: An experimental approach to behavior change.* New York: Guilford.

Hays, P. A. (1995). Multicultural applications of cognitive behavior therapy. *Professional Psychology: Research & Practice, 26,* 309–315.

Hays, P. A. (2001). *Discussing cultural complexities in practice: A framework for clinicians and counselors.* Washington, DC: American Psychological Association.

Hays, P. A. (2006). Cognitive-behavior therapy with Alaska Native people. In P. A. Hays & G. Y. Iwamasa (Eds.), *Culturally responsive cognitive-behavioral therapy: Assessment, practice, and supervision.* Washington, DC: American Psychological Association.

Hays, P. A., & Iwamasa, G. Y. (Eds.). (2006). *Culturally responsive cognitive-behavioral therapy: Assessment, practice, and supervision.* Washington, DC: American Psychological Association.

Hedtke, L. (2000). Dancing with death. *Gecko: A Journal of Deconstruction and Narrative Ideas in Therapeutic Practice, 2,* 5–16.

Heffer, R. W., & Kelley, M. L. (1987). Mothers' acceptance of behavioral interventions for children: The influence of parent race and income. *Behavior Therapy, 2,* 153–163.

Heidegger, M. (1962). *Being and time.* New York: Harper & Row.

Helmeke, K. B., & Sprenkle, D. H. (2000). Clients' perceptions of pivotal moments in couple therapy: A qualitative study of change in therapy. *Journal of Marital and Family Therapy, 26,* 469–483.

Helms, J. (1995). An update of Helm's White and people of color racial identity models. In J. G. Pomeratto, J. M. Casas, I. A. Suzuki, & C. M. Alexander (Eds.), *Handbook of multicultural counseling* (pp. 181–198). Thousand Oaks, CA: Sage.

Hendricks, M. N. (2002). Focusing oriented/experiential psychotherapy. In D. J. Cain & J. Seeman (Eds.), *Humanistic psychotherapies: Handbook of research and practice* (pp. 221–251). Washington, DC: American Psychological Association.

Henggeler, S. W., Melton, G. B., Smith, L. A., Schoenwald, S. K., & Hanley, J. H. (1993). Family preservation using multisystemic treatment: Long-term follow-up to a clinical trail with serious juvenile offenders. *Journal of Child and Family Studies, 2,* 283–292.

Hermann, J. A., de Montes, A. I., Dominguez, B., Montes, F., & Hopkins, B. L. (1973). Effects of bonuses for punctuality on the tardiness of industrial workers. *Journal of Applied Behavior Analysis, 6,* 563–570.

Herring, R. D. (1999). *Counseling with Native American Indians and Alaskan Natives: Strategies for helping professionals.* Thousand Oaks, CA: Sage.

Herring, R. D., & Runion, K. B. (1994). Counseling ethnic children and youth from an Adlerian perspective. *Journal of Multicultural Counseling and Development, 22,* 215–226.

Hill, R., & Rogers, R. H. (1964). The developmental approach. In H. Christensen (Ed.), *Handbook of marriage and family therapy* (pp. 171–209). Chicago: Rand McNally.

Hines, P. (1989). Climbing up the rough side of the mountain. In M. McGoldrick (Ed.), *Revisioning family therapy: Race, culture and gender in clinical practice.* New York: Guilford.

Hines, P., & Boyd-Franklin, N. (1996). African American families. In M. McGoldrick, J. Giodano, & J. K. Pearce (Eds.), *Ethnicity and family therapy* (2nd ed.). New York: Guilford.

Hinton, D. E. (2006). Special issue: Culturally sensitive CBT. *Cognitive and Behavioral Practice, 13,* 246–248.

Hiss, H., & Kozak, M. J. (1991). Exposure treatment of obsessive-compulsive disorder in the mentally retarded. *The Behavior Therapist, 14,* 163–167.

Ho, M., & Settles, A. (1984). The use of popular music in family therapy. *Social Work, 29,* 65–67.

Ho, M. K., Rasheed, J. M., & Rasheed, M. N. (2004). *Family therapy with ethnic minorities* (2nd ed.). Thousand Oaks, CA: Sage.

Hoffman, E. (1994). *The drive for self: Alfred Adler and the founding of individual psychology.* Reading, MA: Addison-Wesley.

Hoffman, I. Z. (1983). The patient as interpreter of the analyst's experience. *Contemporary Psychoanalysis, 19,* 389–422.

Hoffman, I. Z. (1991). Toward a social-constructivist view of the psychoanalytic situation. *Psychoanalytic Dialogues, 1,* 74–105.

Hoffman, I. Z. (1998). *Ritual and spontaneity in psychoanalysis.* Hillsdale, NJ: The Analytic Press.

Hoffman, L. (1990). Constructing realities: An art of lenses. *Family Process, 29,* 1–12.

Hoffman, S. G. (2006). The importance of culture in cognitive and behavioral practice. *Cognitive and Behavioral Practice, 13,* 243–245.

Hollon, S. D., & Beck, A. T. (1986). Research on cognitive therapies. In S. L. Garfield & A. E. Bergin (Eds.), *Handbook of psychotherapy and behavior change* (3rd ed., pp. 443–482). New York: Wiley.

Hollon, S. D., & Beck, A. T. (1994). Cognitive and cognitive behavioral therapies. In A. E. Bergin & S. L. Garfield (Eds.), *Handbook of psychotherapy and behavior change* (4th ed., pp. 428–466). New York: Wiley.

Hollon, S. D., Shelton, R. C., & Davis, D. D. (1993). Cognitive therapy for depression: Conceptual issues and clinical efficacy. *Journal of Consulting and Clinical Psychology, 61*, 270–275.

Holroyd, J. C., & Brodsky, A. M. (1980). Does touching patients lead to sexual intercourse? *Professional Psychology, 11*, 807–811.

Hong, G. K., & Ham, M. D. (1992). Impact of immigration on the family life cycle: Clinical implications for Chinese Americans. *Journal of Family Psychotherapy, 3*(3), 27–40.

Horne, A. M., & Matson, J. L. (1977). A comparison of modeling, desensitization, flooding, skills, and control groups for reducing test anxiety. *Behavior Therapy, 8*, 1–8.

Hubble, M. A., Duncan, B. L., & Miller, S. D. (1999). Directing attention to what works. In M. A. Hubble, B. L. Duncan, & S. D. Miller (Eds.), *The heart and soul of change* (pp. 407–447). Washington, DC: American Psychological Association.

Hughes, C., & Rusch, F. R. (1989). Teaching supported employees with severe mental retardation to solve problems. *Journal of Applied Behavior Analysis, 22*, 365–372.

Hurlburt, D., & Apt, C. (1993). Female sexuality: A comparative study between women in homosexual and heterosexual relationships. *Journal of Sex and Marital Therapy, 19*, 315–327.

Hurlburt, R. T. (1993). *Sampling inner experience in disturbed affect.* New York: Plenum.

Ibrahim, F. A. (1991). Contribution of cultural worldview to generic counseling and development. *Journal of Counseling and Development, 70*, 13–19.

Ibrahim, F. A. (2003). Existential worldview counseling theory: Inception to application. In F. D. Harper & J. McFadden (Eds.), *Culture and counseling: New approaches* (pp. 196–208). Boston: Allyn & Bacon.

Ignatiev, N. (1995). *How the Irish became White.* London: Routledge.

Imber-Black, E. (1988). *Families and larger systems: A family therapist's guide through the labyrinth.* New York: Guilford.

Imber-Black, E. (2004). Of continuities, beginnings and generativities. *Family Process, 43*(1), 1–5.

Ingram, C., & Perlez, A. (2004). The getting of wisdoms. *International Journal of Narrative Therapy and Community Work, 2*, 49–56.

Ivey, A. E. (2000). *Developmental therapy: Theory into practice.* North Amherst, MA: Microtraining Associates.

Ivey, A. E., D'Andrea, M., Ivey, M. B., & Simek-Morgan, L. (2002). *Theories of counseling and psychotherapy: A multicultural perspective.* Boston: Allyn & Bacon.

Ivey, A. E., Ivey, M., Myers, P., & Sweeney, T. (2005). *Developmental counseling and therapy.* Boston: Lahaska Press/Houghton Mifflin.

Ivey, A. E., & Rigazio-DiGilio, S. A. (1994). Developmental counseling and therapy: Can still another theory be useful to you? *Journal for the Professional Counselor, 9*, 23–48.

Jacobsen, J. J. (1986). *Psychiatric sequelae of child abuse: Reconnaissance of child abuse and neglect evaluation, prospects, recommendations.* Springfield, IL: Thomas.

Jacobson, N. (1981). Behavioral marital therapy. In A. S. Gurman & D. P. Kniskern (Eds.), *Handbook of family therapy* (pp. 556–591). New York: Brunner/Mazel.

Jacobson, N. S. (1989). The maintenance of treatment gains following social learning-based marital therapy. *Behavior Therapy, 20,* 325–336.

Jacobson, N. S. (1991, September). *Marital therapy: Theory and treatment considerations.* Workshop sponsored by the Rhode Island Psychological Association, Warwick.

Jacobson, N. S., Christensen, A., Prince, S. E., Cordova, J., & Eldridge, K. (2000). Integrative behavior couple therapy: An acceptance-based, promising new treatment for couple discord. *Journal of Consulting and Clinical Psychology, 68,* 351–355.

Jacobson, N. S., & Margolin, G. (1979). *Marital therapy: Strategies based on social learning and behavior exchange principles.* New York: Brunner/Mazel.

Janov, A. (2000). *The biology of love.* Amherst, NY: Prometheus.

Jay, S. M., Elliott, C. H., Ozolins, M., Olson, R. A., & Pruitt, S. D. (1985). Behavioral management of children's distress during painful medical procedures. *Behaviour Research and Therapy, 23,* 513–520.

Jenkins, A. (1990). *Invitations to responsibility: The therapeutic engagement of men who are violent and abusive.* Adelaide, Australia: Dulwich Centre Publications.

Johansen, T. M. (2005). Applying Individual Psychology to work with clients of the Islamic faith. *Journal of Individual Psychology, 61,* 174–184.

Johnson, N. G., & Remer, P. (1997). Postdoctoral training in feminist psychological practice. In J. Worell & N. G. Johnson (Eds.), *Shaping the future of feminist psychology: Education, research, and practice* (pp. 203–226). Washington, DC: American Psychological Association.

Johnson, P. B. (1976). Women and power: Toward a theory of effectiveness. *Journal of Social Issues, 32,* 99–100.

Johnson, W. G., Corrigan, S. A., & Mayo, L. L. (1987). Innovative treatment approaches to bulimia nervosa. Special issue: Recent advances in behavioral medicine. *Behavior Modification, 11,* 373–388.

Jones, M. C. (1924). A laboratory study of fear: The case of Peter. *Pedagogical Seminar, 31,* 308–315.

Jones, M. L., Eyberg, S. M., Adams, C. D., & Boggs, S. R. (1998). Treatment acceptability of behavioral interventions for children: An assessment by mothers of children with disruptive behavior disorders. *Child & Family Behavior Therapy, 20,* 15–26.

Joshua, J. M., & DiMenna, D. (2000). *Read two books and let's talk next week: Using bibliotherapy in clinical practice.* New York: Wiley.

Jourard, S. M. (1971). *The transparent self: Self disclosure and well-being.* New York: Van Nostrand Reinhold.

Jung, C. G. (1966). Two essays on analytical psychology. In *Collected works of C. G. Jung* (Vol. 7) (R. F. C. Hall, Trans.) (2nd ed.). Princeton, NJ: Princeton University Press.

Kahn, C. H. (1982). Why existence does not emerge as a distinct concept in Greek philosophy. In P. Morewedge (Ed.), *Philosophies of existence: Ancient and medieval* (pp. 7–17). New York: Fordham University Press.

Kaiser, H. (1965). The problems of responsibility in psychotherapy. In B. Fierman (Ed.), *Effective psychotherapy* (pp. 1–13). New York: Free Press. [Reprinted from *Psychiatry, 18* (1955), 205–211.]

Kalichman, S. C., Cherry, C., & Browne-Sperling, F. (1999). Effectiveness of a video-based motivational skills-building HIV-reduction intervention for inner-city African American men. *Journal of Consulting and Clinical Psychology, 67,* 959–966.

Kant, G. L., D'Zurilla, T. J., & Maydeu-Olivares, A. (1997). Social problem solving as a mediator of stress-related depression and anxiety in middle-aged and elderly community residents. *Cognitive Therapy and Research, 21,* 73–96.

Kanz, J. E. (2001). The applicability of Individual Psychology for work with conservative Christian clients. *Journal of Individual Psychology, 57,* 342–353.

Karenga, M. (1996). The nguzo saba (the seven principles): Their meaning and message. In M. K. Asante & A. S. Sbarry (Eds.), *African intellectual heritage* (pp. 543–554). Philadelphia: Temple University Press.

Kasambria, K. P., & Edwards, I. (2000). Counseling and human ecology: A conceptual framework for counselor educators. In *Proceedings of the Eighth International Counseling Conference: Counseling and Human Ecology* (pp. 43–52). San Jose, Costa Rica.

Kaslow, F. W. (2000). History of family therapy: Evolution outside the U.S.A. *Journal of Family Psychotherapy, 11,* 1–36.

Kawulich, B. B., & Curlette, W. L. (1998). Life tasks and the Native American perspectives. *Journal of Individual Psychology, 54,* 359–367.

Kazdin, A. E. (1989). *Behavior modification in applied settings* (4th ed.). Pacific Grove, CA: Brooks/Cole.

Keijsers, G. P. J., Schaap, C. P. D. R., & Hoogduin, C. A. L. (2000). The impact of interpersonal patient and therapist behavior on outcome in cognitive-behavior therapy. *Behavior Modification, 24,* 264–297.

Keller, F. S. (1968). "Good-bye, teacher. . . ." *Journal of Applied Behavior Analysis, 1,* 79–89.

Kempler, W. (1973). *Principles of Gestalt family therapy.* Costa Mesa, CA: Kempler Institute.

Kempler, W. (1981). *Experiential psychotherapy with families.* New York: Brunner/Mazel.

Kendall, P. C. (1989). The generalization and maintenance of behavior change: Comments, considerations, and the "no-cure" criticism. *Behavior Therapy, 20,* 357–364.

Kendall, P. C. (1994). Treating anxiety disorders in children: Results of a randomized clinical trial. *Journal of Consulting and Clinical Psychology, 62,* 100–110.

Kendall, P. C. (1998). Empirically supported psychological therapies. *Journal of Consulting and Clinical Psychology, 66,* 3–6.

Kendall, P. C., & Finch, A. J. (1978). A cognitive-behavioral treatment for impulsivity: A group comparison study. *Journal of Consulting and Clinical Psychology, 46,* 110–118.

Kendall, P. C., & Gerow, M. A. (1995). *Long-term follow-up of a cognitive-behavioral therapy for anxiety-disordered youth.* Unpublished manuscript, Temple University, Philadelphia.

Kern, R. M. (2002). Lifestyle Questionnaire Inventory. In R. Kern, & D. Eckstein (Eds.), *Psychological fingerprints* (pp. 69–70). Dubuque, IA: Kendall Hunt.

Kern, R. M., Yeakle, R., & Sperry, L. (1989). Survey of contemporary Adlerian clinical practices and therapy issues. *Individual Psychology, 45,* 38–47.

Kierkegaard, S. (1949). *Traité du désespoir* [Treatise on hopelessness]. Paris: Gallimard.

Kim, M. S. (2001). The effects of a reality therapy program on locus of control and responsibility of elementary school children. *International Journal of Reality Therapy, 20*(2), 17.

Kingdon, D. G., & Turkington, D. (2005). *Cognitive therapy of schizophrenia*. New York: Guilford.

Kirschenbaum, H. (1979). *On becoming Carl Rogers*. New York: Delacorte.

Kirschenbaum, H., & Jourdan, A. (2005). The current status of Carl Rogers and the person-centered approach. *Psychotherapy: Theory, Research, and Practice, 42*, 37–51.

Kitchener, K. S. (1984). Intuition, critical evaluation and ethical principles: The foundations for ethical decisions in counseling psychology. *The Counseling Psychologist, 12*, 43–55.

Kitchener, K. S. (2000a). *Foundations of ethical practice, research, and teaching in psychology*. Mahwah, NJ: Erlbaum.

Kitchener, K. S. (2000b). Reconceptualizing responsibilities to students: A feminist perspective. In M. M. Brabeck (Ed.), *Practicing feminist ethics in psychology* (pp. 37–54). Washington, DC: American Psychological Association.

Klein, M. (1975). *Envy and gratitude and other works*. New York: Delacorte.

Klesges, R. C., Malott, J. M., & Ugland, M. (1984). The effects of graded exposure and parental modeling on the dental phobias of a four-year-old girl and her mother. *Journal of Behavior Therapy and Experimental Psychiatry, 15*, 161–164.

Kluckhohn, C., & Murray, H. (1959). Personality formation: The determinants. In C. Kluckhohn, H. A. Murray, & D. M. Schneider (Eds.), *Personality in nature, society and culture* (pp. 53–67). New York: Knopf.

Kluckhohn, F. R., & Strodtbeck, F. L. (1961). Variation in value orientations. Evanston, IL: Row, Patterson.

Koch, S. (Ed.). (1959). *Psychology: A study of a science*. New York: McGraw-Hill.

Koder, D.-A., Brodaty, H., & Anstey, K. J. (1996). Cognitive therapy for depression in the elderly. *International Journal of Geriatric Psychiatry, 11*, 97–107.

Koestenbaum, P. (1971). *The vitality of death: Essays in existential psychology and philosophy*. Westport, CT: Greenwood Press.

Kogan, S. M., & Gale, J. E. (1997). Decentering therapy: Textual analysis of a narrative therapy session. *Family Process, 36*, 101–126.

Kohlenberg, R. J., & Tsai, M. (1991). *Functional analytic psychotherapy: Creating intense and curative therapeutic relationships*. New York: Plenum.

Kohlenberg, R. J., & Tsai, M. (1994). Functional analytic psychotherapy: A radical behavioral approach to treatment and integration. *Journal of Psychotherapy Integration, 4*, 175–201.

Kohlenberg, R. J., & Tsai, M. (1995). Functional analytic psychotherapy: A behavioral approach to intensive treatment. In W. T. O'Donohue & L. Krasner (Eds.), *Theories of behavior therapy: Exploring behavior change* (pp. 637–658). Washington, DC: American Psychological Association.

Kohlenberg, R. J., Tsai, M., Parker, C., Bolling, M., & Kanter, J. (1999). The client-therapist interaction: The core of a behavioral approach. *European Psychotherapie, 1*, 21–29.

Kohn, A. (1993). *Punished by rewards*. Boston: Houghton-Mifflin.

Kopec, A. M., Beal, D., & DiGiuseppe, R. [A.] (1994). Training in RET: Disputational strategies. *Journal of Rational-Emotive & Cognitive-Behavior Therapy, 12,* 47–60.

Kottler, J. A. (2001). *Theories in counseling and therapy: An experiential approach.* Boston: Allyn & Bacon.

Kotzé, E., & Kotzé, D. (2001). *Telling narratives.* Pretoria, South Africa: Ethics Alive.

Krop, H., & Burgess, D. (1993). The use of covert modeling in the treatment of a sexual abuse victim. In J. R. Cautela & A. J. Kearney (Eds.), *Covert conditioning casebook* (pp. 153–158). Pacific Grove, CA: Brooks/Cole.

Kuehlwein, K. T. (1992). Working with gay men. In A. Freeman & F. M. Dattilio (Eds.), *Comprehensive casebook of cognitive therapy* (pp. 249–255). New York: Plenum.

Lahav, R., & de Venza Tillmanns, M. (Eds.). (1995). *Essays on philosophical counseling.* Lanham, MD: University Press of America.

Laing, R. D. (1969). *The divided self.* Middlesex, UK: Penguin.

Lambert, M. J. (1992). Psychotherapy outcome research: Implications for integrative and eclectic therapists. In J. C. Norcross & M. R. Goldfried (Eds.), *Handbook of psychotherapy integration* (pp. 94–129). New York: Basic Books.

Lappin, J. (1982). On becoming a culturally-conscious family therapist. In C. J. Falicov (Ed.), *Cultural perspectives in family therapy* (pp. 51–67). Rockville, MD: Aspen Systems.

Lask, B., & Matthew, D. (1979). Childhood asthma: A controlled trial of family psychotherapy. *Archives of Diseases in Childhood, 55,* 116–119.

Latner, J. (1986). *The Gestalt therapy book.* Highland, NY: Gestalt Journal Press.

Law, I. (1999). A discursive approach to therapy with men. In I. Parker (Ed.), *Deconstructing psychotherapy* (pp. 115–131). London: Sage.

Lawrence, D. (2004). The effects of reality therapy group counseling on the self-determination of persons with developmental disabilities. *International Journal of Reality Therapy, 23*(2), 9–16.

Lazarus, A. A. (1959). The elimination of children's phobias by deconditioning. *Medical Proceedings, 5,* 261–265.

Lazarus, A. A. (1961). Group therapy of phobic disorders by systematic desensitization. *Journal of Abnormal and Social Psychology, 63,* 505–510.

Lazarus, A. A. (1976). *Multimodal behavior therapy.* New York: Springer.

Lazarus, A. A. (Ed.). (1985). *Casebook of multimodal therapy.* New York: Guilford.

Lazarus, A. A. (1989a). *The practice of multimodal therapy.* Baltimore: Johns Hopkins University Press.

Lazarus, A. A. (1989b). The practice of rational-emotive therapy. In M. E. Bernard & R. [A.] DiGiuseppe (Eds.), *Inside rational-emotive therapy: A critical appraisal of the theory and therapy of Albert Ellis* (pp. 95–112). San Diego: Academic Press.

Lazarus, A. A. (1995). Different types of eclectism and integration: Let's be aware of the dangers. *Journal of Psychotherapy Integration, 5,* 27–39.

Lazarus, A. A. (1996). The utility and futility of combining treatments in psychotherapy. *Clinical Psychology: Science and Practice, 3,* 59–68.

Lazarus, A. A., & Abramovitz, A. (1962). The use of "emotive imagery" in the treatment of children's phobias. *Journal of Mental Science, 108,* 191–195.

Lazarus, A. A., Beutler, L. E., & Norcross, J. C. (1992). The future of technical eclecticism. *Psychotherapy, 29,* 11–20.

Lazarus, R. S., & Folkman, S. (1984). *Stress, appraisal, and coping.* New York: Springer.

Lebow, J. L. (1987). Training psychologists in family therapy in family institute settings. *Journal of Family Psychology, 1,* 219–231.

Lebow, J. [L.] (1997). The integrative revolution in couple and family therapy. *Family Process, 36,* 1–18.

Lee, E. (Ed.). (1997). *Working with Asian Americans: A guide for clinicians.* New York: Guilford.

Lee, R. M., & Ramirez M., III (2000). The history, current status, and future of multicultural psychotherapy. In I. B. Cuellar & F. A. Paniagua (Eds.), *Handbook of multicultural mental health: Assessment and treatment of diverse populations* (pp. 279–309). San Diego: Academic Press.

Lee, S. K. (2001). A study on a counseling program for decrease of aggression through reality therapy. *International Journal of Reality Therapy, 20*(2), 20–21.

Lehman, N. S. (1993). Pleasure heals: The role of social pleasure—love in its broadest sense—in medical practice. *Archives of Internal Medicine, 153,* 929–934.

Lerner, J., Franklin, M. E., Meadows, E. A., Hembree, E., & Foa, E. B. (1998). Effectiveness of a cognitive-behavioral treatment program for trichotilomania: An uncontrolled evaluation. *Behavior Therapy, 29,* 157–171.

Levendusky, P. G., & Hufford, M. R. (1997). The application of cognitive behavior therapy to the treatment of depression and related disorders in the elderly. *Journal of Geriatric Psychiatry, 30,* 227–238.

Lewin, K. (1951). *Field theory in social science: Selected theoretical papers.* (D. Cartwright, Ed.). New York: Harper & Row.

Lewinsohn, P. M., Clarke, G. N., & Rohde, P. (1994). Psychological approaches to the treatment of depression in adolescents. In W. M. Reynolds & H. F. Johnston (Eds.), *Handbook of depression in children and adolescents* (pp. 309–344). New York: Plenum.

Lewinsohn, P. M., & Graf, M., (1973). Pleasant activities and depression. *Journal of Consulting and Clinical Psychology, 41,* 261–268.

Lewinsohn, P. M., Hoberman, H., Teri, L., & Hautzinger, M. (1985). An integrative theory of depression. In S. Reiss & R. R. Bootzin (Eds.), *Theoretical issues in behavior therapy.* New York: Academic Press.

Lewinsohn, P. M., & Teri, L. (1983). *Clinical geropsychology.* New York: Pergamon.

Lewis, J. A., Lewis, M., Daniels, J. A., & D'Andrea, M. J. (2002). *Community counseling.* Belmont, CA: Wadsworth.

Liberman, R. P., Wallace, C. J., Blackwell, G., Eckman, T. A., Vaccaro, J. V., & Kuehnel, T. G. (1993). Innovations in skills training for the seriously mentally ill: The UCLA social and independent living skills modules. *Innovations and Research, 2,* 43–60.

Lichtenberg, P. A., Kimbarrow, M. L., Morris, P., & Vangel, S. J., Jr. (1996). Behavioral treatment of depression in predominantly African-American medical patients. *Clinical Gerontologist, 17,* 15–33.

Liddell, A., Di Fazio, L., Blackwood, J., & Ackerman, C. (1994). Long-term follow-up of treated dental phobics. *Behaviour Research and Therapy, 32,* 605–610.

Liddle, H. A., & Rowe, C. L. (2004). Advances in family therapy research. In M. Nichols & R. Schwartz (Eds.), *Family therapy: Concepts and methods* (6th ed., pp. 395–345). Boston: Allyn & Bacon.

Lindauer, M. S. (1998). The phenomenal method. In R. J. Corsini & A. J. Auerbach (Eds.), *Concise encyclopedia of psychology.* New York: Wiley.

Lindsley, O. R. (1956). Operant conditioning methods applied to research in chronic schizophrenia. *Psychiatric Research Reports, 5,* 118–139.

Lindsley, O. R. (1960). Characteristics of the behavior of chronic psychotics as revealed by free-operant conditioning methods. *Diseases of the Nervous System* (Monograph Supplement), *21,* 66–78.

Lindsley, O. R. (1963). Free-operant conditioning and psychotherapy. *Current Psychiatric Therapies, 3,* 47–56.

Linehan, M. M. (1993). *Cognitive-behavioral treatment of borderline personality disorder.* New York: Guilford.

Lochman, J. E., & Curry, J. F. (1986). Situational social problem-solving skills and self-esteem of aggressive and nonaggressive boys. *Journal of Abnormal Child Psychology, 14,* 605–617.

Locke, D. (1990). A not so provincial view of multicultural counseling. *Counselor Education and Supervision, 30,* 18–25.

Locke, D. C. (1998). *Increasing multicultural understanding: A comprehensive model* (2nd ed.). Thousand Oaks, CA: Sage.

Loomis, L. R. (Ed.). (1943). *Aristotle: On man in the universe.* Roslyn, NY: Black.

Lopez, M. A., & Silber, S. (1991). Stress management for the elderly: A preventive approach. *Clinical Gerontologist, 10,* 73–76.

Lovaas, O. I. (1977). *The autistic child: Language development through behavior modification.* New York: Irvington.

Lovaas, O. I. (1987). Behavioral treatment and normal educational and intellectual functioning in young autistic children. *Journal of Consulting and Clinical Psychology, 55,* 3–9.

Luborsky, L. (2001). The meaning of *empirically supported treatment* research for psychoanalytic and other long-term therapies. *Psychoanalytic Dialogues, 11*(4), 583–604.

Lumley, V. A., Miltenberger, R. G., Long, E. S., Rapp, J. T., & Roberts, J. A. (1998). Evaluation of a sexual abuse prevention program for adults with mental retardation. *Journal of Applied Behavior Analysis, 31,* 91–101.

Lutgendorf, S. K., Antoni, M. H., Ironson, G., Starr, K., Costello, N., Zuckerman, M., et al. (1998). Changes in cognitive coping skills and social support during cognitive behavioral stress management intervention and distress outcomes in symptomatic human immunodeficiency virus (HIV)-seropositive gay men. *Psychosomatic Medicine, 60,* 204–214.

Lutgendorf, S. K., McCabe, P., Antoni, M. H., Ironson, G., Klimas, N., Fletcher, et al. (1997). Cognitive-behavioral stress management decreases dysphoric mood and herpes simplex virus-Type 2 antibody titers in symptomatic HIV-seropositive gay men. *Journal of Consulting and Clinical Psychology, 65,* 31–43.

Macaskill, A. (1999). Personal therapy as a training requirement: The lack of supporting evidence. In C. Feltham (Ed.), *Controversies in psychotherapy and counseling* (pp. 142–154). Thousand Oaks, CA: Sage.

MacDougall, C. (2002). Rogers' person-centered approach: Considerations for use in multicultural counseling. *Journal of Humanistic Psychology, 42*(2), 48–65.

MacKenzie-Keating, S. E., & McDonald, L. (1990). Overcorrection: Reviewed, revisited, and revised. *The Behavior Analyst, 13,* 39–48.

MacMillan, V., Guevremont, D. C., & Hansen, D. J. (1989). Problem-solving training with a multi-distressed abusive mother. *Journal of Family Violence, 3,* 69–81.

Madanes, C. (1981). *Strategic family therapy.* San Francisco: Jossey-Bass.

Madsen, C. K., Greer, R. D., & Madsen, C. H. (1975). *Research in music behavior: Modifying music behavior in the classroom.* New York: Teachers College Press.

Mahler, M., Pine, F., & Bergman, A. (1975). *The psychological birth of the human infant.* New York: Basic Books.

Mahoney, M. J. (1991). *Human change processes.* New York: Basic Books.

Maisel, R., Epston, D., & Borden, A. (2004) *Biting the hand that starves you: Inspiring resistance to anorexia/bulimia.* New York: Norton.

Manaster, G. (1989). Clinical issues in brief therapy: A summary and conclusion. *Individual Psychology, 45,* 243–247.

Manaster, G., & Corsini, R. (1982). *Individual psychology.* Chicago: Adler School.

Maniacci, M. (1999). Clinical therapy. In R. E. Watts & J. Carlson (Eds.), *Interventions and strategies in counseling and psychotherapy* (pp. 59–85). Philadelphia: Taylor & Francis.

Mann, R. A. (1972). The behavior-therapeutic use of contingency contracting to control an adult behavior problem: Weight control. *Journal of Applied Behavior Analysis, 5,* 99–109.

Mann, R. A. (1976). The use of contingency contracting to facilitate durability of behavior change: Weight loss maintenance. *Addictive Behaviors, 1,* 245–249.

Mansager, E. (2000). Individual psychology and the study of spirituality. *Journal of Individual Psychology, 56,* 371–388.

Mansager, E., Cold, L., Griffith, B., Kai, E., Manaster, G., McArter, G., et al. (2002). Spirituality in the Adlerian forum. *Journal of Individual Psychology, 58,* 177–196.

Mansdorf, I. J., Calapai, P., Caselli, L., Burstein, Y., & Dimant, J. (1999). Reducing psychotropic medication usage in nursing home residents: The effects of behaviorally oriented psychotherapy. *The Behavior Therapist, 22,* pp. 21–23, 29.

Marinoff, L. (1999). *Plato, not Prozac!* New York: HarperCollins.

Marks, I. M., Goldfried, M. R. (Moderators), Sungur, M., Newman, M. G., Moore, K., & Stricker, G. (Panelists). (2005, November). *Towards a common language in psychotherapy.* Panel discussion presented at the annual meeting of the Association for Behavioral and Cognitive Therapies, Washington, DC.

Marlatt, G. A., & Donovan, D. M. (Ed.). (2005). *Relapse prevention: Maintenance strategies in the treatment of addictive behaviors* (2nd ed.). New York: Guilford.

Marlatt, G. A., & Gordon, J. R. (Eds.). (1985). *Relapse prevention: Maintenance strategies in the treatment of addictive behaviors.* New York: Guilford.

Matteson, D. R. (1995). Counseling with bisexuals. *Journal of Individual Psychology, 51,* 144–159.

Maturana, H. R., & Varela, F. J. (1997*). The tree of knowledge: The biological roots of human understanding.* Boston: Shambala.

May, R. (1958). *Existence: A new dimension in psychiatry and psychology.* New York: Simon & Schuster.

May, R. (1961). *Existential psychology.* New York: Random House.

May, R. (1964). Existential basis of psychotherapy. In M. Friedman (Ed.). *The worlds of existentialism: A critical reader* (pp. 440–462). Chicago: University of Chicago Press.

May, R. (1975). *The courage to create.* New York: Norton.

May, R. (1981). *Freedom and destiny.* New York: Dell.

May, R. (1991). Existence: A new dimension in psychiatry and psychology. In J. Ehren-Wald (Ed.), *The history of psychotherapy* (pp. 388–393). Northvale, NJ: Aronson.

May, R., Angel, E., & Ellenberger, H. F. (Eds.). (1958). *Existence: A new dimension in psychiatry and psychology.* New York: Basic Books.

May, R., & Yalom, I. (1984). Existential psychotherapy. In R. J. Corsini (Ed.), *Current psychotherapies* (3rd ed., pp. 354–391). Itasca, IL: Peacock.

McDowell, T. (2004). Listening to the racial experiences of graduate trainees: A critical race theory perspective. *American Journal of Family Therapy, 32*(4), 305–324.

McDowell, T., Fang, S., Brownlee, K., Gomez Young, C., & Khanna, A. (2002). Transforming a MFT program: A model for enhancing diversity. *Journal of Marital and Family Therapy, 28*(2), 179–191.

McDowell, T., Fang, S., Gomez Young, C., Brownlee, K., Khanna, A., & Sherman, B. (2003). Making space for racial dialogue in MFT education. *Journal of Marital and Family Therapy, 29*(2), 179–194.

McDowell, T., & Jeris, L. (2004). Talking about race using critical race theory: Recent trends in the *Journal of Marital and Family Therapy. Journal of Marital and Family Therapy, 30*(1), 81–94.

McGill, D. W. (1987). Language, cultural psychology and family therapy: Japanese example from an international perspective. *Contemporary Family Therapy, 9*(4), 283–292.

McGinn, L. K., & Young, J. E. (1996). Schema-focused therapy. In P. M. Salkovskis (Ed.), *Frontiers of cognitive therapy* (pp. 182–207). New York: Guilford.

McGoldrick, M. (2002). *Re-visioning family therapy: Race, culture, and gender in clinical practice.* New York: Guilford.

McGoldrick, M., Gerson, R., & Shellenberger, S. (1999). *Genograms: Assessment and intervention* (2nd ed.). New York: Norton.

McGoldrick, M., Pearce, J., & Giordano, J. (1996). *Ethnicity and family therapy* (2nd ed.). New York: Guilford.

McIntosh, J. L., Santos, J. F., Hubbard, R. W., & Overholser, J. C. (1994). *Elder suicide: Research, theory, and treatment.* Washington, DC: American Psychological Association.

McIntosh, P. (1986). *Unpacking the invisible knapsack.* Wellesley, MA: Stone Center Working Papers.

McIntyre, A. (2000). Antiracist pedagogy in the university: The ethical challenges of making Whiteness public. In M. M. Brabeck (Ed.), *Practicing feminist ethics in psychology* (pp. 55–74). Washington, DC: American Psychological Association.

McKenzie, W., & Monk, G. (1997). Learning and teaching narrative ideas. In G. Monk, J. Winslade, K. Crocket, & D. Epston (Eds.), *Narrative therapy in action: The archaeology of hope* (pp. 82–117). San Francisco: Jossey-Bass.

McNair, L. D. (1996). African American women and behavior therapy: Integrating theory, culture, and clinical practice. *Cognitive and Behavioral Practice, 3,* 337–349.

McNamee, S., & Gergen, K. (2000). *Social construction and the therapeutic process* (2nd ed.). Newbury Park, CA: Sage.

Medley, S. (2000). *Effect of self-persuasion on date rape prevention.* Lexington: University of Kentucky Press.

Meek, C. R. (1985). *Existence, culture, and psychotherapy.* New York: Philosophical Library.

Meeks, S., & Depp, C. A. (2002). Pleasant events-based behavioral intervention for depression in nursing home residents: A conceptual and empirical foundation. *Clinical Gerontologist, 25,* 125–148.

Meharg, S. S., & Woltersdorf, M. A. (1990). Therapeutic uses of videotape self-modeling: A review. *Advances in Behaviour Research and Therapy, 12,* 85–99.

Meichenbaum, D. [H.] (1971). Examination of model characteristics in reducing avoidance behavior. *Journal of Personality and Social Psychology, 17,* 298–307.

Meichenbaum, D. [H.] (1974). Self-instructional training: A cognitive prosthesis for the aged. *Human Development, 17,* 273–280.

Meichenbaum, D. [H.] (1977). *Cognitive-behavior modification: An integrative approach.* New York: Plenum.

Meichenbaum, D. H. (1985). *Stress inoculation training.* Elmsford, NY: Pergamon.

Meichenbaum, D. [H.], & Cameron, R. (1972). *Stress inoculation: A skills training approach to anxiety management.* Unpublished manuscript, University of Waterloo, Ontario.

Meichenbaum, D. [H.], & Cameron, R. (1973). Training schizophrenics to talk to themselves: A means of developing attentional controls. *Behavior Therapy, 4,* 515–534.

Meichenbaum, D. H., & Deffenbacher, J. L. (1988). Stress inoculation training. *The Counseling Psychologist, 16,* 69–90.

Meichenbaum, D. [H.], & Goodman, J. (1971). Training impulsive children to talk to themselves: A means of developing self-control. *Journal of Abnormal Psychology, 77,* 115–126.

Melamed, B. G., & Siegel, L. J. (1975). Reduction of anxiety in children facing hospitalization and surgery by use of filmed modeling. *Journal of Consulting and Clinical Psychology, 43,* 511–521.

Meyer, R. G. (1975). A behavioral treatment of sleepwalking associated with test anxiety. *Journal of Behavior Therapy and Experimental Psychiatry, 6,* 167–168.

Meyers, A., Mercatoris, M., & Sirota, A. (1976). Use of covert self-instruction for the elimination of psychotic speech. *Journal of Consulting and Clinical Psychology, 44,* 480–483.

Middleton, M. B., & Cartledge, G. (1995). The effects of social skills instruction and parental involvement on the aggressive behaviors of African American males. *Behavioral Medicine, 19,* 192–210.

Miller, C., & LeLieuvre, R. B. (1982). A method to reduce chronic pain in elderly nursing home residents. *The Gerontologist, 22,* 314–317.

Miller, J. (1976). Toward a new psychology of woman. Boston, MA: Beacon.

Miller, J. B. (1988). *Connections, disconnections, and violations* (Work in Progress No. 33). Wellesley, MA: Stone Center Working Paper Series.

Miller, P. (1993). *Theories of developmental psychology* (3rd ed.). New York: W. H. Freeman.

Miller, S. D., Duncan, B. L., & Hubble, M. A. (1997). *Escape from Babel.* New York: Norton.

Miltenberger, R. G., Roberts, J. A., Ellingson, S., Galensky, T., Rapp, J. T., Long, E. S., et al. (1999). Training and generalization of sexual abuse prevention skills for woman with mental retardation. *Journal of Applied Behavior Analysis, 32,* 385–388.

Miltenberger, R. G., & Thiesse-Duffy, E. (1988). Evaluation of home-based programs for teaching personal safety skills to children. *Journal of Applied Behavior Analysis, 21*, 81–87.

Minuchin, S. (1974). *Families and family therapy.* Cambridge, MA: Harvard University Press.

Minuchin, S. (1998). Where is the family in narrative family therapy? *Journal of Marital and Family Therapy, 24*, 397–408.

Miranda, A. O., & Fraser, L. D. (2002). Culture-bound syndromes: Initial perspectives from individual psychology. *Journal of Individual Psychology, 58*, 422–433.

Miranda, A. O., Frevert, V. S., & Kern, R. M. (1998). Life-style differences between bi-cultural, and low and high acculturation level Latinos. *Individual Psychology, 54*, 119–134.

Miranda, J., Azocar, F., Organista, K. C., Munoz, R. F., & Lieberman, A. (1996). Recruiting and retaining low-income Latinos in psychotherapy research. *Journal of Consulting and Clinical Psychology, 64*, 868–874.

Mishara, B. L., Robertson, B., & Kastenbaum, R. (1974). Self-injurious behavior in the elderly. *The Gerontologist, 14*, 273–280.

Mitchell, S. A. (1993). *Hope and dread in psychoanalysis.* New York: Basic Books.

Mohr, D. C., Likosky, W., Bertagnolli, A., Goodkin, D. E., Van Der Wende, J., Dwyer, P., et al. (2000). Telephone-administered cognitive-behavioral therapy for the treatment of depressive symptomology in multiple sclerosis. *Journal of Consulting and Clinical Psychology, 68*, 356–361.

Monk, G., & Drewery, W. (1994). The impact of social constructionist thinking on eclecticism in counsellor education: Some personal thoughts. *New Zealand Journal of Counselling, 16*(1), 5–14.

Monk, G., & Gerhart, D. (2003). Sociopolitical activist or conversational partner? Distinguishing the position of the therapist in narrative and collaborative therapies. *Family Process, 42*, 19–30.

Montalvo, B., & Gutierrez, M. (1983). A perspective for the use of the cultural dimension in family therapy. In C. J. Falicov (Ed.), *Cultural perspetives in family therapy* (pp. 2–15). Rockville, MD.: Aspen Systems.

Moore, N. (1965). Behavior therapy in bronchial asthma: A controlled study. *Journal of Psychosomatic Research, 9*, 257–276.

Morales, E. (1996). Gender roles among Latino gay and bisexual men: Implications for family and couple relationships. In J. Laird & R. Green (Eds.), *Lesbians and gays in couples and families: A handbook for therapists* (pp. 272–297). San Francisco: Jossey-Bass.

Morano, D. V. (1973). *Existential guilt: A phenomenological study.* Assen, The Netherlands: Van Gorcum.

Morgan, A. (2000). *What is narrative therapy? An easy-to-read introduction.* Adelaide, Australia: Dulwich Centre Publications.

Morin, C. M., Colecchi, C., Stone, J., Sood, R., & Brink, D. (1999). Behavioral and pharmacological therapies for late-life insomnia: A randomized controlled trial. *Journal of the American Medical Association, 281*, 991–999.

Morin, C. M., Kowatch, R. A., Barry, T., & Walton, E. (1993). Cognitive-behavior therapy for late-life insomnia. *Journal of Consulting and Clinical Psychology, 61*, 137–146.

Morrison, A. P., Renton, J., Williams, S., & Dunn, H. (1999). *An effectiveness study of cognitive therapy for psychosis: Preliminary findings.* Paper presented at the 3rd International Conference on Psychological Treatment of Schizophrenia, Oxford, UK.

Mosak, H. H. (2000). Adlerian psychotherapy. In R. J. Corsini & D. Wedding (Eds.), *Current psychotherapies* (6th ed., pp. 54–98). Itasca, IL: Peacock.

Mosak, H. H. (2005). Adlerian psychotherapy. In R. J. Corsini & D. Wedding (Eds.), *Current psychotherapies* (7th ed., pp. 52–95). Belmont, CA: Brooks/Cole.

Mosak, H. H., & Maniacci, M. (1999). *A primer of Adlerian psychology: The analytic-behavioral-cognitive psychology of Alfred Adler.* Philadelphia: Accelerated Development/Taylor & Francis.

Mounier, E. (1947). *Introduction aux existentialisms* [Introduction to existentialism]. Paris: Société des éditions Denoël.

Murdock, N. (2004). *Theories of counseling and psychotherapy: A case approach.* Upper Saddle River, NJ: Merrill/Prentice Hall.

Napier, A. Y., & Whitaker, C. A. (1972). *The family crucible.* New York: Harper & Row.

Nasr, S. H. (2002). *The heart of Islam.* New York: HarperCollins.

Neal-Barnett, A. M., & Smith, J. M., Jr. (1996). African American children and behavior therapy: Considering the Afrocentric approach. *Cognitive and Behavioral Practice, 3,* 351–369.

Negy, C. (2000). Limitations of the multicultural approach to psychotherapy with diverse clients. In I. B. Cuellar & F. A. Paniagua (Eds.), *Handbook of multicultural mental health: Assessment and treatment of diverse populations* (pp. 439–453). San Diego: Academic Press.

Neimeyer, G., & Neimeyer, R. A. (1994, January 11). Constructivist methods of marital and family therapy: A practical precis. *Journal of Mental Health Counseling,* 85–104.

Neisser, U. (1967). *Cognitive psychology.* New York: Appleton-Century-Crofts.

Nelson, M. L. (1993). *A feminist perspective on individuation: Implications for therapy boundary management.* Presented at the annual meeting of the American Psychological Association, Toronto, Ontario, Canada.

Newman, C. F., & Haaga, D. A. F. (1995). Cognitive skills training. In W. O'Donohue & L. Krasner (Eds.), *Handbook of psychological skills training: Clinical techniques and applications* (pp. 119–143). Boston: Allyn & Bacon.

Nezu, A. M., Nezu, C. M., D'Zurilla, T. J., & Rothenberg, J. L. (1996). Problem-solving therapy. In Kantor, J. S. (Ed.), *Clinical depression during addiction recovery: Processes, diagnosis, and treatment* (pp. 187–219). New York: Marcel Dekker.

Nezu, C. M., Nezu, A. M., & Houts, P. S. (1993). Multiple applications of problem-solving principles in clinical practice. In K. T. Kuehlwein & H. Rosen (Eds.), *Cognitive therapies in action: Evolving innovative practice* (pp. 353–378). San Francisco: Jossey-Bass.

Nichols, M. P. (1987). *The self in the system.* New York: Brunner/Mazel.

Nicholson, N. L., & Blanchard, E. B. (1993). A controlled evaluation of behavioral treatment of chronic headache in the elderly. *Behavior Therapy, 24,* 395–408.

Nielsen, S. L. (2001). Accommodating religion and integrating religious material during rational emotive behavior therapy. *Cognitive and Behavior Practice, 8,* 34–39.

Noda, S. J. (2000). The concept of holism in Individual Psychology and Buddhism. *Journal of Individual Psychology, 56,* 285–295.

Noddings, N. (1984). *Caring: A feminine approach to ethics and moral education.* Berkeley: University of California Press.

Norcross, J. C. (2001). Purposes, processes, and products of the task force on empirically supported therapy relationships. *Psychotherapy: Theory, Research, and Practice, 38,* 345–356.

Norcross, J. C. (2005). A primer on psychotherapy integration. In J. C. Norcross & M. R. Goldfried (Eds.), *Handbook of psychotherapy integration* (2nd ed.). New York: Oxford University Press.

Norcross, J. C., & Goldfried, M. R. (Eds.). (2005). *Handbook of psychotherapy integration* (2nd ed.). New York: Oxford University Press.

Norcross, J. C., Hedges, M., & Prochaska, J. O. (2002). The face of 2010: A Delphi poll on the future of psychotherapy. *Professional Psychology: Research and Practice, 33,* 316–322.

Norcross, J. C., Karpiak, C. P., & Lister, K. M. (2005). What's an integrationist? A study of self-identified integrative and (occasionally) eclectic psychologists. *Journal of Clinical Psychology, 61,* 1587–1594.

Novaco, R. W. (1975). *Anger control: The development and evaluation of an experimental treatment.* Lexington, MA: Lexington Books.

Novaco, R. [W.] (1977a). A stress-inoculation approach to anger management in the training of law enforcement officers. *American Journal of Community Psychology, 5,* 327–346.

Novaco, R. [W.] (1977b). Stress inoculation: A cognitive therapy for anger and its application to a case of depression. *Journal of Consulting and Clinical Psychology, 45,* 600–608.

Nunes, D. L., Murphy, R. J., & Ruprecht, M. L. (1977). Reducing self-injurious behavior of severely retarded individuals through withdrawal-of-reinforcement procedures. *Behavior Modification, 1,* 499–516.

O'Callaghan, M. E., & Couvadelli, B. (1998). Use of self-instructional strategies with three neurologically impaired adults. *Cognitive Therapy and Research, 22,* 91–107.

O'Connor, R. D. (1969). Modification of social withdrawal through symbolic modeling. *Journal of Applied Behavior Analysis, 2,* 15–22.

Office of Inspector General. (1996, May). *Mental health services in nursing facilities* (Publication OEI-02-91-00860). Washington, DC: Department of Health and Human Services.

Ogden, T. (1986). *The matrix of the mind.* Northvale, NJ: Jason Aronson.

Okonji, J. (1995). Counseling style preference and perception of counselors by African American male students. *Dissertation Abstracts, B 55/09, 3811.*

Okonji, J., Ososkie, J., & Pulos, S. (1996). Preferred style and ethnicity of counselors by African American males. *Journal of Black Psychology, 22,* 329–339.

Okun, B. (1996). *Understanding diverse families.* New York: Guilford.

Olafson, F. A. (1967). Merleau-Ponty, Maurice (1908–1961). In P. Edwards (Ed.), *The encyclopedia of philosophy* (Vol. 5, pp. 279–282). New York: Macmillan/Free Press.

O'Leary, K. D., & Turkewitz, H. (1978). Marital therapy from a behavioral perspective. In T. J. Paolino & B. S. McCrady (Eds.), *Marriage and marital therapy: Psychoanalytic, behavioral and systems theory perspectives* (pp. 240–297). New York: Brunner/Mazel.

Ollendick, T. H., Hagopian, L. P., & King, N. J. (1997). Specific phobias in children. In G. C. L. Davey (Ed.), *Phobia: A handbook of theory, research, and treatment* (pp. 201–224). New York: Wiley.

O'Neill, M. (2004). Researching 'suicidal thoughts' and archiving young people's insider knowledges. *International Journal of Narrative Therapy and Community Work, 3,* 41–42.

Organista, K. C., & Muñoz, R. F. (1996). Cognitive behavioral therapy with Latinos. *Cognitive and Behavioral Practice, 3,* 255–270.

Ornish, D. (1998). *Love & survival: The scientific basis for the healing power of intimacy.* New York: HarperCollins.

Otto, M. W., & Gould, R. A. (1995). Maximizing treatment-outcome for panic disorder: Cognitive-behavioral strategies. In M. H. Pollack, M. W. Otto, & J. F. Rosenbaum (Eds.), *Challenges in psychiatric treatment: Pharmacological and psychosocial strategies* (pp. 113–140). New York: Guilford.

Otto, M. W., Pava, J. A., & Sprich-Buckminster, S. (1995). Treatment of major depression: Applications and efficacy of cognitive-behavior therapy. In M. H. Pollack, M. W. Otto, & J. F. Rosenbaum (Eds.), *Challenges in psychiatric treatment: Pharmacological and psychosocial strategies* (pp. 31–52). New York: Guilford.

Pace, T. M., & Dixon, D. N. (1993). Changes in depressive self-schemata and depressive symptoms following cognitive therapy. *Journal of Counseling Psychology, 40,* 288–294.

Pachuta, D. M. (1989). Chinese medicine: The law of five elements. In A. A. Sheikh & K. S. Sheikh (Eds.), *Eastern and Western approaches to healing* (pp. 64–90). New York: Wiley.

Pack-Brown, S. P., & Williams, C. B. (2003). Ethics in a multicultural context. Thousand Oaks, CA: Sage.

Paniagua, F. A. (2005). *Assessing and treating culturally diverse clients: A practical guide* (3rd ed.). Thousand Oaks, CA: Sage.

Parham, T. A. (2002). Counseling African Americans: The current state of affairs. In T. A. Parham (Ed.), *Counseling persons of African descent: Raising the bar of practitioner competence* (pp. 1–9). Thousand Oaks, CA: Sage.

Parham, T. A., White, J. L., & Ajamu, A. (2000). *The psychology of Blacks: An African-centered perspective* (3rd ed.). Upper Saddle River, NJ: Prentice

Parker, I. (1991). *Discourse dynamics.* London: Routledge.

Patterson, C. H. (1980). *Theories of counseling and psychotherapy* (3rd ed.). New York: Harper & Row.

Patterson, C. H. (1996). Multicultural counseling: From diversity to universality. *Journal of Counseling and Development, 74,* 227–231.

Patterson, G. R. (1975). *Families: Applications of social learning to family life.* Champaign, IL: Research Press.

Patterson, G. R., & Gullion, M. E. (1976). *Living with children: New methods for parents and teachers.* Champaign, IL: Research Press.

Paul, G. L. (1966). *Insight vs. desensitization in psychotherapy.* Stanford, CA: Stanford University Press.

Paul, G. L., & Shannon, D. T. (1966). Treatment of anxiety through systematic desensitization in therapy groups. *Journal of Abnormal Psychology, 71,* 124–135.

Pavlov, I. P. (1927). *Conditioned reflexes.* New York: Liveright.

Payne, M. (2006). *Narrative therapy: An introduction for counsellors* (2nd ed.). London: Sage.

Pedalino, E., & Gamboa, V. U. (1974). Behavior modification and absenteeism: Intervention in one industrial setting. *Journal of Applied Psychology, 59,* 694–698.

Pedersen, P. B. (1991a). Multiculturalism as a generic approach to counseling. *Journal of Counseling & Development, 70,* 6–12.

Pedersen, P. B. (Ed.). (1991b). Multiculturalism as a fourth force in counseling [Special issue]. *Journal of Counseling and Development, 70.*

Pedersen, P. B., Lonner, W., & Draguns, J. (1976). (Eds.). *Counseling across cultures.* Honolulu: University Press of Hawaii.

Peeks, A. L. (1999). Conducting a social skills group with Latina adolescents. *Journal of Child and Adolescent Group Therapy, 9,* 139–153.

Perkins-Dock, R. E. (2005). The application of Adlerian family therapy with African American families. *Journal of Individual Psychology, 61,* 233–249.

Perls, F. S. (1947). *Ego, hunger and aggression: A revision of psychoanalysis.* New York: Random House.

Perls, F. S. (1969). *Gestalt therapy verbatim.* Lafayette, CA: Real People Press.

Perls, F. S., Hefferline, R. F., & Goodman, P. (1951). *Gestalt therapy: Excitement and growth in the human personality.* New York: Julian Press.

Peterson, A., Chang, C., & Collins, P. (1997). The effects of reality therapy on locus of control among students in Asian universities. *Journal of Reality Therapy, 16*(2), 80–87.

Peterson, A., Chang, C., & Collins, P. (1998). Taiwanese university students meet their basic needs through studying choice theory/reality therapy. *Journal of Reality Therapy, 17*(2), 27–29.

Peterson, L., & Ridley-Johnson, R. (1980). Pediatric hospital response to survey on prehospital preparation for children. *Journal of Pediatric Psychology, 5,* 1–7.

Piaget, J. (1954). *Intelligence and affectivity: Their relationship during child development.* Palo Alto, CA: Annual Review.

Piaget, J. (1965). *The moral judgment of the child.* New York: Free Press.

Picchioni, A., & Bonk, E. (1983). *A comprehensive history of guidance in the United States.* Austin: Texas Association of Counseling and Guidance.

Pilalis, J. (1987). Letting gender secrets out of the bag. *Australia and New Zealand Journal of Family Therapy, 8,* 205–211.

Pilalis, J., & Anderton, J. (1984). Feminism and family therapy. *Journal of Family Therapy, 8,* 99–114.

Pina, A. A., Silverman, W. K., Fuentes, R. M., Kurtines, W. M., & Weems, C. F. (2003). Exposure-based cognitive-behavioral treatment for phobic and anxiety disorders: Treatment effects and maintenance for Hispanic/Latino relative to European-American youths. *Journal of the American Academy of Child & Adolescent Psychiatry, 42,* 1179–1187.

Pinderhughes, E. (1989). *Understanding race, ethnicity and power: The key to efficacy in clinical practice.* New York: Free Press.

Pine, F. (1983). *Developmental theory and clinical process.* New Haven, CT: Yale University Press.

Pinkerton, S. S., Hughes, H., & Wenrich, W. W. (1982). *Behavioral medicine: Clinical applications.* New York: Wiley.

Pinsof, W. (1994). An overview of integrative problem-centered therapy: A synthesis of family and individual psychotherapies. *Journal of Family Therapy, 16,* 103–120.

Pinsof, W., & Wynne, L. (1995). The efficacy of marital and family therapy: An empirical overview, conclusions, and recommendations. *Journal of Marital and Family Therapy, 21,* 585–613.

Pinsof, W., & Wynne, L. (2000). Toward progess research: Closing the gap between family therapy practice and research. *Journal of Marital and Family Therapy, 26,* 1–8.

Pinsof, W., Wynne, L., & Hambright, A. (1996). The outcomes of couples and family therapy: Findings, conclusions, and recommendations. *Psychotherapy, 33,* 321–331.

Pipes, R. B., Holstein, J. E., & Aguirre, M. G. (2005). Examining the personal-professional distinction: Ethics codes and the difficulty of drawing a boundary. *American Psychologist, 60,* 325–334.

Planells-Bloom, D. (1992). Latino cultures: Framework for understanding the Latina adolescent and assertive behavior. In I. Fodor (Ed.), *Adolescent assertiveness and social skills training: A clinical handbook.* New York: Springer.

Poche, C., Brouwer, R., & Swearingen, M. (1981). Teaching self-protection to young children. *Journal of Applied Behavior Analysis, 14,* 169–176.

Poche, C., Yoder, P., & Miltenberger, R. (1988). Teaching self-protection to children using television techniques. *Journal of Applied Behavior Analysis, 21,* 253–261.

Polster, E., & Polster, M. (1973). *Gestalt therapy integrated: Contours of theory and practice.* New York: Brunner/Mazel.

Pope, K. S., & Vasquez, M. J. T. (1998). *Ethics in psychotherapy and counseling: A practical guide* (2nd ed.). San Francisco: Jossey-Bass.

Poser, E. G. (1970). Toward a theory of behavioral prophylaxis. *Journal of Behavior Therapy and Experimental Psychiatry, 1,* 39–43.

Poser, E. [G.], & King, M. (1975). Strategies for the prevention of maladaptive fear responses. *Canadian Journal of Behavioural Science, 7,* 279–294.

Powell, J. (2004). Five stages to responsible human behavior. *International Journal of Reality Therapy, 23*(2), 27–30.

Powers, R. L., & Griffith, J. (1987). *Understanding lifestyle: The psycho-clarity process.* Chicago: AIAS.

Powers, W. (1973). *Behavior: The control of perception.* New York: Aldine Press.

Preciado, J. (1999). Behavior therapy's commitment to cultural diversity: The case of Hispanics. *the Behavior Therapist, 22,* pp. 199–200, 207.

Prenzlau, S. (2006) Using reality therapy to reduce PTSD-related symptoms. *International Journal of Reality Therapy, 24*(2), 23–29.

Prochaska, J. O., & Norcross, J. C. (2007). *Systems of psychotherapy: A transtheoretical analysis* (7th ed.). Pacific Grove, CA: Brooks/Cole.

Propst, L. R., Ostrom, R., Watkins, P., Dean, T., & Mashburn, D. (1992). Comparative efficacy of religious and nonreligious cognitive-behavioral therapy for the treatment of clinical depression in religious individuals. *Journal of Consulting and Clinical Psychology, 60,* 94–103.

Prouty, G. (1999). Pre-therapy and pre-symbolic experiencing: Evolutions in person-centered/experiential approaches. In L. S. Greenberg, J. C. Watson, & G. Lietaer (Eds.), *Handbook of experiential psychotherapy* (pp. 388–409). New York: Guilford.

Pryor, D. B., & Tollerud, T. R. (1999). Applications of Adlerian principles in school settings. *Professional School Counseling, 2,* 299–304.

Raabe, P. B. (2001). *Philosophical counseling.* Westport, CT: Praeger.

Rachman, S. (1959). The treatment of anxiety and phobic reactions by systematic desensitization psychotherapy. *Journal of Abnormal and Social Psychology, 58,* 259–263.

Rachman, S. (1967). Systematic desensitization. *Psychological Bulletin, 67,* 93–103.

Rachman, S., & Eysenck, H. J. (1966). Reply to a "critique and reformulation" of behavior therapy. *Psychological Bulletin, 65,* 165–169.

Rachman, S. J., & Wilson, G. T. (1980). *The effects of psychological therapy* (2nd enlarged ed.). Oxford: Pergamon.

Radley, M., Redston, C., Bates, F., & Pontefract, M. (1997). Effectiveness of group anxiety management with elderly clients of a community psychogeriatric team. *International Journal of Geriatric Psychiatry, 12,* 79–84.

Raimy, V. (1950). *Training in clinical psychology.* New York: Prentice-Hall.

Rao, N., Moely, B. E., & Lockman, J. J. (1987). Increasing social participation in preschool social isolates. *Journal of Clinical Child Psychology, 16,* 178–183.

Raue, P. J., Castonguay, L. G., & Goldfried, M. R. (1993). The working alliance: A comparison of two therapies. *Psychotherapy Research, 3,* 197–207.

Raue, P. J., & Goldfried, M. R. (1994). The therapeutic alliance in cognitive-behavior therapy. In A. O. Horvath & L. S. Greenberg (Eds.), *The working alliance: Theory, research, and practice* (pp. 131–152). New York: Wiley.

Rawlings, E. I., & Carter, D. K. (1977). *Psychotherapy for women.* Springfield, IL: Thomas.

Red Horse, J. (1980). Family structure and value orientation in American Indians. *Social Casework, 61,* 490–493.

Red Horse, J. (1982). Clinical strategies for American Indian families in crisis. *Urban and Social Change Review, 15*(2), 17–20.

Reddy, I., & Hanna, F. J. (1995). The life-style of the Hindu woman: Conceptualizing female clients of Indian origin. *Journal of Individual Psychology, 51,* 216–230.

Redstone, A. (2004). Researching people's experience of narrative therapy: Acknowledging contribution of the 'client' to what works in counselling conversations. *International Journal of Narrative Therapy and Community Work, 2,* 63–67.

Reese, W. L. (1980). *Dictionary of philosophy and religion.* Atlantic Highlands, NJ: Humanities Press.

Reimer, C. S. (1999). *Counseling the Inupiat Eskimo.* Westport, CT: Greenwood Press.

Remer, P., & Rostosky, S. (2001). Practice talk: Fears of labeling ourselves feminist practitioners. *The Feminist Psychologist, 28*(4), pp. 30, 32.

Remer, P., & Rostosky, S. (2002). Practice talk: Challenges in implementing feminist egalitarian relationships. *The Feminist Psychologist, 29*(3), 25–26.

Remer, P., Rostosky, S., & Comer-Wright, M. L. (2001). Counseling women from a feminist perspective. In E. R. Welfel & R. W. Ingersoll (Eds.), *Mental health desk reference: A sourcebook for counselors and therapists* (pp. 341–350). New York: Wiley.

Remer, P., & University of Kentucky Counseling Psychology Date Rape Prevention Team (2004, April). *Preventing date rape: Research and treatment challenges.* Symposium presented at University of Kentucky, Lexington, KY.

Remer, P., Worell, J., & Remer, R. (2005, January). *Feminist psychological practice strategies for exploring the intersection of multicultural identities.* Workshop presented at the National Multicultural Conference and Summit, Hollywood, CA.

Renik, O. (2002). Defining the goals of a clinical psychoanalysis. *Psychoanalytic Quarterly, 71*, 117–123.

Rennie, D. L. (2002). Experiencing psychotherapy: Grounded theory studies. In D. J. Cain & J. Seeman (Eds.), *Humanistic psychotherapies: Handbook of research and practice* (pp. 117–144). Washington, DC: American Psychological Association.

Rice, L. N. (1974). The evocative function of the therapist. In D. A. Wexler & L. N. Rice (Eds.), *Innovations in client-centered therapy* (pp. 289–311). New York: Wiley.

Richard, J. (1995). Behavioral treatment of an atypical case of obsessive compulsive disorder. *the Behavior Therapist, 18*, 134–135.

Richardson, L., & St. Pierre, E. (2005). Writing: A method of inquiry. In N. Denzin & Y. Lincoln (Eds.), *The Sage handbook of qualitative research* (3rd ed., pp. 959–978). Thousand Oaks, CA: Sage.

Ricken, F. (1991). *Philosophy of the ancients* (E. Watkins, Trans.). Notre Dame, IN: University of Notre Dame Press.

Rieckert, J., & Moller, A. T. (2000). Rational-emotive behavior therapy in the treatment of adult victims of childhood sexual abuse. *Journal of Rational-Emotive & Cognitive-Behavior Therapy, 18*, 87–101.

Rietveld, C. M. (1983). The training of choice behaviours in Down's Syndrome and nonretarded preschool children. *Australia and New Zealand Journal of Developmental Disabilities, 9*, 75–83.

Rigazio-DiGilio, S. A. (1997). From microscopes to holographs: Client development within a constructivist paradigm. In T. Sexton & B. Griffin (Eds.), *Constructivist thinking in counseling practice, research, and training* (pp. 74–100). New York: Teachers College Press.

Rigazio-DiGilio, S. A. (2000). Reconstructing psychological distress and disorder from a relational perspective: A systemic coconstructive-developmental framework. In R. Neimeyer & J. Raskin (Eds.), *Constructions of disorder* (pp. 309–332). Washington, DC: American Psychological Association.

Rigazio-DiGilio, S. A. (2001). Postmodern theories of counseling. In D. C. Locke, J. E. Myers, & E. L. Herr (Eds.), *The handbook of counseling.* Thousands Oaks, CA: Sage.

Rigazio-DiGilio, S. A. (in press). Family counseling and therapy: Theoretical foundations and issues of practice. In A. Ivey, M. D'Andrea, M. Ivey, & L. Simek-Morgan (Eds.), *Theories of counseling and psychotherapy: A multicultural perspective* (6th ed.). Needham Heights, MA: Allyn & Bacon.

Rigazio-DiGilio, S. A., Gonçalves, O. F., & Ivey, A. E. (1996). From cultural to existential diversity: The impossibility of an integrative psychotherapy within a traditional framework. *Applied and Preventative Psychology: Current Scientific Perspectives, 5*, 235–248.

Rigazio-DiGilio, S. A., & Ivey, A. E. (1993). Systemic cognitive-developmental therapy: An integrative framework. *Family Journal: Counseling and Therapy for Couples and Families*, 208–219.

Rigazio-DiGilio, S. A., & Ivey, A. E. (1995). Individual and family issues in intercultural counselling and therapy: A culturally-centered perspective. *Canadian Journal of Counseling, 29*, 244–261.

Rigazio-DiGilio, S. A., Ivey, A. E., Kunkler-Peck, K. P., & Grady, L T. (2005). *Community genograms: Using individual, family and cultural narratives with clients.* New York: Teacher's College Press.

Rigazio-DiGilio, S., Ivey, A., & Locke, D. (1997). Continuing the post-modern dialogue: Enhancing and contextualizing multiple voices. *Journal of Mental Health Counseling, 19,* 233–255.

Rimm, D. C., deGroot, J. C., Boord, P., Heiman, J., & Dillow, P. V. (1971). Systematic desensitization of an anger response. *Behaviour Research and Therapy, 9,* 273–280.

Ritter, B. (1968a). Effect of contact desensitization on avoidance behavior, fear ratings, and self-evaluative statements. *Proceedings of the American Psychological Association, Annual Convention* (pp. 527–528). Washington, DC: American Psychological Association.

Ritter, B. (1968b). The group desensitization of children's snake phobias using vicarious and contact desensitization procedures. *Behaviour Research and Therapy, 6,* 1–6.

Rivett, M., & Street, E. (2003). *Family therapy in focus.* London: Sage.

Robb, H. B. (2001). Facilitating rational emotive behavior therapy by including religious beliefs. *Cognitive and Behavioral Practice, 8,* 29–34.

Robbins, B. S. (1939). Neurotic disturbances in work. *Psychiatry, 2,* 333–342.

Roberts, R. L., Harper, R., Caldwell, R., & Decora, M. (2003). Adlerian life-style analysis of Lakota women: Implications for counseling. *Journal of Individual Psychology, 59,* 15–29.

Roberts, R. L., Harper, R., Tuttle Eagle Bull, D., & Heideman-Provost, L. M. (1998). The Native American medicine wheel and individual psychology: Common themes. *Journal of Individual Psychology, 54,* 135–145.

Robinson, D., & Worell, J. (1991). *The Therapy with Women Scale (TWS).* Unpublished manuscript, University of Kentucky, Lexington, KY.

Rogers, C. R. (1939). *Clinical treatment of the problem child.* New York: Houghton Mifflin.

Rogers, C. R. (1942). *Counseling and psychotherapy: Newer concepts in practice.* Boston: Houghton Mifflin.

Rogers, C. R. (1951). *Client-centered psychotherapy.* Boston: Houghton Mifflin.

Rogers, C. R. (1957). The necessary and sufficient conditions of therapeutic personality change. *Journal of Consulting and Clinical Psychology, 21,* 95–103.

Rogers, C. R. (1959). A theory of therapy, personality and interpersonal relationships as developed in the client-centered framework. In S. Koch (Ed.), *Formulations of the person and the social context* (pp. 184–256). New York: McGraw-Hill.

Rogers, C. R. (1961). *On becoming a person.* Boston: Houghton Mifflin.

Rogers, C. R. (1967). The interpersonal relationship: The core of guidance. In C. R. Rogers & B. Stevens (Eds.), *Person to person: The problem of being human; a new trend in psychology* (pp. 89–103). Walnut Creek, CA: Real People Press.

Rogers, C. R. (1970). *Carl Rogers on encounter groups.* New York: Harper & Row.

Rogers, C. R. (1972). My personal growth. In A. Burton (Ed.), *Twelve therapists* (pp. 28–77). San Francisco: Jossey-Bass.

Rogers, C. R. (1977). *Carl Rogers on personal power.* New York: Delacorte.

Rogers, C. R. (1980). *A way of being.* Boston: Houghton Mifflin.

Rogers, C. R. (1986). A comment from Carl Rogers. *Person-Centered Review, 1,* 3–5.

Rogers, C. R., & Dymond, R. (1954). *Psychotherapy and personality change.* Chicago: University of Chicago Press.

Rogers, C. R., & Sanford, R. C. (1989). Client-centered psychotherapy. In H. I. Kaplan & B. J. Sadock (Eds.), *Comprehensive textbook of psychiatry* (Vol. 5, pp. 1482–1501). Baltimore: Williams & Wilkins.

Rohner, R. P. (2004). The parental acceptance-rejection syndrome: Universal correlates of perceived rejection. *American Psychologist, 59,* 830–840.

Rojahn, J., Hammer, D., & Kroeger, T. L. (1997). Stereotypy. In N. N. Singh (Ed.), *Prevention and treatment of severe behavior problems: Models and methods in developmental disabilities* (pp. 199–216). Pacific Grove, CA: Brooks/Cole.

Rojano, R. (2004). The practice of community family therapy. *Family Process, 43*(1), 59–78.

Roland, A. (1988). *In search of self in India and Japan: Toward a cross-cultural psychology.* Princeton, NJ: Princeton University Press.

Rolland, J. S. (1994). In sickness and in health: The impact of illness on couples' relationships. *Journal of Marital and Family Therapy, 20,* 327–347.

Rosenberg, L. (2000). *Living in the light of death: On the art of being truly alive.* Boston: Shambhala.

Rossello, J., & Bernal, G. (1999). The efficacy of cognitive-behavioral and interpersonal treatments for depression in Puerto Rican adolescents. *Journal of Consulting and Clinical Psychology, 67,* 734–745.

Rothbaum, B. O., Meadows, E. A., Resick, P., & Foy, D. W. (2000). Cognitive-behavioral therapy. In E. B. Foa, T. M. Keane, & M. J. Friedman (Eds.), *Effective treatments for PTSD* (pp. 60–83). New York: Guilford.

Rusch, F. R., Hughes, C., & Wilson, P. G. (1995). Utilizing cognitive strategies in the acquisition of employment skills. In W. O'Donohue & L. Krasner (Eds.), *Handbook of psychological skills training: Clinical techniques and applications* (pp. 363–382). Boston: Allyn & Bacon.

Rusch, F. R., Martin, J. E., Lagomarcino, T. R., & White, D. M. (1987). Teaching task sequencing via verbal mediation. *Education and Training in Mental Retardation, 22,* 229–235.

Rusch, F. R., Morgan, T. K., Martin, J. E., Riva, M., & Agran, M. (1985). Competitive employment: Teaching mentally retarded employees self-instructional strategies. *Applied Research in Mental Retardation, 6,* 389–407.

Russell, S., & Carey, M. (2003). Feminism, therapy and narrative ideas: Exploring some not so commonly asked questions. *International Journal of Narrative Therapy and Community Work,* (2), 67–91.

Rychlak, J. F. (1981). *Introduction to personality and psychotherapy: A theory-construction approach.* Boston: Houghton Mifflin.

Sachse, R., & Elliot, R. (2001). Process-outcome research on humanistic therapy variables. In D. J. Cain & J. Seeman (Eds.), *Humanistic psychotherapies: Handbook of research and practice* (pp. 83–116). Washington, DC: American Psychological Association.

Safren, S., Otto, M. & Worth, J. (1999). Life-steps: applying cognitive-behavioral therapy to patient adherence to HIV medication treatment. *Cognitive and Behavioral Practice, 6,* 332–341.

Safren, S. A. (2001). Prevalence of childhood ADHD among patients with generalized anxiety disorder and a comparison condition, social phobia. *Depression and Anxiety, 13,* 190–191.

Safren, S. A., Hollander, G., Hart, T. A., & Heimberg, R. G. (2001). Cognitive-behavioral therapy with lesbian, gay, and bisexual youth. *Cognitive and Behavioral Practice, 8,* 215–223.

Sahakian, W. S., & Sahakian, M. L. (1966). *Ideas of the great philosophers.* New York: Barnes & Noble.

Saigh, P. A. (1987). *In vivo* flooding of an adolescent's posttraumatic stress disorder. *Journal of Clinical Child Psychology, 16,* 147–150.

Salkovskis, P. M. (Ed.). (1996). *Frontiers of cognitive therapy.* New York: Guilford.

Samoilov, A., & Goldfried, M. R. (2000). Role of emotion in cognitive-behavior therapy. *Clinical Psychology: Science and Practice, 7,* 373–385.

Sander, F. M. (1979). *The self in the system.* New York: Brunner/Mazel.

Sanders, P. (Ed.). (2004). *The tribes of the person-centered nation.* Ross-on-Wye, UK: PCCS Books.

Sanderson, W. C. (2003). Why empirically supported psychological treatments are important. *Behavior Modification, 27,* 290–299.

Santiago-Rivera, A. L., Arredondo, P., & Gallardo-Cooper, M. (2002). *Counseling Latinos and la familia.* Thousand Oaks, CA: Sage.

Sapp, M. (1996). Irrational beliefs that can lead to academic failure for African American middle school students who are academically at-risk. *Journal of Rational-Emotive & Cognitive-Behavior Therapy, 14,* 123–134.

Sapp, M. (1997). *Counseling and psychotherapy: Theories, associated research, and issues.* Lanham, MD: University Press of America.

Sapp, M. (2006). The strength-based model for counseling at-risk youths. *The Counseling Psychologist, 34,* 108–117.

Sapp, M., McNeely, R. L., & Torres, J. B. (1998). Rational emotive behavior therapy in the process of dying: Focus on aged African Americans and Latinos. *Journal of Human Behavior in the Social Environment, 1,* 305–321.

Sartre, J.-P. (1953). *Being and nothingness* (H. E. Barnes, Trans.). New York: Washington Square Books.

Sartre, J.-P. (1970). *L'existentialisme est un humanisme* [Existentialism is humanism]. Paris: Les éditions Nagel.

Sartre, J.-P. (1983). *Cahiers pour une morale* [Guidelines for a morality]. Paris: Gallimard.

Sartre, J.-P. (1992). *Notebooks for an ethics* (D. Pellauer, Trans.). Chicago: University of Chicago Press.

Satir, V. (1964) *Conjoint family therapy.* Palo Alto, CA: Science & Behavior Books.

Saunders, D. G. (1976). A case of motion sickness treated by systematic desensitization and *in vivo* relaxation. *Journal of Behavior Therapy and Experimental Psychiatry, 7,* 381–382.

Schaap, C., Bennun, I., Schindler, L., & Hoogduin, K. (1993). *The therapeutic relationship in behavioural psychotherapy.* New York: Wiley.

Scheler, M. (1954). *The nature of sympathy* (P. Heath, Trans.). New Haven, CT: Yale University Press.

Schneider, K. J., & May, R. (1995). *The psychology of existence: An integrative clinical perspective.* New York: McGraw-Hill.

Schoenwald, S., Sheidow, A., & Letourneau, E. (2003). Transportability of Multisystemic Therapy: Evidence for multilevel influences. *Mental Health Services Research, 5,* 223–239.

Scholing, A., & Emmelkamp, P. M. G. (1993a). Cognitive and behavioural treatments of fear of blushing, sweating or trembling. *Behaviour Research and Therapy, 31,* 155–170.

Scholing, A., & Emmelkamp, P. M. G. (1993b). Exposure with and without cognitive therapy for generalized social phobia: Effects of individual and group treatment. *Behaviour Research and Therapy, 31,* 667–681.

Schraff, D. E., & Schraff, J. S. (1987). *Object relations family therapy.* Northvale, NJ: Aronson.

Schuster, S. C. (1991). Philosophical counseling. *Journal of Applied Philosophy, 8,* 219–223.

Schuster, S. C. (1999). *Philosophy practice: An alternative to counseling and psychotherapy.* Westport, CT: Praeger.

Schwartzman, J. (1983). Family ethnography: A tool for clinicians. In C. J. Falicov (Ed.), *Cultural perspectives in family therapy* (pp. 137–149). Rockville, MD: Aspen Systems.

Scott, C. S., Scott, J. L., Tacchi, M. J., & Jones, R. H. (1994). Abbreviated cognitive therapy for depression: A pilot study in primary care. *Behavioural and Cognitive Psychotherapy, 22,* 57–64.

Scrivner, R., & Eldridge, N. S. (1995). Lesbian and gay family psychology. In R. H. Mikesell, D.-D. Lusterman, & S. H. McDaniel (Eds.), *Integrative family therapy: Handbook of family psychology and systems theory* (pp. 5–26). Washington, DC: American Psychological Association.

Seaburn, D., Landau-Stanton, J., & Horwitz, S. (1995). Core techniques in family therapy. In R. H. Mikesell, D.-D. Lusterman, & S. H. McDaniel (Eds.), *Integrative family therapy: Handbook of family psychology and systems theory.* Washington, DC: American Psychological Association.

Seeman, J. (1965). Perspectives in client-centered therapy. In B. B. Wolman (Ed.), *Handbook of clinical psychology* (pp. 1215–1229). New York: McGraw-Hill.

Seeman, J. (1988). Self-actualization: A reformulation. *Person-Centered Review, 3*(2), 304–315.

Seeman, J. (2002). Looking back, looking ahead: A synthesis. In D. J. Cain & J. Seeman (Eds.), *Humanistic psychotherapies: Handbook of research and practice* (pp. 617–636). Washington, DC: American Psychological Association.

Seligman, L. (2001). *Systems, strategies, and skills of counseling and psychotherapy.* Upper Saddle River, NJ: Prentice-Hall.

Sells, S. P., Smith, T. E., & Moon, S. (1996). An ethnographic study of client and therapist perceptions of therapy effectiveness in a university-based training clinic. *Journal of Marital and Family Therapy, 22,* 321–342.

Seltzer, W. J., & Seltzer, M. R. (1983). Material, myth and magic: A cultural approach to family therapy. *Family Process, 22,* 3–14.

Selvini-Palazzoli, M., Boscolo, L., Cecchin, G. F., & Prata, G. (1978). *Paradox and counterparadox: A new model in the therapy of the family in schizophrenic transaction.* New York: Aronson.

Serketich, W., & Dumas, J. E. (1996). The effectiveness of behavioural parent training to modify antisocial behaviour in children: A meta-analysis. *Behavior Therapy, 27,* 171–186.

Servan-Schreiber, J.-L. (1987). *The return of courage* (F. Frenaye, Trans.). New York: Addison-Wesley.

Sexton, T. L., & Alexander, J. F. (1999). Family-based empirically supported intervention programs. *Family Digest, 12*(2), 1–14.

Shadish, W. R., Ragsdale, K., Glaser, R. R., & Montgomery, L. M. (1995). The efficacy and effectiveness of marital and family therapy: A perspective from meta-analysis. *Journal of Marital and Family Therapy, 21*, 345–360.

Shaffer, H., Beck, J., & Boothroyd, P. (1983). The primary prevention of smoking onset: An inoculation approach. *Journal of Psychoactive Drugs, 15*, 177–184.

Shannon, H. D., & Allen, T. W. (1998). The effectiveness of a REBT training program in increasing the performance of high school students' mathematics. *Journal of Rational-Emotive & Cognitive-Behavior Therapy, 16*, 197–209.

Shapiro, D. A., Rees, A., Barkham, M., Hardy, G., Reynolds, S., & Startup, M. (1995). Effects of treatment duration and severity of depression on the maintenance of gains after cognitive-behavioral and psychodynamic-interpersonal psychotherapy. *Journal of Consulting and Clinical Psychology, 63*, 378–387.

Shea, M. T. (Panelist). (1990, November). In K. S. Dobson (Moderator), *Cognitive therapy and interpersonal therapy: What do the collaborative study results tell us and where do we go from here?* Panel discussion presented at the annual meeting of the Association for Advancement of Behavior Therapy, San Francisco.

Shepard, M. (1975). *Fritz.* Sagaponack, NY: Second Chance Press.

Sherman, R., & Dinkmeyer, D. (1987). *Systems of family therapy: An Adlerian integration.* New York: Brunner/Mazel.

Shipley, R. H., Butt, J. H., Horwitz, B., & Farbry, J. E. (1978). Preparation for a stressful medical procedure: Effect of stimulus pre-exposure and coping style. *Journal of Consulting and Clinical Psychology, 46*, 499–507.

Shipley, R. H., Butt, J. H., & Horwitz, E. A. (1979). Preparation to re-experience a stressful medical examination: Effect of repetitious videotape exposure and coping style. *Journal of Consulting and Clinical Psychology, 47*, 485–492.

Shorkey, C., & Himle, D. P. (1974). Systematic desensitization treatment of a recurring nightmare and related insomnia. *Journal of Behavior Therapy and Experimental Psychiatry, 5*, 97–98.

Shulman, B. H. (1973). *Contributions to individual psychology.* Chicago: Alfred Adler Institute.

Shulman, B. H., & Mosak, H. H. (1988). *Manual for life-style assessment.* Muncie, IN: Accelerated Development.

Skinner, B. F. (1953). *Science and human behavior.* New York: Macmillan.

Skinner, B. F. (1954). A new method for the experimental analysis of the behavior of psychotic patients. *Journal of Nervous and Mental Disease, 120*, 403–406.

Skinner, B. F., Solomon, H. C., & Lindsley, O. R. (1953, November 30). *Studies in behavior therapy: Status Report I.* Waltham, MA: Metropolitan State Hospital.

Slavik, S. (2006). Models, theories, and research in individual psychology. In S. Slavik & J. Carlson (Eds.), *Readings in the theory of Individual Psychology* (pp. 3–14). New York: Taylor & Francis.

Slavik, S., & Carlson, J. (2006). *Readings in the theory of individual psychology.* New York: Routledge.

Sliep, Y. (2005). A narrative theatre approach to working with communities affected by trauma, conflict, and war. *International Journal of Narrative Therapy and Community Work, 2*, 47–52.

Slipp, S. (1984). *Object relations: A dynamic bridge between individual and family therapy.* Northvale, NJ: Aronson.

Sluzki, C. E. (1979). Migration and family conflict. *Family Process, 18,* 379–390.

Smart, N. (1999). *World philosophers.* New York: Routledge.

Smith, A. J., & Douglas, M. A. (1990). Empowerment as an ethical imperative. In H. Lerman & N. Porter (Eds.), *Feminist ethics in psychotherapy* (pp. 43–50). New York: Springer.

Smith, C. (1997). Introduction: Comparing traditional therapies with narrative approaches. In C. Smith & D. Nyland (Eds.), *Narrative therapies with children and adolescents* (pp. 1–52). New York: Guilford.

Smith, D. (1982). Trends in counseling and psychotherapy. *American Psychologist, 37,* 802–809.

Smith, D. E., Marcus, M. D., & Eldredge, K. L. (1994). Binge eating syndromes: A review of assessment and treatment with an emphasis on clinical application. *Behavior Therapy, 25,* 635–658.

Smith, E. W. (1970). *The growing edge of Gestalt therapy.* Secaucus, NJ: The Citadel Press.

Smith, J. C. (2001). Seok Chan Bang's study of ABC relaxation training as a treatment for depression for the Korean elderly. In J. C. Smith (Ed.), *Advances in ABC relaxation: Applications and inventories* (pp. 205–208). New York: Springer.

Smith, M. L., Glass, G. V., & Miller, T. I. (1980). *The benefits of psychotherapy.* Baltimore: John Hopkins University Press.

Sowers, J., Rusch, F. R., Connis, R. T., & Cummings, L. E. (1980). Teaching mentally retarded adults to time manage in a vocational setting. *Journal of Applied Behavior Analysis, 13,* 119–128.

Speck, R. V., & Attneave, C. L. (1973). *Family networks.* New York: Pantheon.

Speedy, J. (2004). Living a more peopled life: Definitional ceremony as inquiry into psychotherapy 'outcomes.' *International Journal of Narrative Therapy and Community Work,* (3), 43–53.

Sperry, L., & Carlson, J. (Eds.). (1996). *Psychopathology and psychotherapy: From DSM-IV diagnoses to treatment* (2nd ed.). Washington, DC: Accelerated Development.

Spiegler, M. D. (1971, May). *The use of a school model and contingency management in a day treatment program for psychiatric outpatients.* Paper presented at the annual meeting of the Rocky Mountain Psychological Association, Denver.

Spiegler, M. D. (1973). Classroom approach teaches patients independence skills. *Hospital and Community Psychiatry, 24,* 216–221.

Spiegler, M. D. (1980, November). Behavioral primary prevention: Introduction and overview. In M. D. Spiegler (Chair), *Behavioral primary prevention: A challenge for the 1980s.* Symposium presented at the annual meeting of the Association for Advancement of Behavior Therapy, New York.

Spiegler, M. D. (1983). *Contemporary behavioral therapy.* Palo Alto, CA: Mayfield.

Spiegler, M. D., & Agigian, H. (1977). *The Community Training Center: An educational-behavioral-social systems model for rehabilitating psychiatric patients.* New York: Brunner/Mazel.

Spiegler, M. D., Cooley, E. J., Marshall, G. J., Prince, H. T., II, Puckett, S. P., & Skenazy, J. A. (1976). A self-control versus a counterconditioning paradigm for systematic desensitization: An experimental comparison. *Journal of Counseling Psychology, 23,* 83–86.

Spiegler, M. D., & Guevremont, D. C. (1993). *Contemporary behavior therapy* (2nd ed.). Pacific Grove, CA: Brooks/Cole.

Spiegler, M. D., & Guevremont, D. C. (1994, November). *The relationship between behavior therapy practice and research*. Paper presented at the annual meeting of the Association for Advancement of Behavior Therapy, San Diego.

Spiegler, M. D., & Guevremont, D. C. (1998). *Contemporary behavior therapy* (3rd ed.). Pacific Grove, CA: Brooks/Cole.

Spiegler, M. D., & Guevremont, D. C. (2003). *Contemporary behavior therapy* (4th ed.). Belmont, CA: Wadsworth.

Spiegler, M. D., Liebert, R. M., McMains, M. J., & Fernandez, L. E. (1969). Experimental development of a modeling treatment to extinguish persistent avoidance behavior (pp. 45–51). In R. D. Rubin & C. M. Franks (Eds.), *Advances in behavior therapy, 1968*. New York: Academic Press.

Stagoll, B. (2000). Interactions not factions [Contribution to dialogues of diversity in therapy: A virtual symposium]. *Australia and New Zealand Journal of Family Therapy, 21*, 124–126.

Staniforth, M. (1964). *Marcus Aurelius: Meditations* (M. Staniforth, Trans.). New York: Penguin.

Stanton, D. (1981). Strategic approaches to family therapy. In A. Gurman & D. Kniskern, (Eds.), *Handbook of family therapy* (pp. 361–402). New York: Brunner/Mazel.

Stanton, M. D., & Shadish, W. R. (1997). Outcome, attrition, and family-couples treatment for drug abuse: A meta-analysis and review of the controlled, comparative studies. *Psychological Bulletin, 122*, 170–190.

Star, T. Z. (1986). Group social skills training: A comparison of two coaching programs. *Techniques, 2*, 24–38.

Stein, H. F. (1985). Therapist and family values in a cultural context. *Counseling and Values 30*(1), 35–46.

Stein, H. T., & Edwards, M. E. (1998). Alfred Adler: Classical theory and practice. In P. Marcus & A. Rosenberg (Eds.), *Psychoanalytic versions of the human condition: Philosophies of life and their impact on practice* (pp. 64–93). New York: New York University Press.

Steinmark, S. W., & Borkovec, T. D. (1974). Active and placebo treatment effects on moderate insomnia under counterdemand and positive demand instructions. *Journal of Abnormal Psychology, 83*, 157–163.

Striker, G., & Gold, J. R. (Eds.). (1993). *Comprehensive handbook of psychotherapy integration*. New York: Plenum.

Strümpfel, U. (2004). Research on Gestalt therapy. *International Gestalt Journal, 27*, 9–54.

Sturdivant, S. (1980). *Therapy with women: A feminist philosophy of treatment*. New York: Springer.

Sue, D. W., Ivey, A. E., & Pedersen, P. (1996). *A theory of multicultural couseling and therapy*. Pacific Grove, CA: Brooks/Cole.

Sue, D. W., & Sue, D. (1990). *Counseling the culturally different: Theory and practice* (2nd ed.). New York: Wiley.

Sue, D. W., & Sue, D. (2003). *Counseling the culturally diverse: Theory and practice* (4th ed.). New York: Wiley.

Sue, D. W., & Torino, G. C. (2004). Racial-cultural competence: Awareness, knowledge, and skills. In R. T. Carter (Ed.), *Handbook of racial-cultural psychology and counseling: Training and practice* (Vol. 2, pp. 3–18). New York: Wiley.

Sue, S. (1983). Ethnic minorities in psychology: A reexamination. *American Psychologist, 38*, 583–592.

Sue, S., & Zane, H. (1987). The role of culture and cultural techniques in psychotherapy: A critique and reformulation. *American Psychologist, 39*, 1234–1235.

Suinn, R. M. (2001). The terrible twos—anger and anxiety: Hazardous to your health. *American Psychologist, 56*, 27–36.

Sullivan, H. S. (1947). *Conceptions of modern psychiatry.* Washington, DC: William Alanson White Foundation.

Sullivan, H. S. (1953). *The interpersonal theory of psychiatry.* New York: Norton.

Sullivan, M. A., & O'Leary, S. G. (1990). Maintenance following reward and cost token programs. *Behavior Therapy, 21*, 139–149.

Suzman, K. B., Morris, R. D., Morris, M. K., & Milan, M. A. (1997). Cognitive-behavioral remediation of problem solving deficits in children with acquired brain injury. *Journal of Behavior Therapy and Experimental Psychiatry, 28*, 202–212.

Swaggart, B., Gagnon, E., Bock, S. J., Earles, T. L., Quinn, C. P., Myles, B. S,. et al. (1995). Using social stories to teach social and behavioral skills to children with autism. *Focus on Autistic Behavior, 10*, 1–16.

Sykes, D. K. (1987). An approach to working with black youth in cross-cultural therapy. *Clinical Social Work journal, 15*(3), 260–270.

Taft, J. (1933). *The dynamics of therapy in a controlled relationship.* New York: Macmillan.

Tamasese, K., Waldegrave, C., Tuhaka, F., & Campbell, W. (1998). Furthering conversation about partnerships of accountability. *Dulwich Centre Journal, 4*, 50–62.

Tanner, S., & Ball, J. (1989). *Beating the blues.* Sidney: Doubleday.

Taylor, D. W. A. (1971). A comparison of group desensitization with two control procedures in the treatment of test anxiety. *Behaviour Research and Therapy, 9*, 281–284.

Teasdale, J. D., Segal, Z., & Williams, J. M. G. (1995). How does cognitive therapy prevent depressive relapse and why should attention control (mindfulness) training help? *Behaviour Research and Therapy, 33*, 25–39.

Teri, L. (1991). Behavioral assessment and treatment of depression in older adults. In P. A. Wisocki (Ed.), *Handbook of clinical behavior therapy with the elderly client* (pp. 225–243). New York: Plenum Press.

Teri, L., & Gallagher-Thompson, D. (1991). Cognitive-behavioral interventions for treatment of depression in Alzheimer patients. *The Gerontologist, 31*, 413–416.

Teri, L., & Uomoto, J. M. (1991). Reducing excess disability in dementia patients: Training caregivers to manage patient depression. *Clinical Gerontologist, 10*, 49–63.

Thomlison, B. (2002). *Family assessment handbook.* Pacific Grove, CA: Brooks/Cole.

Thompson, C. D., & Born, D. G. (1999). Increasing correct participation in an exercise class for adult day care clients. *Behavioral Interventions, 14*, 171–186.

Thompson, L. W., Gallagher-Thompson, D., & Breckenridge, J. (1987). Comparative effectiveness of psychotherapies for depressed elders. *Journal of Consulting and Clinical Psychology, 55*, 385–390.

Thorndike, E. L. (1911). *Animal intelligence: Experimental studies.* New York: Macmillan.

Thorndike, E. L. (1931). *Human learning.* New York: Century.

Thorndike, E. L. (1933). *An experimental study of rewards.* New York: Teachers College Press.

Toman, W. (1976). *Family constellation: Its effects on personality and social behavior.* New York: Springer.

Tomm, K. (1989). Foreword. In M. White & D. Epston, *Literate means to therapeutic ends* (pp. 5–8). Adelaide, Australia: Dulwich Centre Publications.

Tootell, A. (2004). Decentering research practice. *International Journal of Narrative Therapy and Community Work, 3,* 54–60.

Trepper, T. S. (2005). Family therapy around the world—An introduction. *Family Therapy Magazine, 4,* 10–13.

Tryon, G. S. (1979). A review and critique of thought stopping research. *Journal of Behavior Therapy and Experimental Psychiatry, 10,* 189–192.

Turk, D. [C.] (1975). *Cognitive control of pain: A skill training approach.* Unpublished manuscript, University of Waterloo, Ontario.

Turk, D. [C.] (1976). *An expanded skills training approach for the treatment of experimentally induced pain.* Unpublished doctoral dissertation, University of Waterloo, Ontario.

Ungersma, A. J. (1961). *The search for meaning: A new approach in psychotherapy and pastoral psychology.* Philadelphia: Westminster.

U.S. Department of Health and Human Services. (2001). *Mental health: Culture, race, and ethnicity—A supplement to mental health: A report of the Surgeon General.* Rockville, MD: U.S. Department of Health and Human Services, Substance Abuse and Mental Health Services Administration, Center for Mental Health Services.

Vaccaro, F. J. (1992). Physically aggressive elderly: A social skills training program. *Journal of Behavior Therapy and Experimental Psychiatry, 23,* 277–288.

Valdez, J. N. (2000). Psychotherapy with bicultural Hispanic clients. *Psychotherapy, 37,* 240–246.

Van Deurzen-Smith, E. (1988). *Existential counseling in practice.* Beverly Hills, CA: Sage.

van Oppen, P., & Arntz, A. (1994). Cognitive therapy for obsessive-compulsive disorder. *Behaviour Research and Therapy, 32,* 79–87.

van Oppen, P., de Hann, E., van Balkom, A. J. L. M., Spinhoven, P., Hoogduin, K., & van Dyck, R. (1995). Cognitive therapy and exposure *in vivo* in the treatment of obsessive-compulsive disorder. *Behaviour Research and Therapy, 33,* 379–390.

Vasquez, M. J. T. (2005). Independent practice settings and the multicultural guidelines. In M. G. Constantine & D. W. Sue (Eds.), *Strategies for building multicultural competence in mental health and educational settings* (pp. 91–108). Hoboken, NJ: Wiley.

Vernon, D. T. A. (1974). Modeling and birth order in responses to painful stimuli. *Journal of Personality and Social Psychology, 29,* 794–799.

Visher, E. (1996) *Therapy with step families.* New York: Brunner/Mazel.

von Bertalanffy, L. (1950). An outline of general system theory. *British Journal of the Philosophy of Science, 1,* 134–165.

von Bertalanffy, L. (1968). *General systems theory.* New York: Braziller.

Vontress, C. E. (1979). Cross-cultural counseling: An existential approach. *Personnel and Guidance Journal, 58,* 117–122.

Vontress, C. E. (1985). Theories of counseling: A comparative analysis. In R. J. Samuda & A. Woolfgang (Eds.), *Intercultural counseling and assessment: Global perspectives* (pp. 19–31). Toronto: Hogrefe.

Vontress, C. E. (1988). An existential approach to cross-cultural counseling. *Journal of Multicultural Counseling and Development, 16,* 73–83.

Vontress, C. E. (1991). Traditional healing in Africa: Implications for cross-cultural counseling. *Journal of Counseling and Development, 70,* 242–249.

Vontress, C. E. (2003). On becoming an existential cross-cultural counselor. In F. D. Harper & J. McFadden (Eds.), *Culture and counseling: New approaches* (pp. 20–30). Boston: Allyn & Bacon.

Vontress, C. E., Johnson, J. A., & Epp, L. R. (1999). *Cross-cultural counseling: A casebook.* Alexandria, VA: American Counseling Association.

Wachtel, P. (1997). *Psychoanalysis, behavior therapy, and the relational world.* Washington, DC: American Psychological Association.

Waldegrave, C. (1990). Just therapy. *Dulwich Centre Newsletter, 1,* 6–46.

Waldegrave, C. (2000). Therapy as metaphorical reflection. *Gecko: A Journal of Deconstruction and Narrative Ideas in Therapeutic Practice, 3,* 3–12.

Walsh, F. (1998). *Strengthening family resilience.* New York: Guilford.

Walsh, W. (2002). *Essentials of family therapy* (2nd ed.). Denver, CO: Love.

Walsh, W. M., & McGraw, J. A. (2002). *Essentials of family therapy.* Denver, CO: Love.

Wampler, L. D., & Strupp, H. H. (1976). Personal therapy for students in clinical psychology: A matter of faith? *Professional Psychology: Research and Practice, 7,* 195–201.

Wampold, B. E. (2000). Outcomes of individual counseling and psychotherapy: Empirical evidence addressing two fundamental questions. In S. D. Brown & R. W. Lent (Eds.), *Handbook of counseling psychology* (3rd ed.). Hoboken, NJ: Wiley.

Watson, J. B. (1914). *Behavior: An introduction to comparative psychology.* New York: Holt.

Watson, J. C. (2001). Revisioning empathy: Theory, research, and practice. In D. J. Cain & J. Seeman (Eds.), *Humanistic psychotherapies: Handbook of research and practice* (pp. 445–473). Washington, DC: American Psychological Association.

Watson, J. C., Greenberg, L. S., & Lietaer, G. (1998). The experiential paradigm unfolding. In L. S. Greenberg, J. C. Watson, & G. Lietaer (Eds.), *Handbook of experiential psychotherapy* (pp. 1–27). New York: Guilford.

Watson, T. S., & Kramer, J. J. (1995). Teaching problem solving skills to teachers-in-training: An analogue experimental analysis of three methods. *Journal of Behavioral Education, 5,* 295–317.

Watts, A. (1975). *Psychotherapy: East and West.* New York: Vintage.

Watts, A. (1995a). *The Tao of philosophy.* Boston: Tuttle.

Watts, A. (1995b). *The philosophies of Asia: The edited transcripts.* Boston: Tuttle.

Watts, A. (1996). *Buddhism: The religion of no-religion: The edited transcripts.* Boston: Tuttle.

Watts, R. E. (1998). The remarkable similarity between Rogers' core conditions and Adler's social interest. *Journal of Individual Psychology, 54,* 4–9.

Watts, R. E. (2000a). Entering the new millennium: Is Individual Psychology still relevant? *Journal of Individual Psychology, 56,* 21–30.

Watts, R. E. (2000b). Biblically based Christian spirituality and Adlerian psychotherapy. *Journal of Individual Psychology, 56,* 316–328.

Watts, R. E. (Ed.). (2003). *Adlerian, cognitive, and constructivist psychotherapies: An integrative dialogue.* New York: Springer.

Watts, R. E., & Carlson, J. (Eds.). (1999). *Interventions and strategies in counseling and psychotherapy.* Philadelphia: Accelerated Development/Taylor & Francis.

Watzlawick, P., Beavin, J., & Jackson, D. (1967). *Pragmatics of human communication.* New York: Norton.

Weidner, F. (1970). *In vivo* desensitization of a paranoid schizophrenic. *Journal of Behavior Therapy and Experimental Psychiatry, 1,* 79–81.

Weiner, N. (1948). *Cybernectics or control and communication in the animal and machine.* Cambridge, MA: Tecnnology Press.

Weingarten, K. (1992). Consultations to myself on a work/family dilemma: A post-modern feminist reflection. *Journal of Feminist Family Therapy, 4*(1), 3–29.

Weingarten, K. (1997). *The mother's voice: Strengthening intimacy in families.* New York: Guilford.

Weingarten, K. (1998). The small and ordinary: The daily practice of a postmodern narrative therapy. *Family Process, 37,* 3–15.

Weingarten, K. (2003). *Common shock: Witnessing violence in everyday life.* New York: Dutton.

Weinhardt, L. S., Carey, M. P., Carey, K. B., & Verdecias, R. N. (1998). Increasing assertiveness skills to reduce HIV risk among woman living with a severe and persistent mental illness. *Journal of Consulting and Clinical Psychology, 66,* 680–684.

Weiss, J. (1993). *How psychotherapy works: Process and technique.* New York: Guilford.

Weisz, J. R., Weersing, V. R., & Henggeler, S. W. (2005). Jousting with straw men: Comment on Westen, Novotny, and Thompson-Brenner (2004). *Psychological Bulletin, 131,* 418–426.

Welwood, J. (2002). *Toward a psychology of awakening.* Boston: Shambhala.

Westbury, E., & Tutty, L. M. (1998). *Child Abuse and Neglect, 23,* 31–44.

Wetherell, J. L. (1998). Treatment of anxiety in older adults. *Psychotherapy: Theory, Research, and Practice, 35,* 444–457.

Wetherell, J. L. (2002). Behavior therapy for anxious older adults. *The Behavior Therapist, 25,* 16–17.

Wheeler, S. (1991). Personal therapy: An essential aspect of counselor training, or a distraction from focusing on the client? *International Journal for the Advancement of Counseling, 14,* 193–202.

Whitaker, C. A. (1967). The growing edge. In J. Haley & L. Hoffman (Eds.), *Techniques of family therapy.* New York: Basic Books.

White, M. (1989). *Selected papers.* Adelaide, Australia: Dulwich Centre Publications.

White, M. (1991). Deconstruction and therapy. *Dulwich Center Newsletter, 3,* 21–40.

White, M. (1993). Commentary: The histories of the present. In S. Gilligan & R. Price (Eds.), *Therapeutic conversations* (pp. 121–135). New York: Norton.

White, M. (1995). *Re-authoring lives: Interviews and essays.* Adelaide, Australia: Dulwich Centre Publications.

White, M. (1997). *Narratives of therapists' lives.* Adelaide, Australia: Dulwich Centre Publications.

White, M. (2000). *Reflections on narrative practice: Essays and interviews.* Adelaide, Australia: Dulwich Centre Publications.

White, M. (2001). Folk psychology and narrative practice. *Dulwich Centre Journal, 2,* 3–37.

White, M. (2004). *Narrative practice and exotic lives: Resurrecting diversity in everyday life.* Adelaide, Australia: Dulwich Centre Publications.

White, M. (2005). Statement of position maps 1 & 2. In Workshop notes. Available at www.dulwich.centre.com.au

White, M., & Epston, D. (1989). *Literate means to therapeutic ends*. Adelaide, Australia: Dulwich Centre Publications.

White, M., & Epston, D. (1990). *Narrative means to therapeutic ends*. New York: Norton.

Williams, K. E., & Chambless, D. L. (1994). The results of exposure-based treatment in agoraphobia. In S. Friedman (Ed.), *Anxiety disorders in African Americans* (pp. 149–165). New York: Springer.

Wilson, G. T. (1997). Behavior therapy at century close. *Behavior Therapy, 28,* 18–23.

Winnicott, D. W. (1965). *The maturational processes and the facilitating environment*. New York: International Universities Press.

Winnicott, D. W. (1975). *Through pediatrics to psychoanalysis*. New York: Basic Books.

Winslade, J., Crocket, K., & Monk, G. (1997). The therapeutic relationship. In G. Monk, J. Winslade, K. Crocket, & D. Epston (Eds.), *Narrative therapy in action: The archaeology of hope* (pp. 53–81). San Francisco: Jossey-Bass.

Winslade, J., & Smith, L. (1997). Countering alcoholic narratives. In G. Monk, J. Winslade, K. Crocket, & D. Epston (Eds.), *Narrative therapy in action: The archaeology of hope* (pp. 158–192). San Francisco: Jossey-Bass.

Wolf, M. M., Braukmann, C. J., & Ramp, K. A. (1987). Serious delinquent behavior as part of a significantly handicapping condition: Cures and supportive environments. *Journal of Applied Behavior Analysis, 20,* 347–359.

Wolfe, J. L. (1992). Working with gay women. In A. Freeman & F. M. Dattilio (Eds.), *Comprehensive casebook of cognitive therapy* (pp. 257–265). New York: Plenum.

Wolpe, J. (1958). *Psychotherapy by reciprocal inhibition*. Stanford, CA: Stanford University Press.

Woo, A. (1998). A developmental study of a group social work program using reality therapy. Unpublished doctoral dissertation, Department of Social Work, Yonsei University, Seoul, Korea.

Wood, B. L. (1995). A developmental biopsychosocial approach to the treatment of chronic illness in children and adolescents. In R. Mikesell, D.-D. Lusterman, & S. McDaniel (Eds.), *Integrating family therapy* (pp. 37–55). Washington, DC: American Psychological Association.

Woodward, L. J., & Fergusson, D. M. (2001). Life course outcomes of young people with anxiety disorders in adolescence. *Journal of the American Academy of Child and Adolescent Psychiatry, 40,* 1086–1093.

Word, C., Zanna, M., & Cooper, J. (1974). The non-verbal mediation of self-fulfilling prophecies in inter-racial interaction. *Journal of Experimental Social Psychology, 10,* 109–120.

Worell, J. (1980). New directions in counseling women. *Personnel and Guidance Journal, 58,* 477–484.

Worell, J. (2001). Feminist interventions: Accountability beyond symptom reduction. *Psychology of Women Quarterly, 25,* 335–343.

Worell, J., & Chandler, R. (1999). *The Personal Progress Scale, Revised (PPS-R)*. Unpublished manuscript, University of Kentucky, Lexington, KY.

Worell, J., Chandler, R., Robinson, D., & Blount, A. (1996, August). Measuring beliefs and behaviors of feminist therapists. In J. Worell (Chair), *Evaluating process and outcomes in feminist therapy and counseling*. Symposium presented at the annual meeting of the American Psychological Association, Toronto, Ontario, Canada.

Worell, J., & Johnson, N. G. (1997). *Shaping the future of feminist psychology: Education, research, and practice.* Washington, DC: American Psychological Association.

Worell, J., & Remer, P. (1992). *Feminist perspectives in therapy: An empowerment model for women.* Chichester, England: Wiley.

Worell, J., & Remer, P. (2003). *Feminist perspectives in therapy: Empowering diverse women.* Hoboken, NJ: Wiley.

Wubbolding, R. (1996). *Employee motivation: What to do when what you say isn't working.* Knoxville, TN: SPC Press.

Wubbolding, R. (2000). *Reality therapy for the 21st century.* Philadelphia: Brunner/Routledge.

Wubbolding, R. (2002). Reality therapy. In M. Hersen & W. Sledge (Eds.), *The encyclopedia of psychotherapy* (Vol. 2, pp. 482–494). New York: Elsevier.

Wubbolding, R. (2003). Reality therapy theory. In D. Capuzzi & D. Gross (Eds.), *Counseling and psychotherapy: Theories and interventions* (3rd ed., pp. 255–282). Upper Saddle River, NJ: Merrill/Prentice Hall.

Wurtele, S. K. (1990). Teaching personal safety skills to four-year-old children: A behavioral approach. *Behavior Therapy, 21,* 25–32.

Wurtele, S. K., Currier, L. L., Gillispie, E. I., & Franklin, C. F. (1991). The efficacy of a parent-implemented program for teaching preschoolers personal safety skills. *Behavior Therapy, 22,* 69–83.

Wurtele, S. K., Marrs, S. R., & Miller-Perrin, C. J. (1987). Practice makes perfect? The role of participant modeling in sexual abuse prevention programs. *Journal of Consulting and Clinical Psychology, 55,* 599–602.

Wyche, K. F., & Rice, J. K. (1997). Feminist therapy: From dialogue to tenets. In J. Worell & N. G. Johnson (Eds.), *Shaping the future of feminist psychology: Education, research, and practice* (pp. 57–72). Washington, DC: American Psychological Association.

Yalom, I. D. (1980). *Existential psychotherapy.* New York: Basic Books.

Yalom, I. [D.]. (1989). *Love's executioner.* New York: Basic Books.

Yalom, I. D. (2003). *The gift of therapy: An open letter to a new generation of therapists and their patients.* New York: HarperCollins (Perennial).

Yellow Bird, M. J. (2001). Critical values and First Nations peoples. In R. Fong & S. Furuto (Eds.), *Culturally competent practice: Skills, interventions, and evaluations* (pp. 61–74). Needham Heights, MA: Allyn & Bacon.

Yontef, G. (1993). *Awareness, dialogue, and process: Essays on Gestalt therapy.* Highland, NY: Gestalt Journal Press.

Young, J. E. (1994). *Cognitive therapy for personality disorders: A schema-focused approach* (Rev. ed.). Sarasota, FL: Professional Resource Press.

Zahm, S. (1998). Therapist self disclosure in the practice of Gestalt therapy. *The Gestalt Journal, 21,* 21–52.

Zimmerman, J., & Dickerson, V. (1996). *If problems talked: Narrative therapy in action.* New York: Guilford.

Zimring, F. M., & Raskin, N. J. (1992). Carl Rogers and client/person-centered therapy. In D. K. Freedheim (Ed.), *History of psychotherapy* (pp. 629–656). Washington, DC: American Psychological Association.

Name Index

Abbott, J., 113
Abrahms, J. L., 334
Abramowitz, A., 280
Abramowitz, J. S., 304
Abrams, M., 327
Ackerman, C., 342
Ackerman, N., 443, 456
Adamowicz, J., 291
Adams, C. D., 296
Adams, M. V., 92
Adler, A., 93–97, 103–115, 443
Agigian, H., 285, 308, 310
Agran, M., 338
Aguiree, M. G., 30
Ajamu, A., 14
Al-Rashidi, B., 389n
Alberti, R., 357
Alexander, J., 461, 476
Alexopoulos, P., 291
Alferi, S. M., 334
Alford, B. A., 334
Aljure, J. P., 389n
Allen, K. D., 315
Allen, T. W., 327
Altman, N., 15, 41, 51, 52–55, 92
Alvarez, M. F., 327
Anderson, H., 446
Anderson, S. A., 446, 448, 455
Andersson, G., 309
Anderton, J., 492
Angel, E., 2
Angelo, M., 363
Ansbacher, H. L., 97, 104, 105, 107–109, 113, 125, 134, 135, 138
Ansbacher, R. R., 138
Anstey, K. J., 336
Anton, W. D., 300
Antoni, M. H., 334, 342
Antoninus, M. A., 361
Aponte, H. J., 445
Arciniega, G. M., 100
Arean, P. A., 340
Ariel, S., 480
Aristotle, 141, 153, 369

Arkowitz, H., 281
Armstrong, K. J., 296
Arnold, M. S., 480
Arntz, A., 334
Aron, L., 92
Arredondo, P., 480
Asante, M. K., 480
Asarnow, J. R., 338
Asay, T. P., 219
Asen, E., 477
Attneave, C., 480
Attneave, C. L., 480
Aubrey, R. F., 480
Aurelius, M., 155, 361, 367
Aydin, G., 336
Ayim, M., 410
Ayllon, T., 279, 358
Azocar, F., 307
Azrin, N. H., 279, 296

Bagarozzi, D., 446, 448
Baker, F. M., 306
Baker, J., 146
Baker, M., 500
Ball, J., 336
Ballard, K. D., 308
Balter, R., 327
Bandura, A., 280, 284, 315
Bankart, C. P., 96
Barkham, M., 335
Barnhill, L. H., 452
Barry, T., 292
Baruth, L. G., 99
Bates, F., 301
Baucom, D. H., 334, 477
Beal, D., 326
Beauvoir, S. de, 152
Bechet, S., 146
Beck, A. T., 3, 280, 328–335, 358
Beck, J., 340
Becker, W., 281
Becvar, D., 446, 476
Becvar, R., 446, 476
Bedford, M., 156

Beels, C. C., 444
Beidel, D. C., 307
Beisser, A., 248
Bell, J., 442
Bell-Dolan, D. J., 329
Bemak, F., 99
Bennun, I., 343
Bergman, A., 51
Bernal, G., 327
Bernard, M. E., 324, 326, 328
Bernstein, D. A., 357
Beutler, L. E., 17, 262
Bhabha, H., 50
Bigelow, K. M., 294
Biggam, F. H., 338
Bingham, R., 27
Binswanger, L., 143, 144, 148, 149, 152, 161, 170
Bird, J., 494, 528
Bird, M., 291
Black, D., 340
Black, M. J., 92
Blackwell, G., 285
Blackwood, J., 342
Bloom, J. W., 5
Blount, A., 434
Bock, S. J., 315
Boddington, S. J. A., 305
Boggs, S. R., 296
Bogolepov, S., 389n
Bohart, A. C., 214
Boisvert, J., 340
Bollas, C., 72
Bolling, M., 349
Bonaventura, S. H., 297
Bonk, E., 2
Boord, P., 300
Boothroyd, P., 340
Bootzin, R. R., 292, 301
Borden, A., 496, 497
Borkovec, T. D., 300, 357
Born, D. G., 291
Boscolo, L., 444
Boss, M., 143, 159
Boszormenyi-Nagy, I., 443, 444, 456
Boudin, H. M., 296
Bowen, M., 443, 444, 456, 457–460
Bowers, W. A., 333
Bowlby, J., 442
Boyd-Franklin, N., 113, 445, 480
Boyers, A. E., 334
Bozarth, J., 214, 226
Braaten, L. S., 297
Brabeck, M. M., 24, 27, 29
Braswell, L., 340
Breckenridge, J., 336

Breuer, J., 41, 42, 81
Breunlin, D., 446, 448
Brickell, J., 389n, 395, 396
Brickman, J., 423
Brink, D., 336
Brodaty, H., 336
Broder, M. S., 323
Brodsky, A. M., 36, 399
Brofenbrenner, U., 467
Brouwer, R., 308
Broverman, D. M., 418
Broverman, I. K., 418
Brown, G. K., 335
Brown, L., 24, 25
Browne-Sperling, F., 313
Brownlee, K., 450
Bryan, H., 180
Buber, M., 143, 159, 241
Bugental, J. F. T., 144
Bujold, A., 340
Burck, C., 478
Burgess, D., 312
Burgio, L. F., 294
Burns, D., 329, 358
Burr, V., 498, 499
Burstein, Y., 309
Burt, V., 533
Busch, R., 525
Butt, J. H., 315

Cain, D. J., 177, 192–193, 220, 226, 227
Calamari, J. E., 305
Calapai, P., 309
Caldwell, R., 99
Callan, J. W., 338
Cameron, R., 338, 342
Campbell, T. J., 480
Campbell, W., 492
Camus, A., 142, 152
Capuzzi, D., 135
Carey, G., 480
Carey, K. B., 313
Carey, M., 492
Carey, M. P., 297, 313
Cariaga, J., 294
Carkhuff, R., 495
Carlson, J., 99, 130, 134
Carlson, J. D., 93, 94, 96, 99, 101–102, 105–109, 106, 112, 116, 121, 125, 130, 132, 135, 139
Carlson, J. M., 99, 121
Carmin, C. N., 305
Carr, A., 477
Carstensen, L. L., 294, 310
Carter, B., 445, 453
Carter, D. K., 399

Cartledge, G., 308
Caselli, L., 309
Cass, V., 412
Cassell, P., 98
Castonguay, L. G., 343
Cecchin, G. F., 444
Chambless, D. L., 288, 289, 306, 345
Chandler, C. K., 99
Chandler, R., 434
Chang, C., 389
Chang, E. C., 338
Charlop, M. H., 308
Chasin, R., 425
Cheatham, H., 480
Chemtob, C. M., 334
Cherry, C., 313
Cheshire, A., 522
Chessick, R. D., 149, 187
Cheston, S. E., 99
Chorpita, B. F., 351
Christensen, A., 468
Christian, J. L., 142, 153, 161
Christopher, F., 340
Christophersen, E. R., 281
Chung, R. C., 99
Church, M., 336
Clarke, G. N., 335, 336
Clarkson, F. E., 418
Cloitre, M., 280
Cohen, D. B., 158
Cold, L., 99
Colecchi, C., 336
Collins, J. F., 335
Collins, P., 389
Colvin, C., 305
Combs, G., 494, 526, 532
Comer-Wright, M. L., 397
Congress, E. P., 460
Connis, R. T., 338
Constantine, M. G., 24
Cook, D. A., 433
Cooley, E. J., 300
Cooper, J., 62
Cooper, M., 185
Cordova, J., 468
Corey, G., 39, 132
Cornelius-White, C., 183
Cornelius-White, J., 183
Correia, C. J., 334
Corrigan, S. A., 340
Corsini, R., 132
Costello, N., 342
Cotharin, R. L., 301
Couvadelli, B., 338
Creswell, J. W., 264

Crews, W. D., 297
Crits-Christoph, P., 345
Croce, B., 161
Crocket, K., 489, 495–498, 506, 510, 522, 524, 527, 533
Crooks, T. J., 308
Cross, W. E., 412
Cruess, D. G., 334
Culver, J. L., 334
Cummings, L. E., 338
Cunningham, P., 450
Curlette, W. L., 99
Currier, L. L., 308
Curry, J. F., 338

Daiuto, A. D., 477
D'Andrea, M., 14n, 453
Danforth, J. S., 315
Daniels, J. A., 453
Danto, E. A., 51
Dattilio, F. M., 334
Davies, B., 501
Davies, J. M., 56
Davies, W. H., 342
Davis, D. D., 335
Davis, S., 301, 476
Davison, G. C., 281, 327
Dawson, B., 340
de Armas, A., 340
de Beauvoir, S., 146
de Hann, E., 334
de Montes, A. I., 281
de Shazer, S., 526
de Venza Tillmanns, M., 171
Dean, T., 336
DeBarry, S., 301
Decora, M., 99
Deegear, J., 263
Deffenbacher, J. L., 338, 342
deGroot, J. C., 300
DeMaria, R., 460
Deming, W. E., 362, 363
Denborough, D., 533
Depp, C. A., 293
Derrida, J., 49
D'Haene, M. T., 433
Di Fazio, L., 342
Di Giuseppe, R., 324, 328
Dias, F., 389n
Dick-Siskin, L. P., 329, 330
Dickerson, V., 494, 533
DiGuseppe, R. A., 326
Diller, A., 410
Dillow, P. V., 300
Dimant, J., 309
DiMenna, D., 5

Dinkmeyer, D. C., 98, 105, 111, 112, 125, 139, 444
Dixon, D. N., 335
Dobson, K. S., 335
Dominguez, B., 281
Donohue, B., 290
Donovan, D. M., 350
Douglas, M. A., 28
Downing, N. W., 412
Dowrick, P. W., 309
Drabman, R. S., 296, 315
Dreikurs, R., 3, 97, 98, 105, 109, 112, 139
Drewery, W., 491, 492, 498, 524
Droit, R.-P., 142
Dryden, W., 324, 327
Dubois, P., 361
Dumas, J. E., 477
Duncan, B. L., 213, 218
Dunn, H., 334
Dupree, L., 323
Durant, L. E., 297
Durant, W., 156
Durie, M., 492
Duvall, E. M., 452
D'Zurilla, T. J., 338, 340, 358

Earles, T. L., 315
Eckman, T. A., 285
Ecrement, E. R., 99
Edelman, R. E., 289
Edens, J. L., 342
Edwards, I., 467
Edwards, M. E., 107, 477
Egel, A. L., 308
Einstein, A., 372
Eissler, K., 85
Eldredge, K. L., 306
Eldridge, K., 468
Eldridge, N. S., 480
Elkin, I., 335
Ellenberger, H., 2
Ellingson, S., 308
Elliot, R., 215
Elliott, C. H., 315
Elliott, R., 184
Ellis, A., 3, 99, 133, 280, 322, 323, 324, 326, 327, 358
Ellis, C. R., 297
Emery, G., 333, 334
Emmelkamp, P. M. G., 327
Englar-Carlson, M., 93, 102–103
Engle-Friedman, M., 301
Enns, C. Z., 398, 400–404, 414, 423
Enns, E. Z., 440
Epp, L. R., 151, 161, 162
Epstein, D., 292
Epstein, N., 334

Epstein, R., 95
Epston, D., 467, 491, 493, 496, 497, 498, 500, 502, 506, 507, 522, 524, 528, 533
Erikson, E., 55, 56, 58–59
Eyberg, S. M., 296
Eysenck, H. J., 279, 280
Ezra, E., 306

Faber, S. D., 305
Faccini, L., 338
Fairbairn, R., 48, 56, 71
Fairbairn, W. R. D., 74
Falicov, C., 445, 480
Fall, K. A., 133, 134
Fang, S., 450
Fanon, F., 50
Farbry, J. E., 315
Farrell, S. P., 342
Fassinger, R. E., 415
Fenichel, O., 46
Ferguson, E. D., 105
Fergusson, D. M., 305
Fernandez, L. E., 284, 315
Feske, U., 307
Finch, A. J., 338
Fink, C. M., 307
Fisch, R., 443
Fisher, J. E., 294, 310
Fitzgerald, L. F., 400
Fleece, L., 343
Flew, A., 142
Flores, M. T., 480
Flynn, W., 294
Foa, E. B., 323, 332, 334, 342
Foerster, F. S., 263
Folkman, S., 341
Fonagy, P., 84
Forsyth, A. D., 297
Forsyth, J. P., 281
Foucault, M., 49, 493, 500
Foxx, R. M., 296
Foy, D. W., 342
Fraenkel, P., 445, 478, 523
Frame, C. L., 309
Frame, M., 460
Framo, J., 456
Frank, J. B., 32
Frank, J. D., 32
Frank, R., 308
Frankl, V., 142–143, 158, 367
Franklin, C. F., 308
Franklin, M. E., 323
Franks, C., 281
Fraser, L. D., 108
Freedman, J., 494, 526, 532

Freeman, A., 335
Freidman, M., 242
Freire, P., 450
Freud, A., 41, 45, 46, 55, 56
Freud, S., 41–45, 48, 49, 50–51, 58, 64–66, 67, 81, 83, 85, 96, 106
Frevert, V. S., 104, 107, 108, 110, 113
Frew, J., 1, 228, 236–238, 264
Frey, D. H., 187
Friedman, M., 187, 217, 219
Friedman, S., 305, 352
Frye, A. A., 338
Fudge, R. C., 327
Fuentes, R. M., 305

Gaddis, S., 524
Gagnon, E., 315
Gale, J. E., 478
Galensky, T., 308
Gallagher, K. T., 148, 151
Gallagher-Thompson, D., 293, 336
Gallardo-Cooper, M., 480
Gamboa, V. U., 281
Gambrill, E., 308, 310, 313
Garcia-Preto, N., 480
Garfield, S. L., 262
Gaston, L., 343, 344
Gehart, D., 478
Gehin, J. M., 297
Gendlin, E., 181, 184, 216
Gendlin, G., 101
Gergen, K., 446, 492, 499, 533
Gerhart, D., 526
Gerow, M. A., 340
Gerson, R., 460
Gil, K. M., 342
Gilbert, L. A., 414
Gill, M., 74
Gilligan, C., 24, 30, 49
Gillispie, E. I., 308
Gillock, K. L., 305
Gilman, S., 51
Glaser, R. R., 477
Glass, D. C., 371
Glass, G. V., 130
Glasser, W., 3, 360, 361, 362, 364, 369, 392, 395
Gleason, J. R., 297
Gold, J., 5, 18
Goldfried, M. R., 18, 281, 321, 338, 343, 344
Goldman, R. N., 227
Goldstein, H., 308
Gomez Young, C., 450
Gonzales, R., 301
Goodman, D., 403, 410, 441
Goodman, J., 337, 338

Goodman, L. A., 404, 414, 441
Goodman, P., 2, 229, 240
Goodman, S. H., 338
Goolishian, H., 446
Gorenstein, E. E., 291, 305, 306
Goss, S., 523
Gould, R.A., 335
Grady, L. T., 460, 469
Graf, M., 293
Grant, B., 183
Greaves, D., 327
Green, J. B., 477, 478
Greenberg, J., 47, 66, 73
Greenberg, L. S., 184, 185, 214, 215, 217, 263, 343, 344
Greene, B., 413
Greenspan, M., 399, 415, 418
Greer, R. D., 461
Griffith, B., 99
Griffith, E. H., 306
Griffith, J., 104
Gross, D. M., 334
Gross, D. R., 135
Grunebaum, H., 425
Guba, E. G., 478
Guevremont, D. C., 279, 281, 287–289, 295, 305, 335, 338, 339, 340, 346, 357
Gullion, M. E., 281
Gumpel, T. P., 308
Gurman, A., 445, 476

Haaga, D. A. F., 323, 327
Hagopian, L. P., 338
Hains, A. A., 342
Haley, J., 443, 444, 452, 461
Hall, C., 14
Hall, M. L., 358
Hall, R. V., 358
Halpern, B., 305
Ham, M. D., 480
Hamada, R. S., 334
Hambright, A., 476
Hammer, D., 287
Hammond, W., 368
Handlbauer, B., 96
Hanley, J. H., 477
Hanly, C., 154
Hanna, F. J., 99, 108
Hansen, D. J., 340
Hardy, G., 335
Hardy, K. V., 460, 480
Hare-Mustin, R. T., 399, 445, 492, 512
Harel-Hochfeld, M., 389n
Harper, R., 99
Harrington, G. L., 362
Harris, S. L., 297

Hart, T. A., 342
Hartmann, D. P., 460
Hartmann, H., 46, 56
Harway, M., 399
Hatch, M. L., 352
Hayes, S. C., 281
Hays, P. A., 344, 352
Hazlett-Stevens, H., 357
Hedges, M., 133
Hedtke, L., 522
Heffer, R. W., 296
Hefferline, R., 2, 229
Heidegger, M., 142, 241
Heideman-Provost, L. M., 99
Heiman, J., 300
Heimberg, R. G., 342
Helmeke, K. B., 478
Helms, J., 404, 412, 414, 441
Hembree, E., 323
Hendricks, M. N., 216
Henggeler, S. W., 345, 477
Henriques, G. R., 335
Herlihy, B., 39
Hermann, J. A., 281
Herring, R. D., 14, 99
Heslet, F. E., 187
Hill, L. K., 327
Hill, R., 452
Himle, D. P., 300
Hines, P., 480
Hinton, D. E., 352
Hiss, H., 305
Hitsman, B. L., 305
Ho, M. K., 480
Hof, L., 460
Hoffman, E., 95, 139
Hoffman, I. Z., 50, 56, 67
Hoffman, L., 526, 528
Hoffman, S. G., 352
Holden, J. M., 133, 134
Holford, J., 139
Hollander, G., 342
Hollander, J. E., 335
Hollon, S. D., 288, 328, 334, 335, 345
Holroyd, J. C., 36
Holstein, J. E., 30
Hong, G. K., 480
Hoogduin, C. A. L., 344
Hoogduin, K., 334, 343
Hooper, A., 139
Hopkins, B. L., 281
Horne, A. M., 306
Horney, K., 443
Horvath, A. O., 343, 344
Horwitz, B., 315

Horwitz, E. A., 315
Houston, B., 410
Houts, P. S., 340
Hubbard, R. W., 327, 336
Hubble, M. A., 213, 218
Hufford, M. R., 340
Hughes, C., 338
Hughes, H., 281
Hull, D. B., 338
Hurlburt, R. T., 477
Husserl, E., 142
Huynen, K. B., 294

Ibrahim, F. A., 144, 145
Ignatiev, N., 51
Imber, S. D., 335
Imber-Black, E., 445, 446, 483
Imhof, L., 389n
Ingram, C., 524
Ironson, G., 334, 342
Ivey, A. E., 14n, 447, 448, 460, 469, 471, 478, 480
Ivey, M., 14n, 471
Iwamasa, G. Y., 352

Jacobson, N. S., 340, 351, 444, 468
James, W., 361
Janov, A., 151
Javier, R. A., 92
Jay, S. M., 315
Jenkins, A., 527
Jeris, L., 450
Johansen, T. M., 99
Johnson, D., 434
Johnson, J. A., 151, 161, 162
Johnson, N. G., 29, 401, 403, 414, 441
Johnson, W. G., 340
Jones, M. C., 277
Jones, M. L., 296
Jones, R. H., 335
Jordan, J., 37
Joseph, T. X., 340
Joshua, J. M., 5
Jourard, S. M., 259
Jourdan, A., 223
Jung, C., 46, 50, 58–59

Kahn, C. H., 141
Kai, E., 99
Kaiser, H., 361
Kakitani, M., 378, 389n
Kalichman, S. C., 313
Kant, G. L., 338
Kanter, J., 349
Kanz, J. E., 99
Kasambria, K. P., 467

Kaslow, F. W., 442, 479
Kastenbaum, R., 294
Kawulich, B. B., 99
Kazdin, A. E., 297, 357
Keijsers, G. P. J., 344
Keller, F. S., 281
Kelley, M. L., 296
Kelly, J. A., 340
Kempler, W., 444
Kendall, P. C., 288, 338, 340, 351
Kern, R. M., 104, 113, 134, 340
Khanna, A., 450
Kierkegaard, S., 142, 153, 154, 185
Kilbourn, K. M., 334
Kim, I., 389n
Kim, M. S., 389
Kimbarrow, M. L., 293
King, M., 341
King, N. J., 338
Kingdon, D. G., 334
Kirschenbaum, H., 222, 223, 227
Kirshern, D. P., 476
Kitchener, K., 26
Kitchener, K. S., 21–22, 29–32, 34
Kleber, M. S., 291, 305, 306
Klein, M., 43, 47–48, 56, 59
Klesges, R. C., 313
Klimas, N., 334, 342
Kluckhohn, C., 185
Kluckhohn, F. R., 244
Koder, D.-A., 336
Koegel, R. L., 308
Koestenbaum, P., 154
Kogan, S. M., 478
Kohlenberg, R. J., 344, 349
Kohn, A., 367
Kopec, A. M., 326
Korman, L. M., 215, 217
Kottler, J. A., 97, 131
Kotzé, D., 494, 524
Kotzé, E., 494, 524, 525
Kovel, J., 92
Kowatch, R. A., 292
Kozak, M. J., 305
Kramer, J. J., 480
Kroeger, T. L., 287
Krop, H., 312
Kuehlwein, K. T., 336
Kuehnel, T. G., 285
Kumar, M., 334
Kunkler-Peck, K. P., 460, 469
Kurtines, W. M., 305

Ladouceur, R., 340
Lagomarcino, T. R., 338

Lahav, R., 171
Laing, R. D., 185
Lambert, M. J., 219
Lask, B., 477
Laszloffy, T. A., 460, 480
Latner, J., 250, 273
Latta, R. E., 404, 414, 441
Law, I., 499
Lawrence, D., 389
Lawson, D. M., 263
Lazarus, A., 17, 18, 269, 280, 281, 300, 326, 343
Lazarus, R. S., 341
Lebow, J. L., 444, 478
Lee, E., 480
Lee, R. M., 13, 14
Lee, S. K., 389
Lehman, J. M., 334
Lehman, N. S., 149
LeLieuvre, R. B., 295
Lennon, B., 389n
Lerner, J., 323
Lescoe, F. J., 187
Letourneau, E., 476
Levendusky, P. G., 340
Levine, C., 305
Lewin, K., 240, 478
Lewinsohn, P. M., 293, 301, 335, 336
Lewis, J. A., 453
Lewis, M., 453
Liang, B., 404, 414, 441
Liberman, R. P., 285
Lichtenberg, P. A., 293
Liddell, A., 342
Liddle, H. A., 476
Lidz, T., 443
Lieberman, A., 307
Liebert, R. M., 284, 315
Liese, B. S., 330, 332, 334
Lietaer, G., 185
Lincoln, Y. S., 478
Lindauer, M. S., 190
Lindberg, P., 309
Lindsley, O. R., 279
Linehan, M. M., 350
Lochman, J. E., 338
Lock, A., 525
Locke, D., 14, 469, 478, 480
Lockman, J. J., 308
Lojk, L., 389n
Long, E. S., 308
Longo, D., 452
Loomis, L. R., 153
Lopez, M. A., 343
Losconcy, L. E., 125

Lovaas, O. I., 308
Luborsky, L., 84
Lumley, V. A., 308
Lusk, M., 434
Lutgendorf, S., 334, 342
Lutzker, J. R., 294

Macaskill, A., 7
MacKenzie-Keating, S. E., 296
MacKune-Karrer, B., 446, 448
MacMillan, V., 340
Madanes, C., 461
Madsen, C. H., 461
Madsen, C. K., 461
Mahler, M., 51, 56
Maisel, R., 496, 497
Maisto, S. A., 297
Malott, J. M., 313
Manaster, G., 99, 132, 134
Maniacci, M., 94, 96, 98, 99, 105–109, 109,
    112, 116, 122, 130, 133–135, 135, 139
Mann, R. A., 296
Manning, M. L., 99
Mansager, E., 99, 135
Mansdorf, I. J., 309
Marcel, G., 142
Marcus, M. D., 306
Margolin, G., 340
Marino, G., 187
Marinoff, L., 171
Marks, I. M., 18
Marlatt, G. A., 350
Marquis, A., 133, 134
Marshall, G. J., 300
Martin, D., 294
Martin, J. E., 338
Mashburn, D., 336
Matic, V., 442
Matson, J. L., 306, 309
Matteson, D. R., 99
Matthew, D., 477
Maturana, H. R., 525
May, R., 2, 142, 143, 144, 151, 154–156,
    160, 161, 185
Maydeu-Olivares, A., 338
Mayo, L. L., 340
McArter, G., 99
McCabe, P., 342
McDonald, L., 296
McDowell, T., 442, 449–450, 450
McGinn, L. K., 335
McGoldrick, M., 445, 453, 460, 480, 487
McGrath, M. L., 340
McGraw, J. A., 468
McIntosh, J. L., 327, 336

McIntosh, P., 410
McIntyre, A., 29
McKay, G. D., 105
McKenzie, W., 503, 524
McMains, M. J., 284, 315
McNair, L. D., 307, 352
McNamee, S., 446
McNeely, R. L., 327
Meadows, E. A., 323, 342
Mearns, D., 227
Medley, S., 433
Meek, C. R., 148
Meeks, S., 293
Meharg, S. S., 309
Meichenbaum, D. H., 280, 313, 337, 338,
    341, 342, 359
Melamed, B. G., 315
Melin, L., 309
Melton, G. B., 477
Menlove, F. L., 315
Mercatoris, M., 338
Merleau-Ponty, M., 142
Messina, M., 389n
Meyer, R. G., 301
Meyers, A., 338
Middleton, M. B., 308
Mikulas, W. L., 301
Milan, M. A., 338
Miller, C., 295
Miller, J., 455
Miller, J. B., 32
Miller, S. D., 213, 218
Miller, T. I., 130
Milstein, J. P., 308
Miltenberger, R., 308
Miltenberger, R. G., 308
Minuchin, S., 443, 444, 461–463, 526
Miranda, A. O., 104, 107, 108, 110, 113
Miranda, J., 307
Mishara, B. L., 294
Mitchell, S. A., 47, 56, 66, 83, 92
Moely, B. E., 308
Moller, A. T., 327
Monk, G., 498, 503, 506, 510, 522, 526,
    527, 532, 533
Montes, F., 281
Montgomery, L. M., 477
Moon, S., 478
Moore, K., 18
Moore, N., 300
Morales, E., 480
Morano, D. V., 155
Morgan, A., 505–507, 532
Morgan, K. P., 410
Morgan, T. K., 338

Morin, C. M., 292, 336
Morris, M. K., 338
Morris, P., 293
Morris, R. D., 338
Morrison, A. P., 334
Mosak, H. H., 93, 94, 96, 98, 100, 104,
    107, 109, 110, 112, 114, 116, 122,
    131, 133–135, 139
Moskowitz, M., 92
Mounier, E., 141
Mousetis, L., 308
Mudd, E., 443
Mueser, K. T., 477
Muñoz, R. F., 307, 352
Murdock, N., 390
Murphy, R. J., 294
Murray, H., 185
Myers, P., 471
Myles, B. S., 315

Nagy, T. F., 39
Napier, A. Y., 465
Nasr, S. H., 149
Neal-Barnett, A. M., 352
Neimeyer, G., 446
Neimeyer, R. A., 446
Neisser, U., 282
Nelson, M. L., 25, 33
Nevis, E., 273
Newlon, B. J., 100
Newman, C. F., 323, 330, 332, 334
Newman, M. G., 18
Nezu, A. M., 340, 358
Nezu, C. M., 340
Ng, K., 487
Nielsen, S. L., 327
Nietzsche, F., 142
Noda, S. J., 99
Noddings, N., 24, 30–32
Nolen-Hoeksema, S., 329
Norcross, J. C., 17, 18, 130, 133, 262, 281
Nottingham, E. J., 338
Novaco, R. W., 334, 342
Nunes, D. L., 294
Nutt, R., 400

O'Callaghan, M. E., 338
O'Connor, R. D., 308
Ogden, T., 73
Okonji, J., 389
Okun, B., 480
Olafson, F. A., 142
O'Leary, K. D., 340
O'Leary, S. G., 296
Ollendick, T. H., 338, 345

Olson, R. A., 315
Omar, M., 389n
O'Neill, M., 524
Ong, K., 389n
Organista, K. C., 307, 352
Ornish, D., 151
Ososkie, J., 389
Ostrom, R., 336
Otto, M. W., 329, 334, 335, 340
Overholser, J. C., 327, 336
Ozolins, M., 315

Pace, T. M., 335
Pachuta, D. M., 148
Pack-Brown, S. P., 24
Padesky, C. A., 334
Paivio, S. C., 263
Paniagua, F. A., 131, 132
Papp, L. A., 291, 305, 306
Paradis, C., 305, 352
Parham, T. A., 14, 113
Parker, C., 349
Pascal, B., 142
Patterson, C. H., 143
Patterson, G. R., 281
Patterson, J. M., 480
Paul, G. L., 84, 300
Pava, J. A., 329, 334
Pavio, S. C., 215, 217
Pavlov, I., 277, 279
Payne, M., 494
Payton, C., 30
Pedalino, E., 281
Peeks, A. L., 310
Perez-Foster, R., 92
Perkins-Dock, R. E., 99, 110, 113
Perlez, A., 524
Perls, F., 2, 228–234, 240, 242
Perls, L., 228–231, 234, 240, 242, 273
Perri, M. G., 340
Peterson, A., 389
Peterson, L., 315
Piaget, J., 472, 473
Picchioni, A., 2
Pilalis, J., 492
Pina, A. A., 305
Pinderhughes, E., 445
Pine, F., 51, 68–69
Pinkerton, S. S., 281
Pinsof, W., 446, 476, 477
Pipes, R. B., 30
Planells-Bloom, D., 310
Poche, C., 308
Polster, E., 250
Polster, M., 250

Pontefract, M., 301
Pope, K., 26, 31, 33
Poppe, C. J., 305
Porche-Burke, L., 27
Poser, E. G., 341, 351
Powell, J., 385
Power, K. G., 338
Powers, B., 98
Powers, W., 362
Prata, G., 444
Preciado, J., 352
Prenzlau, S., 389
Prince, H. T., II, 300
Prince, S. E., 468
Prochaska, J. O., 130, 133
Propst, L. R., 336
Pruitt, S. D., 315
Pryor, D. B., 98
Puckett, S. P., 300
Pulos, S., 389

Quinn, C. P., 315

Raabe, P. B., 171
Rachman, S., 280, 315
Radley, M., 301
Ragsdale, K., 477
Raimy, V., 4
Ramirez, M., III, 13, 14
Randall, L., 478
Rao, N., 308
Rapaport, D., 46
Rapp, J. T., 308
Rasheed, J. M., 480
Rasheed, M. N., 480
Rastogi, M., 488
Ratliff, D., 478
Raue, P. J., 343, 344
Rawlings, E. I., 399
Ready, J., 342
Red Horse, J., 480
Reddy, I., 99, 108
Redston, C., 301
Redstone, A., 524
Rees, A., 335
Reese, W. L., 150
Reeve, C., 155
Reinhard, K. E., 301
Remer, P., 397, 400, 403, 405–412, 414, 415, 417,
    420–423, 432, 433, 434, 441
Remer, R., 410, 411
Remley, T. P., 39
Renik, O., 85
Renton, J., 334
Resick, P., 342

Reynolds, S., 335
Rice, J. K., 403, 414–416
Rice, L. N., 184, 263
Richard, J., 306
Richardson, L., 500
Richman, G. S., 308
Richmond, M., 442
Ricken, F., 161
Ricketts, R. W., 297
Ridley-Johnson, R., 315
Rieckert, J., 327
Rietveld, C. M., 308
Rigazio-DiGilio, S. A., 442, 446–449, 460,
    468, 469, 478, 480
Rimm, D. C., 300
Ritter, B., 314
Riva, M., 338
Robb, H. B., 327
Robbins, B. S., 46
Robbins, M., 488
Roberts, J. A., 308
Roberts, R. L., 99
Robertson, B., 294
Robinson, D., 434
Rogers, C., 2, 143, 146, 147, 177–182, 183, 185,
    194–197, 204, 207, 218, 220–222, 227
Rogers, N., 227
Rogers, R. H., 452
Rohde, P., 335, 336
Rohner, R. P., 483
Rojahn, J., 287
Roland, A., 52, 92
Rolland, J. S., 480
Romanczyk, R. G., 297
Romney, D., 368
Rose, S., 523
Rosenberg, L., 154
Rosenkrantz, P. S., 418
Rossello, J., 327
Rostosky, S., 397, 417, 433
Rothbaum, B. O., 332, 334, 342
Rothenberg, J. L., 340
Roush, K. L., 412
Rowe, C. L., 476
Rudolph, W., 113
Runion, K. B., 99
Runyon, M. K., 290
Ruprecht, M. L., 294
Rusch, F. R., 338
Rush, A. J., 333, 334
Russell, S., 492
Rychlak, J. F., 142, 144, 148, 150, 153, 167

Sabatelli, R. M., 455
Sachse, R., 215

Safren, S., 340, 342, 352
Sahakian, M. L., 151
Sahakian, W. S., 151
Salkovskis, P. M., 334
Samoilov, A., 281
Sanders, P., 183
Sandrson, W. C., 345
Sanford, R. C., 204, 207
Santiago-Rivera, A. L., 480
Santos, J. F., 327, 336
Sapp, M., 115, 135, 327
Sartre, J.-P., 152–154, 172
Sartre, J.-P., 142
Satir, V., 443, 444, 465–466
Saunders, D. G., 300
Schaap, C. P. D. R., 343, 344
Scharff, D., 456
Scharff, J., 456
Schein, R. L., 340
Schindler, L., 343
Schneider, K. J., 142, 144
Schoenwald, S., 476, 477
Scholing, A., 327
Schreibman, L., 308
Schuster, S. C., 171
Schwartz, R., 446, 448
Scott, B., 309
Scott, C. S., 335
Scott, J. L., 335
Scrivner, R., 480
Sedway, J., 342
Seeman, J., 217, 219
Segal, Z., 335
Seligman, L., 99
Sells, S. P., 478
Selvini-Palazzoli, M., 444
Serketich, W., 477
Servan-Schreiber, J.-L., 149
Settles, A., 480
Sexton, T., 476, 488
Shadish, W. R., 477
Shaffer, H., 340
Shannon, D. T., 300
Shannon, H. D., 327
Shapiro, D. A., 335
Sharp, H., 192
Shaw, B. F., 333, 334
Shea, M. T., 335
Sheidow, A., 476
Shellenberger, S., 460
Shelton, R. C., 335
Shepard, M., 232
Sherman, B., 450
Sherman, R., 444
Shipley, R. H., 315

Shoham, V., 477
Shorkey, C., 300
Shostrom, E., 227
Shulman, B., 98, 107, 111, 114
Siegel, L. J., 315
Silber, S., 343
Silverman, W. K., 305
Simek-Morgan, L., 14n
Singer, I., 187
Singer, J. E., 371
Singh, N. N., 297
Sirota, A., 338
Skenazy, J. A., 300
Skinner, B. F., 279
Slavik, S., 99, 125, 130, 139
Sleeman, J., 226
Sliep, Y., 522
Slipp, S., 444
Sluzki, C. E., 480
Smart, N., 148, 149
Smith, A. J., 28
Smith, C., 526
Smith, D., 222
Smith, D. E., 306
Smith, E. W., 230
Smith, J. C., 301
Smith, J. M., Jr., 352
Smith, L., 524, 527
Smith, L. A., 477
Smith, L. C., 305
Smith, M. L., 130
Smith, T. E., 478
Socrates, 141, 151, 161, 162
Solomon, H. C., 279
Soltz, V., 98
Sood, R., 336
Sotsky, S. M., 335
Sowers, J., 338
Sparks, E., 404, 414, 441
Speck, R. V., 480
Speedy, J., 523, 524
Sperry, L., 106, 111, 112, 134, 139
Spiegler, M. D., 1, 275, 279, 281, 283–285,
        284, 285, 287–289, 295, 300, 305,
        308, 310, 315, 320, 335, 339, 346, 357
Spinhoven, P., 334
Sprenkle, D. H., 478
Sprich-Buckminster, S., 329, 334
Sprinkle, L., 192
St. Pierre, E., 500
Stagoll, B., 526
Staniforth, M., 155
Stanton, D., 444
Stanton, M. D., 477
Star, T. Z., 308

Starr, K., 342
Startup, M., 335
Stein, H. T., 107
Steinglass, P., 477
Steinmark, S. W., 300
Stewart, J., 480
Stickle, T. R., 477
Stoltz, V., 139
Stone, J., 336
Stricker, G., 18
Strodtbeck, F. L., 244
Strong, T., 525
Strosahl, K. D., 281
Strümpfel, U., 263, 264
Strupp, H., 7, 284
Sturdivant, S., 399, 419
Sue, D., 14, 190, 220, 266
Sue, D. W., 14, 24, 27, 190, 220, 266
Sue, S., 122, 218
Suinn, R. M., 342
Sullivan, H. S., 47, 58, 59, 67, 443
Sullivan, M. A., 296
Sungur, M., 18
Suzman, K. B., 338
Swaggart, B., 315
Swearingen, M., 308
Sweeney, T., 471
Sylvain, C., 340

Tacchi, M. J., 335
Tamasese, K., 492
Tanner, S., 336
Tausch, R., 214, 226
Taylor, D. W. A., 300
Teasdale, J. D., 335
Ten Have, T., 335
Teri, L., 293, 301
Tham, E., 389n
Thevenin, D. H., 290
Thibadeau, S. F., 358
Thiesse-Duffy, E., 308
Thomas, L., 533
Thompson, C. D., 291
Thompson, L. W., 336
Thorndike, E., 279
Thorne, B., 227
Tillich, P., 142, 156, 187, 229
Ting, K., 24, 27, 29
Tishelman, A. C., 338
Tollerud, T. R., 98
Toman, S., 273
Toman, W., 458
Tootell, A., 524
Trepper, T. S., 479
Tryon, A. S., 308

Tryon, G. S., 323
Tsai, M., 344, 349
Tuhaka, F., 492
Turkewitz, H., 340
Turkington, D., 334
Turner, S. M., 307
Tuttle Eagle Bull, D., 99
Tutty, L. M., 433

Ugland, M., 313
Undheim, L. T., 389n
Unger, P., 327
Ungersma, A. J., 155
Uomoto, J. M., 293

Vaccaro, F. J., 308
Vaccaro, J. V., 285
Vaihinger, H., 106
Valdez, J. N., 321
Van Balen, R., 184
van Balkom, A. J. L. M., 334
Van Deurzen-Smith, E., 143, 144
van Dyck, R., 334
Van Houten, R., 358
Van Kaam, A., 187
van Oppen, P., 334
Vangel, S. J., Jr., 293
Varela, F. J., 525
Vasquez, M. J. T., 20, 24, 25–27, 31, 33
Verdecias, R. N., 313
Vernon, D. T. A., 315
Visher, E., 480
Viswanathan, R., 305
Vogel, S. R., 418
von Bertalanffy, L., 443, 450
Vontress, C. E., 141, 144–147, 149, 151,
    161, 162, 171

Wachtel, P., 86
Waldegrave, C., 492
Walker, L., 441
Wallace, C. J., 285
Walsh, F., 445
Walsh, W. M., 468
Walters, R. H., 280
Walton, E., 292
Walz, G. R., 5
Wampler, L. D., 7
Wampold, B. E., 32
Warner, M. S., 227
Watkins, J. T., 335
Watkins, P., 336
Watson, J., 263, 277, 343, 344
Watson, J. C., 185, 214, 227
Watson, T. S., 480

Watts, A., 148, 149, 154, 158
Watts, R. E., 94, 96, 99, 100, 105–109,
    112, 116, 125, 129, 130, 131,
    133, 135, 139
Watzlawick, P., 443
Weakland, J., 443
Weeks, G., 460, 488
Weems, C. E., 305
Weersing, V. R., 345
Weidner, F., 301
Weiling, E., 488
Weingarten, K., 467, 494
Weinhardt, L. S., 313
Weintraub, S. R., 404, 414, 441
Weishaar, M., 329, 331
Weisz, J. R., 345
Welwood, J., 158
Wenrich, W. W., 281
Wertheimer, M., 229
Westbury, E., 433
Wetherell, J. L., 301, 336
Wheeler, S., 7
Whitaker, C., 443, 444, 465
White, D. M., 338
White, J. L., 14
White, M., 491, 493, 494, 495, 497, 498,
    500, 502, 503–506, 508, 511,
    517, 521, 522, 524, 525, 526, 533
Wiegartz, P. S., 305
Williams, C. B., 24
Williams, J. M. G., 335
Williams, K. E., 306
Williams, S., 334
Williamson, E. G., 146
Wilson, G. T., 288, 315
Wilson, J. J., 342
Wilson, K. G., 281
Wilson, P. G., 338
Wilson, T. G., 345
Winnicott, D., 48, 56
Winslade, J., 506, 510, 522, 524, 527, 532, 533
Wisocki, P. A., 358
Woldt, A., 273

Wolfe, J. L., 324
Wolpe, J., 2, 279, 298, 322, 358
Woltersdorf, M. A., 309
Woo, A., 389
Wood, B. L., 480
Wood, J. M., 292
Woodward, L. J., 305
Word, C., 62
Worell, J., 29, 397, 399, 400, 401, 414,
    415, 417, 420–423, 432, 434
Workman, E., 342
Worrell, J., 405–412, 441
Worth, J., 340
Wright, F. D., 330, 332, 334
Wubbolding, R., 360, 361, 363, 365–366,
    373, 375, 384, 390, 391, 395, 396
Wurtele, S. K., 308
Wyche, K. F., 403, 414–416
Wynne, L., 443, 476, 477

Xie, S. X., 335

Yalom, I., 151
Yalom, I. D., 7, 143, 158
Yeakle, R., 134
Yellow Bird, M. J., 480
Yerin, O., 336
Yoder, P., 308
Yontef, G., 231, 245, 274
Young, J. E., 335
Young, J. F., 335
Yunus, U., 305

Zahm, S., 259
Zane, H., 122
Zanna, M., 62
Zarski, J. J., 99
Zimmerman, J., 494, 533
Zimring, F., 226
Zimring, F. M., 214
Zinker, J., 274
Zuckerman, M., 342
Zunin, L., 361

Subject Index

AABT, 281
ABC model, 285–286
ABCT, 281, 356
Ableism, 398
Absent but implicit, 505–506
Absolute (dichotomous) thinking, 324
ACA ethics code, 21
Acceleration target behavior, 294
Acting as if, 127–128
Acting out, 66
Action therapy, 10, 288–289
Active disputing, 326
Activism, 36–37
Activity schedule, 333
Actualizing tendency, 194, 216–217
Adaptive behaviors, 8, 9
Adlerian therapy, 8, 93–140
    acting as if, 127–128
    asking "the question," 126
    assessment stage, 120–121
    basic life tasks, 111–112
    basic mistakes, 110–111
    birth order, 113–115
    blind spots, 131–132
    challenges, 133–134
    change process, 115–117
    client-counselor relationship, 129
    core fears, 111
    crisis of relevance, 136
    cultural differences, 134–135
    early recollections, 110, 118
    emotions, 109–110
    encouragement, 104–106, 125
    evaluation of, 130–131
    family constellation, 115
    faulty logic, 107
    future directions, 134–135
    historical overview, 94–100
    holism, 104
    inferiority, 113
    inferiority complex, 113
    insight and interpretation stage, 122
    key concepts, 103–115, 136
    life goals, 104
    life-style, 107–110
    life tasks, 94, 111–112
    limitations, 132–133
    Midas technique, 128
    mistaken goals, 116
    pleasing someone, 129
    private logic, 106–107
    push-button technique, 126–127
    reframing, 125–126
    relationship stage, 129
    reorientation stage, 122–124
    social interest, 112–113
    subjective or private logic, 106–107
    superiority, 113
    therapeutic strategies, 124–129
    therapy stages, 120–124
Ageism, 398
Alternative story, 489, 504
Anal stage, 58
Analyst in the Inner City, The (Altman), 70
Androcentric, 398
Androgyny, 406
Animism, 144
Antecedents, 285
Anxiety, 68, 69, 154, 186
Anxiety hierarchy, 299
APA ethics code, 20–21
APA Ethics Committee, 20
Arbitrary inference, 329
Archetypes, 46
Asking "the question," 126
Assertion training, 310–313
Assertive behaviors, 309, 310
Assessment stage, 120–121
Assimilation, 245
Association for Advancement of Behavior Therapy
    (AABT), 281
Association for Behavioral and Cognitive Therapies
    (ABCT), 281, 356
Audience and witnessing, 507–508
Authenticity
    in existential theory, 153–154, 160
    in person-centered therapy, 203
Automatic thoughts, 328, 331
Autonomy, 22
Autonomy *vs.* shame and doubt, 60

Avoiding, 109
Awareness, 7, 8, 244, 250

Background, 243
Backup reinforcers, 297
Bad faith, 160
Bad-me, 59
Bad object, 71n
Bartering, 35
Basic life tasks, 111–112
Basic mistakes, 110–111
Becoming, 156, 160
Becoming white, 51
Behavior rehearsal, 307
Behavior therapy, 275–359
    ABC model, 285–286
    acceleration target behavior, 294
    action therapy, as, 288–289
    activity schedule, 333
    antecedents, changing in, 291–292
    assertion training, 310–313
    automatic thoughts, 328, 331
    behavioral rehearsal, 309, 311, 312
    blind spots, 349
    brief/graduated exposure therapy, 298–302
    challenges, 350–351
    client-counselor relationship, 343–344
    cognitive-behavioral, 277, 282, 320–343. *See also*
        Cognitive-behavioral therapy
    cognitive-behavioral rehearsal, 309
    cognitive distortions, 329
    cognitive modeling, 337
    cognitive participant modeling, 337
    cognitive restructuring, 321
    cognitive restructuring therapies, 321–336
    cognitive therapy, 280, 328–336
    common characteristics, 289–290
    consequences, changing in, 292–298
    decatastrophizing, 332
    deceleration target behavior, 294
    defining themes, 288–289
    differential reinforcement, 294
    differential relaxation, 301
    diversity, issues of, 305–307, 335–336, 343,
        348–349, 352
    effectiveness, 345–347
    evaluation of, 344–349
    exposure therapy, 298–307
    extinction, 295
    flooding, 302–305
    follow-up assessments, 286
    future directions, 351–352
    graded task assignments, 333–334
    historical overview, 277, 279–283
    in vivo exposure therapy, 301–302
    irrational beliefs, common, 324

    learning focus, 288, 289
    length of, 290
    limitations, 350
    maintaining conditions, 286
    mastery and pleasure ratings, 333
    measurement in, 286
    modeling therapy, 307–316
    organization of, 277, 278
    overcorrection, 296–297
    participant modeling, 314–315
    physically aversive consequences, 294, 297
    Premack principle, 293
    present focus, 288, 289, 349
    process of, 287
    prolonged/intense exposure therapy, 302–303
    prompts, 291
    psychoanalysis, compared with, 283
    punishment, 294
    rational emotive behavior therapy (REBT), 280,
        323–327, 328
    reinforcement, 292–294, 295
    relapse prevention, 342, 350
    relaxation training, 301
    response cost, 295–296
    response prevention, 303–305
    scientific approach, 288
    scope, 347–348
    setting events, 291–292
    shaping, 293–294
    skills training, 308–313
    social skills training, 309–313
    steps in, 286–287
    step-wise progression, 290
    stimulus control, 291–292
    systematic desensitization, 280, 298–301
    target behavior, defined, 286
    terminology, 276, 279
    theory of change, 286, 320
    thought diary, 331–332
    thought stopping, 322–323
    time out from positive reinforcement, 295
    token economy, 279, 297–298
    traditional, 277, 282, 290–316
    treatment package, 290
    vicarious consequences, 307
    vicarious extinction, 313–315
Behavioral avoidance test, 303
Behavioral medicine, 281
Behavioral prompt, 291
Behaviorism, 277, 280, 282
Being and Nothingness (Sartre), 152
Being good, 110
Being socially useful, 110
Belonging and love needs, 368
Beneficence, 22
Bibliotherapy, 5, 424–425

Birth order, 113–115
Book, overview, 18–19
Boundaries, 451, 462, 463
Brief/graduated exposure therapies, 298–302
Brief therapy, *See* Short-term therapy

Cahiers pour une Morale (Sartre), 172
Carl Rogers on Encounter Groups (Rogers), 181
Catastrophizing, 324
Change process/theory of change
    Adlerian therapy, 115–117
    behavior therapy, 286, 320
    cognitive-behavioral/interactional family approach,
      461–462
    existential-humanistic family therapy, 465
    family therapy, 470–471
    feminist therapy, 425–426
    Gestalt therapy, 248–249, 261
    person-centered therapy, 197–200
    psychoanalytic therapy, 62–64
    psychodynamic/historical family systems, 456–457
    reality therapy, 372–373
Change strategy, 7–9
    adaptive behaviors, engaging in, 9
    awareness, increasing, 8
    changing cognitions, 8–9
    insight, developing, 8
    systemic change, creating, 9
Changing cognitions, 8–9. *See also*
    Cognitive-behavioral therapy
Children: The Challenge (Dreikurs/Stolz), 98
Choice theory, 367–371
Choosing a therapy approach, 15–17
Classical conditioning, 277
Classical psychoanalytic therapy, 64–66
Classism, 398
Client-centered therapy, 178, 180–184. *See also*
    Person-centered therapy
Client-Centered Therapy (Rogers), 2, 180
Client-counselor relationship, 10
    Adlerian therapy, 129
    behavior therapy, 343–344
    existential therapy, 192
    feminist therapy, 424
    Gestalt therapy, 257–261
    narrative therapy, 521–522
    person-centered therapy, 200, 201
    psychoanalytic therapy, 56–57, 64
    reality therapy, 374–375
Client freedom, 201
Clients, demographic patterns 1, 12–13
Clinical Treatment of the Problem Child (Rogers), 178
Closure, 244
Coaching environment, 474
Cognitive-behavioral/interactional family therapy,
    461–464

Cognitive-behavioral therapy, 8–9, 280, 281, 320–343.
    See also Behavior therapy
    cognitive-behavioral coping skills therapies, 9, 336–343
    cognitive restructuring therapies, 321–336
    cognitive therapy, 328
    problem-solving therapy, 338–341
    rational emotive behavior therapy (REBT), 323–327, 328
    schema-based cognitive therapy, 335
    self-instructional training, 281, 337–338
    stress inoculation training, 281, 341–343
    thought stopping, 322–323
Cognitive modeling, 337
Cognitive participant modeling, 337
Cognitive restructuring, defined, 321
Cognitive restructuring therapies, 321–336
Cognitive therapy, 280, 328–336
Collaborating environment, 475
Collaborative empiricism, 331
Collective unconscious, 46
Common Language of Psychotherapy Procedures, 18
Community genogram, 469
Compassion, 31
Condensation, 43
Conditions of worth, 196
Confidentiality, 22, 23
Confluence, 252
Confrontation, 231, 233, 252
Congruence, 195, 203, 222
Conscious, 43
Consciousness-raising, 399
Consciousness-raising groups, 423–424
Consent, 23
Consequences, 285
Consulting environment, 474–475
Consulting your consultants, 524
Contact, 245, 250–251
Contact boundary, 251
Contact boundary disturbances, 251–253
Control theory, 362
Coping model, 313
Core fears, 111
Coresearch, 494, 509, 510, 511–512, 514–515, 517,
    520–522
Counseling, defined, 4–5
Counseling and Psychotherapy: Newer Concepts in Practice
    (Rogers), 179, 180
Counterstory, 504
Countertransference. *See* Transference/countertransference
Courage, 155–156, 160
Covert self-instructions, 337
Covert self-modeling, 309
Creative adjustment, 246–247
Cross-cultural issues. *See* Diversity/cultural diversity
Cultural analysis, 420–421
Cultural diversity. *See* Diversity/cultural diversity
Cultural feminist counselors, 402, 403

Cultural identity, 189
Cultural mutuality, 31–32
Cultural theorists, 49
Culturally competent, 13, 14
Culturally relative perspective, 14
Culturally universal perspective, 14
Culture, as a meaning-making system, 81
Curious questioning, 503
Cybercounseling, 5
Cycle of awareness and contact, 245–246

Dasein, 142
Death, 160
Death drive, 43, 66
Decatastrophizing, 332
Deceleration target behavior, 294
Defense mechanism, 45–46, 69
Deflection, 252
Denial, 45
Denial of one's basic worth, 111
Depression, 129, 152, 158, 186
Depressive position, 73
Dereflection, 143
Derivatives, 64
Deuxième Sexe (de Beauvoir), 146
Developmental therapy (DT), 471–475
Dialectic, 161–162
Dialogue, 241–242, 259
Dichotomous thinking, 324, 329
Differential reinforcement, 294
Differential relaxation, 301
Differentiation of self, 457
Discipline without Tears (Dreikurs/Cassell), 98
Discouragement, 105
Discourse/discursive practices, 499
Discursive listening, 501, 512–513
Displacement, 43
Dissociation, 68
Diversity/cultural diversity, 3, 13–15, 29. *See also* Feminist
    multicultural ethics; Race/racism
    defined, 1
    in Adlerian therapy, 134–135
    in behavior therapy, 305–307, 335–336, 343,
        348–349, 352
    in existential therapy, 162–66, 170–172
    in exposure therapy, 305–307
    in family therapy, 455, 479–480
    in feminist multicultural ethics, 24–37
    in feminist therapy, 436–437
    in Gestalt therapy, 234, 266
    in narrative therapy, 492, 528–529
    in person-centered therapy, 185–190, 219–222
    in psychoanalytic therapy, 68–69, 74–78, 80–81, 85, 87
    in reality therapy, 363, 389, 391–392
Dominant discourses, 500
Dominant story, 489

Dream analysis, 43
Dreams, role of, 65
Drive models, 47

Early recollections, 110, 118
Eclectism, 17
Effectiveness of therapy, 11–12
EFT, *See* Emotionally focused therapy
Ego, 44, 69
Ego and the Mechanisms of Defense, The (Freud), 45
Ego, Hunger and Aggression: A Revision of Psychoanalysis
    (Perls/Perls), 229
Ego integrity *vs.* despair, 61
Ego psychology, 45–46, 51–52, 56–57, 80
Ego strength, 51–52
Eigenwelt, 148, 150
Electra complex, 44, 45, 46, 47, 48, 58
Emotional insight, 8
Emotionally focused therapy (EFT), 184, 407–419
Emotions
    Adlerian therapy, 109–110
    family therapy, 454–455
    life-style, 109–110
    person-centered therapy, 215–216
Empathic listening, 201–202
Empathy, 197, 214–215, 222
Empirical research, 82, 130, 433
Empirically supported treatments (ESTs), 262, 345
Empowerment, 409
Empowerment feminist therapy (EFT), 407–419
Empowerment of clients, 28–29
Empty chair technique, 232, 281, 321
Enactments, 464
Encouragement, 104–106, 125
Energic model, 42–43
Environment, defined, 228
Environmental field, 230
Environmental prompt, 291
Environmental structuring environment, 474
Erikson's theory of psychosocial development, 58–59, 60–61
Eros, 43
Essence, 150–151
Ethics, 20–40. *See also* Feminist multicultural ethics
    ACA ethics code, 21
    APA ethics code, 20–21
    confidentiality, 23
    informed consent, 23
    moral principles, 22
Ethics in Counseling and Psychotherapy: A Practical Guide
    (Vasquez/Pope), 26
Ethic of care, 30–31
Ethnocentrism, 398
Exciting object, 71
Existence, 150–151
Existence: A New Dimension in Psychiatry and Psychology
    (May et al.), 2

Existential anxiety, 154
Existential-humanistic family therapy, 465–467
Existential therapy, 8, 141–176
    anxiety, 154
    authenticity, 153–154
    becoming, 156
    blind spots, 169
    challenges, 170
    client-counselor relationship, 159–160
    courage, 155–156
    cross-cultural counseling, 162–166, 170–172
    dereflection, 143
    diagnosis, 160–161
    dialectic, 161–162
    Eigenwelt, 143, 150
    evaluation of, 167–168
    existence and essence, 150–151
    existential anxiety, 154
    freedom, 154–155
    future directions, 170–172
    historical overview, 141–145
    I-Thou, 143, 159
    intervention procedures, 160–161
    limitations, 169–170
    logotherapy, 143
    love, 151–152
    meaning in life, 143, 158
    Mitwelt, 143, 149–150
    object, 149
    paradoxical intention, 143
    psychotherapeutic eros, 143
    responsibility, 152–153
    self-knowledge, 151
    Socratic dialogue, 160–161
    subject, 149
    theoretical principles, 148–158
    Uberwelt, 143, 164
    Umwelt, 143, 148–149
    unfolding, 156–158
Existentialism, 141–145, 169–172
Experiential family therapy (Whitaker/Satir), 465–467
Experiment, 253–256
Exposure therapy, 298–307
Expressions of care, 35–36
Extended family, 446, 447
External factors, emphasis on, 9–10
External locus of control, 384
Externalizing conversations, 496, 502–503
Externalizing language, 502
Extinction, 295

Family constellation, 115
Family culture, 454–455
Family development, 452–453
Family ego mass, 457

Family functioning, 455
Family genogram, 460
Family hierarchy, 463
Family map, 462, 463
Family myths, 466
Family projection process, 457–458
Family sculpting, 466
Family structure, 445, 453–454
Family systems approach (Bowen), 457–461
Family therapy, 3–4, 9, 442–488
    blind spots/limitations, 481–483
    Bowen's family system approach, 457–461
    cognitive-behavioral/interactional approaches, 461–464
    contemporary, 467–475
    diversity, issues in, 455, 479–480
    evaluation of, 475–480
    existential-humanistic approaches, 465–467
    families as systems, 450–452
    family culture, 454–455
    family development, 452–453
    family functioning, 455
    family structure, 453–454
    future directions, 483–484
    historical overview, 442–447
    idiographic research, 477–478
    idiothetic research, 478–479
    Minuchin's structural family therapy, 462–464
    nomothetic research, 475–476
    psychodynamic/historical approaches, 456–461
    traditional, 455–467
    Whitaker and Satir's experiential family therapy 465–467
Faulty logic, 107
Faulty values, 111
Feedback loops, 451
Feminist counseling orientations, 402, 403
Feminist multicultural ethics, 24–37
    activism, 36–37
    answering client's questions, 33, 34
    attending life transitional events, 34–35
    bartering, 35
    boundary setting, 33–36
    empowerment of clients, 28–29
    ethics of care, 30–31
    expressions of care, 35–36
    gift giving/receiving, 35
    hugs, 35–36
    moral principles, 32
    mutuality, 31–32
    nonsexual touching, 35–36
    people of color, 27, 30
    self-disclosure, 33–34
    social justice, 29–30
    social roles, 34–35
    sociopolitical context, 27–28

verbal boundaries, 33–34
women, 27, 30
Feminist perspective, 50
Feminist therapy, 3, 9, 397–441
   bibliotherapy, 424–425
   blind spots/limitations, 434–435
   challenges, 435–436
   consciousness-raising groups, 423–424
   counseling approaches, 402
   cultural analysis, 420–421
   diversity, issues in, 436–437
   empowerment feminist therapy (EFT), 407–419
   evaluation of, 432–434
   foundational values and worldviews, 408–409
   future directions, 436–437
   gender-role analysis, 421–422
   historical overview, 398–404
   intrapsychic sources of client problems, 432
   long-term *vs.* short-term therapy, 426
   oppression, 397, 430–431
   power analysis, 422–423
   reframing, 425
   relabeling, 425
   self-disclosure, 424
   self-involving responses, 424
   social change, 430
   social identities analysis, 420, 421
   strengths/weaknesses, 429–432
   theory of change, 425–426
   values, 431–432
Fidelity, 22
Field, 240
Field theory, 240–241
Figure, 229
Figure formation and destruction, 243–244
Figure/ground image, 229
Film and video modeling, 315
Flooding, 302–305
Focusing-oriented psychotherapy, 184, 216
Free association, 43, 65
Freedom, 154–155
Freedom and independence needs, 368
Friendship task, 94
Fun and enjoyment needs, 368

Gemeinschaftsgefühl, 112
Gender-role analysis, 421–422
Generativity *vs.* stagnation, 61
Genital stage, 58
Genogram, 460, 469
Gestalt, 229
Gestalt psychology, 229
Gestalt therapy, 8, 228–274
   assimilation, 245
   awareness, 244, 250

basic tenet concepts, 247
blind spots, 267
boom-boom-boom style, 231
challenges, 268–270
change process, 248–249, 261
client-counselor relationship, 257–261
confluence, 252
confrontation, 231, 233, 252
contact, 245, 250–251
contact boundary disturbances, 251–253
creative adjustment, 246–247
cycle of awareness and contact, 245–246
dialogue, 241–242, 259
diversity, issues in, 234, 266
evaluation of, 262
experiment, 253–256
field theory, 240–241
figure formation and destruction, 243–244
future directions, 270
historical overview, 228–236
I-Thou, 241–242
idiographic evaluation, 264–266
limitations, 267–268
long-term *vs.* short-term application, 261–262
misconception about, 268–269
nomothetic evaluation, 263–264
organismic self-regulation, 242–243
Perls's method of practice, 233
phenomenological inquiry, 238, 258
phenomenology, 241
philosophical foundations, 240–242
present moment, 244
qualitative research, 264
resistance, 256–257
self, 239, 240
self-disclosure, 259–260
theoretical concepts, 242–247
theory of change, 248–249
Gestalt Therapy: Excitement and Growth in the Human Personality (Perls et al.), 2, 229
Gift giving/receiving, 35
Goals, false or impossible, 110
Good-me, 59
Good object, 71n
Graded task assignments, 333
Ground, 229
Guided discovery, 330
Guidelines for Psychological Practice with Girls and Women, 400–401

Health Book for the Tailoring Trade (Adler), 95
Heterosexism, 398
Holism, 93, 104
Holistic, 144, 230, 269, 481
Homework assignment, 288

Hugs, 35–36
Humorous deflection, 252

I-It, 241–242
I-Thou, 143, 159, 241–242
Id, 44, 69
Ideal self, 194
Identification, 45
Identity development models, 412
Identity *vs.* role confession, 61
Idiographic evaluation, 11, 130, 264–266, 347, 477–478, 524–525
Idiographic family therapy research, 477–478
Idiothetic family therapy research, 478–479
Imaginal flooding, 302
In-session *vs.* in vivo continuum, 10
In vivo, 10, 289
In vivo exposure therapy, 301
In vivo flooding, 303–305
Incongruence, 195
Industry *vs.* inferiority, 60
Inferiority complex, 113
Informed consent, 23
Initiative *vs.* guilt, 60
Inner world, 48
Insider knowledges, 497
Insight, 7, 8
Insight and interpretation stage, 122
Instrumental (operant) conditioning, 279
Integration, psychotherapy, 18, 281
Intellectual insight, 8
Intellectual midwife, 162
Interactionist, 397
Internal factors, emphasis on, 9
Internal frame of reference, 197
Internal locus of control, 384
Internal object relations, 71n
Internal objects, 48
Interpretation of Dreams (Freud), 94, 96
Interpretation, 50, 68, 122
Intimacy *vs.* isolation, 61
Intrapsychic, 397, 432
Introjection, 251

Jungian psychology, 46
Just therapy, 492
Justice, 22

La Peste (Camus), 152
Latency period, 58
Laughter, 369
Length of therapy, 11
L'Etranger (Camus), 142
Level of commitment, 383–384
Liberal feminist counselors, 402, 403
Libido, 42

Life goals, 104
Life-style, 107–110
Life-style inventory, 110
Life-style types, 109
Life tasks, 94, 111–112
Life transitional events, 34–35
Literate Means to Therapeutic Ends (White/Epston), 493
Live modeling, 313
Local knowledges, 493
Locus of control, 384
Locus of evaluation, 196
Logic, subjective or private, 106–107
Logotherapy, 143
Long-term therapy, 11, 86, 348
Love, 151–152
Love or intimacy task, 94

Maieutic method, 162
Maintaining conditions, 285
Maori, defined, 492
Mastery and pleasure ratings, 333
Meaning (in life), 143, 158, 160Midas technique, 128
Middle child, 114–115
Minuchin's structural family therapy, 462–464
Misperceptions of life and life's demands, 111
Missed appointments, 69–73, 80
Mistaken goals, 116
Mitwelt, 143, 149–150
Modeling therapy, 307–316
Moral principles, 22, 32
Multicultural counseling/therapy, 13–14. *See also* Diversity/cultural diversity
Multigenerational transmission process, 458
Multimodal therapy, 280
Musterbation, 324
Mutuality, 31–32

Narrative Means to Therapeutic Ends (White/Epston), 493
Narrative therapy, 3, 4, 9, 489–533
    absent but implicit, 505–506
    accountability, 523–525
    alternative story, 489, 503–504, 510, 514–515
    asking permission, 510
    audience and witnessing, 507–508
    blind spots, 525–526
    challenges, 528
    client-counselor relationship, 521–522
    consulting your consultants, 524
    context of counseling, 508–509
    coresearching, 494, 509, 510, 511–512, 514–515, 517, 520–522
    curiosity, counselor's, 494
    curious questioning, 503
    discourse/discursive practices, 499, 512–513
    discursive listening, 512–513
    diversity, 492, 528–529

dominant discourses, 500
dominant story, 489
effects of coresearch, 520–521
evaluation of, 523–525
evaluation of justification, 515–517
external language, 502
externalizing conversations, 502–503
future directions, 528–529
hearing/using a distinction, 510–511
historical overview, 491–495
key practices, 491
knowledge claims, 490, 500
language, use of, 491, 502, 527
limitations, 526–528
links with community of others, 513–514
long-term *vs.* short-term application, 522–523
metaphor of story, 489, 491
normalizing judgment, 500–501
permission-power relations, 510
philosophical foundations, 499–500
problem story, 489, 503–504
remembering conversations, 507
response-listening for storylines, 509–510
scaffolding of inquiry, 504–505
starting points (ethics and politics), 509
storying what is implicit, 512
theoretical concepts, 500–502
therapeutic documents, 506–507
thin/thick descriptions, 505, 520
transport, 508
two-way account of therapy, 525
underlying premise, 490
witnessing, 507–508, 516
National Defense Education Act (NDEA), 2
"Necessary and Sufficient Conditions of Therapeutic
      Personality Change, The" (Rogers), 181, 197, 221
Needs, 368–369
Neo-Kleinians, 83
Neurosis, 63
New object, 74
Nomothetic evaluation, 11–12, 263–264, 345–347, 523
Nomothetic family therapy research, 476–477
Nonmaleficence, 22
Nonsexual touching, 35–36
Normalizing judgment, 500–501
Not-me, 59
Notebooks for an Ethics (Sartre), 172
Nuclear family, 447
Nuclear family emotional system, 457

Object, 47, 149
Object relations, 47–48, 56–57, 56–57, 71, 73–74
Object Relations in Psychoanalytic Theory
      (Greenberg/Mitchell), 47
Observational learning, 280, 307
Oedipus complex, 44, 46, 47, 48, 58, 85

Old object, 73–74
Oldest born, 114
On Becoming a Person (Rogers), 181
Only child, 114
Openness to experience, 195
Operant (instrumental) conditioning, 279
Oppression, 398, 408, 430–431
Oral stage, 58
Organismic self-regulation, 230, 242–243, 267
Organismic-valuing process, 196–197
Overcorrection, 296–297
Overgeneralizing/overgeneralization, 110, 324, 329
Overt self-instructions, 337
Overview of book, 18–19

Pain behaviors, 295
Pakeha, defined, 492
Paradoxical intention, 143
Paradoxical theory of change, 248
Paranoid-schizoid position, 73
Parental subsystem, 463
Participant modeling, 314
Participant observer, 67
Pasifka, defined, 492
Patriarchal, 402
Penis envy, 49
Person-centered therapy, 8, 177–227
      actualizing tendency, 194, 216–217
      authenticity, 203
      blind spots, 216–217
      challenges, 218–219
      change process, 197–200
      client-centered therapy, 178, 180–184
      client-counselor relationship, 200
      client freedom, 201
      conditions of worth, 196
      congruence, 195
      diversity, issues in, 185–190, 219–222
      duration of treatment, 213–214
      emotion, 215–216
      emotionally focused therapy (EFT), 184
      empathic listening, 201–202
      empathy, 197, 214–215
      essential terms, 194–197
      evaluation of, 214–216
      existential influences, 185
      focusing-oriented psychotherapy, 184, 216
      future directions, 219–222
      historical overview, 177–191
      ideal self, 194
      incongruence, 195
      internal frame of reference, 197
      limitations, 217–218
      locus of evaluation, 196
      openness to experience, 195
      organismic-valuing process, 196–197

Person-centered therapy (*continued*)
    phenomenology, 190
    positive regard, 196
    process-experiential psychotherapy, 184
    psychological adjustment, 195
    psychological maladjustment, 195–196
    relational attitudes in action, 201
    Rogers's formal statement of this theory (1959), 183
    Rogers's life story, 177–182
    self, 194–195
    self-actualization, 194, 217
    therapist qualities, 221–222
    unconditional positive regard, 177, 196, 197, 222
Personal growth, as goal of therapy, 6, 7
Personal worthlessness, 324
Personalization, 329
Phallic stage, 58
Phenomenological inquiry, 238, 258
Phenomenology, 190, 241
Philosophy of "As If," The (Vaihinger), 106
Physical prompt, 291
Physically aversive consequences, 297
Pleasing someone, 129
Positive psychology movement, 134
Positive regard, 196
Postcolonialism, 50
Postmodernism, 49–50, 500, 501
Power, 422
Power, achievement, and inner control needs, 368
Power analysis, 422–423
Preconscious, 43
Premack principle, 293
Present moment, 244
Prevention, 7, 351
Primary process, 43
Private logic, 106–107
Privilege, 423, 430–431
Problem-solving therapy, 338–341
Problem story, 489, 503
Process, defined, 230
Process-experiential psychotherapy, 184
Professional ethics, 20–40. *See also* Ethics
Progressive relaxation, 298, 299, 301
Projection, 45, 251
Projective identification, 59, 61
Prolonged/intense exposure therapies, 302–305
Prompts, 291
Psychoanalytic therapy, 8, 41–92, 279
    acting out, 66
    anal stage, 58
    behavior therapy, compared with, 283
    change process, 62–64
    classical psychoanalytic therapy, 11, 56–57, 69, 66–74
    client-counselor relationship, 64
    core theoretical concepts, 55, 56–57

    countertransference. *See* Psychoanalytic therapy, transference/countertransference
    cultural diversity, issues in, 68–69, 74–78, 81, 85
    cultural theorists, 49
    ego psychology, 45–46, 56–57, 66, 68
    ego-supportive interventions, 68
    energic model, 42–43
    Erikson's theory of psychosocial development, 58–59, 60–61
    evaluation of, 82–85
    feminist criticism, 49
    free association, 43, 65
    Freud, 42–45, 56–57, 58
    future directions, 87
    genital stage, 58
    historical overview, 42–52
    interpretation, 50, 68, 77
    Jungian psychology, 46
    latency period, 58
    limitations/blind spots, 85
    missed appointments, 69–73, 76, 78
    object relations, 47–48, 56
    one-person model, 66
    oral stage, 58
    outcome research, 84–85
    phallic stage, 58
    postcolonial theorists, 50
    postmodernism, 49–50
    process research, 83
    projection, 77
    projective identification, 59
    psychosexual development, stages of, 58
    purity of technique, 85–87
    racism, 61–62
    relational psychoanalysis, 47–49, 56–57, 69, 66–68
    self, development of, 59
    social constructivism, 50
    structural model, 44–45
    theory of development, 55–62
    topographic model, 43–44
    transference/countertransference, 65, 67, 69, 74–80, 86
    unconscious, 43, 65, 69, 86
Psychodynamic/historical family systems approaches, 456–461
Psychological adjustment, 195
Psychological maladjustment, 195–196
Psychosexual development, 58
Psychotherapeutic eros, 143, 159
Psychotherapy approaches, 5–18
    adopting more than one approach, 17–18
    change strategies, 7–9
    choosing an approach, 15–17
    consumers, 12–13
    cultural differences, 13–15. *See also* Diversity/cultural diversity
    ethics, 20–40. *See also* Feminist multicultural ethics

evaluation of effectiveness, 11–12
internal *vs.* external factors, 9–10
length of therapy, 11
locus of time, 10–11
process, 10–11
purpose or goal, 6–7
theoretical foundation, 6
Psychotherapy by Reciprocal Inhibition (Wolpe), 2
Psychotherapy, defined, 4–5
Psychotherapy integration, 18
Punishment, 294
Push-button technique, 126–127

Qualitative research, 264, 524
Quality world, 369

Race/racism. *See also* Diversity/cultural diversity
    defined, 398
        psychoanalytic explanation, 61–62
        psychoanalytic therapy, and, 78–80
        systematic desensitization for, 298–301
Radical feminist counselors, 402, 403
Rational emotive behavior therapy (REBT), 280,
    323–327, 328
Rationalization, 45
Reaction formation, 43
Reality therapy, 9, 360–396
    belonging and love needs, 368
    blind spots, 390
    challenges, 391
    choice theory, 366–371
    client-counselor relationship, 374–375
    commitment, client's level, 383–384
    control theory, 362
    counseling environment, 373–374
    counselor behaviors, 373–374
    doing (D), 377, 384–385, 384–385
    diversity, 363, 389, 391–392
    evaluation (self), 372, 377, 385–387
    evaluation of, 389–390
    freedom and independence needs, 368
    fun and enjoyment needs, 368–369
    future directions, 391–392
    historical overview, 360–364
    level of commitment, 383–384
    limitations, 391
    locus of control, 384
    long-term *vs.* short-term applications, 388–389
    needs, 368–369
    philosophical foundations, 367
    planning (P), 372, 377, 388, 393
    power, achievement, and inner control needs, 368
    psychiatric drugs, use of, 364, 392
    SAMIC^3, 388
    survival, self-preservation, and physiological needs, 368
    theoretical concepts, 367

theory of change, 372–373
    tonic behaviors, 373
    total behavior, 370, 372
    toxic behaviors, 374
    wants, 369–370, 372, 377, 378–384
    wants and needs (W), 378–384
    wants and needs, 363, 371
    WDEP system, 375–388
Reality Therapy (Glasser), 362
Reattribution of responsibility, 332
REBT, 280, 323–327, 328
Recreation, 368–369
Reductionism, 93
Reframing, 125–126, 425, 462
Regression, 45
Reinforcement, 292–294, 295
Reinforcer, 292
Rejecting object, 71
Relabeling, 425
Relapse prevention, 342, 350
Relational model, 47
Relational psychoanalysis, 47–49, 56–57, 63–68
Relationship stage, 120
Relaxation training, 301
Remembering conversations, 507
Reorientation stage, 122–124
Repression, 43
Resistance, 65–66
Response cost, 295–296
Response prevention, 303–305
Responsibility, 152–153, 161
Retroflection, 252

SAMIC^3, 388
Scaffolding of inquiry, 504–505
Schema, 335
Schema-based cognitive therapy, 335
Schools Without Failure, 362
Second born, 114
Secondary process, 43
Seduction theory, 42
Selective abstraction, 329
Self
    Bowen's family systems approach, 457–461
    Gestalt therapy, 239, 240
    person-centered therapy, 194–195
    psychoanalytic therapy, 59
Self-actualization, 194, 217, 364, 466
Selfconcept, 105
Self-disclosure, 33–34
    feminist therapy, 424
    Gestalt therapy, 259–260
Self-ideal, 105
Self-instructional training, 337–338
Self-involving responses, 424
Self-knowledge, 151, 160

Self-modeling, 309
Self-talk, 321
Setting events, 291–292
Sexism, 398, 399
Shaping, 293–294
Short-term therapy, 11, 134, 213–214, 261–262, 348, 426, 522
Sibling position, 458
Sibling subsystem, 463
Skills training, 308–313
Social change, 430
Social cognitive theory, 280
Social constructionism, 498, 499, 523, 527
Social constructivism, 50, 82
Social identities, 409, 410
Social identities analysis, 421
Social interest, 112–113
Social justice, 29–30
Social learning theory, 280
Social locations, 410
Social locations exercise, 411
Social roles, 34–35
Social skills, 309
Social skills training, 309–310
Society for Exploration of Psychotherapy Integration, 18
Socratic dialogue, 160–161
Socratic method, 330
Spousal subsystem, 463
Stimulus control, 291–292
Stoics, 141
Storytelling, in modeling therapy, 315
Strategic family therapy, 461
Stress inoculation training, 341–343
Structural family therapy, 462–464
Structural model, in psychoanalysis, 44–45
Stuckness, 156–158
Style matching, 474
Sublimation, 45
Subsystem, 462
Superego, 44, 69
Superiority, 113
Survival, self-preservation, and physiological needs, 368
Symbolic modeling, 313
Systematic desensitization, 298–301
Systemic change, 8, 9
Systemic cognitive development therapy (SCDT), 471–475

Target behavior, 286
Technical eclecticism, 17
Technique, 232
Theoretical eclecticism, 17
Theoretical orientation, 6
Theory of change. *See* Change process/theory of change
Therapeutic documents, 506–507

Therapeutic empathy, 214–215
Thick descriptions, 505
Thin descriptions, 505
Thought diary, 331–332
Thought stopping, 322–323
Time limited therapy, 11
Time out from positive reinforcement, 295
Token economy, 297–298
Tonic behaviors, 373
Top dog-underdog dialogue, 232
Topographic model, 43–44
Total behavior, 370, 372
Touching, 35–36
Toxic behaviors, 374
Traditional behavior therapy, 290–316. *See also* Behavior therapy
Traditional family therapy, 455–457
Training of counselors, 7
Transference, 65, 67, 69, 74–80
Transference-countertransference interaction, 65, 67, 69, 74–80, 86
Transference neurosis, 65
Transitional space, 48
Transport, 508
Treatment package, 290
Triangles and triangulation, 458
Tribes of the Person-Centered Nation, The (Sanders), 183
Trust *vs.* mistrust, 60
Two-way account of therapy, 525

Uberwelt, 143, 164
Umwelt, 143, 148–149
Unconditional positive regard, 177, 196, 197, 222
Unconscious, 43, 65, 69, 86
Understanding Human Nature (Adler), 94
Undifferentiated ego mass, 457
Unfolding, 156–158

Verbal prompt, 291
Verbal therapy, 10
Veterans Administration, role in counseling profession, 2
Vicarious consequences, 307
Vicarious extinction, 313–315
Vicarious reinforcement, 313
Victimized, 110
Video modeling, 315
Video self-modeling therapy, 309, 315

Wants, 369–370, 372, 377, 378–384
WDEP system, 375–389
Well behaviors, 295
Witnessing, 507–508
Women of Color feminist counselors, 402, 403

Youngest born, 115